# AUTOIMMUNE DISORDERS – CURRENT CONCEPTS AND ADVANCES FROM BEDSIDE TO MECHANISTIC INSIGHTS

Edited by **Fang-Ping Huang**

**Autoimmune Disorders – Current Concepts and Advances from Bedside to Mechanistic Insights**
Edited by Fang-Ping Huang

**Published by InTech**

Janeza Trdine 9, 51000 Rijeka, Croatia



**Publishing Process Manager** Alenka Urbancic

**Technical Editor** Teodora Smiljanic

**Cover Designer** InTech Design Team

Additional hard copies can be obtained from orders@intechopen.com

Autoimmune Disorders – Current Concepts and Advances from Bedside to Mechanistic Insights, Edited by Fang-Ping Huang
p. cm.
ISBN 978-953-307-653-9

For EU product safety concerns:
IN TECH d.o.o., Prolaz Marije Krucifikse Kozulić 3, 51000 Rijeka, Croatia,
info@intechopen.com or visit our website at intechopen.com.

# Meet the editor

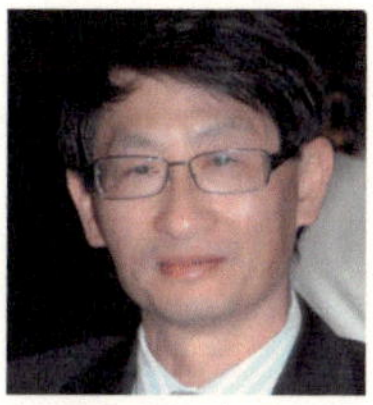

Dr. Huang received his initial medical education in China (Shantou, 1977-82). He was later awarded the Li Ka Shing Academic Foundation Scholarship to undertake postgraduate training in the UK (1987-90), and subsequently became engaged in active immunology research and teaching at the Universities of Glasgow (1990-7), Oxford (1997-2000) and Hong Kong (2000-7). He is currently a Senior Lecturer affiliated to the Imperial College London (since 2007). Immunology has been his major field of research, with a focus on immune regulation in autoimmune diseases. His current research focuses on the roles of dendritic cells (DC), regulatory T (Treg) and B (Breg) cells in systemic autoimmunity (lupus). Based on their findings, he and his research group members are trying to understand how the immune system is normally regulated, why dysregulation of which may cause diseases, and whether the so-called "self-reactivity" (autoimmunity) can be alternatively switched on, and then effectively redirected for cancer treatment (anti-tumour immunity).

# Contents

# Preface

*Every coin has two sides.* The immune system, which protects us from diseases otherwise, can itself directly and evidently cause diseases. Due to failure in the process of tolerance induction and regulation, immune responses, when mistakenly directed against body's own components ('self' antigens), can result in long lasting and recurrent pathological damages to the targeted organs and tissues. These are collectively known as autoimmune disorders, ranging from various organ-specific ones, to those systemic in nature.

The term autoimmunity signifies the presence of self-reactive immune responses with antigen specificity and immunological memory, two key features of the adaptive immunity. Autoimmune responses however, are detected not only in patients with autoimmune diseases, but frequently in healthy individuals as well. The pathological consequence of these reactions depends, often due to lack of certain protective mechanisms, on the type of the responses induced. Some of these autoimmune reactions can even be beneficial; for example, in removing or dumping off various unwanted or aged tissue components. There is also convincing evidence indicating that such responses are involved into fight against tumors, i.e. the 'altered self'. The basis of autoimmunity is still far from being fully understood, although both genetic and environmental factors are believed to often contribute to the pathogenesis together. A good understanding of the autoimmune mechanisms is therefore important for effective diagnosis, as well as better treatment of many autoimmune diseases, and even further beyond.

In this book, thanks to many experts in the field who have made their valuable contributions as authors, updated information is gathered on various autoimmune disorders. These include some of the most classical and unique disease phenotypes, such as Hashimoto's thyroiditis, Type 1 diabetes, rheumatoid arthritis, systemic lupus erythematosus, primary Sjogren syndrome, Sweet syndrome, multiple sclerosis and various other neurological and hematological disorders. Importantly, the book focuses on current advances and new concepts based on cutting-edge findings from both clinical and basic scientific studies. A total of 29 chapters are divided into 5 main sections according to the emphasis of their contents: (I) Disease phenotypes (Chapters 1-7), (II) Diagnostics & prognostics (Chapters 8-11), (III) Therapeutic interventions

(Chapters 12-20), (IV) Pathogenesis & underlying mechanisms (Chapters 21-25), and (V) Other conceptual advances & new insights (Chapters 26-29).

The primary aim of this book is to provide most up-to-date information in the 5 defined aspects as stated above, and in the form of Open Access in particular, to be freely available to both clinicians and basic scientists regarding current advances in the areas. The readers are also recommended to read another upcoming book with a closely related theme and title, i.e. "Autoimmune Disorders – Pathogenic Aspects", edited by Dr Clio Mavragani (ISBN 978-953-308-70-9). I sincerely hope that many of them will find the books useful and inspiring for their future applications in clinical practice and research studies into autoimmunity. Through the editing process, it has been hugely beneficial for me to have the opportunity to learn about the subject in more updated details, and in a systemic way.

I would like to express my sincere gratitude and appreciation to our InTech Publishing Process Manager, Ms Alenka Urbancic, her devoted team, and my associate Dr Susanne Sattler, for their generous support and intellectual input during the editing process. I would also like to thank my family for their constant support and understanding. I dedicate this book respectfully to many of my mentors, particularly Professor Zhong-Ying Shen, Professor Henry HY Wong, Dr Jocelyn W Dow, Dr George BM Lindop, Dr Fiona Miller, Professor Donald Cambell, Professor Laurence C Hunter, Professor David I Stott, Professor Eddy FY Liew, and Professor G Gordon MacPherson. I also acknowledge the generous funding supports received, especially those from the MacFeat Bequest (Glasgow), the Hong Kong Research Grant Committee (Hong Kong), and the Arthritis Research UK (UK). Finally, and specially, I wish to acknowledge the Shantou University Medical College where I received my initial medical education (1977-82), and the Li Ka Shing Academic Foundation which has been generously supporting it, and me in the past.

**Fang-Ping Huang**
*MBBS, MSc, MUA, PhD*
Division of Immunology & Inflammation,
Department of Medicine, Imperial College,
Hammersmith Hospital, London,
UK

# Part 1

# Disease Phenotypes

# 1

# Autoimmune Disorders Associated to Type 1 Diabetes Mellitus in Children and Adolescents

Giuseppe d'Annunzio and Chiara Russo,
Ramona Tallone and Renata Lorini
*Pediatric Clinic, University of Genoa, IRCCS G. Gaslini Institute, Genoa*
*Italy*

## 1. Introduction

Autoimmune diseases occur when an individual develops an immune response targeted against specific organ or number of organs. Genetic susceptibility and environmental factors are the main responsible of the development of the autoimmune process leading to a clinically evident disease.

The majority of organ-specific autoimmune diseases are characterized by an initial infiltration by lymphocytes and macrophages, of the organ, with impaired activity of the organ followed by atrophy. This progressive autoimmune process takes time, and is T cell mediated. Antibodies against specific antigens of the involved gland are detectable in the blood before the clinical onset of the specific disease, so they represent a risk marker and their screening and follow-up allow precocious diagnosis and treatment of autoimmune-related disease in genetically susceptible individuals (Allen et al., 2008).

Genetic factors and autoimmunity are closely related since the developmental maturation of T cells occurs through an interaction between HLA antigen and T cell receptor. In genetically susceptible individuals, disease-prone HLA molecules are ineffective at binding and presenting peptides from tissue-specific antigens, therefore auto-reactive T cells can survive and trigger a poorly regulated immune response thereafter (Van den Driessche, 2009).

Patients affected by type 1 diabetes mellitus are at increased risk of developing other autoimmune conditions like celiac disease, autoimmune thyroid disease, adrenal insufficiency, atrophic gastritis, autoimmune hepatitis, primary ovarian failure.

The frequency of organ specific autoimmunity in patients with type 1 diabetes might be due to multiple immunologic abnormalities, i.e an imbalance in B and T lymphocytes, or a tendency to react against specific antigens, or poor ability to develop immune tolerance.

## 2. Type 1 diabetes mellitus

### 2.1 Background

Type 1 diabetes mellitus is the most common endocrinopathy to have clinical onset in childhood or adolescence, with varied pathogenesis, clinical appearance and outcome, and seriously affects patients' and families' life. A combination of genetic, environmental and immunological factors exerts to a T-cell mediated autoimmune process targeted against insulin-producing β-cells in the pancreatic islet of Langerhans (Daneman, 2006).

### 2.2 Epidemiology

The incidence of Type 1 diabetes is increasing worldwide and may double the burden of the disease in youngest children by 2020. Large collaborative studies like DiaMond and EURODIAB Registries demonstrated that one century ago childhood diabetes was rare and fatal, while at the end of the century a steady increase in several parts of the world has been observed. In particular, DiaMond Project reported the trend in incidence of Type 1 diabetes from 1990 to 1999; over this period the average annual increase in incidence was 2.8%, with a slight higher rate in the last 5 year-period as compared to the first 5-year period. Similarly, EURODIAB Study reported a 3.9% annual increase from 1989-2003 (Vehil & Dabelea, 2011). The rising incidence of Type 1 diabetes over the past decades is too quick to be attributed to an increased genetic susceptibility, since the proportion of newly-diagnosed patients carrying the highest-risk HLA genotype (HLA DR3/DR4) seems unchanged.

### 2.3 Pathogenesis

*Genetic susceptibility* plays an important pathogenetic role in type 1 diabetes mellitus, with the HLA -DR and –DQ genes explaining about 50% of the risk. The different penetrance of these genes can partially explain the role of environmental factors. Whereas differences in incidence between populations may be due to genetic susceptibility or protection genes, the increasing incidence is to be ascribed to environmental factors. Studies aimed to analyze the temporal changes in the frequency of genotypes associated with type 1 diabetes susceptibility reported a decreasing frequency of those higher-risk HLA genotypes (DRB1 03-DQA1*0501-DQB1*0201/DRB104-DQA1*0301-DQB1*0302) between recently diagnosed patients as compared to those diagnosed 50 years before (Hermann et al., 2003). Therefore the increasing incidence of type 1 diabetes could be explained by a more permissive environment, exerting in increased penetrance of low/moderate risk genotypes or in interplay between environmental factors and other non-HLA genes (Nejentsev et al., 2007, Todd et al., 2007). On the other hand, several environmental factors such as dietary habits, sedentary lifestyle, climate changes, pollution, viral (also maternal) and other infectious disease frequency and type, have changed over the past years and deserve attention (Oikarinen et al., 2011).

The *immune-mediated β-cell destruction* occurs over several years and exerts in progressive insulin deficiency, leading to various degrees of hyperglycemia up to severe metabolic derangement , i.e. diabetic ketoacidosis (Devendra et al., 2004).

Studies in both humans and animal models are trying to clarify the specific antigenic targets involved in the islet cell autoimmunity. Islet cell antibodies (ICA) detected by immunofluorescence, were firstly isolated in patients with diabetes mellitus and autoimmune polyglandular syndrome (Bottazzo et al., 1974). These autoantibodies are transient, being observed in 70-80% of newly-diagnosed cases and tend to disappear thereafter. Their positivity in subjects at risk of diabetes (i.e. first-degree relatives) represents a useful means to predict the future development of the disease.

Anti-insulin autoantibodies (IAA) can be detected both by radioimmunoassay (RIA) or by ELISA, but the first method is recommended. IAA positivity is inversely related to age at diabetes diagnosis (81% in patients younger than 10 and 61% in older ones), and is higher and adolescent males (Williams et al., 2003). IAA are the first autoantibodies to became positive, and they can later decline. Interestingly, substitutive insulin therapy can be followed by an immune response against itself, and this subtype of insulin antibodies can be distinguished from anti-insulin autoantibodies.

In 1990 Baekkeskov and co-workers reported that the 64,000 M (R) molecule previously defined as an antigenic target of Type 1 diabetes was the GABA-synthesizing enzyme glutamic acid decarboxylase (GAD) (Baekkeskow et al., 1990). GAD is not expressed exclusively on β-cells, but also in other islet cells. Anti-GAD autoantibodies (GADA) can be detected both by RIA or by ELISA. The prevalence of anti-GAD autoantibodies positivity is 84%, and is positively related to age and female sex. Their peak level can be reached after diabetes diagnosis and persist longer than anti-islet cell antibodies, making them a useful marker especially for adult patients.

In 1994 a cDNA coding a 548 aminoacid protein named ICA-512 was described as a major target of humoral immunity by screening an islet c-DNA expression library with patients' sera (Rabin et al., 1994). Moreover it has been reported that IA-2, a 979 aminoacid transmembrane protein of the tyrosine phosphatase family, is a major autoantigen in type 1 diabetes. IA-2 is a intrinsic membrane protein of secretory granules neuroendocrine cells, like pancreatic islets. IA-2 autoantibodies (IA-2A) can be detected by RIA as well as by ELISA. Recently a not radio-isotopic method (time-resolved immunofluorometric assay (TR-IFMA) showed comparable results with RIA. The prevalence of IA-2A has been reported about 73%, and no correlation with age was found (Tsirogianni et al., 2009).

Recently the cation efflux transporter 8 (ZnT8) has been identified as a novel target auto-antigen in patients with type 1 diabetes. Autoantibodies to ZnT8 (ZnT8 A) are detectable in about 70% of newly diagnosed patients, independent of age (Achenbach et al., 2009). Patients presenting with a single islet cell autoantibody were also positive for ZnT8 A, suggesting that they could be a marker for type 1 diabetes risk stratification. Three variants of ZnT8 A have been recognized: 1) ZnT8RA (arginine 325 zinc transporter 8 autoantibody), 2) ZnT8WA (tryptophan 325 zinc transporter 8 autoantibody), 3) ZnT8QA (glutamine 325 zinc transporter 8 autoantibody). These 3 ZnT8 variants precede T1DM clinical onset and are all detectable by radio-binding assay (Andersson et al., 2011).

### 2.4 Diagnosis and treatment

Diagnosis of type 1 diabetes is based on symptoms of hyperglycemia: polyuria, polydipsia, with mild symptoms up to severe ketoacidosis. After intravenous fluid, insulin and salt replacement for metabolic imbalance recovery, treatment of type 1 diabetes consists of lifelong substitutive subcutaneous insulin therapy, together with correct dietary habits, self-management of the disease and regular physical activity, as result of a prolonged educational intervention starting at the time of clinical diagnosis (Maffeis & Pinelli, 2008, Bangstad et al., 2007). Recognition, management and prevention of hypoglycemic episodes as well as hyperglycemic spikes is mandatory. Continuous education implementation starting at the time of clinical diagnosis, designed for children, adolescents and their parents, is necessary thereafter (Weinzimer et al., 2005).

### 2.5 Follow-up

The most serious problem related to pediatric type 1 diabetes is the risk, even in young adulthood, of microvascular and macrovascular complications, i.e. retinopathy, nephropathy, neuropathy, cardiovascular and cerebrovascular diseases (Donaghue et al., 2007). The key role of good glycaemic control to prevent diabetes-related complications has been firmly established by the Diabetes Control and Complications Trial Study, which demonstrated the protective role of intensive insulin treatment (DCCT, 1993). Sustained chronic hyperglycaemia and acute blood glucose fluctuations have a deleterious effect on the metabolic mechanisms involved in the development of microangiopathy, such as protein glycation and oxidative stress. In particular, glucose variability from peaks to nadir, with upward as in the postprandial periods, and nadirs, as in the interprandial periods activates the oxidative stress (Monnier & Colette, 2008). As regards pediatric diabetes, despite better insulin preparations and strict self-management of the disease few children and adolescents maintain mean glycated hemoglobin A1c (HbA1c) levels within the normal ranges, with serious impact on metabolic control and subjects' caregiver quality of life (Rewers et al, 2009).

## 3. Celiac disease

### 3.1 Background and epidemiology

Celiac disease is an immune-mediated disorder, the only one with a well-established causal agent, resulting from a permanent gluten intolerance triggered by the ingestion of the gliadin fraction of wheat gluten and similar alcohol-soluble proteins named prolamines of barley and rye (Di Sabatino & Corazza, 2009). Gluten intolerance exerts a chronic inflammatory lesion characterized by flattened villi of the small bowel mucosa and sub-mucosa, with a diverse clinical heterogeneity ranging from asymptomatic disease to severe malabsorption syndrome in genetically susceptible individuals (Branski et al., 2006).

Once considered a rare childhood disorder, celiac disease is now known to be a very common condition, even if it remains widely unrecognized and underdiagnosed worldwide both in children and in adults. Availability of new very sensitive and specific serological markers (initially anti-gliadin and anti-reticulin antibodies, and thereafter anti-endomysial and anti-transglutaminase antibodies) allowed more efficient screening, independently from classical clinical picture. Thanks to these serological markers, celiac disease has been identified in a high proportion of children adolescents and adults who did not previously received a correct clinical diagnosis. The prevalence of celiac disease was dramatically increased, and defined as 1 case in 99 schoolchildren in Finland (Mäki et al., 2003), and 1 in 106 in Italy (Tommasini et al., 2004).

### 3.2 Pathogenesis

Celiac disease develops from the interplay between a well-defined environmental factor and genetic susceptibility, with the participation of other causative cofactors (drugs like interferon-α, infectious agents like intestinal rotavirus, modifications in infant-feeding timing) (Di Sabatino & Corazza, 2009).

*The causal agent,* for CD are specific immunogenic peptides present exclusively in the dietary gluten proteins, from wheat and other cereals like rye and barley. Gluten proteins can be divided into 2 fractions, gliadins and glutenins, both characterized by immunogenicity and by toxicity. Among gluten immunostimolatory peptides, some are more active than others. In particular, a 33 aminoacid immuno-dominant peptide identified from an α-gliadin fraction has functional properties attributable to many proline and glutamine residues. Proline increases the peptide resistance to gastrointestinal proteolysis, with more strength binding with HLA-DQ2 and HLA-DQ8 molecules on antigen presenting cells. Glutamine residues are a preferred substrate for transglutaminase-mediated deamination, with subsequent increased immunogenicity (Shan et al., 2002).

*Genetic factors* play an important pathogenetic role, as demonstrated by a concordance rate of 85% in monozygotic twins and by familiar aggregation. HLA-DQ genes, in particular DQ2 variant (alleles DQA1*05/DQB1*02) and DQ8 variant (alleles DQA1*03/DQB1*0302) are strongly associated to CD. Beside the HLA genes (i.e. COELIAC 1, on chromosome p21), other non-HLA genes are recognized to confer additional susceptibility: COELIAC 2, on chromosome 5q31-33, which contains cytokine gene clusters; COELIAC 3, on chromosome 2q33, which codes the negative co-stimulatory molecule CTLA4; COELIAC 4, on chromosome 19p13.1, which contains the myosin IXB gene variant encoding a myosin that alters actin remodeling (Di Sabatino & Corazza, 2009).

As regards *pathophysiology* od CD, it has been demonstrated that gluten peptides, which are resistant to digestion by gastric and pancreatic enzymes, after crossing intestinal epithelium, are deaminated by tissue transglutaminase and then presented by DQ2+ or DQ8+ antigen-presenting cells to gluten-specific CD4+ T cells. These cells once activated drive a Th1 response, characterized by production of pro-inflammatory cytokines, and responsible for the development of celiac lesions, i.e. lamina propria infiltration of inflammatory cells, crypt hyperplasia and villous atrophy (Di Sabatino & Corazza, 2009).

### 3.3 Clinical presentation and diagnosis

The clinical range of celiac disease has a wide spectrum, from asymptomatic to severe malnutrition, with gastrointestinal and extra-intestinal manifestations. The most common feature of celiac disease includes gastrointestinal symptoms (i.e. abdominal pain, increased frequency of bowel movements), weight loss, bone disease, various degree of anemia and weakness.

Different subtypes of celiac disease have been described. Symptomatic or classic celiac disease means typical gastrointestinal symptoms with severe malabsorption syndrome. The term atypical celiac disease is applied to cases with mild or absent gastrointestinal symptoms (colitis or irritable bowel), and characterized by extra-intestinal manifestations, including iron deficient anemia, osteoporosis, failure to thrive. In both cases villous atrophy in observed during endoscopy or intestinal biopsies (Alaedini & Green, 2005). More recently it has been suggested to define celiac disease as silent, minor or major. Silent celiac disease is referred to asymptomatic subjects, sometimes relatives of patients with known celiac disease, or subjects eventually found to be positive at screening procedures. Minor celiac disease is referred to subjects with transient symptoms (dyspepsia, irritable bowel syndrome without malabsorption), anemia, cryptic hypertransaminasemia, infertility, peripheral and central neurological disorders, osteoporosis, dental enamel defects, failure to thrive, dermatitis herpetiformis. Major celiac disease is referred to patients with major gastrointestinal symptoms (Di Sabatino & Corazza, 2009).

The mechanism underlying the severity of clinical presentation at present remains unknown. Researchers have shown that neither the degree of duodenal villous atrophy nor the extent of visible enteropathy assessed by capsule endoscopy correlates with presentation (Di Sabatino & Corazza, 2009).

The recognition of a pre-celiac disease state is usually retrospective and this condition has been termed latent celiac disease.

*Potential celiac disease* is characterized by positive antibodies but normal mucosa; there is no evidence to support managing these patients with a gluten-free diet. A higher prevalence of potential CD was found in patients with type 1 diabetes, and this observation may be ascribed to the routine screening preformed in these patients, although the influence of genetic factors cannot be excluded. (Franzese et al., 2011).

*Refractory celiac disease* is relatively rare complication occurring approximately from 2% to 5% of patients. It is classified as persistent or recurrent symptoms of malabsorption and enteropathy. Refractory celiac disease is divided into two key categories, type I and type II.

As regards celiac disease diagnosis, it has been demonstrated that case-finding by serological markers detection followed by histological confirmation on duodenal biopsy is an accurate, cost-effective and valid approach for diagnosis, in particular for high-risk subjects, like those affected by other autoimmune conditions, like type 1 diabetes mellitus.

Celiac disease is associated with circulating antibodies against gliadin and endomysial tissue. Anti-endoMysial antibodies showed higher specificity and sensitivity than anti-gliadin antibodies, and represent a useful means for screening procedures. Anti-reticulin antibodies screening showed less sensibility and it has been replaced by anti-endomysial antibodies. In 1997 the transglutaminase 2 enzyme was found to be the autoantigen for anti-endomysial antibodies. Both anti-endomysial and anti-transglutaminase antibodies belong to the IgA class. The first are detected by immunofluorescence staining antibodies and results are qualitative or semiquantitative, while anti-transglutaminase antibodies are detected by an enzyme linked immunosorbent assay (ELISA) or radioimmunoprecipitation, and the results are quantitative. Testing for IgG anti-transglutaminase and antibodies and, more recently for IgG anti-deaminated gliadin peptides are a useful alternative for patients with IgA deficiency (Di Sabatino & Corazza, 2009).

In subjects with serological markers of celiac disease, a small intestinal biopsy is the "gold standard" for diagnosis. The finding of histological picture of villous atrophy with increased number of intraepithelial lymphocytes makes sure diagnosis of celiac disease, irrespective of serological markers result. The Marsh criteria (Marsh et al., 2005) are commonly used for histological staging.

### 3.4 Treatment

The only proven treatment for celiac disease is lifelong gluten-free diet. Foods containing gluten from wheat, rye, barley and their derivatives must be avoided since also small amounts of gluten are harmful. It has been reported that no more than 10 mg of gluten ingested can be tolerated.

Compliance to gluten-free diet is sometimes difficult, particularly during adolescence and for patients with silent celiac disease diagnosed by means of screening procedures. Dietary compliance can be evaluated through anti-endomysial and anti-deaminated gliadin antibodies detection. Complications of celiac disease are frequently observed in patients with delayed diagnosis and with poor compliance and include non-Hodgkin lymphoma, probably due to accumulation in the intestinal epithelium of aberrant and clonal intraepithelial lymphocytes (Al-Toma et al., 2007). Other complications include refractory celiac disease and ulcerative jejunoileitis (Rubio-Tapia et al., 2009).

### 3.5 Celiac disease and type 1 diabetes mellitus

That celiac disease prevalence is higher in patients with type 1 diabetes mellitus as compared to general population is universally accepted. After autoimmune thyroiditis, the second most commonly reported autoimmune disease in type 1 diabetes is celiac disease (Van den Driessche, 2009).

Gluten consumption could be a common causative factor, as confirmed by the possible diagnosis of both diseases at the same time (Frisk et al. 2008). Moreover the duration of gluten exposure seems to increase the risk of other autoimmune diseases (Ventura et al.., 1999). Dietary gluten could act as a modifier rather than a determinant causative factor, facilitating the progression of other dietary antigens to the small bowel lamina propria, where they can activate the immune response against β-cells. Based on this hypothesis, the removal of gluten from diet has been proposed in subjects at risk as prevention trial to reduce the progression to type 1 diabetes mellitus (Pastore et al., 2003). A six-month of gluten-free diet in subjects at risk of type 1 diabetes did not influence β-cells autoantibody titer, but only improved endogenous insulin secretion (Pastore et al., 2003).

Recently, in samples from the small bowel mucosa from patients with celiac disease and type 1 diabetes a low expression of tight junction protein 1 (TJP1) mRNA has been observed, indicating an increase in intestinal permeability that might represent a causative factor. Furthermore, the highest expression of Forkhead box P3 (FoxP3) mRNA, a marker of regulatory T cells was observed, suggesting an increased immunoregolatory mechanisms (Uibo et al., 2011).

The mean prevalence of celiac disease in type 1 diabetes is about 8%, with an extremely variable range (from 1% up to 11%) (Kakleas et al., 2010), almost 10-20 fold higher than observed in general pediatric population (Maki et al., 2003). The different prevalence data could be due to different screening procedures and diagnostic tests used. The prevalence of celiac disease in type 1 diabetes increased over recent decade as compared to the past (Salardi et al., 2008), and seems to be related to changes in environmental factors like dietary habits or infectious diseases. Another possible explanation of this high association could be the same genotypes involved in both diseases.. Three celiac disease loci, i.e. RGS1 on chromosome 1q31, IL18RAP on chromosome 2q12 and TAGAP on chromosome 6q25 were associated with type 1 diabetes mellitus. Moreover, the 32-bp insertion-deletion variant on chromosome 3p21, the PTPN2 on chromosome 18p11 and CTLA4 on chromosome 2q33 and SH2B3 on chromosome 12q24 are shared by both diseases (Smyth et al., 2008). Younger age at diabetes clinical onset, female gender, and coexistence of another autoimmune disease are predictive factors for celiac disease development (Cerutti et al, 2004)

In the majority of patients with type 1 diabetes clinical presentation of celiac disease is usually silent, and thanks to screening procedure is diagnosed (Holmes, 2001, Barera et al, 2002). On the other hand, a detailed medical history allows to identify several signs or symptoms attributable to celiac disease. Extra-intestinal manifestations such as failure to thrive, delayed puberty, iron-deficiency anemia, increased levels of liver enzyme tests, bleeding tendency, precocious osteoporosis, and unexplained hypoglycemic episodes are frequently reported. Gastrointestinal symptoms, i.e. diarrhea and abdominal pain, are reported in 28% and 14% of patients, respectively (Bhadada et al., 2011). Symptoms attributable to celiac disease are more common in children than in adolescents or adults (Larsson et al., 2008).

Type 1 diabetes precedes celiac disease diagnosis (Holmes, 2001); in a small proportion (up to 25%) of cases type 1 diabetes develops in already diagnosed celiac patients (Valerio et al., 2002).

In the majority of cases type 1 diabetes precedes celiac disease diagnosis (Holmes, 2001); in a small proportion of cases (up to 25%) type 1 diabetes develops in patients with already diagnosed celiac disease (Valerio et al., 2002).

Positivity for disease-related antibodies allows identification of patients with suspected celiac disease who must undergo intestinal biopsy. IgA-transglutaminase antibodies show the highest sensitivity and allow to identify around 98% of patients with celiac disease, while their specificity is lower, especially at a low titer (Salardi et al., 2008). IgA-anti-endomysial antibodies show lower sensitivity (98%) but higher specificity. Fluctuating positivity for anti-endomysial antibodies at a low titer can be detected at time of diabetes clinical onset, and in absence of signs or symptoms related to celiac disease only periodical screening is recommended .

Total IgA screening is mandatory before celiac disease-related antibodies detection. Patients with IgA deficiency benefit from IgG anti-transglutaminase antibody detection (Lenhardt et al., 2004) and, as recently reported, by IgG anti-deaminated gliadin peptides (Volta et al., 2010). IgA deficiency deserves attention, since this condition is more frequent in patients with celiac disease (1.7%) as compared to control population (0.25%)(Cataldo et al., 1997).

As regards timing of screening, it has been reported that the serological screening of celiac disease allows diagnosing 1% of patients with celiac disease. The frequency of diagnoses increases to 5% when screening is performed in the next 5 years after diabetes diagnosis (Larsson et al., 2008). It has been reported that up to 85% of cases of celiac disease is diagnosed 2-5 years after type 1 diabetes clinical onset (Saukkonen et al., 1996). Markers of celiac disease can appear within 10 years, so it is recommended to perform screening yearly for the first 4 years after diabetes diagnosis, and every 2 years in the following 6 years (Kordonouri et al., 2009).

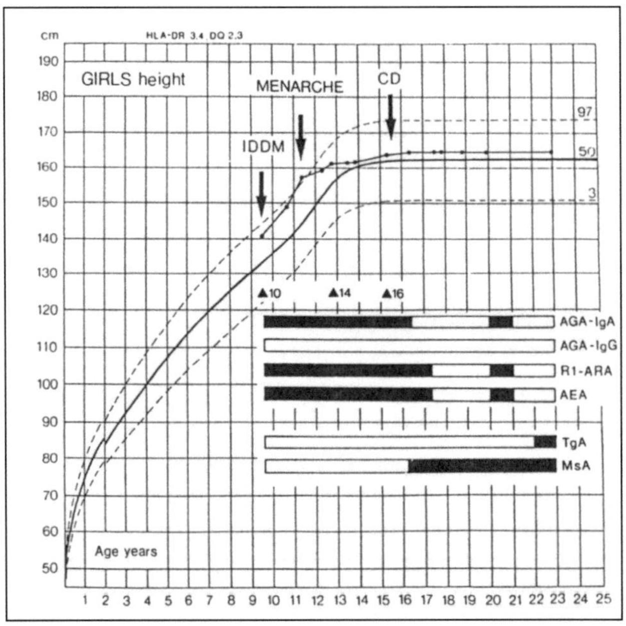


Fig. 1. Linear growth in a girl with type 1 diabetes and concomitant celiac disease, who developed autoimmune thyroiditis

Diagnosis of celiac disease by intestinal biopsy requires a lifelong gluten-free diet. Major problems related to gluten-free diet include quality of life, impairment of social life, poor compliance especially in adolescents and in patients with silent celiac disease diagnosed through screening procedures. Moreover, gluten-free diet can exert an increased insulin requirement since persistent hyperglycemia can occur. Gluten-free diet exerts in increased weight and height (Goh et al., 2010), as well as serum ferritin and hemoglobin (Hansen et al., 2006). Moreover improvement of bone status in patients with type 1 diabetes and adherence to gluten-free diet has been reported (Valerio et al., 2008).

## 4. Autoimmune thyroid disease

### 4.1 Hashimoto's thyroiditis

#### 4.1.1 Background and genetic susceptibility

Autoimmune thyroid diseases include many thyroid gland disorders, with different histological and clinical pictures ranging from the hypothyroidism of chronic lymphocytic thyroiditis to the hyperthyroidism of Graves' disease.

As other autoimmune diseases, **chronic lymphocytic thyroiditis** (also defined Hashimoto's thyroiditis from the physician who firstly described this condition) derives from a combination of genetic susceptibility and some environmental trigger factors (Pearce et al, 2003).

Hashimoto's thyroiditis is more frequent in females than in males (3.5 cases/1000 people/year versus 0.8 cases/1000 people/year, respectively), and global prevalence is increasing with age.

Hashimoto thyroiditis is the most common cause of acquired hypothyroidism in children and adolescents (formerly called "adolescent" or "simple" goiter), and usually presents itself during early adolescence or among schoolchildren, with or without gout, with a prevalence of 1% among schoolchildren (Lorini et al, 2003).

Susceptibility to Hashimoto's thyroiditis is determined by individual genetic background, including both major histocompatibility complex (MHC) and non-MHC genes.

Associations have been reported between Hashimoto's thyroiditis and HLA- DR3, HLA-DR4, or HLA-DR5. Furthermore, in children and adolescents paternal alleles and antibodies status have been shown to influence susceptibility to autoimmune thyroid disease. The expression of HLA-DR antigens on thyroid cells have a potential role in perpetuating the immune response, related to certain HLA-DR subtypes. As regards non-HLA susceptibility genes, several studies demonstrated the association between a polymorphism of the CTLA-4 gene and autoimmune thyroid disease (Barker, 2006).

In literature are reported linkage with loci on the X chromosome and on chromosome 20 or 14. Observations in twins are correlated with a genetic predisposition to thyroid autoimmunity. There are several cases of identical twins where one twin showed Graves' disease and the others Hashimoto's thyroiditis. It is common to find family clusters with HT and the incidence in parents or siblings of patient with HT can reach about 25% (Lorini et al., 2003).

#### 4.1.2 Pathogenesis

There is no evidence that a clear infectious agent is responsible for autoimmune thyroiditis. However, long-term follow-up of patients with subacute thyroiditis showed a possible reaction to viral infection with signs of persistence thyroid autoimmune disease. To this purpose, hepatitis C can act as a trigger for the development of autoimmune thyroiditis through thyroid follicular cell apoptosis. Potential mechanisms of infectious triggers include cell damage with the release of auto-antigens, expression of new antigens and molecular mimicry mechanisms.

Drugs containing iodine or supplementary dietary iodine can trigger an autoimmune thyroiditis in subjects at risk, although the mechanism is still unknown. Accumulation of iodine in animal models leads to iodination of thyroglobulin which triggers an immune reaction because T-cell-reactive peptides can be more antigenic when iodinated. Moreover dietary supplementation of iodine in the population of iodine-deficient regions such as the use of drugs rich in iodine (i.e. amiodarone) induce cases of thyroiditis, and a significant increase in lymphocytic infiltration by thyroid-specific auto-antibodies. Furthermore, patients treated with cytokines such as IL-1 or α-interferon can trigger an autoimmune thyroiditis, which is more frequent in patients with pre-existing positivity for anti-thyroid auto-antibodies.

Hashimoto's thyroiditis is an organ-specific autoimmune disease, characterized histologically by a lymphocytic infiltration of the thyroid gland, initially characterized by hyperplasia and subsequently by infiltration of lymphocytes and plasma cells between follicles, then resulting in a follicle atrophy. Lymphocytic infiltration is composed of B lymphocytes, about 30%, and T-lymphocytes, about 60%, including CD4+ helper and CD 8+ suppressor. Autoimmune thyroiditis is characterized by thyroid cell apoptosis leading to follicular destruction, rather than thyroid stimulation and cellular hyperplasia. Thyroid gland is infiltrated by B- and T-lymphocytes, the later are capable of destroying thyroid cells, which express Fas, via apoptosis and release several cytokines that increase the damage. The process is exacerbated by the action of auto-antibodies directed against several thyroid antigens, like thyroid peroxidase antibodies (TPO-Abs), detectable in 90% of patients with Hashimoto's thyroiditis, previously considered non-pathogenic, but now their role has been shown. They inhibit enzyme activity and stimulate cytotoxicity by natural killer. Anti-thyroglobulin antibodies (TgA) are detectable in a small percentage of patients, while high levels of thyrotropin receptor-blocking antibodies are often present, particularly in patients who develop autoimmune hypothyroidism.

#### 4.1.3 Clinical picture

Hashimoto's thyroiditis is the most common cause of acquired hypothyroidism in the pediatric population, occurring in about 1% of children and adolescents. Goiter is the hallmark of this autoimmune disease, and often may appear either insidiously or variable in size, however is usually enlarged with accentuation of the normal lobular architecture. Occasionally goiter gives the sensation of local pressure or causes difficulty in swallowing. Hashimoto's thyroiditis is more frequent in girls than in boys (four to seven times), with onset at 3 years but often sharply to 6 years with a peak incidence during adolescence.

The most common clinical symptoms are related to hypothyroidism, and include deceleration in the rate of growth, although some children are apparently asymptomatic, and show abnormal values in laboratory tests only. A few children complain clinical signs and symptoms of thyroid hyperfunction, such as nervousness, irritability, agitation, hot intolerance, weight loss. Eventually patient with Hashimoto's thyroiditis can show ophthalmopathy in absence of Graves' disease. The most frequent symptom in Hashimoto's thyroiditis is goiter, followed by menstrual disorders, short stature, and nervousness in girls, while constipation and exophthalmos are more frequently reported in boys. Other signs are hot and cold intolerance, weight loss or weight gain and sweating. The clinical course of Hashimoto's thyroiditis is quite variable. In fact, the goiter may reduce or disappear, or persist unchanged for years, while the patient remains euthyroid or progressively develops hypothyroidism. Spontaneous remission is frequent in adolescents (Lorini et al, 2003).

#### 4.1.4 Laboratory findings

In patients with autoimmune thyroiditis high serum levels of thyroid antibodies are present, therefore their detection is mandatory. Anti-thyroglobulin antibodies have been reported in 60% of patients with diffuse goiter or hypothyroidism or both while anti-thyroid peroxidase antibodies are detectable in 95% of cases so they represent a more sensitive marker. In 20% of cases there are significant antibody titers in the absence of thyroiditis, while lower titer are related to other thyroid diseases and in normal population.
Subclinical hypothyroidism means altered values of thyroid hormones in presence of a slightly or moderately elevated TSH. Many children with HT have normal level of TSH because the goiter is caused by lymphocytic infiltrations or growth-stimulating immunoglobulin.

#### 4.1.5 Imaging

On imaging studies, the thyroid gland shows enlargement without specific characteristics. High resolution ultrasound may show hypoechogenic micronodules (Fig. 2). Scintigraphic findings are variable; in some patients with Hashimoto's thyroiditis have thyroid gland enlarged with dysomogeneous distribution of tracer, in other cases the thyroid scan is normal but in most patients the uptake of radioiodine is decreased or increased. The perclorate washout is positive in 60% of patients. Often children and adolescents, evaluated at diagnosis, show a thyroid ultrasound picture altered. The definitive diagnosis of HT is confirmed by a biopsy of the thyroid, that confirmed the elevated titers of thyroid autoantibodies in the serum. High serum TSH concentration can be found in 30-40% of cases, associated with low serum T4, with normal or near-normal serum T3 concentration. Thyroid scan exclude thyroid dysgenesis. Elevated level of TSH clarifies if hypothyroidism is originated from pituitary or thyroid disease.

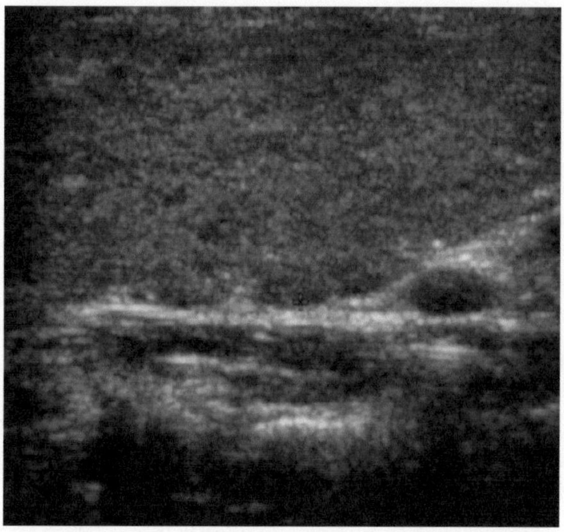

Fig. 2. Hashimoto's thyroiditis: thyroid ultrasound showing hypoechogenicity

#### 4.1.6 Treatment

The treatment of autoimmune thyroid follows the guidelines of congenital hypothyroidism. If the TSH level is greater than 10 µU/ml, L-thyroxin is the drug of choice. The initial dose is related on patient's age and on patient's clinical status from 25 µg/day to 100-150 µg/day. The therapy required periodic reevaluation, in particular when prominent nodules persist despite suppressive therapy, because there is a greater risk of cancer in patients with lymphocitic thyroiditis.

### 4.2 Graves' disease

Graves' disease is the most important cause of thyrotoxicosis in pediatrics and affects about 0.02% in children and adolescents. Its frequency increases with age: it is rare before the four years, gradually rises, reaching a peak during adolescence, with a preponderance for female gender (Kaguelidou et al, 2009). The aim of therapy is to reduce the excessive hormone production. First, this can be done with anti-thyroid drugs, as tionamides, with side effects especially after long-term therapy. Secondly, can be used thyroidectomy; however this surgical procedure may be complicated by several problems, such as hypoparathyroidism or recurrent nerve injury. Third method, is based on the use of radioiodine, that has not been yet universally accepted in children. Initial treatment, is medication and in the second instance, surgery or radioiodine. The goal of treatment is to maintain euthyroidism for a period at least 24 month and then discontinue the medical therapy. The positive results, with pharmacological treatment alone reaches 25% of cases. In *adults* the disease control is accomplished through the use of radioactive iodine or with drug for short periods. In *children*, however, use the medication for long periods, and then radioiodine, is just as an alternative option. The average age of onset is at 11 years (from 2.5 to 19 years), with preponderance in girls and with more cases of exophthalmos, low BMI, and higher height SDS. The goal of treatment is to limit the biosynthesis of thyroid hormones and maintain euthyroidism by maintaining a check on lab tests. Adverse effects are recorded in 5-32% of cases with skin rashes, transient neutropenia and agranulocytosis. Children have more adverse effects but less severe, often reversible spontaneously or with therapy change. Alternatively, using radioiodine in patients with hyperthyroidism resistant to drug treatment of 4.5 years, there was more remission (about 25% between 2-4 years of follow up). Most side-effect of the therapy is a permanent hypothyroidism, which can be treated with replacement therapy. The problem of this method is a potential carcinogenic risk (thyroid cancer and leukaemia), that declines with age, genetic damage, and a possible damage to reproduction. Radioiodine for safety, low cost and morbidity, could be the definitive treatment of Graves' disease in older children and young adolescents, but no in children younger than 5 years old (Gruneiro-Papendich et al, 2003).

### 4.3 Autoimmune thyroid disease and type 1 diabetes

Autoimmune thyroid disease is frequently reported in patients with type 1 diabetes mellitus, sometimes associated with celiac disease (Ergur et al, 2010). Serological screening studies aimed to evaluate the prevalence of thyroid involvement have gained momentum in recent years (Kadiyala et al. 2010). The prevalence of thyroid autoimmunity in patients with type 1 diabetes has been reported to be two to four times more frequent than in control population.

In control population the prevalence of thyroid autoimmunity ranges from 2.9% to 3.2%, while in young patients with type 1 diabetes the prevalence is higher, ranging from 19% to 23.4% (Kakleas et al., 2009). In children and adolescents with type 1 diabetes, risk factors for developing thyroid autoimmunity are quite similar to those reported in adult population, and include mainly female gender and increasing age. The role of anti-glutamic acid decarboxylase antibody persistence, age at diabetes diagnosis and duration of diabetes remains unclear. At-risk haplotypes for autoimmune thyroiditis include HLA-DQA1*0301 (linked to DR4), DQB1*0301 (linked to DR5) and DQB1*0201 (linked to DR3), which is associated with autoimmune hyperthyroidism, while the HLA-DQA1*0501 is associated with autoimmune hypothyroidism. The HLA haplotype DR3-DQB1*0201 confers the genetic susceptibility to type 1 diabetes mellitus, autoimmune thyroiditis and autoimmune polyendocrine syndrome type II. Finally, the HLA-haplotype DQB1*05 seems to be protective for autoimmune thyroid disease development (Kakleas et al., 2009). Other loci, i.e. VNTR and CTLA-4 may influence disease phenotype and severity (Van Driessche et al., 2009).

A symmetric, painless goitre is usually the first presentation of autoimmune thyroid disease, while atrophic thyroid gland is observed in 10% of patients. A subclinical hypothyroidism has been reported up to 58% of patients with thyroid autoantibodies. Early recognition and treatment of hypothyroidism is important, since the decrease in basal metabolism may exert weight gain, dyslipidemia, atheroscleroticheart disease, sometimes goiter, and may negatively affect metabolic control. Hypothyroidism is confirmed by low free thyroxin and high TSH levels. Compensated hypothyroidism mean normal thyroxine levels with increased TSH. Substitutive L-thyroxin treatment exerts normalization of TSH levels and goitre regression when present. Treatment with L-thyroxin in patients with type 1 diabetes, thyroid autoantibodies and thyroid enlargement is safe and effective to reduce thyromegaly, with no effect on thyroid autoantibodies titer (Brown, 2007, Kordonouri et al, 2007, Karges et al. 2007).

Autoimmune thyroid disease and type 1 diabetes mellitus are sometimes associated with chronic urticaria, also in young patients, as a possible consequence of thyroid chronic inflammations. However the mechanisms underlying this association have not yet been defined, but this association emphasizes the need for a routine screening (Hyman et al., 2008).

In young patients with type 1 diabetes mellitus overt hyperthyroidism is rarely encountered. It may be expression of Graves' disease or the transient hyperthyroid phase of Hashimoto's thyroiditis. Unstable metabolic control despite strict compliance, weight loss despite regular food intake, agitation, tremors, tachycardia, insomnia, heath intolerance, thyroid enlargement and characteristic eye signs are the main clinical features. Treatment is based on anti-thyroid drugs like propylthiuracil and metimazole.During acute thyrotoxicosis beta-adrenergic blockers agents are indicated. Persistent hyperthyroidism requires surgery or radioiodine (Kordonouri et al, 2009).

## 5. Atrophic gastritis

### 5.1 Background

While the association between type 1 diabetes and celiac disease and/or thyroid autoimmunity is clearly documented, particularly in young patients, few data are available about the frequency of other autoimmune diseases, like autoimmune gastritis and pernicious anemia.

Autoimmune gastritis, firstly described by Thomas Addison in 1849, is characterized by autoantibodies directed against gastric parietal cells, atrophy of gastric corpus and fundus, hypochlorhydria/achlorhydria, hypergastrinemia, iron deficiency anemia and pernicious anemia.
In *adult* general population the frequency of autoimmune gastritis is about 1-2%, and is 3-5 fold increased in patients with type 1 diabetes (De Block et al, 2008). As regards *children, adolescents* and *young adults* with type 1 diabetes, the frequency of parietal cells antibodies is 15.8%, with a close association with older age and duration of disease (De Block et al, 2008, Warncke et al, 2010). Female gender association is controversial.

### 5.2 Pathogenesis

Antibodies against parietal cells (PCA) and their secretory product Intrinsic Factor (AIF) are serological markers for autoimmune gastritis and are targeted towards H+, K+-ATPase of gastric parietal cells and denote autoimmune gastritis, characterized by atrophy of corpus and fundus. The chronic auto-aggression to the proton pump exerts in hypochlorhydria/achlorhydria and hypergastrinemia and iron-deficiency anemia as a consequence of impaired gastric secretion and iron absorption. Moreover PCA are responsible for the reduced intrinsic factor secretion with subsequent pernicious anemia due to vitamin 12 deficiency. PCA and AIF are detectable not only in serum, but also in gastric juice. PCA titer is positively related to severity of gastric atrophy and negatively related to concentration of parietal cells. Low serum levels of pepsinogen I, as a consequence of chief cell destruction, represent another early marker of autoimmune gastritis and pernicious anemia. Both pernicious anemia and autoimmune gastritis may predispose to gastric cancer. Gastric adenocarcinomas are reported on 1-10 % of adult patients with autoimmune gastritis through intestinal meta/dysplasia. (De Block et al., 2003) Helicobacter Pylori infection has been reported as a risk factor for autoimmune gastritis, by stimulating granulocytes to produce oxygen radicals, which are mutagenic and lead to corpus atrophy (D'Elios et al., 2004). Molecular mimicry and/or T-helper l-induced expression of HLA-class II and co-stimulatory molecules on gastric epithelial cells are considered as pathogenic mechanisms for Helicobacter Pylori induced autoimmunity (Lahner et al., 2011). The evidence of a link between pernicious anemia and particular HLA haplo/genotypes is not strong. As regards type 1 diabetes, a weak association between PCA positivity and the HLA-DQA1*0501-B1*0301 haplotype, linked to HLA-DR5, has been observed. In mouse models, four distinct genetic regions that confer susceptibility to autoimmune gastritis have been identified: two loci, located on distal chromosome 4, are called *Gasa1* and *Gasa2;* two other loci, located on chromosome 6, are called *Gasa3* and *Gasa4,* respectively. Interestingly, three out of these four susceptibility loci are non-major histocompatibility complex genes which co-localize with those of type 1 diabetes. This is the strongest concordance identified between any two autoimmune disease so far (De Block et al., 2008).

### 5.3 Diagnosis

Parietal cell antibodies are measured using immunoblotting or enzyme linked immunoassay (ELISA), which are more sensitive than indirect immunofluorescence technique. Iron deficiency anemia is defined as microcytic hypochromic anemia with a transferrine saturation of less than 20% and low iron and ferritin levels. Pernicious anemia is defined as macrocytic anemia with subnormal vitamin B12 levels and positive levels of PCAs

Diagnosis of AG requires gastroscopy with at least two biopsies from gastric antrum and gastric body. Atrophy of the gastric body mucosa is defined as focal or complete oxyntic gland loss and/or replacement by metaplastic pylori or intestinal glands. To each graded variable, the scores usually employed are: 0 = absence; 1 = mild; 2 = moderate; 3 = severe (Bordi et al., 1997).

### 5.4 Treatment

Therapy of autoimmune gastritis includes supplementation of iron or vitamin B12 or removal of pre-malignant gastric lesions. Patients with PCA antibodies and high gastrin levels should undergo endoscopy with biopsies.

Determining risk factors for and early diagnosis of autoimmune gastritis is mandatory to prevent and treat iron-deficiency anemia, pernicious anemia and pre-malignant gastric lesions. In all PCA positive patients gastroscopy with multiple biopsies should be performed and subsequent clinical and endoscopic close follow-up are mandatory.

### 5.5 Autoimmune gastritis and type 1 diabetes

Autoimmune gastritis is rarely encountered in children and adolescents with type 1 diabetes, since the prevalence of parietal cell antibodies increases with age and with longer duration of disease. It is noteworthy that even young patients with type 1 diabetes are positive for parietal cell antibodies, with a frequency about 4%, which is higher than in controls (1.9%) (De Block et al., 2008). On the other hand, autoimmune gastritis is more frequent in children and adolescents with autoimmune thyroid disorder (Fig. 3 ).

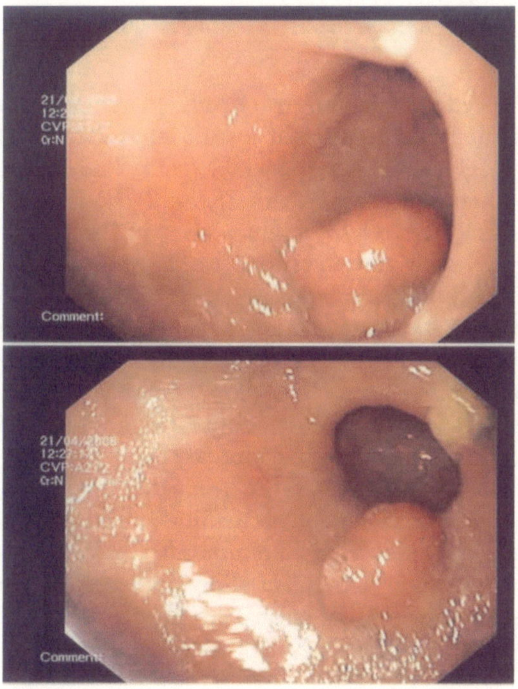


Fig. 3. Atrophic gastritis and sessile antral polyp with signs of esophageal candidiasis (personal data)

## 6. Addison's disease

### 6.1 Background

In 1849 Thomas Addison firstly described a group of patients characterized by anemia and disease of adrenal glands. Addison's disease is an insidious, chronic disorder of the adrenal cortex resulting in decreased production of glucocorticoids, mineralocorticoids, and androgens. There is a concomitant increased secretion of ACTH from the pituitary gland aimed to stimulate the adrenal gland. In developed countries an autoimmune process is recognized as the most common etiological factor of adrenal gland insufficiency (70-90%); the second cause is tuberculosis of the adrenal gland (10 to 20%). Three clinical forms of adrenal insufficiency are recognized: Addison disease within syndromes characterized by autoimmune involvement of several organs and named Autoimmune Polyendocrine Syndromes (APS-1 and APS-2), and Addison disease as an isolated condition.

### 6.2 Pathogenesis

Genetically predisposed individuals develop autoantibodies toward the 21-hydroxylase enzyme and eventually lose the ability to produce cortisol. Autoantibodies against 21-hydroxylase are present in the majority of recently diagnosed patients. Susceptibility is conferred through the genes encoding the class II Major Histocompatibility Complex. Similarly as for type 1 diabetes mellitus, there is a strong association with the DR3 haplotype. The highest risk genotype, occurring in 30% of patients with Addison's disease, is represented by DR3/4, DQ2/DQ8 and the DRB1*0404 /DQ8-DRB1*0301/DQ2 genotype occurs at an increased frequency in individuals with isolated AD and in those with AD and type 1 diabetes mellitus (El Fassi et al., 2007).

### 6.3 Diagnosis

Addison's disease is preceded by a long prodromic, asymptomatic period, followed by subtle clinical manifestations up to adrenal insufficiency. Main symptoms are persistent vomiting, anorexia, hypoglycemia, unexplained weight loss, malaise, ill-defined fatigue, muscular weakness, hypotension, and craving for salt. The most specific sign of primary adrenal insufficiency is generalized hyperpigmentation of the skin and mucosal surfaces, as a consequence of high plasma concentrations of melanocyte stimulating activity of β-lipotropin, which origins from the same precursor as ACTH. Laboratory tests can aid in the diagnosis: hypoglycemia, hyponatriemia, hyperkaliemia, acidosis, high levels of ACTH and a deficiency of cortisol. Furthermore, adrenal antibodies represent a useful marker, with a higher predictive value in younger than in adult patient, being present in more than 90% of patients with autoimmune Addison disease. Antibodies are directed against steroidogenic enzymes (CYP21A2 and 21 hydroxylase) or adrenal cortex (Adrenal cortex autoantibodies, ACA). In addition, hypocorticism may cause frequent hypoglycemic events (Van den Driessche et al 2009). We recommend screening patients with type 1A diabetes, hypoparathyroidism, and polyendocrine autoimmunity for 21-hydroxylase autoantibodies. If present, yearly monitoring with an ACTH stimulation test is performed to allow early diagnosis and prevent an adrenal crisis (Aaron et al., 2008).

### 6.4 Treatment

Addison's disease treatment consists of urgent lifelong glucocorticoids replacement, with clear counseling about the need for stress dose steroids for illnesses and prior to surgical procedures (Aaron et al., 2008). In some cases supplementation with mineralcorticoids in mandatory.

### 6.5 Addison's disease and type 1 diabetes

In adolescents with type 1 diabetes Addison's disease is rarely encountered, and symptoms are sometimes aspecific. Addison's disease usually follows type 1 diabetes diagnosis, being more frequently observed within the Autoimmune Polyendocrine Syndrome type 1 and type 2 (Kordonouri et al., 2009). Correct diagnosis of Addison's disease requires a high degree of clinical suspicion and since the disease is a life-threatening condition, several investigators recommend periodical screening of Addison's disease in all young patients since type 1 diabetes diagnosis (Brewer et al., 1997). In an adolescent with type 1 diabetes, Addison's disease should be suspected in case of recurrent hypoglycemic episodes, unexplained decrease of insulin requirement and improvement of metabolic control, fatigue, weight loss, hyponatriemia and hyperkaliemia. Diagnosis confirmation requires low cortisol levels after ACTH stimulation test. Screening procedures allow to detect asymptomatic children and adolescents with positive adrenal antibodies; where raised ACTH levels suggest the presence of adrenal insufficiency. Risk factors for Addison's disease in patients with type 1 diabetes include a history of other autoimmune conditions, in particular thyroid disease, and a positive family history for autoimmunity, as reported in a case series of 4 adolescents with pre-existing type 1 diabetes who developed Addison disease (Thomas et al., 2004). Three out of 4 patients showed unexplained hypoglycemia and the other one showed unawareness hypoglycemia; all cases reported unexplained improvement in diabetes control. Two out of 4 patients reported skin hyperpigmentation. In all 4 patients a positive personal and family history of other autoimmune conditions has been reported, in particular celiac and/or thyroid autoimmune diseases and Autoimmune Polyendocrine Syndrome type 2. A more recent study in 491 newly diagnosed children with type 1 diabetes aimed to define the prevalence of additional autoimmune conditions reported 1% positivity of antibodies to 21-hydroxylase, while overt Addison's disease was found only in 20% of the positive patients (Triolo et al.; 2011). Noteworthy, all young patients with type 1 diabetes and adrenal autoantibodies develop Addison's disease during the follow-up period, with a progression to overt adrenal failure much more rapid than in adults, indicating that different autoimmune responses may be evoked at different age periods (Betterle et al., 1997).

## 7. The Autoimmune Polyglandular Syndromes (APS)

From the time of Addison's original description of his disease onwards, it has been apparent that multiple autoimmune endocrine disease can affect individual patients and their families in recognizable clinical clusters.

Twenty years ago, the autoimmune polyglandular syndromes (APS) were classified into three basic types based on the patient's age at onset, their clinical associations with specific endocrinopathies and HLA typing.

**Type I APS**, called also APECED (Autoimmune PolyEndocrinopathy-Candidiasis-Ectodermal Dystrophy) is a rare autosomal recessive disorder originally identified through the typical association of mucocutaneous candidiasis with Addison's disease and hypoparathyroidism. These symptoms usually constitute the first manifestation of the disease in early childhood; other endocrine and non-endocrine disorders can be associated: thyroiditis, autoimmune hypogonadism, hypophysitis, chronic active hepatitis, atrophic gastritis, pernicious anemia, alopecia, vitiligo and ectodermal dystrophy (Mazza et al., 2011). The disease results from the inheritance of recessive genes (AIRE gene) mapping to 21q22.3 and it is not linked to genes within the HLA-DR/DQ genetic region of chromosome 6.

**Type II APS** is more common than type 1 APS, the prevalence is 1/20,000 with a female preponderance (male/female ratio = 1/3) and has a peak incidence between the ages of 20 and 60 years, mostly in the third or fourth decade (Van den Driessche et al., 2009). It is defined by the association of Addison's disease with thyroid autoimmunity, type 1 diabetes and sometimes pernicious anemia, vitiligo and hypogonadism. Type II APS is HLA-associated (DQB1*0302/0201), while Hashimoto's thyroiditis itself is associated with HLA-DQB1*0301. Multiple antigens have now been identified for the component disease of type II APS ie: thyroperoxydase and thyroglobulin in Hashimoto's thyroiditis; TSH receptors I Graves' disease; insulin, GAD and IA-2 and IA-2B in type 1 diabetes mellitus; 21 hydroxylase in Addison's disease; 17 hydroxylase and SCC (all p450 enzymes) in hypogonadism; tyrosine in vitiligo; H+K+ATPase an intrinsic factor in pernicious anemia and the calcium sensing receptor (CaSR) in hypoparathyroidism. Indeed the autoantibody that reacts to CaSR does so through its external domain, suggesting that the respective autoimmunity (hypoparathyroidism) may be antibody dependent. In mice, such immune responses proceeded through a T cell helper-2 (Th2) pathway; whereas those that results in cell mediated pancreatic β-cell loss are though to occur through a Th1 pathway. It could be that APS I results from an inherited defective Th1 responsiveness resulting in uninhibited Th2 overactivity. On the other hand, APSII/III appears to results from Th1 autoimmunity, perhaps explaining why APS-I does not co-exist with APS-II or III.

CD4+ T helper (Th) cells play important roles in regulating immune responses including that of immunological tolerance to self. When these regulatory processes go away, one or more organ-specific autoimmune disease may develop. One prevailing theory developed in the mice is that immunoresponsiveness follows at least two polarized pathways. While one track (Th1) promotes cellular immune responses, the other (Th2) pathway favours antibody or allergic immunoresponsiveness. Such differentiated Th cells can be distinguished based upon their cytokine phenotypes.

## 8. Conclusions

It is now established that patients with type 1 diabetes are at increased risk of other autoimmune diseases as compared to general populations (Michels & Eisenbarth, 2010). Besides islet-cell autoantibodies, other antibodies against numerous non β-cell antigens have been frequently reported. Clinically-evident diseases are rarely observed in young patients with type 1 diabetes, and can be considered as the tip of the iceberg. Latent forms of these autoimmune-associated diseases, characterized by the presence of circulating autoantibodies with mild or no symptoms, are more frequent. Early detection of antibodies and latent organ-specific dysfunction are advocated to alert physicians to take appropriate actions aimed to prevent full-blown disease. Moreover patients and their relatives should be instructed to recognize subclinical signs and symptoms attributable to these autoimmune-associated diseases. Several risk factors have been identified for a group of autoimmune diseases like genetic background, gender, age, age at clinical onset and duration of diabetes.

## 9. References


Achenbach, P.; Lampasona, V.; Landherr, U.; Koczwara, K.; Krause, S.; Grallert, H.; Winkler, C.; Pfuger, M.; Illig, T.; Bonifacio, E. & Ziegler, A. (2009). Autoantibodies to zinc transporter 8 and SLC30A8 genotype stratify type 1 diabetes. *Diabetologia*, Vol.9, No.52, pp. 1881-1888

Alaedini, A. & Green, PHR. (2005). Narrative review: celiac disease: understanding a a complex auotimmune disorder. *Ann Intern Med*, Vol 142, pp. 289-298

Allen, S.; Huber, J. & Devendra, D. (2008). Prevalence of organ-specific autoantibodies in childhood- and adult-onset type 1 diabetes. *Ann N Y Acad Sci.*, Vol.1150, pp. 260-262

Al-Toma, A.; Verbeek, WH.; Hadithi, M.; von Blomberg, BM. & Mulder, CJ. (2007). Survival in refractory celiac disease and enteropathy-associated T-cell lymphoma: retrospective evaluation of a single-centre experience. *Gut*, Vol. 56, No.10, pp. 1373-1378

Andersson C.; Larsson, K.; Vaziri-Sani, F.; Lynch, K.; Carlsson, A.; Cedervall, E.; Jönsson, B.; Neiderud, J.; Månsson, M.; Nilsson, A.; Lernmark, A.; Elding Larsson, H. & Ivarsson, SA. (2011). The three ZNT8 autoantibody variants together improve the diagnostic sensitivity of childhood and adolescent type 1 diabetes. *Autoimmunity*, early online pp. 1-12

Baekkeskov, S.; Aanstoot, HJ.; Christgau, S.; Reetz, A.; Solimena, M.; Cascalho, M.; Folli, F.; Richter-Olesen, H. & De Camilli, P. (1990). Identification of the 64K autoantigen in insulin-dependent diabetes as the GABA-synthesizing enzyme glutamic acid decarboxylase. *Nature*, Vol.6289, No.13, pp. 151-156

Bangstad, HJ.; Danne, T.; Deeb, LC.; Jarosz-Chobot, P.; Urakami, T. & Hanas, R. (2007). International Society for Pediatric and Adolescent Diabetes. ISPAD Clinical Practice Consensus Guidelines 2006-2007. Insulin treatment. *Pediatr Diabetes*, Vol.8, No.2, pp. 88-102

Barera, G.; Bonfanti, R.; Viscardi, M.; Bazzigaluppi, E.; Calori, G.; Meschi, F.; Bianchi, C. & Chiumello, G. (2002). Occurrence of celiac disease after onset of type 1 diabetes: a 6-year prospective longitudinal study. *Pediatrics*, Vol.109, No.5, pp. 833-838

Barker, JM (2006). Type 1 diabetes-associated autoimmunity: natural history, genetic associations, and screening. *J Clin Endocrinol Metab*, Vol. 91, N.4, pp. 1210-1217

Betterle, C.; Volpato, M.; Rees Smith, B.; Furmaniak, J.; Chen, S.; Zanchetta, R.; Greggio, N.; Pedini, B.; Boscaro, M. & Presotto F. (1997). Adrenal cortex and steroid 21-hydroxylase autoantibodies in children with organ-specific autoimmune diseases: markers of high progression to clinical Addison's disease. *J Clin Endocrinol Metab*, Vol.82, No.3, pp 939-942

Bhadada, SK.; Kochhar, R.; Bhansali, A; Dutta, U.; Kumar, PR.; Poornachandra, KS.; Vaiphei, K.; Nain, CK. & Singh K. (2011). Prevalence of clinical profile of celiac disease in type 1 diabetes mellitus in North India. *J Gastroenetrol Hepatol*, Vol.26, No.2, pp. 378-381

Bordi, C.; Annibale, B.; Azzoni, C.; Marignani, M.; Ferraro, G.; Antonelli, G.; D'Adda, T.; D'Ambra, G. & Delle Fave, G. (1997). Endocrine cell growths in atrophic body gastritis. Critical evaluation of a histological classification. *J Pathol*, Vol.3, No 182, pp. 339-346

Bottazzo, GF.; Florin-Christensen, A. & Doniach, D. (1974). Islet-cell antibodies in diabetes mellitus with autoimmune polyendocrine deficiencies. *Lancet*, Vol.7892, No.2, pp. 1279-1283

Bransky, D.; Fasano, A. & Troncone, R. (2006). Latest developments in the pathogenesis and treatment of celiac disease. *J Pediatr,* Vol.149, pp. 295-300

Brewer, KW.; Parziale, WS. & Eisenbarth GS. (1997). Screening patients with insulin dependent diabetes mellitus for adrenal insufficiency. N Engl J Med Vol. 237, pag. 202

Brown, RS. (2007). Euthyroid autoimmune thyroiditis in children and adolescents with type 1 diabetes mellitus: to treat or not to treat?. *Pediatr Diabetes,* Vol.8, No.4, pp. 177-179

Cataldo, F.; Marino, V.; Bottaro, G.; Greco, P. & Ventura A. (1997). Celiac disease and selective immunoglobulin A deficiency. *J Pediatr,* Vol.131, No.2, pp. 306-308

Cerutti, F.; Bruno, G.; Chiarelli, F.; Lorini, R.; Meschi, F.; Sacchetti, C. & the Diabetes Study Group of Italian Society of Pediatric Endocrinology and Diabetology (2004). Younger age at onset and sex predict celiac disease in children and adolescents with type 1 diabetes: an Italian multicenter study. *Diabetes Care,* Vol.27, No.6, pp.1294-1298

Daneman, D. (2006). Type 1 diabetes. *Lancet*, Vol.367, No.9513, pp. 847-858

D'Elios, MM.; Bergman, MP.; Amedei, A.; Appelmelk, BJ. & Del Prete G. (2004). Helicobacter pylori and gastric autoimmunity. *Microbes Infect,* Vol.6, No.15, pp. 1395-401

De Block, CEM.; De Leeuw, IH.; Bogers, JJPM.; Pelckmans, PA.; Ieven, MM.; Van Marck, EAE.; Van Acker, KL. & Van Gaal, LF. (2003) Autoimmune gastropathy in type 1 diabetic patients with parietal cell antibodies. *Diabetes Care*, Vol.26, No.1, pp. 82-88

De Block, CE.; De Leeuw, IH. & Van Gaal, LF. (2008). Autoimmune gastritis in type 1 diabetes: a clinically oriented review. *J Clin Endocrinol Metab,* Vol.93, No.2, pp. 363-371

Devendra, D.; Liu, E. & Eisenbarth, GS. (2004). Type 1 diabetes: recent developments. *BMJ*, Vol.328, No.7442, pp. 750-754

Di Sabatino, A. & Corazza, GR. (2009). Coeliac disease. *Lancet,* Vol.373, No. 9673, pp. 1480-1493

Donaghue, K.; Chiarelli, F.; Trotta, D.; Allgrove, J. & Dahl Jorgensen, K. (2007) Microvascular and macrovascular complications. *Pediatr Diabetes,* Vol.10, Supplement 12, pp. 195-203

El Fassi, D.; Nielsen, CH.; Bonnema, SJ.; Hasselbalch, HC. & Hegedüs, L. (2007). B lymphocyte depletion with the monoclonal antibody rituximab in Graves' disease: a controlled pilot study. *J Clin Endocrinol Metab*, Vol.92, No.5, pp. 1769-1772

Ergür, AT.; Oçal, G.; Berberoğlu, M.; Adıyaman, P.; Sıklar, Z.; Aycan, Z.; Evliyaoğlu, O.; Kansu, A.; Girgin, N. & Ensari, A. (2010). Celiac disease and autoimmune thyroid disease in children with type 1 diabetes mellitus: clinical and HLA-Genotyping Results. *J Clin Res Pediatr Endocrinol*, Vol.2, No.4, pp. 151-154

Franzese, A.; Iafusco, D.; Spadaro, R.; Cavaliere, O.; Prisco, F.; Auricchio, R.; Troncone, R. & Valerio, G. (2011). The Study-Group on Diabetes of Italian Society of Pediatric Endocrinology and Diabetology (ISPED). Potential celiac disease in type 1 diabetes: A multicenter study. *Diab Res Clin Pract*, Vol.14

Frisk, G.; Hansson, T.; Dahlbom, I. & Tuvemo, T. (2008). A unifying hypothesis on the development of type 1 diabetes and celiac disease: gluten consumption may be a shared causative factor. *Med Hypotheses* Vol.70, No.6, pp. 1207-1209

Goh, VL.; Estrada, DE.; Lerer, T.; Balarezo, F. & Sylvester, FA. (2010). Effect of gluten-free diet on growth and glycemic control in children with type 1 diabetes and asymptomatic celiac disease. *J Pediatr Endocrinol Metab*, Vol.23, No.11, pp. 1169-1173

Green, PH.; Rostami, K. & Marsh, MN. (2005). Diagnosis of coeliac disease. *Best Pract Res Clin Gastroenterol*, Vol.19, No.3, pp. 389-400

Gruneiro-Papendieck, L.; Chiesa, A.; Finkielstain, G. & Heinrich, JJ. (2003). Pediatric Graves' disease: outcome and treatment. *J Pediatr Endocrinol Metab*, Vol 16, No. 2, pp. 1249-1255

Hansen, D.; Brock-Jacobsen, B.; Lund, E.; Bjørn, C.; Hansen, LP.; Nielsen, C.; Fenger, C.; Lillevang, ST. & Husby, F. (2006). Clinical benefit of a gluten-free diet in type 1 diabetic children with screening-detected celiac disease. *Diabetes Care*, Vol 29, N. 11, pp. 2452-2456

Hermann, R.; Knip, M.; Veijola, R.; Simell, O.; Laine, AP.; Akerblom, HK.; Groop, PH.; Forsblom, C.; Pettersson-Fernholm, K.; Ilonen, J. & FinnDiane Study Group. (2003). Temporal changes in the frequencies of HLA genotypes in patients with Type 1diabetes--indication of an increased environmental pressure? *Diabetologia*, Vol.3, No.46, pp. 420-425

Holmes, G. (2001). Celiac disease and type 1 diabetes mellitus - the case for screening. *Diabet Med* Vol. 18, N. 3, pp 169-177.

Hyman, SJ.; Shreffler, WG. & Rapaport, R. (2008). Type 1 diabetes, autoimmune thyroid disease, and chronic urticaria. *Pediatr Diabetes*, Vol.9, No.5, pp. 508-511

Kadiyala, R.; Peter, R.& Okosieme OE. (2010). Thyroid dysfunction in patients with diabetes: clinical implications and screening strategies. *Int J Clin Pract*, Vol.64, No.8, pp. 1130-1139

Kaguelidou, F.; Carel, JC. & Léger, J. (2009). Graves' disease in childhood: advances in management with antithyroid drug therapy. *Horm Res*, Vol.71, No.6, pp. 310-317

Kakleas, K.; Paschali, E.; Kefalas, N.; Fotinou, A.; Kanariou, M.; Karayianni, C. & Karavanaki, K. (2009). Factors for thyroid autoimmunity in children and adolescents with type 1 diabetes mellitus. *Ups J Med Sci*, Vol.114, No.4, pp. 214-220

Kakleas, K.; Karayianni, C.; Critselis, E.; Papathanasiou, A.; Petrou, V.; Fotinou, A. & Karavanaki, K. (2010). The prevalence and risk factors for coeliac disease among children and adolescents with type 1 diabetes mellitus. *Diab Res Clin Pract*, Vol.90, No.2, (September 2010), pp. 202-208

Karges, B.; Muche, R.; Knerr, I.; Ertelt, W.; Wiesel, T.; Hub, R.; Neu, A.; Klinghammer, A.; Aufschild, J.; Rapp, A.; Schirbel, A.; Boehm, BO.; Debatin, KM.; Heinze, E. & Karges, W. (2007). Levothyroxine in euthyroid autoimmune thyroiditis and type 1 diabetes: a randomized, controlled trial. *J Clin Endocrinol Metab.* Vol.92, No.5, pp. 1647-1652

Kordonouri, O.; Hartmann, R.; Riebel, T. & Liesenkoetter KP. (2007). Early treatment with L-thyroxine in children and adolescents with type 1 diabetes, positive thyroid antibodies, and thyroid gland enlargement. *Pediatr Diabetes*, Vol.8, No.4, pp. 180-184

Kordonouri, O.; Maguire, AM.; Knip, M.; Schober, E.; Lorini, R.; Holl, RW. & Donaghue, KC. (2009). Other complications and associated conditions with diabetes in children and adolescents. *Pediatr Diabetes*, Vol.12, No.10, pp. 204-210

Lahner, E.; Bernardini, G.; Possenti, S.; Renzone, G.; Scaloni, A.; Santucci, E. & Annibale, B. (2011). Immunoproteomics of Helicobacter Pylori infection in patients with atrophic body gastritis, a predisposing condition of gastric cancer. *Int J Med Microbiol*, Vol.301, No.2, pp. 125-132

Larsson, K.; Carlsson, A.; Cederwall, E.; Jönsson, B.; Neiderud, J.; Jonsson, B.; Lernmark, A. & Ivarsson, SA. Skåne Study Group (2008). Annual screening detects celiac disease in children with type 1 diabetes. *Pediatr Diabetes*, Vol.9, No.4, pp. 354-359

Lenhardt, A.; Plebani, A.; Marchetti, F.; Gherarduzzi, T.; Not, T.; Meini, A.; Villanacci, V.; Martelossi, S. & Ventura, A. (2004). Role of human tissue transglutaminase IgG and anti-gliadin IgG antibodies in the diagnosis of celiac disease in patients with selective IgA deficiency. *Dig Liv Dis*, Vol. 36, pp. 730-734

Lorini, R.; Gastaldi, R.; Traggiai, C. & Polo Perucchin, P. (2003). Hashimotos's thyroiditis. *Ped Endocrinol Rev*, Vol. 1, Supplement 2, pp. 205-211

Maffeis, C. & Pinelli, L. (2008). Teaching children with diabetes about adequate dietary choices. *Br J Nutr*, Vol.99, Supplement 1, pp. 33-39

Mäki, M.; Mustalahti, K.; Kokkonen, J.; Kulmala, P.; Haaplahti, M.; Karttunen, T.; Ilonen, J.; Laurila, K.; Dahlbom, I.; Hansson, T.; Höpfl, P. & Knip, M. (2003). Prevalence of celiac disease among children in Finland. *N Engl J Med*, Vol. 348, pp. 2517-2524

Mazza, C.; Buzi, F.; Ortolani, F.; Vitali, A.; Notarangelo, LD.; Weber, G.; Bacchetta, R.; Soresina, A.; Lougaris, V.; Greggio, A.; Taddio, A.; Pasic, S.; de Vroede, M.; Pac, M.; Kilic, SS.; Ozden, S.; Rusconi, R.; Martino, S.; Capalbo, D.; Salerno, M.; Pignata, C.; Radetti, G.; Maggiore, G.; Plebani, A.; Notarangelo, LD. & Badolato, R. (2011). Clinical heterogeneity and diagnostic delay of autoimmune polyendocrinopathy-candidiasis-ectodermal dystrophy syndrome. *Clin Immunol*, Vol.139, No.1, pp. 6-11

Michels, AW. & Eisenbarth GS. (2010). Immunologic endocrine disorders. *J Allergy Clin Immunol.*, Vol.125, No.2, pp. 226-237

Monnier, L. & Colette, C. (2008) Glycemic variability: should we and can we prevent it? *Diabetes Care*, Vol.31, Supplement 2, pp. 150-154

Nejentsev, S.; Howson, JM.; Walker, NM.; Szeszko, J.; Field, SF.; Stevens, HE.; Reynolds, P.; Hardy, M.; King, E.; Masters J.; Hulme, J.; Maier, LM.; Smyth, D.; Bailey, R.; Cooper, JD.; Ribas, G.; Campbell, RD.; Clayton, DG. & Todd, JA. (2007). Localization of type 1 diabetes susceptibility to the MHC class I gens HLA-B and HLA-A. *Nature*, Vol.7171, No.450, pp. 887-892

Oikarinen, S.; Martiskainen, M.; Tauriainen, S.; Huhtala, H.; Ilonen, J.; Veijola, R.; Simell, O.; Knip, M.& Hyoty, H. (2011). Enterovirus RNA in blood is linked to the development of type 1 diabetes. *Diabetes*, Vol.60, No. 1, pp. 276-279

Pearce, EN.; Farwell, AP. & Braverman, L. (2003). Thyroiditis. *N Engl J Med* Vol. 348, N. 26, pp. 2646-2655

Pastore, MR.; Bazzigaluppi, E.; Belloni, C.; Arcovio, C.; Bonifacio, E. & Bosi E. (2003). Six months of gluten-free diet do not influence autoantibody titers, but improve insulin secretion in subjects at high risk for type 1 diabetes. *J Clin Endocrinol Metab*, Vol.88, No.1, pp.162-165

Rabin, DU.; Pleasic, SM.; Shapiro, JA.; Yoo-Warren, H.; Oles, J.; Hicks, JM.; Goldstein, DE. & Rae, PM. (1994). Islet cell antigen 512 is a diabetes-specific islet autoantigen related to protein tyrosine phosphatases. *J Immunol*, Vol.6, No.152, pp. 3183-3188

Rewers, M.; Pihoker, C.; Donaghue, K.; Hanas, R.; Swift, P. & Klingensmith, GJ. (2009). Assessment and monitoring of glycemic control in children and adolescents with diabetes. *Pediatr Diabetes*. Vol.10, Supplement 12, pp. 71-81

Rubio-Tapia, A.; Kelly, DG.; Lahr, BD.; Dogan, A.; Wu, TT. & Murray JA. (2009). Clinical staging and survival in refractory celiac disease: a single center experience. *Gastroenterology*, Vol. 136, No.1, pp. 99-107

Salardi, S.; Volta, U.; Zucchini, S.; Fiorini, E.; Maltoni, G.; Vaira, B. & Cicognani, A. (2008). Prevalence of celiac disease in children with type 1 diabetes mellitus in the mid-1990s: an 18-year longitudinal study based on anti-endomysial antibodies. *J Pediatr Gastroenterol Nutr*, Vol.46, No.5, pp. 612-614

Saukkonen, T.; Savilahti, E.; Reijonen, H.; Ilonen, J.; Tuomilehto-Wolf, E. & Ackerblom, HK. (1996). Coeliac disease: frequent occurrence after clinical onset of insulin-dependent diabetes mellitus. Childhood diabetes in Finland Study Group. *Diabet Med*, Vol 13, No.5, pp. 464-470

Shan, L.; Molberg, Ø.; Parrot, I.; Hausch, F.; Filiz, F.; Gray, GM.; Sollid, LM. & Khosla C. (2002) Structural basis for gluten intolerance in celiac sprue. *Science*, Vol.297, No.5590, pp. 2275-2279.

Smyth, DJ.; Plagnol, V.; Walker; NM., Cooper, JD.; Downes, K.; Phil, M.; Yang, JHM.; Howson, JMM.; Stevens, H.; McManus, R.; Wijmenga, C.; Heap, GA.; Dubois, PC.; Clayton, DG.; Hunt, KA.; van Heel, DA.; Phil, D. & Todd, JA. (2008). Shared and distinct genetic variants in type 1 diabetes and celiac disease. *N Engl J Med*, Vol.359, No.26, (December 2008) pp. 2767-2777

The Diabetes Control and Complications Trial Research Group. (1993). The effect of intensive treatment of diabetes on the development and progression of long-term complications in insulin-dependent diabetes mellitus. *N Engl J Med*, Vol.14, No. 329, pp. 977-986

Thomas, JB.; Petrovsky, N. & Ambler JR. (2004). Addison's disease presenting in four adolescents with type 1 diabetes. *Pediatr Diab* Vol. 5, pp. 207-211

Todd, JA.; Walker, NM.; Cooper, JD., Smyth, DJ.; Downes, K.; Plagnol, V.; Bailey, R.; Nejentsev, S.; Field, SF.; Payne, F.; Lowe, CE.; Szeszko, JS.; Hafler, JP.; Zeitels, L.; Yang, JH.; Vella, A.; Nutland. S.; Stevens, HE.; Schuilenburg, H.; Coleman, G.; Maisuria, M.; Meadows, W.; Smink, LJ.; Healy, B.; Burren, OS.; Lam, AA.; Ovington, NR.; Allen, J.; Adlem, E.; Leung, HT.; Wallace, C.; Howson, JM.; Guja, C. & Ionescu-Tîrgovişte, C. (2007). Robust association of four new chromosome regions from genome-wide analyses of type 1 diabetes. *Nat Genet*, Vol.7, No.39, pp. 857-864

Tommasini, A.; Not, T.; Kiren, V.; Baldas, V.; Santon, D.; Trevisiol, C.; Berti, I.; Neri, E.; Gerarduzzi, T.; Bruno, I.; Lenhardt, A.; Zamuner, E.; Spanò, A.; Crovella, S.; Martellossi, S.; Torre, G.; Sblattero, D.; Marzari, R.; Bradbury, A.; Tamburlini, G. & Ventura A. (2004). Mass screening for coeliac disease using antihuman transglutaminase antibody assay. *Arch Dis Child*, Vol.89, No.6, pp. 512-515

Triolo, TM.; Armstrong, TK.; McFann, K.; Rewers, MJ.; Klingensmith, GJ.; Eisenbarth, GS & Barker, JM. (2011). One-third of patients have evidence of an additional autoimmune disease at type 1 diabetes diagnosis. *Diabetes Care*

Tsirogianni, A.; Pipi, E. & Soufleros, K. (2009). Specificity of islet cell autoantibodies and coexistence with other organ specific autoantibodies in type 1 diabetes mellitus. *Autoimmunity Reviews*, Vol.8, No.8, pp. 687-691

Uibo, R.; Panarina, M.; Teesalu, K.; Talja I.; Sepp, E.; Utt, M.; Mikelsaar, M.; Heilman, K.; Uibo, O. & Vorobjova, T. (2011). Celiac disease in patients with type 1 diabetes: a condition with distinct changes in intestinal immunity? *Cell Mol Immunol*, Vol 8, No.2, pp. 150-156

Valerio, G.; Maiuri, L.; Troncone, R.; Buono, P.; Lombardi, F.; Palmieri, R. & Franzese A. (2002). Severe clinical onset of diabetes and increase prevalence of other autoimmune diseases in children with coeliac disease diagnosed before diabetes mellitus. *Diabetologia*, Vol.45, No.12, pp. 1719-1722

Valerio, G.; Spadaro, R.; Iafusco, D.; Lombardi, F.; del Puente, A.; Esposito, A.; De Terlizzi F.; Prisco, F.; Troncone, R. & Franzese, A. (2008). The influence of gluten free diet on quantitative ultrasound of proximal phalanxes in children and adolescents with type 1 diabetes mellitus and celiac disease. *Bone*, Vol.2, No. 43, pp. 322-326

Van den Driessche, A.; Eenkhoorn, V.; Van Gaal, L. & De Block, C. (2009). Type 1 diabetes and autoimmune polyglandular syndrome: a clinical review. *Neth J Med*, Vol.67, No.11, pp. 376-387

Vehil, K. & Dabelea, D. (2011). The changing epidemiology of type 1 diabetes: why is it going through the roof? *Diabet Metab Res Rev*, Vol.1, No.27, pp. 3-13

Ventura, A.; Magazzù, G. & Greco L. (1999). Duration of exposure to gluten and risk for autoimmune disorders in patients with celiac disease. SIGEP Study Group for Autoimmune Disorders in Celiac Disease. *Gastroenterology*, Vol.117, No.2, pp. 297-303

Volta, U.; Fabbri, A.; Parisi, C.; Piscaglia, M.; Caio, G.; Tovoli, F. & Fiorini E. (2010). Old and new serological tests for coeliac disease screening. *Expert Rev Gastroenterol Hepatol*, Vol.4, No.1, pp. 31-35

Warncke, K.; Frohlic-Reiterer, EE.; Thon, A.; Hofer, SE. Wiemann, D. & Holl EW on behalf of DPV. (2010). Polyendocrinopathy in children, adolescents, and young adults with type 1 diabetes. *Diabetes Care*, Vol.9, No.33, pp. 2010-2012

Williams, AJ.; Norcross, AJ.; Dix, RJ.; Gillespie, KM.; Gale, EA. & Bingley, PJ. (2003). The prevalence of insulin autoantibodies at the onset of Type 1 diabetes is higher in males than females during adolescence. *Diabetologia*, Vol.10, No.46, pp.1354-1356

Weinzimer, SA.; Doyle, EA. & Tamborlane, WV Jr. (2005). Disease management in the young diabetic patient: glucose monitoring, coping skills, and treatment strategies. *Clin Pediatr (Phila)*, Vol.5, No.44, pp. 393-403

# 2

# Hashimoto's Thyroiditis in Children and Adolescents

Erkan Sarı, Abdulbaki Karaoglu and Ediz Yeşilkaya
*Gülhane Military Medical Academy Department of Pediatric Endocrinology, Ankara, Turkey*

## 1. Introduction

Hashimoto's thyroiditis (HT) is an autoimmune disease with genetic background. It is also named as autoimmune thyroiditis or chronic lymphocytic tiroiditis. Hashimoto's thyroiditis is the most common cause of thyroid diseases in children and adolescents and it is also the most common cause of acquired hypothyroidism with or without goiter. Hashimoto's thyroiditis was first described in 1912 by Hakura Hashimoto in a series of patients with diffusely enlarged, firm thyroid glands with distinct pathologic features, classified as chronic lymphocytic thyroiditis (1). The characteristic histologic features include diffuse lymphocytic infiltration, atrophic follicles, well-developed germinal centers, and fibrosis.

Hashimoto's thyroiditis is the most important cause of hypothyroidism in children and adolescents. In an American population with age between 11 and 18 years, five new cases were detected out of 1,000 adolescents screened every year. It is more common among girls, varying from 4:1 to 8:1 depending on the geographical region. Although the disease can be seen before three years of age, it is usually seen after six years of age and its peak ages are 10 and 11 years (2). The prevelance of Hashimoto's thyroiditis between 6-18 years old is 3% in Japan. Thirty-40% of the cases have familial history of thyroid disease. It occurs far more often in women than in men (between 10:1 and 20:1), and is most prevalent between 45 and 65 years old.

Autoimmune thyroid disease (AITD) has two clinical forms: a goitrous form more common in young age groups, in whom goiter may be the only clinical expression (3), often referred to as classical Hashimoto's disease, and an atrophic one often called atrophic thyroiditis (4). Both are characterized by circulating thyroid autoantibodies and varying degrees of thyroid dysfunction, differing only by the presence or absence of goiter.

The prognosis is not known very well, and studies reporting about long-term outcome of the disease are scarce (3,5). Thyroid function tests show variations at the time of diagnosis; mostly euthyroid or hypothyroid and rarely hyperthyroid. Hypothyroidism is thought to be a permanent sequelae of HT. Patients with overt hypothyroidism may have been recommended lifelong levothyroxine (LT4) therapy but it should be checked after puberty if LT4 therapy is still necessary or not.

## 2. Etiology

Hashimoto's thyroiditis is influenced by both genetic and environmental factors (6). Family and twin studies support the evidence for genetic susceptibility (7-9). Dittmar et al. (10) have

shown the increased familial risk especially for the first-degree relatives and females. In particular, children and siblings of patients with Hashimoto's thyroiditis had a 32-fold and 21-fold increased risk, respectively, for developing immunthyroiditis. In comparison, the risk for developing Graves' disease has been enhanced 7-fold in both children and siblings (10). The high prevalence of AITD in first degree, foremost female, and relatives of patients with AITD demonstrates the importance of family history for developing AITD. This genetic susceptibility shows necessity of familial regular screening.
Candidate gene analysis, whole-genome linkage screening, genome-wide association studies, and whole-genome sequencing are the major technologies that have advanced this field, leading to the identification of at least seven genes whose variants have been associated with AITD (11). Using these techniques, 6 AITD susceptibility genes have been identified and confirmed, HLA-DR, CD40, CTLA-4, PTPN22, Thyroglobulin (Tg) and TSH receptor. The AITD susceptibility genes identified so far can be divided into two broad groups: immune modulating genes and thyroid specific genes. The first group includes the HLA-DR, CD40, CTLA-4, and PTPN22 genes, while the second group includes the Tg and TSH reseptor genes (12). In our previous study, we have studied an association of three polymorphic markers of CTLA-4 gene, namely, C(-318)T, A49G, and (AT)n dinucleotide repeat, which is known the relation with Graves' disease and we reported that A49G polymorphism may increase the susceptibility for Hashimoto's thyroiditis (13).
It is clear that additional genes contribute to the genetic susceptibility to AITD, as well as to the different phenotypes of AITD, disease severity, and, possibly, response to therapy but HLA-DR and Tg genes have stronger relation with HT than the others (14).
Several environmental and non-genetic triggers have been implicated in the etiology of HT. These include smoking, stress, iodine excess, medications, bacterial, and viral infections, irradiation, pollutants, and pregnancy. The mechanisms by which certain environmental agents induce thyroid disease could involve interference with thyroid function, direct toxic effects on thyrocytes, or immune stimulation, as well as other effects. It is often difficult to directly link an environmental exposure with thyroid autoimmunity, as disease may be associated with a combination of factors and can manifest over a long period of time. When an environmental exposure triggers HT in individuals with pre-existing thyroid autoantibodies, this may indicate gene-environment interaction, as the presence of thyroid antibodies is usually a surrogate marker of genetic susceptibility (15).

## 3. Iodine

Iodine is one of the most important precipitants of thyroid dysfunction. Although essential for normal thyroid function, excess iodine supplementation can be associated with the onset of thyroid autoimmunity. Potential mechanisms by which iodine can induce autoimmunity in the thyroid include direct stimulation of immune responses to the thyroid, increased immunogenicity of highly iodinated Tg, and direct toxic effects of iodine on thyrocytes via free oxygen radicals generation (16). A few studies have demonstrated increased incidence of autoimmune thyroiditis in regions where iodine consumption is high according to regions with low consumption (16-18).

## 4. Selenium

Selenium is a trace element that plays an essential role in thyroid hormone synthesis, because two enzymes involved in thyroid hormone production are selenoproteins: the deiodinases and glutathione peroxidase. Selenium influences the immune system probably by enhancing plasma glutathione peroxidase and thioredoxin reductase activity and by decreasing toxic concentrations of hydrogen peroxide and lipid hydroperoxides, resulting from thyroid hormone synthesis (19,20). A deficit of selenium results in increased intrathyroidal levels of hydrogen peroxide, which possibly increase the activity and immunogenicity of Thyroid Peroxidase (TPO) (21). Low selenium blood levels cause increased thyroid volume and thyroid hypoechogenicity, a marker for lymphocytic infiltration (22).

## 5. Medication

Several medications may play a role in the development of HT. Interferon-α, interleukin-2, lithium, amiodarone, and highly active antiretroviral therapy are the agents most commonly associated with thyroid dysfunction (23).

## 6. Infections

Several infections have been implicated in the pathogenesis of HT including Helicobacter pylori, Borrelia burgdorferi, Yersinia enterocolitica, Coxsackie virus, and retroviruses. Furthermore, recent studies but not all have substantiated a strong association between HT and HCV (24,25).

Seasonal and geographic variations also support infection as a trigger of HT (11,23). Various mechanisms have been proposed to explain induction of autoimmunity by infection but it seems that three possibilities may be important in individuals susceptible to developing autoimmune disease: molecular mimicry (perhaps to retroviruses); polyclonal T cell activation (by an endogenous superantigen or an infecting organism); and MHC class II antigen induction (26). Although infections may promote HT, they can also be partially protective, as suggested by the hygiene hypothesis. According to this hypothesis, the immune system builds tolerance to repeated infectious exposures, and this may explain a lower prevalence of thyroid antibodies in those of lower socioeconomic class (27).

### 6.1 Environmental toxins

Many environmental pollutants, such as polyaromatic hydrocarbons, perfluorinated chemicals, phthalates, and bisphenol A, have been shown to be toxic to thyroid cells and promote the onset of HT (15). These chemicals are widely used in various industrial and consumer products and may specifically have thyroid-disrupting properties (28,29). Polyaromatic hydrocarbons, including polychlorinated biphenyls and polyhalogenated biphenyls, are organic compounds produced from coal and found in air and water, and they can possibly trigger thyroiditis. Polyhalogenated biphenyls are commonly used compounds in products including adhesives, lubricants, and flame retardants, while polychlorinated biphenyls are found in plasticizers. A high prevalence of hypothyroidism was observed in individuals exposed to polyhalogenated biphenyls with an associated elevation in antimicrosomal antibodies and anti-Tg antibodies (30). In view of the evidence that many of these chemicals can interfere with thyroid function, there is a growing concern about their effects on neurological development during embryonic life (15,29). Exposure during pregnancy, for example, which itself is a risk factor for HT, can have hazardous effects on the developing fetus in which normal thyroid hormone levels are crucial for normal growth and brain development. It is important, therefore, to be aware of environmental triggers of HT and to monitor thyroid functions closely in susceptible women during pregnancy (15,23).

## 7. Pathogenesis

The activation of CD4 T-lymphocytes specific for thyroid antigens is believed to be the first step in pathogenesis. Once activated, self-reactive CD4 T cells recruit cytotoxic CD8 T cells as well as autoreactive B cells into the thyroid. T cells play a crucial role in disease pathogenesis by reacting with thyroid antigens and secreting inflammatory cytokines. Besides the others, mutations in the Tg gene and CTLA-4 are associated with HT (31,32).

The three main targets of thyroid antibodies are Tg, TPO, and the TSH receptor. It is believed that these autoantibodies are secondary to thyroid follicular cell damage induced by T cells Anti-TPO antibodies have been shown to inhibit the activity of the enzyme in vitro, but direct cytotoxicity by CD8 T cells is believed to be the main mechanism of hypothyroidism in vivo. Thyroid peroxidase is the major autoantigen and autoantibodies to TPO are closely associated with disease activity. Although this has not been proven in children Anti-TSH receptor antibodies of the blocking type may contribute to hypothyroidism in a minority of adult patients with the atrophic form of autoimmune thyroiditis. Histologically, HT is characterized by diffuse lymphocytic infiltration with occasional germinal centers. Thyroid follicles may be reduced in size and contain sparse colloid. Individual thyroid cells are often enlarged with oxyphilic cytoplasm. In contrast, the gland of atrophic autoimmune thyroiditis is small, with lymphocytic infiltration and fibrous replacement of the parenchyma (5).

## 8. Clinical manifestation

Hashimoto's thyroiditis is one of the most common organ specific autoimmune diseases (33). Weetman (34) reported clinical HT prevalence rate at 1 in 182 or 0.55% in the US. In the UK, Tunbridge et al (35) reported an overall HT prevalence of 0.8%. However, diagnosis based fine needle aspiration biopsy study; the cytology of HT seems to be much more prevalent, at 13.4% (36). This difference may be partially explained by the fact that for diagnosing clinical HT, abnormally elevated TSH, low thyroid hormones (34,35) and the confirmatory presence of thyroid autoantibodies are usually accounted for.

The most common clinical manifestations are goiter and hypothyroidism related findings. The goiter may appear insidiously and may be small or large. In most patients, the thyroid is diffusely enlarged, firm, and nontender. In about 30% of patients, the gland is lobular and may seem to be nodular (37). Most of the affected children are clinically euthyroid and asymptomatic; some may have symptoms of pressure in the neck. Some children have clinical signs of hypothyroidism, but others who appear clinically euthyroid have laboratory evidence of hypothyroidism. A few children have manifestations suggestive of hyperthyroidism, such as nervousness, irritability, increased sweating, and hyperactivity, but results of laboratory studies are not necessarily those of hyperthyroidism (37). In one study from iodine replete area with 140 patients with HT, the most common complaint was goiter (55%). Upon admission, 18.6% of patients had complaints related to hypothyroidism (7.4% growth retardation, 4.9% weight gain and 6.3% other complaints related to hypothyroidism). Eighteen patients (11.1%) were diagnosed incidentally upon detection of goiter during routine examination (38). Staii et al. reviewed 761 patients for which ultrasound guided thyroid fine needle aspiration biopsy were performed for nodule. The HT cohort consisted of 102 (13.4%) patients (659 out of 761 did not have cytological Hashimoto's diagnosis) for which 46 (6%) were identified as having clinical disease (i.e. diagnosed hypothyroid on thyroid hormone replacement and with cytological Hashimoto's diagnosis), 9 (1.2%) as having subclinic hypothyroidism and 47 (6.2%) as having euthyroid autoimmunity (36). Occasionally, the disorder may coexist with Graves's disease. Ophthalmopathy may occur in lymphocytic thyroiditis in the absence of Graves's disease.

Hashimoto's encephalopathy is a rare condition and the estimation of incidence and prevalence is difficult. One prospective study examining cases of unexplained encephalopathy that had detectable antithyroid antibodies, estimated a prevalence of 2.1/100 000 subjects (39). Adequate information is not available about the frequency of Hashimoto's encephalopathy in children (40). The clinical picture of a relapsing and remitting encephalopathy in a female characterised by seizures, stroke-like episodes, neurological signs such as myoclonus and tremor, cognitive disturbance and hallucinations, and other psychotic symptoms is highly suggestive of Hashimoto's encephalopathy (41). Normal routine investigations, nonspecific neuroimaging and CSF findings (apart from elevated protein), and encephalopathic EEG can be supportive of the diagnosis. Thyroid hormone studies are not helpful, but may identify subclinical thyroid dysfunction (41). Detection of antithyroid (in particular anti-TPO) antibodies confirms the diagnosis. As anti-TPO antibodies are detected in as many as 10 % of the general population, (42) high titres (usually over 100-fold normal (43)) of these antibodies in conjunction with the clinical features of Hashimoto's encephalopathy are necessary before a diagnosis can be made. Thyroid antibody levels should be measured even in the setting of normal thyroid function and the diagnosis of Hashimoto encephalopathy has to be considered in patients with Down syndrome who present with rapid cognitive decline, particularly in association with myoclonus and an abnormal EEG result (44). Corticosteroid responsiveness can also support the diagnosis (45).

## 9. Related disorders

HT may be the initial presentation of an autoimmune polyglandular syndrome, and the possibility of coexisting autoimmune diseases such as type I diabetes, celiac disease, Addison's disease, and pernicious anemia must be addressed by the past medical history (46). In a study performed on 268 children with type I diabetes mellitus, the percentage of those who presented with circulating thyroperoxidase and Tg antibodies was significantly higher than those with celiac disease (47). In another study performed in Bratislava, 40-50% of patients with different types of diabetes had autoimmune thyroiditis (48). The incidence of histologic findings of autoimmune thyroid disease in diabetic patients increases with age (49). Several other studies have confirmed the coincidence of autoimmune thyroiditis and latent or overt diabetes (50) and relatives of patients with type I diabetes have an increased incidence of HT (51). In a recent study, genetic susceptibility between autoimmune thyroiditis and diabetes was investigated among 448 individuals. Three loci in chromosomes 2q, 6p and Xp were identified (52).

Hashimoto's thyroiditis sometimes may be associated with connective tissue, cutaneous, hematologic (pernicious anemia, idiopathic thrombocytopenic purpura), gastrointestinal (autoimmune liver disease, celiac disease), genetic (autoimmune polyglandular syndrome type II/III, ovarian failure, Down syndrome, Klinefelter's syndrome, Turner's syndrome), infectious (Hepatitis C infection), neurologic (Miller Fisher syndrome, Guillain-Barre´ syndrome, multiple sclerosis, myasthenia gravis) and renal diseases (minimal change glomerular disease) (53).

The coexistence of papillary thyroid carcinoma and HT is not known exactly, but it is reported to range from 10% to 58% in various studies (54,55). The prevalence of HT in patients with papillary thyroid carcinoma has been reported to be significantly higher than with benign thyroid tumours (56). Patients with HT are suggested to be at higher risk for papillary thyroid carcinoma compared with patients without HT (57)

## 10. Laboratory findings

Although the level of TSH may be slightly or even moderately raised in some individual's thyroid function tests are often normal, termed subclinical hypothyroidisms (37). In a study from iodine-replete area, twenty-four patients (21%) were euthyroid, 48 (42%) had compensated hypothyroidism, and 42 (37%) had hypothyroidism (including two patients with transient hyperthyroidism reversed to hypothyroidism within weeks). There was no difference in clinical symptoms of hypothyroidism by thyroid status, except for a higher rate of constipation in the hypothyroid group (38). The fact that many children with lymphocytic thyroiditis do not have elevated levels of TSH indicates that the goiter may be caused by the lymphocytic infiltrations or by thyroid growth-stimulating immunoglobulins.

In normal individuals, positive anti-TPO were detected in 13.0 ± 0.4%, and positive Anti-Tg was detected in 11.5 ± 0.5%. The prevalence of positive antibodies was lower in the disease-free population: Anti-TPO, 11.3 ± 0.4% and Anti-Tg, 10.4 ± 0.5%. The prevalence of positive Anti-TPO and positive Anti-Tg in the total and disease-free population was higher in females than males ($P < 0.001$) and increased with age, especially among females. Approximately 18% of the disease-free population had detectable Anti-Tg or Anti-TPO of those with positive Anti-Tg, 69.9% also had positive Anti-TPO; and of those with positive Anti-TPO, 54.5% also had positive Anti-Tg. Anti-TPO was positive alone in 4.4%, and Anti-Tg was positive alone in 3.4%. Anti-TPO and Anti-Tg were detected together in 6.9% (59).

Almost all young children with HT have serum antibody titres to TPO, but the anti-Tg test for thyroid antibodies is positive in fewer than 50%. Antibodies to TPO and Tg are found equally in adolescents with HT. When both tests are used, approximately 95% of patients with thyroid autoimmunity are detected. Levels in children and adolescents are lower than those in adults with HT, and repeated measurements are indicated in questionable instances because titres may increase later in the course of the disease (37). Results about decreasing Anti-TPO under LT4 treatment have been found variable with 10% and 90% after a follow-up of 6 to 24 months (60,61). Decreasing Anti-TPO under LT4 treatment appears to depend on time, a 45 % decrease after 1 year and a 70% decrease after 5 years (62).

## 11. Imaging

Thyroid ultrasonography is a useful tool to support the diagnosis, and classical sonographic findings are present in 20-95% of affected individuals (63). Furthermore, their presence is related to subclinical hypothyroidism and levels of thyroid autoantibodies (64,65), and ultrasonography has been used for the follow-up of patients (66). Thyroid ultrasonography is usually heterogeneous because of fibrosis and hypoechogenic areas, it is not necessary for diagnosis but it is recommended to confirm the presence of a thyroid nodule, solitary or multiple nodule can be detected both hypothyroid or euthyroid patients. During disease progression, reduced echo levels develop gradually, reflecting either reduction of colloid content and increased intrathyroidal blood flow or lymphocytic tissue infiltration, which induces diffuse fibrosis (64). The appearance of thyroid gland on ultrasonography may be normal at diagnosis, but characteristic changes evolve over time. Vlachopapadopoulou et al. studied 105 children, the time needed for 30%, 50%, and 70% of children to demonstrate an abnormal thyroid sonographic pattern has been detected 4, 7, and 14 months, respectively. Important factors accelerating sonographic changes have been demonstrated as goiter, hypothyroidism, and seropositivity for both anti-TPO and anti-Tg autoantibodies (67).

## 12. Diagnosis

Hashimoto's thyroiditis is diagnosed based on findings of seropositivity for Tg autoantibodies and/or TPO autoantibodies, accompanied by at least one of the following: abnormal thyroid function; enlarged thyroid gland; morphological changes on thyroid ultrasound. If anti-TPO antibodies are absent, less common etiologies of primary hypothyroidism should be considered for example transient hypothyroidism due to postsubacute thyroiditis, hypothyroidism related to external irradiation (69) and consumptive hypothyroidism due to the inactivation of thyroid hormone by the paraneoplastic expression of type III iodothyronine deiodinase, mostly in vascular tumors (70).

The typical patient with hypothyroidism secondary to HT has an elevated TSH, a low fT4, and positive anti-TPO antibodies. In early stages of the disease, TSH may be normal and anti-TPO antibodies may be positive with or without goiter. Later, TSH elevation becomes modest (5-10 IU/mL) with a normal fT4 (biochemical or subclinical hypothyroidism). Up to 90% of patients with hypothyroidism secondary to HT have positive anti-TPO antibody (46). If HT is suggested and thyroid autoantibodies are negative, they should be controlled later. It is possible to raise in follow-up.

## 13. Treatment

Most of these patients are asymptomatic, but studies in the adult population suggest that individuals with the combined risk factors of TSH level above the normal limit and positive thyroid antibodies (anti-Tg or anti-TPO) are at high risk for progression to overt hypothyroidism. For this reason, thyroid hormone replacement is recommended in all patients with TSH values >10 IU/mL or with TSH values >5 IU/mL in combination with goiter or thyroid autoantibodies (71). Levothyroxine is the replacement therapy of choice. There are almost no adverse reactions; its good intestinal absorption and its long half life of 5-7 days allow oral administration once a day. Although very rare, the development of pseudotumor cerebri associated with the initiation of LT4 has been described in a few school-age children (72). Alternatively, a starting dose can be estimated based upon the patient's age and ideal body weight (73). The medication's long half-life insures a gradual equilibration over the course of 5 – 6 weeks, and dosing should be individualized based on biochemical monitoring (73). TSH normalization (0.5-2 micro IU/mL) is the goal of replacement. This will usually be associated with an fT4 in the upper half of the normal range. Thyroid function tests should be obtained about 6-8 weeks after the beginning or next adjustment of the LT4 dosage. Very high TSH levels at diagnosis can be associated with thyrotroph hypertrophy and gradual suppression over the first year of treatment (74,75). Once biochemical euthyroidism has been achieved, TSH can be monitored every 4-6 months in the growing child and yearly up to the attainment of final height. If poor compliance is suspected as the cause of treatment failure, fT4 should be measured.

Levothyroxine should be administered at least 20 min, before eating or ingestion of any medication known to impair its absorption, such as calcium and iron supplements, sucralfate, potassium-binding resins, antacids containing aluminium, and bile-acids binding resins. All other medications should be checked for interactions, particularly with antidepressants and seizure medications.

Growth and sexual development should be followed systematically as in any pediatric patient. Parents of children with HT should be advised that the hypothyroidism is likely to be permanent and monitoring of thyroid function for all patients should be life long. The prognosis for recovering lost linear growth depends on the duration of the hypothyroidism as well as the age at which treatment is started. If hypothyroidism is long-standing, thyroid replacement will not recover all lost stature. Similarly, if the diagnosis is made around puberty, there may be limited time for recovering the growth spurt before attaining final height. If the onset of childhood hypothyroidism occurs after age 3 years, no permanent intellectual damage or neurologic deficit is probable.

Surgical therapy for HT most commonly is recommended in case of malignancy or for relief of compressive symptoms in patients who develop a nodular or diffuse goiter. Patients may have an associated firm nodule in the thyroid gland and the thyroid gland may be adherent to adjacent structures with associated enlarged lymph nodes, mimicking thyroid cancer. Large goiter with HT can cause local compressive symptoms such as dysphagia, coughing or choking spells, dyspnea, and hoarseness that may require surgery for relief of compression (76). Thirty-two (15%) of 216 patients with HT were referred with thyroid enlargement and compressive symptoms; 25 (78%) had an associated nodule and 12 (38%) had retrosternal extension. Symptom resolution occurred in 30 (94%) and improvement occurred in 2 (6%) patients after total thyroidectomy in 21 (66%) and thyroid lobectomy in 11 (34%) patients. The only complication was transient hypocalcemia in 12 (38%) patients. One patient had an incidental thyroid lymphoma (77).

## 14. Follow-up

Although a percentage of patients acquire hypothyroidism gradually within months or years, most children who are euthyroid at presentation remain euthyroid. Over several years, about half of children with subclinical hypothyroidism revert to euthyroidism, while the other half develops overt hypothyroidism. In a multicentre study Radetti et al. investigated the outcome of euthyroid children with HT and showed that 64.8% of them remained euthyroid, 9.5% progressed to subclinical hypothyroidism and 25.7% to overt hypothyroidism after 5 years (78).

Few studies have examined the spontaneous evolution of the disease (80,81). A recent Italian retrospective study described the outcome of 160 children affected with HT followed for up to 32.6 years in 20 pediatric endocrine clinics (78). In compatible with other reports (80,81), TSH concentrations have showed large fluctuations overtime. The presence of associated diseases has not worsened the prognosis, because at the end of the follow-up no difference has been found in the frequency of abnormally elevated TSH between the groups with or without associated diseases. In agreement with previous findings in children (82,83) and in contrast with adults (84), the TSH level at baseline was not a useful marker to predict disease evolution. Both thyroid antibodies were significantly higher at the last visit in the group with deteriorating thyroid function; however, whereas anti-Tg antibodies were already higher at baseline, anti-TPO antibodies increased progressively with time. This finding suggests that anti-TPO antibodies might represent a marker of deteriorating thyroid function, in agreement with a previous report showing a good correlation between anti-TPO antibodies levels and lymphocytic infiltration of the gland (85). The evaluation of patients, according to their final outcome, revealed that subjects with deteriorating thyroid function had significantly higher anti-Tg antibodies, TSH concentrations, and greater thyroid volume at presentation. Nonetheless, these findings were not helpful in individual patients. On the other hand, it should be remarked that at 5 years of followup, more than 50% of the patients remained or became euthyroid. Ikemoto investigated 199 adult patients with HT and reported a recovery rate from hypothyroidism of 40% within 10.5 years of follow-up. In the same study elevated titres for thyroid autoantibody, age above 50 years and the presence of a stony-hard goitre were the best predictive factors for permanent hypothyroidism (86). In children the presense of predictive factors for permanent hypothyroidism are controversial. In the current study, initial TSH levels and thyroid volume at presentation, duration of levothyroxine therapy and anti-TPO Ab titre were not predictive for permanent hypothyroidism (79). Previously it was shown that iodine supplementation is associated with increased incidence of HT (87,88). In addition, it has been suggested that patients with HT are prone to develop hypothyroidism following iodine administration. Daily iodine supplementation over 1 mg has been shown to potentially contribute to underlying thyroid pathology in those with HT or Graves' disease. Exacerbation of nodularities in euthyroid individuals may occur if daily intake exceeds 20 mg iodine or iodide (89,90).

It is usually offered a trial of LT4 therapy to adolescents, after the completion of growth and puberty. Thyroid function is retested 6–8 weeks after the stop of medication, to determine if hypothyroidism is permanent and potentially restart therapy.

## 15. References

[1] Hashimoto H. Zur kenntniss der lymphomatosen veranderung der schilddruse (struma lymphomatosa). Arch Klin Chir 1912; 97: 219-248.

[2] Setian NS. Hypothyroidism in children: diagnosis and treatment. Jornal de Pediatria 2007; 83: 209-216.

[3] Rallison ML, Dobyns BM, Keating FR, Rall JE, Tyler FH. Occurrence and natural history of chronic lymphocytic thyroiditis inchildhood. Journal of Pediatrics 1975; 86: 675-682.

[4] Brown RS: Thyroid disease in infancy, childhood and adolescence. In: Braverman LE (ed). Contemporary Endocrinology. Totowa, Humana Press, 1997, 81-102.

[5] Dayan CM, Daniels GH. Chronic autoimmune thyroiditis. New England Journal of Medicine 1996; 335: 99-107.

[6] Weetman AP. Autoimmunity and endocrinology. Exp Clin Endocrinol Diabetes 1999; 107: 63-66.

[7] Villanueva R, Greenberg DA, Davies TF, Tomer Y. Sibling recurrence risk in autoimmune thyroid disease. Thyroid 2003; 13: 761-764.

[8] Hall R, Stanbury JB. Familial studies of autoimmune thyroiditis. Clin Exp Immunol 1967; 2: 719-725.
[9] Segni M, Wood J, Pucarelli, Toscano V, Toscano R, Pasquino AM. Clustering of autoimmune thyroid diseases in children and adolescents: a study of 66 families. J Ped Endocrinol Metab 2001; 14: 1271-1297.
[10] Dittmar M, Libich C, Brenzel T, Kahaly GJ. Increased Familial Clustering of Autoimmune Thyroid Diseases. Horm Metab Res 2011; 43: 200-204.
[11] Yaron T, Amanda H. The etiology of autoimmune thyroid disease: A story of genes and environment. Journal of Autoimmunity 2009; 32: 231-239.
[12] Lander E, Kruglyak L. Genetic dissection of complex traits: guidelines for interpreting and reporting linkage results. Nat Genet 1995; 11: 241-247.
[13] Yeşilkaya E, Koç A, Bideci A, Camurdan O, Boyraz M, Erkal O, Ergun MA, Cinaz P. CTLA-4 gene polymorphisms in children and adolescents with autoimmune thyroid diseases. Genet Test 2008; 12: 461-464.
[14] Deirdre CE, Alia H, Yaron T, Cutting E. The Etiology of Autoimmune Thyroid Diseases. Curr Opin Endocrinol Diabetes Obes 2010; 17: 437-439.
[15] Brent GA. Environmental exposures and autoimmune thyroid disease. Thyroid 2010; 20; 755-761.
[16] Papanastasiou L, Vatalas L, Koutras DA, Mastorakos G. Thyroid autoimmunity in the current iodine environment. Thyroid 2007; 17: 729-739.
[17] Teng W, Shan Z, Teng X, Guan H, Li Y, Teng D, Jin Y, Yu X, Fan C, Chong W, Yang F, Dai H, Yu Y, Li J, Chen Y, Zhao D, Shi X, Hu F, Mao J, Gu X, Yang R, Tong Y, Wang W, Gao T, Li C. Effect of iodine intake on thyroid diseases in China. N Engl J Med 2006; 354: 2783-2793.
[18] Doufas AG, Mastorakos G, Chatziioannou S, Tseleni-Balafouta S, Piperingos G, Boukis MA, Mantzos E, Caraiskos CS, Mantzos J, Alevizaki M, Koutras DA. The predominant form of non-toxic goiter in Greece is now autoimmune thyroiditis. Eur J Endocrinol 1999; 140: 505-511.
[19] Beckett GJ, Arthur JR. Selenium and endocrine systems. J Endocrinol 2005; 184: 455-465.
[20] Duntas LH. The role of selenium in thyroid autoimmunity and cancer. Thyroid 2006; 16: 455-460.
[21] Caturegli P, Kimura H, Rocchi R, Rose NR. Autoimmune thyroid diseases. Curr Opin Rheumatol 2007; 19: 44-48.
[22] Klecha AJ, Barreiro Arcos ML, Frick L, Genaro AM, Cremaschi G. Immune-Endocrine Interactions in Autoimmune Thyroid Diseases. Neuroimmunomodulation 2008; 15: 68-75.
[23] Tanda ML, Piantanida E, Lai A, Lombardi V, Dalle Mule I, Liparulo L, Pariani N, Bartalena LThyroid autoimmunity and environment. Horm Metab Res 2009; 41: 436-442.
[24] Menconi F, Hasham A, Tomer Y. Environmental triggers of thyroiditis: Hepatitis C and interferon-α J Endocrinol Invest 2011; 34: 78-84.
[25] Mori K, Yoshida K. Viral infection in induction of Hashimoto's thyroiditis: a key player or just a bystander? Curr Opin Endocrinol Diabetes Obes 2010; 17: 418-424.
[26] Tomer Y, Davies TF. Infections and autoimmune endocrine disease. Bailli eres Clin Endocrinol Metab 1995; 9: 47-70.
[27] Desailloud R, Hober D. Viruses and thyroiditis: an update. Virol J 2009; 12: 6: 5.

[28] Andrade LJ, Atta AM, D'Almeida Junior A, Paraná R Thyroid dysfunction in hepatitis C individuals treated with interferon-alpha and ribavirin—a review. Braz J Infect Dis 2008; 12:144-148.
[29] Boas M, Main KM, Feldt-Rasmussen U. Environmental chemicals and thyroid function: an update. Curr Opin Endocrinol Diab Obes 2009; 16: 385-391.
[30] Bahn AK, Mills JL, Snyder PJ, Gann PH, Houten L, Bialik O, Hollmann L, Utiger RD. Hypothyroidism in workers exposed to polybrominated biphenyls. N Engl J Med 1980; 302: 31-33.
[31] Ban Y, Greenberg DA, Concepcion E, Skrabanek L, Villanueva R, Tomer Y. Amino acid substitutions in the thyroglobulin gene is associated with susceptibility to human and murine autoimmune thyroid disease. Proc Natl Acad Sci USA 2003; 100: 15119-15124.
[32] Ban Y, Davies TF, Greenberg DA, Kissin A, Marder B, Murphy B, Concepcion ES, Villanueva RB, Barbesino G, Ling V, Tomer Y. Analysis of the CTLA-4, CD28, and inducible costimulator (ICOS) genes in autoimmune thyroid disease. Genes Immun 2003; 4: 586-593.
[33] Hay ID. Thyroiditis: A clinical update. Mayo Clin Proc 1985; 60: 836-843.
[34] Weetman AP: Thyroid disease. In: the Autoimmune Disease. Rose NR, Mackay IR (eds). 2006; 467-482.
[35] Tunbridge WM, Evered DC, Hall R, Appleton D, Brewis M, Clark F, Evans JG, Young E, Bird T, Smith PA. The spectrum of thyroid disease in a community: The Whickham survey. Clin Endocrinol (Oxf) 1977; 7: 481-493.
[36] Staii A, Mirocha S, Todorova-Koteva K, Glinberg S, Jaume JC. Hashimoto thyroiditis is more frequent than expected when diagnosed by cytology which uncovers a pre-clinical state. Thyroid Research 2010, 3: 11.
[37] Kliegman RM: Disorder of thyroid gland. In: Kliegman RM, Behrman RH, Jenson HB, Stanton BMD (eds). Nelson Textbook of Pediatrics. 18th ed, Sounders, 2007.
[38] Demirbilek H, Kandemir N, Gonc E.N, Ozon A, Alikasifoglu A, and Yordam N. Hashimoto's Thyroiditis in Children and Adolescent: A Retrospective Study on Clinical Epidemiological and Laboratory Properties of the Disease. Journal of Pediatric Endocrinology & Metabolism 2007; 20:1199-1205.
[39] Ferracci F, Bertiato G, Moretto G. Hashimoto's encephalopathy: epidemiologic data and pathogenetic considerations. J Neurol Sci 2004; 217: 165-168.
[40] Gayatri NA, Whitehouse WP. Pilot survey of Hashimoto's encephalopathy in children. Dev Med Child Neurol 2005; 47: 556-558.
[41] Mocellin R, Walterfang M, Velakoulis D. Hashimoto's Encephalopathy Epidemiology, Pathogenesis and Management. CNS Drugs 2007; 21: 799-811.
[42] Hollowell JG, Staehling NW, Flanders WD, Hannon WH, Gunter EW, Spencer CA, Braverman LE. Serum TSH T(4), and thyroid antibodies in the United States population (1988 to 1994): National Health and Nutrition Examination Survey (NHANES III). J Clin Endocrinol Metab 2002; 87: 489-499.
[43] Kothbauer-Margreiter I, Sturzenegger M, Komor J, Baumgartner R, Hess CW. Encephalopathy associated with Hashimoto thyroiditis. J Neurol 1996: 243: 585-593.
[44] Brodtmann A. Hashimoto encephalopathy and Down syndrome. Arch Neurol 2009; 66: 663-666.

[45] Chong JY, Rowland LP. What's in a NAIM? Hashimoto encephalopathy, steroid-responsive encephalopathy associated with autoimmune thyroiditis, or nonvasculitic autoimmune meningoencephalitis? Arch Neurol 2006; 63: 175-176.

[46] Cappa M, Bizzarri C, Crea F. Autoimmune Thyroid Diseases in Children. Journal of Thyroid Research 2010; 2011:675-703.

[47] Körner A, Tóth-Heyn P, Dezsofi A, Veres G, Madácsy L, Arató A. Incidence of thyroid autoimmunity in children with type 1 diabetes mellitus. Orv Hetil 2008; 149: 4012-4406.

[48] Schroner Z, Lazurova I, Petrovicova J. Autoimmune thyroid disease in patients with diabetes mellitus. Bratisl Lek List 2008; 109: 125-129.

[49] Sharifi F, Ghasemi L, Mousavinasab N. Thyroid function and antithyroid antibodies in Iranian patients with type 1 diabetes mellitus: influence of age and sex. Iran J Allergy Asthma Immunol 2008; 31: 6-10.

[50] Araujo J, Brandão LA, Guimarães RL, Santos S, Falcão EA, Milanese M, Segat L, Souza PR, de Lima-Filho JL, Crovella S. Prevalence of autoimmune thyroid disease and thyroid dysfunction in young Brazilian patients with type 1 diabetes. Pediatr Diabetes 2008; 9: 272-276.

[51] Payami H, Joe S, Thomas G. Autoimmune thyroid disease type 1 diabetic families. Genet Epidemiol 1989; 6: 137-143.

[52] Villano MJ, Huber AK, Greenberg DA, Golden BK, Concepcion E, Tomer Y. Autoimmune thyroiditis and diabetes: dissecting the joint genetic susceptibility in a large cohort of multiplex families. J Clin Endocrinol Metab 2009; 94: 1458-1466.

[53] Ai J, Leonhardt JM, Heymann WR. Autoimmune thyroid diseases: Etiology, pathogenesis, and dermatologic manifestations. J Am Acad Dermatol 2003; 48: 641-659.

[54] Tamimi DM. The association between chronic lymphocytic thyroiditis and thyroid tumors. Int J Surg Pathol 2002; 10: 141-146.

[55] Schäffler A, Palitzsch KD, Seiffarth C, Höhne HM, Riedhammer FJ, Hofstädter F, Schölmerich J, Rüschoff J. Coexistent thyroiditis is associated with lower tumour stage in thyroid carcinoma. Eur J Clin Invest 1998; 28: 838-844.

[56] Okayasu I, Fujiwara M, Hara Y, Tanaka Y, Rose NR. Association of chronic lymphocytic thyroiditis and thyroid papillary carcinoma. A study of surgical cases among Japanese, and white and African Americans. Cancer 1995; 76: 2312-2318.

[57] Holm LE, Blomgren H, Lowhagen T. Cancer risks in patients with chronic lymphocytic thyroiditis. N Engl J Med 1985; 312: 601-604.

[58] Saravanan P, Dayan CM. Thyroid autoantibodies. Endocrinology and Metabolism Clinics of North America 2001; 30: 315-337.

[59] Hollowell JG, Staehling NW, Flanders WD, Hannon WH, Gunter EW, Spencer CA, Braverman LE. Serum TSH, T(4), and thyroid antibodies in the United States population (1988 to 1994): National Health and Nutrition Examination Survey (NHANES III). J Clin Endocrinol Metab 2002; 87: 489-499.

[60] Aksoy DY, Kerimoglu U, Okur H, Canpinar H, Karaagaoglu E, Yetgin S, Kansu E, Gedik O. Effects of prophylactic thyroid hormone replacement in euthyroid Hashimoto's thyroiditis. Endocr J 2005; 52: 337-343.

[61] Hegedu's L, Hansen JM, Feldt-Rasmussen U, Hansen BM, Hoier-Madsen M. Influence of thyroxine treatment on thyroid size and anti-thyroid peroxidase antibodies in Hashimoto's thyroiditis. Clin Endocrinol 1991; 35: 235-238.

[62] Schmidt M, Voell M, Rahlff I, Dietlein M, Kobe C, Faust M, Schicha H. Long-term follow-up of antithyroid peroxidase antibodies in patients with chronic autoimmune thyroiditis (Hashimoto's thyroiditis) treated with levothyroxine. Thyroid 2008; 18: 755-760.

[63] Pedersen OM, Aardal NP, Larssen TB, Varhaug JE, Myking O, Vik-Mo H. The value of ultrasonography in predicting autoimmune thyroid disease. Thyroid 2000; 10: 251-259.

[64] Schiemann U, Avenhaus W, Konturek J, Gellner R, Hengst K, Gross M. Relation of clinical features and laboratory parameters to thyroid echogenicity measured by standardized grey scale ultrasonography in patients with Hashimoto's thyroiditis. Med Sei Monit 2003; 9: 49-53.

[65] Raber W, Gessl A, Nowotny P, Vierhapper H. Thyroid ultrasound versus antithyroid peroxidase antibody determination: a cohort study of four hundred fifty-one subjects. Thyroid 2002; 12: 725-731.

[66] Loy M, Cianchietti ME, Cardia F, Melis A, Boi F, Mariotti S. Correlation of computerized gray-scale sonographic findings with thyroid function and thyroid autoimmune activity in patients with Hashimoto's thyroiditis. J Clin Ultrasound 2004; 32: 136-140.

[67] Vlachopapadopoulou E, Thomas D, Karachaliou F, Chatzimarkou F, Memalai L, Vakaki M, Kaldrymides P, Michalacos S. Evolution of Sonographic Appearance of the Thyroid Gland in Children with Hashimoto's Thyroiditis. Journal of Pediatric Endocrinology & Metabolism 2009; 22: 339-344.

[68] Alos N, Huot C, Lambert R, Van Vliet G. Thyroid scintigraphy in children and adolescents with Hashimoto disease. J Pediatr 1995; 127: 951-953.

[69] Hancock SL, McDougall IR, Constine LS. Thyroid abnormalities after therapeutic external radiation. Int J Radiat Oncol Biol Phys. 1995; 31: 1165-1170.

[70] Bessho K, Etani Y, Ichimori H, Miyoshi Y, Namba N, Yoneda A, Ooue T, Chihara T, Morii E, Aoki T, Murakami M, Mushiake S, Ozono K. Increased type 3 iodothyronine deiodinase activity in a regrown hepatic hemangioma with consumptive hypothyroidism. Eur J Pediatr. 2010; 169: 215-221.

[71] Mandel SJ, Brent GA, Larsen PR. Levothyroxine therapy in patients with thyroid disease. Ann Intern Med 1993; 119: 492-502.

[72] Van Dop C, Conte FA, Koch TK, Clark SJ, Wilson-Davis SL, Grumbach MM. Pseudotumor cerebri associated with initiation of levothyroxine therapy for juvenile hypothyroidism. N Engl J Med 1983; 308: 1076-1080.

[73] Lafranchi S. Thyroiditis and acquired hypothyroidism. Pediatr Ann 1992; 21: 32-39.

[74] Kuroiwa T, Okabe Y, Hasuo K, Yasumori K, Mizushima A, Masuda K. MR imaging of pituitary hypertrophy due to juvenile primary hypothyroidism: a case report. Clinical Imaging 1991; 15: 202–205.

[75] Ahmed M, Banna M, Sakati N, Woodhouse N. Pituitary gland enlargement in primary hypothyroidism: a report of 5 cases with follow-up data. Hormone Research 1989; 32: 188-192.

[76] Shih ML, Lee JA, Hsieh CB, Yu JC, Liu HD, Kebebew E, Clark OH, Duh QY. Thyroidectomy for Hashimoto's thyroiditis: complications and associated cancers. Thyroid 2008; 18: 729-734.
[77] Wormer BA, McHenry CR. Hashimoto's thyroiditis: Outcome of surgical resection for patients with thyromegaly and compressive symptoms. The American Journal of Surgery 2011; 201: 416-419.
[78] Radetti G, Gottardi E, Bona G, Corrias A, Salardi S, Loche S; Study Group for Thyroid Diseases of the Italian Society for Pediatric Endocrinology and Diabetes (SIEDP/ISPED). The natural history of euthyroid Hashimoto's thyroiditis in children. Journal of Pediatrics 2006; 149: 827-832.
[79] Demirbilek H, Kandemir N, Gonc E.N, Ozon A, Alikasifoglu A. Assessment of thyroid function during the long course of Hashimoto's thyroiditis in children and adolescents. Clinical Endocrinology 2009; 71: 451-454.
[80] Gopalakrishnan S, Marwaha RK. Juvenile autoimmune thyroiditis. J Pediatr Endocrinol Metab 2007; 20: 961-970.
[81] Gopalakrishnan PK, Chugh M, Chhillar VK, Ambardar MS, Sankar R. Goitrous autoimmune thyroiditis in a pediatric population: a longitudinal study. Pediatrics 2008; 122: 670-674.
[82] Jaruratanasirikul S, Leethanaporn K, Khuntigij P, Sriplung H. The clinical course of Hashimoto's thyroiditis in children and adolescents: 6 years longitudinal follow-up. Journal of Pediatric Endocrinology and Metabolism 2001; 14: 177-184.
[83] Wasniewska M, Salerno M, Cassio A, Corrias A, Aversa T, Zirilli G, Capalbo D, Bal M, Mussa A, De Luca F. Prospective evaluation of the natural course of idiopathic subclinical hypothyroidism in childhood and adolescence. Eur J Endocrinol 2009; 160: 417-421.
[84] D´ıez JJ, Iglesias P. Spontaneous subclinical hypothyroidism in patients older than 55 years: an analysis of natural course and risk factors for the development of overt thyroid failure. Journal of Clinical Endocrinology and Metabolism 2004; 89: 4890-4897.
[85] Yoshida H, Amino N, Yagawa K, Uemura K, Satoh M, Miyai K, Kumahara Y. Association of serum antithyroid antibodies with lymphocytic infiltration of the thyroid gland: studies of seventy autopsied cases. J Clin Endocrinol Metab 1978; 46: 859-862.
[86] Ikemoto K. A long-term follow-up study of patients with goitrous Hashimoto's disease - prognosis and its predictive factors. Nippon Naibunpi Gakkai Zasshi 1990; 66: 619-635.
[87] Konno N, Makita H, Yuri K, Iizuka N, Kawasaki K. Association between dietary iodine intake and prevalence of subclinical hypothyroidism in the coastal regions of Japan. J Clin Endocrinol Metab 1994; 78: 393-397.
[88] Yoon SJ, Choi SR, Kim DM, Kim JU, Kim KW, Ahn CW, Cha BS, Lim SK, Kim KR, Lee HC, Huh KB. The effect of iodine restriction on thyroid function in patients with hypothyroidism due to Hashimoto's thyroiditis. Yonsei Med J 2003; 44: 227-235.
[89] Dunn JT, Semigran MJ, Delange F. The prevention and management of iodine-induced hyperthyroidism and its cardiac features. Thyroid 1998; 8: 101-106.
[90] Robison LM, Sylvester PW, Birkenfeld P, Lang JP, Bull RJ. Comparison of the effects of iodine and iodide on thyroid function in humans. J Toxicol Environ Health A 1998; 55: 93-106.

3

# Primary Sjögren's Syndrome: Current Pathophysiological, Diagnostic and Therapeutic Advances

Christine Delporte[1], Jason Perret[1] and Muhammad S. Soyfoo[1,2]
[1]*Laboratory of Biological Chemistry and Nutrition, Université Libre de Bruxelles, Brussels,*
[2]*Division of Rheumatology, Erasme University Hospital Brussels,*
*Belgium*

## 1. Introduction

Sjogren's syndrome (SS) is a chronic autoimmune disease characterized by the lymphocytic infiltration of exocrine glands, mainly the salivary and lachrymal glands entailing the classical sicca syndrome of xerostomia (Sjögren, 1933) and xeropthalmia. Lymphocytic infiltration of other organs results in systemic manifestations. SS is classified as either primary (pSS), when occurring alone, or secondary (sSS), when occurring in addition to other autoimmune diseases such as rheumatoid arthritis, systemic lupus erythematosus or myositis. As one of the most frequent autoimmune disease, affecting approximately 0.5% of the world population, SS is often associated with other diseases such as Hashimoto thyroiditis, coeliac disease, Biermer's disease or systemic sclerosis. SS evolves as a slow, insidious disease affecting predominantly middle-aged women (female to male ratio of 9:1), SS lies at the cross roads of autoimmune diseases characterized by both cellular and humoral abnormalities. The disease typically affects middle-aged women around their fourth and fifth decades with extremes ranging from to 2 to 83 years. The morbidity of patients suffering from SS is incapacitating ranging from severe fatigue to evolving arthralgia. Even if the patients suffering from SS have a mortality rate comparable to the general population, they present an increased risk of developing lymphoma. The diagnosis of SS is based upon defined criteria according to the American-European consensus encompassing subjective and objective clinical signs and symptoms as well as immunological alterations. The pathogenesis of SS is complex and involves many components taking part in the autoimmune destruction of exocrine glands: pro-inflammatory cytokines secretion, apoptosis, matrix metalloproteases upregulation, autoantibody formation, as well as T and B cell proliferation. In SS, the classical histological findings in exocrine glands comprise focal inflammatory infiltrates, cell destruction and fibrosis in later stages of the disease. So far, SS treatment has been mainly symptomatic, consisting in relieving the clinical signs. However, recent pathophysiological findings have led to the development of new treatments.

## 2. Diagnostic criteria

The diagnosis of SS is currently essentially based on the American-European criteria. These criteria, 6 in total, include 2 subjective and 4 objective criteria. The subjective criteria are

ocular and oral symptoms, while the objective criteria are ocular signs, histopathology, salivary gland involvement, and autoantibodies. Experts have recommended making the diagnosis of SS when 4 of the 6 criteria are present, as long as histopathology or serology is positive, or when 3 of any of the 4 objective criteria are present (Vitali et al., 2002).
It necessary to bear in mind that the most frequent symptoms of SS include the triad of fatigue, polyarthralgia and sicca symptoms, which are often commonly found in the general population and aging population. Many drugs have anti-cholinergic properties, which complicate the diagnostic process of SS. Exclusion criteria for the diagnosis of SS include the presence of hepatitis C and HIV viruses, sarcoidosis, prior cervical radiation, lymphoma, graft versus host disease and the use of anti-cholinergic drugs (Vitali et al., 2002).

### 2.1 Ocular symptoms

Ocular symptoms are taken into consideration when patients complain about troublesome dry eyes, recurrent sensation of sand or gravel in the eye, or the use of tear substituent.

### 2.2 Oral symptoms

Oral symptoms are considered pertinent when patients experience daily feeling of dry mouth, recurrent or persistent swollen salivary glands, or frequent drinking to facilitate dry food swallowing.

### 2.3 Ocular signs

Evidence of ocular involvement relies on positive Schirmer's test (<5mm/min) or positive ocular dye score (score > 4 according to the van Bijsterveld score; Van Bijsterveld, 1969).

### 2.4 Histopathology

A histological sign is considered positive when minor salivary gland biopsy show a focus score >1 (more than 50 lymphocytes per 4 $mm^2$ of tissue).

### 2.5 Salivary gland involvement

Objective evidence of salivary gland involvement relies on low unstimulated saliva flow (< 1.5ml/15 min), abnormal sialography, or altered salivary scintigraphy.

### 2.6 Autoantibodies

Serological signs are considered positive when the presence of antibodies to either Ro (SSA) or La (SSB) or both are detected in the serum.

### 2.7 New diagnostic tools

To prevent excessive prescriptions of exams for establishing diagnosis of SS, newer diagnostic tools have been validated. However, these tools have not yet been included in the American-European diagnosis criteria of SS. For example, ultrasonography of salivary glands might prove to be useful to detect anatomical changes in parotid and submandibular glands, with similar diagnostic ability to sialography. Detection of hypoechoic areas, echogenic streaks, cysts and irregular gland margins are highly suggestive of SS (Tagaki et al., 2010). Parotid MRI can also prove to be an adjunct diagnostic tool to detect heterogeneity in salivary glands and specific cystic lesions (Roberts et al., 2008).

## 3. Pathophysiology of SS

The pathophysiology of SS is highly complex. Despite tremendous progress made to unearth the different mechanistic processes underlying the autoimmune abnormality, the etiology of the disease still remains to be discovered. It is actually held that in patients with predisposed genetic background, the combination of viral infections and/or environmental stress leads to epithelial cell activation and upregulation of toll-like receptors(TLR). Initiation of disease is favored by alterations of glandular architecture such as modification of extracellular matrix and cell-cell interactions (that may lead to gene expression reprogramming by epigenetic gene modifications triggered by mecanotransduction). Activation of innate immunity through TLR, leads to T cell activation and secretion of pro-inflammatory cytokines. Moreover, following epithelial cell activation, there is an upregulation of pro-apoptotic molecules and autoantigen processing resulting in the formation of exosomes, activation of dendritic cells (secretion of IFNα) and further activation of T cells. In advanced stages of the disease, following BAFF activation, B-cell proliferation, and aberrant lymphocyte homing favoring diseased gland destruction and the formation of germinal centers and ensuing lymphoma (Figure 1).

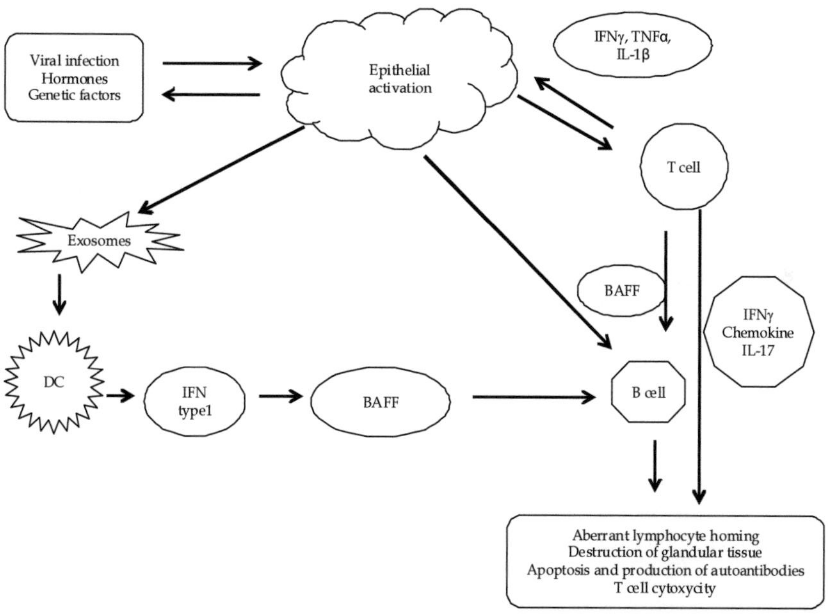


Fig. 1. Mechanisms underlying the pathogenesis of SS. Hormones, viral infections and environmental factors in appropriate genetic background are believed to trigger initial events in SS. Epithelial cells are activated resulting in T and B cell activation. T cells produce pro-inflammatory cytokines, which in turn perpetuates activation of epithelial cells, and stimulates B cell activation and proliferation resulting in aberrant lymphocyte homing, autoantibodies production, germinal ectopic centers and tissue destruction. Following epithelial cell activation, production of exosomes activates dendritic cells to produce type 1 IFN and thus BAFF secretion. BAFF stimulates aberrant B-cell maturation resulting in the production of self-reactive B cells synthesising autoantibodies. BAFF: B-cell activating factor; DC: dendritic cells; IFN: interferon; Il-1β: interleukin-1 β; TNF-α: tumor necrosis factor α.

## 3.1 Environmental factors

### 3.1.1 Viral infections

Ebstein-barr, Human T Lymphotropic Virus-1 and hepatitis C have been proposed to be associated with SS. However, the link between these viral infections and SS remains weak (Pflugfelder et al., 1993; Green et al., 1989, Haddad et al., 1992; Iwakiri et al., 2009). Coxsackie virus was found to be increased in SS salivary glands, but these findings have been the subject of some controversies (Triantafyllopoulou et al., 2004, Gottenberg et al., 2006a). Innate immunity is classically stimulated by infectious agents, which results in type I interferon production. Upon viral infection, the activation of the interferon pathway can be perpetuated by the formation of immune complexes containing viral RNA, thereby leading to plasmacytoid dendritic cell activation and production of interferon-$\alpha$.

### 3.1.2 Stress

Stress has been advocated as being a forerunner of SS, since pSS patients experienced a high degree of stress prior to the onset of disease (Karaiskos et al., 2009).

## 3.2 Endocrine factors

### 3.2.1 Sexual hormones

The high female to male predominance of SS clearly delineates the role of hormones in the pathogenesis of SS. Estrogenic action is largely imputed in the high female predominance in several autoimmune diseases, including SS (Whitacre, 2001). Estrogens and androgens are thought to respectively contribute or protect to autoimmunity. Onset of SS generally occurs around menopause, when modification of the androgen-estrogen ratio occurs. Patients with SS have been shown to possess lower systemic concentrations of dehydroepiandrosterone (DHEA) than matched aged-controls (Valtysdottir et al., 2001). Furthermore, decreased salivary DHEA levels, reduced cystein-rich secretory protein (CRISP-3, a protein upregulated by DHEA) expression, alteration of CRISP-3 polarized expression in acini, altered and decreased conversion of DHEA, and abnormal expression of steroidogenesis enzymes were detected in SS patients (Laine et al., 2007, Porola et al., 2008; Spaan et al., 2009). Women's local salivary gland dihydrotestosterone production is totally dependent on DHEA conversion, rendering them highly vulnerable to local androgen deficiency.

Estrogens play a cardinal role in targeting salivary epithelial cell and stimulating apoptosis through a Fas-mediated mechanism (Ishimaru et al., 1999). Retinoblastoma-associated protein 48 (RbAp48) induces tissue specific apoptosis in salivary glands depending on the level of estrogen deficiency (Ishimaru et al., 2008). More recently, the presence of functional estrogen receptors has been observed in salivary epithelial cells (Tsinti et al., 2009). In the latter study, estrogen was shown to block expression of ICAM-1, an adhesion molecule displaying increased expression in salivary glands of SS patients. It may therefore be speculate that estrogen deficiency might lead to increased innate immunity.

Prolactin, a pro-inflammatory hormone, stimulates estrogen activity and inhibits estrogen production, high level T cell proliferation, IL2 receptor expression, IFN-$\gamma$ production and stimulation of antibody production (Taiym et al., 2004). Higher levels of prolactin are detected in SS patients, and may be involved with the production of autoantibodies involved in SS (Taiym et al., 2004).

### 3.3 Genetic factors

#### 3.3.1 Genetic variation

Genetic predisposition is widely accepted as being an important etiological factor in many autoimmune diseases (Hewagama & Richardson, 2009). Several studies support the existence of predisposition to SS (Jonsson et al., 2007). Alleles within the major histocompatibility complex class II gene region, predominantly the HLA-DR and HLA-DQ (Loiseau et al., 2001), are implicated in the pathogenesis of SS. Susceptibility alleles in SS patients may also vary according to ethnic origin (Bolstad and Jonsson, 2005).

An increasing body of evidence for the implication of other gene variants outside the HLA locus association is being put forth recently. Gene polymorphisms of IRF-5 and STAT-4 genes, two transcription factors of pivotal importance in interferon pathway, have been associated with various autoimmune diseases (Martinez et al., 2008), as well as with SS (Miceli-Richard et al., 2007; Korman et al., 2008; Miceli-Richard et al., 2009; Nordmark et al., 2009, Gestermann et al., 2010). The most significantly associated single nucleotide polymorphism (SNP) of the IRF5 gene was a 4 fold repetition, instead of three, of a sequence within the promoter region (Nordmark et al., 2009). An association between this polymorphism and high levels of IRF5 mRNA was demonstrated in PBMCs and in cultured salivary epithelial cells after viral infection (Miceli-Richard et al., 2009). STAT4 polymorphism was also associated with SS (Nordmark et al., 2009; Korman et al., 2008; Gestermann et al., 2010; Palomino-Morales et al., 2010).

MECP2 and IL2-IL21 polymorphisms have also been associated with SS (Cobb et al., 2010; Maiti et al., 2010). Gene polymorphisms in IL-10, IL-6, IL-1 receptor antagonist, IL-4 receptor α, TNF-α, IFN-γ and TGF-β1 have also been associated with pSS (Cobb et al., 2008).

PTPN22 (protein tyrosine phosphatase nonreceptor 22), primarily expressed in lymphoid tissues, has been suggested to have prominent roles in T-cell signaling. The 1858 T allele of PTPN22 has been shown to be a risk factor for SS in one Columbian study whilst other studies did not find any significant association with SS (Gomez et al., 2005; Ittah et al., 2005).

PTEN, a tumour suppressor gene, displayed a rare mutations shown to be associated concomitantly with SS and Cowden disease (Raizis et al., 1998) and may be associated, in diseases, with the latter occurrence of non-Hodgkin lymphoma.

Very recently, a large Swedish-Norwegian study has associated potentially muscarinic receptor-3 gene variant with SS (Appel et al., 2011). In this study, focus scores, abnormal Schimer's test and autoantibody presence were associated with muscarinic receptor-3 SNPs.

Recent data have suggested an increased association between immune system genes and the pathogenesis of primary SS. Indeed, an increase in the copy number of 2 genes linked to immune regulation-FCGR3B and CCL3L1-that can confer susceptibility to SS (Mamtani et al., 2010). A similar study revealed, besides confirming association of STAT4 and IRF5/TNPO3, three new loci as being associated as well with SS. However, the SNPs studied were not associated with the presence of anti-SSA/anti-SSB antibodies; though they are all involved in B-cell differentiation and activation (Nordmark et al., 2011).

Finally, in contrast one polymorphic variant, 168His of the minor histocompatibilty antigen HA-1, has been described as protective, lowering the risk of pSS (Harangi et al., 2005).

#### 3.3.2 Epigenetic control

Epigenetic mechanisms are currently and increasingly being associated in disease processes, including autoimmune diseases such as rheumatoid arthritis, systemic lupus erythematosus,

systemic sclerosis and SS (Pan and Sawalha., 2009; Richardson, 2007; Hewagama & Richardson, 2009; Brooks et al., 2010). In salivary glands from SS patients undergoing extracellular matrix remodelling, mechanotransduction may convey organ structural modifications that will inturn affect epigenetic control of gene expression (Gonzalez et al., 2011a). Indeed, the global DNA methylation of salivary glands from SS patients appears to be decreased, while specific genes appear to be hypermethylated (Gonzalez et al., 2011b).
MicroRNAs (miRNA) are an emerging field of epigenetic gene expression control, with potential involvement in autoimmune diseases (Dai & Ahmed, 2011; Alevizos & Illei, 2010a). miRNAs are small (20-22 nucleotides RNAs), resulting from a complex cellular processing, leading to RNA sequestration or destruction. miRNAs 17 & 92 have been shown to be associated with SS (Alevizoz et al., 2011a). Another study showed that over-expression of 2 miRNAs (miR-574 and miR-768-3p) participates to the epigenetic control of gene expression in salivary glands from SS patients (Alevizos et al., 2011b). These two micro-RNAs were associated with a high degree of inflammation and correlated with the histological focus score. As such, they could represent future biomarkers of inflammation in SS patients (Alevizos & Illei, 2010b, 2011). In animal model of SS, upregulation of miRNA 150 and 146 in PBMC and target tissue was observed (Lu et al., 2010). Furthermore, miR23A is highly expressed in salivary glands from SS patients and may regulate CUL3 expression (Gonzalez et al., 2011a).

### 3.4 Immune system alterations

The innate immune system plays a fundamental role in the pathogenesis of SS. Following viral infection, an increase in the expression of Toll-like receptors (TLR) has been shown in the salivary glands of SS patients. The functional TLR 2, 3, 4 as well as myeloid differentiation factor 88 (MYD88) are expressed in the labial salivary glands of SS patients (Kawakami et al., 2007). Following TLR activation in salivary glands, an increase in CD54 (ICAM-1) expression and IL-6 production, as well as upregulation of CD54, MHC class I and CD40 have been observed (Spachidou et al., 2007). Upregulation of TLR3 in salivary glands of female new Zealand/WF1 female mice, in response to polyinosinic:polycytidylic acid (a TLR3 ligand) resulted in activation of cytokine pathways and severe loss of glandular function (Deshmukh et al., 2009). These data underline increased TLR signaling pathways in salivary glands of SS patients leading to production of proinflammatory cytokines, T cell activation and a T helper type 1 driven immune response.
Upregulated expression of human leukocyte antigen (HLA) molecules occurs in epithelial cells of salivary glands from SS patients and may be involved in antigen presentation, leading to destruction of the tissue by CD4+ T cells as well as cytokine production and stimulation of B cells proliferation and differentiation (Jonsson et al., 2002).
Several cytokines have been implicated in the pathogenesis of SS. Increased expression of IFN-regulated genes has been shown in salivary glands from SS patients (Gottenberg et al., 2006; Hjelmervik et al., 2005), as well as in PBMC and whole blood (Emamian et al., 2009). Increased serum levels of IFN-$\alpha$ and $\beta$ have been observed in pSS patients. Circulating PDC express high levels of CD40 (a marker of cellular activation), which correlate with the expression level of several type 1 IFN-induced genes in monocytes (Wildenberg et al., 2008). Type-1 IFN activation and secretion result in activation of immature dendritic cells, BAFF secretion, stimulation of Fas ligand expression and increased apoptosis, increased T cell proliferation and survival, induction of several chemokines and favoring Th1 responses

(Mavragani and Crow., 2010). Increased expression of TNF-α, IL-1, IL-12, IL-18, and IFN-α has also been shown in SS patients (Vougarelis and Tzioufas, 2010, Becker et al., 2010). Recently, the role of IL-17 producing cells (Th17) has been underlined in the pathogenesis of SS (Nguyen et al., 2008; Espinosa et al., 2009). The IL-23/Th17 pathway triggers autoimmune exocrinopathy and systemic autoimmunity. Mice lacking Ro 52 antigen are characterized by increased proinflammatory cytokines, tissue inflammation and systemic inflammation. Loss of IL-23 and IL-17 in Ro52 null mice, results in protection from systemic autoimmunity (Espinosa et al., 2009). Elevated serum levels of IL-17 and Th17 cells in patients with SS and related cytokines are predominant in salivary glands and strongly correlate with histological focus score (Katsifis et al., 2009).

Once T-cell infiltration of epithelial cells is established, CD4+ T cells and PDC produce B-cell targeted cytokines and other survival factors such as B-cell-activating factor of the tumor necrosis factor family (BAFF, also known as BLYS) and APRIL (Lavie et al., 2004). Ectopic germinal centre-like structures are a hallmark of B cell activation and proliferation and occur in about 20% of patients with pSS (Garcia-Carrasco et al., 2002). B cell hyperactivity has been found in SS patients (Kassan and Moutsopoulos, 2004). BAFF promotes B-cell survival and antibody secretion. BAFF-transgenic mice develop clinical features of SS, polyarthritis and lupus (Mackay and Schneider, 2009). SS patients display increased BAFF serum levels correlating with decreased BAFF-R expression on B-cells and disease activity (Sellam et al., 2007). BAFF secretion is induced by type 1-IFN in monocytes and dendritic cells, type 1 IFN in monocytes and salivary epithelial cells (Ittah et al., 2006), virus or double stranded DNA in salivary epithelial cells (Ittah et al., 2008). BAFF can be released by the epithelial salivary cells and B cells. B cell dysregulation plays a crucial role in perpetuating inflammation and tissue damage (Pers et al., 2007). Decreased levels of apoptosis among BAFF-expressing cells in salivary epithelial cells result in increased levels of BAFF expression, which in turn amplifies B cell signaling and proliferation and increased production of antibody-producing plasma cells (Mariette et al., 2003; Groom et al., 2002; Jonsson et al., 2005).

### 3.5 Autonomic system

Autonomic system dysfunction is also considered as a central feature in the pathogenesis of SS (Fox and Stern, 2002; Dawson et al., 2001). It might be responsible for glandular dysfunction and diminished salivary and lachrymal production (Waterman et al., 2000; Humphreys-Beher et al., 1999). The role of autonomic dysfunction in SS pathogenesis is supported by the presence of anti muscarinic M3 receptors (M3R) autoantibodies in SS patients (Naito et al., 2005; Nakamura et al., 2008). In the salivary glands of SS patients, there is an upregulation of M3R, which might be the corollary of antagonistic M3R autoantibodies or impaired release of acetylcholine (Beroukas et al., 2002a) or yet modified epigenetic control on M3R (Appel et al., 2010). Furthermore, M3R Tcells play a fundamental role in autoimmune sialoadenitis (Iizuka et al., 2010). An additional mechanism that could contribute to autonomic dysfunction is elevated levels of acetylcholinesterase in the salivary glands of patients with SS (Dawson et al., 2000). Decreased levels of acetylcholine due to increased cholinesterase levels result in glandular dysfunction and diminished production of saliva (Dawson et al., 2001).

### 3.6 Autoantibodies

Autoantibodies against Ro (SSA) and La (SSB) are found in the serum of pSS and sSS patients (Garcia-Carrascos et al., 2002). They are linked to the onset, severity, duration and extraglandular manifestations of SS (Jonsson et al., 2002; Skopouli et al., 2005). It is still undetermined if these antibodies play a direct pathogenic role in the glandular damage. Nonetheless, there is evidence supporting a role of anti Ro and anti La antibodies in the local autoimmune response. Indeed, autoantibodies to Ro and La have been found in saliva and infiltrating cells of salivary glands in patients with SS. Increased mRNA production of La in acinar epithelial cells and translocation of La protein, resulting in membrane localization, in the conjunctival epithelial cells have been observed in SS patients (Hammi et al., 2005; Tzioufas et al., 1999).

Autoantibodies against α–fodrin, a major constituent of the cytoskeleton, have also been detected in sera from patients with SS. Abnormal location of α-fodrin on the surface of apoptotic-induced cells suggests the role of α-fodrin in SS through apoptotic pathways. Aberrant proteolysis of α-fodrin results in its expression at the surface of apoptotic epithelial cells entailing the autoimmune process (Locht et al., 2008; Willeke et al., 2007).

Autoantibodies to muscarinic M3 receptors, found in the serum of SS patients, induce the inhibition of the synapse between the efferent nerves and the salivary glands, leading to decreased saliva production (Fox and Stern, 2002; Sumida et al., 2010).

More recently, antibodies against carbonic anhydrase II, VI and XIII have been described in relation to renal manifestations of SS (Pertovaara et al., 2011).

### 3.7 Epithelial cells activation

Impaired function and/or architectural destruction of epithelial cells occur in salivary glands from SS patients. Epithelial cells are now considered as playing active roles in immune defenses (Manoussakis and Kapsogeorgou, 2010). Epithelial salivary glands cells, even if not proven to act as antigen-presenting cells possess all the features to do so (Manoussakis et al., 1999; Matsumura et al., 2001). Epithelial cells might act as non-professional antigen-presenting cells, and thereby participate in autoimmune responses leading to the development of SS (Tsunawaki et al., 2002; Xanthou et al., 2001; Dimitriou et al., 2002; Lavie et al., 2004). Proinflammatory cytokines and other factors can induce activation of surrounding epithelial cells (Abu-Helu et al., 2001). Furthermore, as a result of apoptosis and formation of exosomes, epithelial cells present intracellular autoantigens such as the Ro and La autoantigens, further contributing to the autoimmune process. Besides, following type 1 IFN stimulation and viral infection of epithelial cells, the latter releases BAFF thereby activating B cells (Kapsogeorgou et al., 2005; Ittah et al., 2009).

### 3.8 Apoptosis

A pivotal role for apoptosis as a pathogenic mechanism in SS-related glandular damage has been demonstrated. Increased apoptosis of the ductal and acinar epithelia occurs in pSS patients. Upregulation of the expression of several apoptotic-related molecules has been described in lymphocytes and epithelial cells from salivary glands of patients with SS. Epithelial cell apoptosis contributes to the glandular destructive lesions through the upregulation of molecules leading to the proteolysis of exocrine autoantigens and ensuing glandular damage. Disequilibrium between pro-apoptotic signals and anti-apoptotic mechanisms might act as the basis of epithelial cell destruction of exocrine glands in pSS.

Apoptotic cell death might also function in a specific fashion favoring abnormal exposure of nuclear and cytoplasmic autoantigens thereby providing mechanism of antigen presentation to autoreactive T cells. Furthermore, anti-Ro and anti-La autoantibodies can activate caspase-3 and cleave PARP and trigger apoptosis. Furthermore, these autoantibodies have been shown to also activate extrinsic apoptotic pathways by transcriptional upregulation and activation of caspase-8. Anti-Ro and anti-La autoantibodies could trigger apoptosis resulting into tissue destruction (Ramos-Casals and Font, 2005).

### 3.9 Alterations of proteins involved in glandular function

Aquaporins (AQP) are small transmembrane proteins involved in water flow across cell membranes. Several AQPs are expressed in salivary glands and lachrymal glands (Delporte, 2009). AQP5, expressed on salivary acinar cells, contributes to salivary flow (Ma et al., 1999). A modified distribution of AQP5 expression has been documented in both human salivary and lachrymal glands from pSS patients (Steinfeld et al., 2001; Tsubota et al., 2001) and in SS animal models (Konttinen et al., 2005; Soyfoo et al., 2007, Sasaki et al., 2007; Ohashi et al., 2008). Treatment by rituximab restored apical localization of AQP5 (Ring et al., 2006). A decreased expression of AQP1 in salivary glands of SS patients was observed (Beroukas et al., 2001; Beroukas et al., 2002). Both AQP5 and AQP1 could participate to the pathogenesis of SS, although they can not account for salivary and lachrymal secretory defects.

An active remodelling of the basal lamina is taking place in acinar and ductal cells from SS patients. In normal salivary glands, laminin 5 bridges the basal lamina with epithelial cells by forming adhesion complexes through specific integrin $\alpha6\beta4$ (Velozo et al., 2009). Modified expression of basal laminins, laminins 1 and 5, occurs during different stages of SS (Kwon et al., 2006; Laine et al., 2004). In salivary acinar cells from SS patients, altered distribution of $\alpha6\beta4$ integrin results in the destruction epithelial cell complexes with laminins (Velozo et al., 2009). Tight junction protein levels and distribution of ZO-1, occluding, claudin-1 and claudin-4 were modified in patients with SS (Ewert et al., 2010). Therefore, maintenance of equilibrium between cell-cell and cell-basal lamina attachment is necessary to ensure gland cell survival.

## 4. Clinical manifestations

### 4.1 Xeropthalmia

Xerophtalmia is often less prominent than xerostomia. It is therefore necessary to follow a detailed anamnestic investigation to detect symptoms of ocular dryness. The main complaint of xeropthalmia is foreign-body sensation, but other symptoms such as grittiness, thick rope like secretions at the inner canthus, photosensitivity, burns, and sensation of having a veil before the eyes, absence of tears after irritation or emotion are all frequent features of xerophtalmia. Xerophtalmia is due to the lymphocytic infiltration of lachrymal glands leading to reduced lachrymal flow and tear composition, thereby altering corneal and conjunctival epithelia, characterizing the known condition of keratoconjunctivitis sicca (KCS). In severe disease, functional disability with visual impairment may occur (Fox, 2005).

### 4.2 Xerostomia

More than 90% of patients with SS complain of symptoms resulting from functional alteration of salivary glands. The symptoms range from dry mouth and lips, the need to drink more water when eating, to difficulties in the mastication process. In the early phase of the disease, xerostomia is less obvious for the patients but with disease progression and severe alteration of salivary glands, xerostomia manifests as a painful syndrome with the sensation of permanent mouth burns, taste alteration, fissuring of the tongue, angular cheleitis and ulcers. Further progression of xerostomia leads to multiple complications such as teeth decay, atrophy of lingual papillae, increased incidence of mucosal infections (primarily candidiasis) loss of teeth and ultimately dentition (Fox, 2005).

### 4.3 Systemic manifestations

#### 4.3.1 Musculoskeletal manifestations

More than 70% of patients complain of articular manifestations. Symmetric, non-erosive, polyarthritis affecting the small joints can also be observed and precede the sicca syndrome. Myalgias are also a frequent feature, accompanied with asthenia, fatigue and muscle tenderness, reminiscent of a fibromyalgia-like syndrome (Mavragani and Moutsopoulos, 2010).

#### 4.3.2 Respiratory manifestations

Reduced secretion from nasal epithelial cells results in nasal crusting, epistaxis and recurrent sinusitis. Tracheal dryness results in a dry non-productive cough and dyspnoea. In > 50% of SS patients, dry irritating cough was present without any radiographic abnormalities. Bronchial hyperreactivity might lead to small airways obstruction. Due to lymphocytic hyperplasia, severe airway obstruction can also occur (Parke, 2008).

Interstitial lung disease (ILD) is a classic manifestation of SS. These patients present cough, dyspnea on exertion, bilateral pulmonary infiltrates on plain radiographs and several other abnormalities on computer tomography scanner. Later stages of the disease are characterized by its evolution to fibrosis and neutrophilic alveolitis (Parambil et al., 2006).

Lymphocytic interstitial pneumonia (LIP), previously considered as a hallmark of lung involvement in SS, forms part of the spectrum of ILD. It is a consequence of bronchus associated lymphoid tissue proliferation (BALT) (Parambil et al., 2006).

Patients with SS are at increased risk of developing lymphoma, usually low grade MALT lymphoma and primary pulmonary lymphoma. These patients present few clinical symptoms contrasting with severe radiographic changes (Parke, 2008).

Pulmonary hypertension is a very rare finding in patients with SS. Only 17 cases have been documented in the literature. Prolonged vasospasm and vasculature remodeling have been assigned to contribute to the development of this pathology (Launay et al., 2007).

#### 4.3.3 Renal manifestations

Tubular renal acidosis and glomerulonephritis are two main features of kidney involvement in SS. Distal tubular acidosis is the most frequent renal manifestation of SS occurring in up to 20% of cases. Very often, it is asymptomatic without any clinical or biological impact. Glomerulonephritis is rare in SS, and often due to cryoglobulinemia (Aasarod et al., 2000).

#### 4.3.4 Cutaneous features

Besides the classical features of dry skin, other skin manifestations are present. Purpura is presents as petechia, which are localized in the lower limbs. Histological analysis shows leucocytoclastic vasculitis. The symptoms usually resolve with corticosteroids. Other skin manifestations include erythema nodosa, vitiligo, and digital ulcers (Kittridge et al., 2011).

### 4.3.5 Neurological manifestations

The spectrum of neurological disorders associated with SS is broad ranging from peripheral neuropathy to central nervous involvement. The frequency of neurological involvement in SS is relatively low and might precede the diagnosis of SS (Segal et al., 2008).
The cardinal features of CNS involvement in SS are very much identical to that of systemic lupus erythematosus. As such, the clinical profile includes hemiparesis, cranial neuropathy and more often optic nerve neuropathy, brainstem and cerebellar disorders, movement disorders, epilepsia. Spinal cord syndromes include transverse myelitis, Brown-Sequard syndrome and progressive myelitis. Because of the occurrence of optic neuropathy and myelitis, a diagnosis of multiple sclerosis is often evoked. Furthermore, MRI imaging shows hyperintense lesions in the white matter. Neuromyelitis optica (Devic's disease) is often associated with SS and is characterized by episodes of myelitis and optic neuropathy. The clinical features of neuropsychiatric syndrome include often cognition, anxiety, mood changes, and depression and sleep disorders (Lafitte et al., 2001).
Peripheral neuropathy is much more frequent than CNS involvement and precedes the diagnosis of SS. Sensory neuronopathy is considered to be distinctive of SS but sensorimotor neuropathy, sensory neuropathy, autonomic neuropathy, moneuritis multiplex are amongst other features of peripheral nervous system involvement. Trigeminal neuropathy is one of the most frequent manifestations of neurological invovement in SS (Lafitte et al., 2001). In most of the cases, sensory ataxia, painful sensory neuropathies, and trigeminal neuropathy are related to sensory ganglionitis, whereas mononeuritis multiplex and multiple cranial neuropathies are more closely associated with peripheral nerve vasculitis (Segal et al., 2008).

### 4.3.6 Gastrointestinal features

The manifestations of gastrointestinal tract are not very specific and include oesphageal dysmotility and gastro intestinal reflux. There are no specific liver abnormalities, which can be attributed to SS, but autoimmune hepatitis and primary biliary cirrhosis can be associated diseases (Mavragani and Moutsopoulos, 2010; Fox, 2005).

### 4.3.7 Serological manifestations

Several hematological features such as anemia, leucopenia and thrombopenia can be present. Anemia is a rare feature and when it exists, it is rarely due to inflammation but results from hemodilution due to polyclonal hypergammaglobulinemia. Leucopenia < 4000/mm3 is present in 30% of cases. In certain cases of major hypergammaglobulinemia, a hyperviscosity syndrome can be present. Typical symptoms include headaches, visual impairement and hemorrhages (Fox, 2005).

### 4.4 Lymphoma

Patients with SS have a 20 to 40-fold risk of developing non-hodgkin lymphoma (NHL) as compared to the general population. NHL has a prevalence of about 4% in SS and occurs classically following a median of 7.5 years after its initial diagnosis. The most frequent histological type of NHL is the MALT lymphoma. The histopathological features of MALT lymphoma include reactive lymphoid follicles, small plasma cells, lymphoepithelial lesions and MZ and/or monocytoid B cells. The clinical course of NHL lymphoma is indolent and the clinical characteristics include small tumor burden and good performance status. The most frequent anatomical localizations are the salivary glands but extra nodal sites can be involved, such as stomach or kidneys.The clinical and biological factors heralding imminent are low C4 levels, palpable purpura, high β2-microglobulin levels, CD4 lymphocytopenia, parotid gland swelling and persistent enlargement and hypocaptation on salivary scintigraphy, mixed monoclonal cryoglobulinemia, leg ulcers, splenomegaly and the presence of serum or urine monoclonal bands (Voulgarelis and Moutsopoulos, 2008).

## 5. Therapeutic approaches

Conventional therapy of SS is symptomatic and consists in alleviating of sicca features. As such, treatment consists in the use of artificial saliva and tears, surgical removal of plugs in the lachrymal ducts, the use of topical cyclosporine for ocular symptoms. Cholinergic drugs such as pilocarpine and civemeline are available to increase glandular secretion. Hydroxychloroquine is prescribed for arthralgia and myalgia, but recent studies have shown that it also has slight anticholinesterase properties in improving glandular function (Rihl et al., 2009). The efficacy of steroids is limited and restricted to patients with arthritis and severe extraglandular manifestations. Immunosuppressive treatments such as cyclophosphamide and azathioprine are used for systemic features of SS. More recently, newer immunosuppressive drugs, such as mizoribine and mycophenolate mofetil, have shown promising results. These drugs inhibit inosine monophosphate dehydrogenase, the rate-limiting enzyme for purine synthesis, and have an antiproliferative effect on activated lymphocytes (Becker et al., 2010). An intraoral electrostimulation device showed promising results in alleviating xerostomia and increasing salivary output (Strietzel et al., 2011).

### 5.1 B-cell targeted therapies

Rituximab, a chimeric monoclonal mouse antibody that targets CD20 at the surface of B-cells, is the most studied biologic therapy in SS. Several pilot studies have shown efficacy of rituximab in terms of improvement of fatigue, quality of life and glandular function. A randomized-controlled trial has confirmed these results (Meijer et al., 2010). Epratuzumab is a humanized antibody directed against the B cell antigen CD22. An open labeled trial has shown improvement of sicca symptoms and fatigue scores (Steinfeld et al., 2006).

### 5.2 Inhibition of IFN release

Interferon-α (IFN) plays a pivotal role in the pathogenesis of several autoimmune diseases including SS. Besides antiviral effects, IFN-α has immunomodulating properties. Four pilot studies have shown beneficial effects of oromucosal IFN-α, whereby salivary flow was increased and salivary gland histology after treatment demonstrated reduced lymphocytic infiltrâtes (Cummins et al., 2003; Tobon et al., 2010). A phase III trial performed later, showed an increase in unstimulated salivary flow but the main clinical endpoint, which was improvement of stimulated salivary flow, was not met.

### 5.3 Transplantation of bone-marrow-derived stem cells

Stem cells from the spleen, when harvested and transplanted in NOD mice, an animal model for SS, have been shown to regenerate salivary epithelial cells (Faustman et al., 2010). Current undergoing trials are investigating whether the transplanted adult hematopoietic cells can restore glandular function in patients suffering from SS.

### 5.4 Gene therapy

Gene therapy consists in the introduction of new genetic material in an individual for therapeutic purposes. Several targets for gene therapy include aquaporins, inflammatory mediators, apoptotic molecules and intracellular molecules.

Initial gene therapy studies, using serotype 5 adenoviral vector (Ad5), showed extremely efficient *in vivo* gene transfer to rodent salivary glands (Mastrangeli et al., 1994). Further studies using Ad5 encoding human aquaporin 1 (Ad5hAQP1), a water channel, showed the function and potential utility of this vector to restore impaired saliva flow in rats with irradiated-induced salivary hypofunction (Delporte et al., 1997). The efficacy and scaling studies of this particular gene therapy were then performed in large animal models: rhesus macaques (O'Connell et al., 1999) and miniature pigs (Li et al., 2004). A NIH clinical trial using Ad5hAQP5 has been undertaken to test the safety and efficacy in individuals with irradiation-induced parotid salivary hypofunction.

Gene transfer therapies based on the anti-inflammatory properties of IL-10 and vasoactive intestinal peptide (VIP) have also been proposed as future treatment of SS. Indeed, administration of adenovirus vectors encoding either human IL-10 or VIP to salivary glands from NOD mice, a mouse model for SS, led to significant salivary flow improvement (Kok et al., 2003; Lodde et al., 2006).

Gene transfer has also been used to treat chronic sialadenitis and modulate apoptosis in a murine model of SS: B6-gld/gld mice deficient in Fas ligand. When infected with murine cytomegalovirus, these mice presented chronic sialadenitis similar to SS. Delivery of a recombinant adenovirus vector coding for Fas ligand to the salivary glands of these mice, induced a significant reduction in infiltrating lymphocytes (Fleck et al., 2001).

As IL17A administration to mice salivary glands, using recombinant adenoviral vector, leads to SS-like disease (Nguyen et al., 2011), localized anti-IL-17 might be effective in preventing glandular dysfunction.

### 5.5 Other therapeutic perspectives

BAFF is a cytokine that prevents apoptosis of B-cells and thereby contributes to the hyperreactivity of B cells and their survival. Increased BAFF secretion might explain in part the partial response of rituximab in SS patients. Targeting BAFF might therefore prove to be a future therapeutical approach (Mariette, 2008). In systemic lupus erythematous, an autoimmune disease that shares similar pathogenetic features with SS, in that both diseases are characterized by an interferon signature, Belimumab, an anti-BAFF monoclonal agent, has shown beneficial effects in a randomized controlled trial (Navarra et al., 2011). Atacicept, a fusion protein inhibiting B cell stimulation, could be a promising therapeutic drug in SS (Dorner et al., 2009).

Other therapeutic perspectives for SS also include the restoration of salivary glands function using bone marrow-derived cells (BMDCs) (Tran et al., 2011) and tissue engineering of salivary glands (Kagami et al., 2011). BMDCs transplantation by intravenous injection rescues salivary gland function in mice with head and neck irradiation by preventing apoptosis, increasing tissue vascularization, increasing the number of proliferating cells, and maintaining the putative salivary stem cells (Sumita et al., 2011; Lombaert et al., 2008). Furthermore, BMDCs transplantation into NOD mice treated as well with complete Freund's adjuvant (CFA), led to both qualitative and quantitative saliva restoration, and normoglycemia (Khalili et al., 2010). Tissue engineering of salivary glands utilizes cells, biodegradable scaffold, and signals to regenerate tissues. Since the pioneer work reporting the culture of salivary epithelial cell culture (Brown 1974), several culture procedures have been described (Horie et al., 1996; Aframian et al., 2004; Joraku et al., 2005; Tran et al., 2006). A multipotent stem cell population has been discovered in human adult salivary glands (Okumura et al., 2003; Hisatomi et al., 2004; Kishi et al., 2006), but their potential for engineering salivary glands has not been proven. Developping appropriate scaffold materials will be essential for salivary gland tissue engineering (Kagami et al., 2011).

## 6. Conclusions

SS is one of the most frequent autoimmune diseases, characterized by the dysregulation of cellular and humoral mechanisms, thereby portraying the prototype of autoimmune disorders. Although, the pathogenesis of SS still remains to be discovered, tremendous progress has been made in deciphering the intrinsic abnormalities behind initiation and perpetuation of inflammation and tissue destruction. The herald of new pathophysiological mechanisms such as epigenetic control may prove cardinal in tailoring new treatments providing improved relief to patients with SS.

## 7. Acknowledgements

This work was supported by grant 3.4502.09 from the Fund for Medical Scientific Research (FRSM, Belgium).

## 8. References

Aasarød K, Haga HJ, Berg KJ, Hammerstrøm J & Jørstad S. Renal involvement in primary Sjögren's syndrome.QJM 2000; 93:297-304.

Abu-Helu RF, Dimitriou ID, Kapsogeorgou EK, Moutsopoulos HM & Manoussakis MN. Induction of salivary gland epithelial cell injury in Sjogren's syndrome: in vitro assessment of T cell-derived cytokines and Fas protein expression. J Autoimmun 2001; 17:141-153.

Aframian DJ, David R, Ben-Bassat H, Shai E, Deutsch D, Baum BJ & Palmon A. Characterization of murine autologous salivary gland graft cells: a model for use with an artificial salivary gland. Tissue Eng 2004; 10:914-920.

Alevizos I & Illei GG. MicroRNAs in Sjögren's syndrome as a prototypic autoimmune disease. Autoimmun Rev 2010a; 9:618-21.

Alevizos I & Illei GG. MicroRNAs as biomarkers in rheumatic diseases. Nat Rev Rheumatol 2010b; 6:391-8.

Alevizos I, Alexander S, Turner RJ & Illei GG. MicroRNA expression profiles as biomarkers of minor salivary gland inflammation and dysfunction in Sjögren's syndrome. Arthritis Rheum 2011; 63:535-544.

Appel S, Le Hellard S, Bruland O, Brun JG, Omdal R, Kristjansdottir G, Theander E, Nordmark G, Kvarnström M, Eriksson P, Rönnblom L, Wahren-Herlenius M & Jonsson R. Potential association of muscarinic receptor 3 gene variants with primary Sjogren's syndrome. Ann Rheum Dis 2011; annrheumdis138966, in press.

Becker H, Pavenstaedt H & Willeke P. Emerging treatment strategies and potential therapeutic targets in primary Sjogren's syndrome, Inflamm Allergy Drug Targets 2010; 9:10-19.

Beroukas D, Hiscock J, Jonsson R, Waterman SA & Gordon TP. Subcellular distribution of aquaporin 5 in salivary glands in primary Sjogren's syndrome. Lancet 2001; 358 : 1875-1876.

Beroukas D, Goodfellow R, Hiscock J, Jonsson R, Gordon TP & Waterman SA. Up-regulation of M3-muscarinic receptors in labial salivary gland acini in primary Sjögren's syndrome. Lab Invest 2002a; 82:203–210.

Beroukas D, Hiscock J, Gannon BJ, Jonsson R, Gordon TP & Waterman SA. Selective down-regulation of aquaporin-1 in salivary glands in primary Sjogren's syndrome. Lab Invest 2002b; 82: 1547-1552.

Bolstad AI & Jonsson R. Gene therapeutics in sjogren's syndrome. Expert Opin Biol Ther 2005; 5:763-772.

Bowman SJ, St Pierre Y, Sutcliffe N, Isenberg DA, Goldblatt F, Price E, Hamburger J, Richards A, Rauz S, Regan M, Rigby S, Jones A, Mulherin D & Clarke AE. Estimating indirect costs in primary Sjogren's syndrome. J Rheumatol 2010; 37:1010-1015.

Brooks WH, Le Dantec C, Pers JO, Youinou P & Renaudineau Y. Epigenetics and autoimmunity. J Autoimmun 2010; 34:J207-J219.

Brown AM & Frankel A. Leukocyte mediated cytotoxicity of chemically induced rat salivary gland neoplasms. J Oral Pathol 1974; 3: 239-255.

Cobb BL, Fei Y, Jonsson R, Bolstad AI, Brun JG, Rischmueller M, Lester SE, Witte T, Illei G, Brennan M, Bowman S, Moser KL, Harley JB & Sawalha AH. Genetic association between methyl-CpG binding protein 2 (MECP2) and primary Sjogren's syndrome. Ann Rheum Dis 2010; 69:1731-1732.

Cummins MJ, Papas A, Kammer GM & Fox PC. Treatment of primary Sjögren's syndrome with low-dose human interferon alfa administered by the oromucosal route: combined phase III results. Arthritis Rheum 2003; 49:585–593.

Dai R & Ahmed SA. MicroRNA, a new paradigm for understanding immunoregulation, inflammation, and autoimmune diseases. Transl Res 2011; 157:163-179.

Dawson LJ, Christmas SE & Smith PM. An investigation of interactions between the immune system and stimulus-secretion coupling in mouse submandibular acinar cells. A possible mechanism to account for reduced salivary flow rates associated with the onset of Sjogren's syndrome. Rheumatology 2000; 39:1226-1233.

Dawson LJ, Field EA, Harmer AR & Smith PM. Acetylcholine-evoked calcium mobilization and ion channel activation in human labial gland acinar cells from patients with primary Sjögren's syndrome. Clin Exp Immunol 2001; 124:480–485.

Delporte C, O'Connell BC, He X, Lancaster HE, O'Connell AC, Agre P & Baum BJ. Increased fluid secretion after adenoviral-mediated transfer of the aquaporin-1 cDNA to irradiated rat salivary glands. Proc Natl Acad Sci USA 1997; 94:3268-3273.

Delporte C. Aquaporins in secretory glands and their role Sjögren's syndrome. Hand Exp Phramacol 2009; 190:185-201.

Deshmukh US, Nandula SR, Thimmalapura PR, Scindia YM & Bagavant H. Activation of innate immune responses through Toll-like receptor 3 causes a rapid loss of salivary gland function. J Oral Pathol Med 2009; 38:42–47.

Dimitriou ID, Kapsogeorgou EK, Moutsopoulos HM & Manoussakis MN. CD40 on salivary gland epithelial cells: high constitutive expression by cultured cells from Sjögren's syndrome patients indicating their intrinsic activation. Clin Exp Immunol 2002; 127:386-392.

Dörner T, Radbruch A & Burmester GR. B-cell-directed therapies for autoimmune disease. Nat Rev Rheumatol 2009; 5:433–441.

Emamian ES, Leon JM, Lessard CJ, Grandits M, Baechler EC, Gaffney PM, Segal B, Rhodus NL & Moser KL. Peripheral blood gene expression profiling in Sjögren's syndrome. Genes Immun 2009; 10:285–296.

Espinosa A, Dardalhon V, Brauner S, Ambrosi A, Higgs R, Quintana FJ, Sjöstrand M, Eloranta ML, Ní Gabhann J, Winqvist O, Sundelin B, Jefferies CA, Rozell B, Kuchroo VK & Wahren-Herlenius M. Loss of the lupus autoantigen Ro52/Trim21 induces tissue inflammation and systemic autoimmunity by disregulating the IL-23-Th17 pathway. J Exp Med 2009; 206:1661-1671.

Ewert P, Aguilera S, Alliende C, Kwon YJ, Albornoz A, Molina C, Urzúa U, Quest AF, Olea N, Pérez P, Castro I, Barrera MJ, Romo R, Hermoso M, Leyton C & González MJ. Disruption of tight junction structure in salivary glands from Sjögren's syndrome patients is linked to proinflammatory cytokine exposure. Arthritis Rheum 2010; 62:1280-1289.

Faustman DL & Davis M. Stem cells in the spleen: therapeutic potential for Sjogren's syndrome, type I diabetes, and other disorders. Int J Biochem Cell Biol 2010; 42:1576-1579.

Fleck M, Zhang HG, Kern ER, Hsu HC, Müller-Ladner U & Mountz JD. Treatment of chronic sialadenitis in a murine model of Sjögren's syndrome by local fasL gene transfer. Arthritis Rheum 2001; 44:964-973.

Fox RI & Stern M. Sjogren's syndrome: mechanisms of pathogenesis involve interaction of immune and neurosecretory systems. Scand J Rheumatol Suppl 2002; 116:3-13.

Fox RI. Sjogren's syndrome. Lancet 2005; 366: 321-331.

García-Carrasco M, Ramos-Casals M, Rosas J, Pallarés L, Calvo-Alen J, Cervera R, Font J & Ingelmo M. Primary Sjögren syndrome: clinical and immunologic disease patterns in a cohort of 400 patients. Medicine 2002; 81:270–80.

Gestermann N, Mekinian A, Comets E, Loiseau P, Puechal X, Hachulla E, Gottenberg JE, Mariette X & Miceli-Richard C. STAT4 is a confirmed genetic risk factor for Sjögren's syndrome and could be involved in type 1 interferon pathway signaling. Genes Immun. 2010; 11:432-438.

Gomez LM, Anaya JM, Gonzalez CI, Pineda-Tamayo R, Otero W, Arango A & Martín J. PTPN22 C1858T polymorphism in Colombian patients with autoimmune diseases. Genes Immun 2005; 6:628-631.

González S, Aguilera S, Urzúa U, Quest AF, Molina C, Alliende C, Hermoso M & González MJ. Mechanotransduction and epigenetic control in autoimmune diseases. Autoimmun Rev 2011a; 10:175-179.

González S, Aguilera S, Alliende C, Urzúa U, Quest AF, Herrera L, Molina C, Hermoso M, Ewert P, Brito M, Romo R, Leyton C, Pérez P & González MJ. Alterations in type I hemidesmosome components suggestive of epigenetic control in the salivary glands of patients with Sjögren's syndrome. Arthritis Rheum 2011b; 63:1106-1115.

Gottenberg JE, Cagnard N, Lucchesi C, Letourneur F, Mistou S, Lazure T, Jacques S, Ba N, Ittah M, Lepajolec C, Labetoulle M, Ardizzone M, Sibilia J, Fournier C, Chiocchia G & Mariette X. Activation of IFN pathways and plasmacytoid dendritic cell recruitment in target organs of primary Sjögren's syndrome. Proc Natl Acad Sci USA 2006a; 103:2770–2775.

Gottenberg JE, Pallier C, Ittah M, Lavie F, Miceli-Richard C, Sellam J, Nordmann P, Cagnard N, Sibilia J & Mariette X. Failure to confirm coxsackievirus infection in primary Sjögren's syndrome. Arthritis Rheum 2006b; 54:2026–2028.

Green JE, Hinrichs SH, Vogel J, & Jay G. Exocrinopathy resembling Sjögren's syndrome in HTLV-1 tax transgenic mice. Nature 1989; 341:72–74.

Groom J, Kalled SL, Cutler AH & Jay G. Association of BAFF/BLyS overexpression and altered B cell differentiation with Sjögren's syndrome. J Clin Invest 2002; 109:59–68.

Haddad J, Deny P, Munz-Gotheil C, Ambrosini JC, Trinchet JC, Pateron D, Mal F, Callard P, Beaugrand M. Lymphocytic sialadenitis of Sjögren's syndrome associated with chronic hepatitis C virus liver disease. Lancet 1992; 339:321–323.

Hewagama A & Richardson B. The genetics and epigenetics of autoimmune diseases. J Autoimmun 2009; 33:3-11.

Hammi AR, Al-Hashimi IH, Nunn ME & Zipp M. Assessment of SS-A and SS-B in parotid saliva of patients with Sjogren's syndrome. J Oral Pathol Med 2005; 34:198-203.

Harangi M, Kaminski WE, Fleck M, Orsó E, Margit Zeher4, Kiss E, Szekanecz Z, Zilahi E, Marienhagen J, Aslanidis C, Paragh G, Bolstad A, Jonsson R & SchmitzG. Homozygosity for the 168His variant of the minor histocompatibility antigen HA-1 is associated with reduced risk of primary Sjögren's syndrome. Eur J Immunol 2005, 35:305–317.

Haugen AJ,Peen E, Hultén B, Johannessen AC, Brun JG, Halse AK & Haga HJ. Estimation of the prevalence of primary Sjogren's syndrome in two age-different community-based populations using two sets of classification criteria: the Hordaland Health Study. Scand J Rheumatol 2008; 37:30-34.

Hjelmervik TO, Petersen K, Jonassen I, Jonsson R & Bolstad AI. Gene expression profiling of minor salivary glands clearly distinguishes primary Sjögren's syndrome patients from healthy control subjects. Arthritis Rheum 2005; 52:1534-1544.

Hisatomi Y, Okumura K, Nakamura K, Matsumoto S, Satoh A, Nagano K, Yamamoto T, & Endo F. Flow cytometric isolation of endodermal progenitors from mouse salivary gland differentiate into hepatic and pancreatic lineages. Hepatology 2004; 39:667-675.

Horie K, Kagami H, Hiramatsu Y, Hata K, Shigetomi T & Ueda M. (1996). Selected salivary-gland cell culture and the effects of isoproterenol, vasoactive intestinal polypeptide and substance P. Arch Oral Biol 41: 243-252.

Humphreys-Beher MG, Brayer J, Yamachika S, Peck AB & Jonsson R. An alternative perspective to the immune response in autoimmune exocrinopathy: induction of functional quiescence rather than destructive autoaggression. Scand J Immunol 1999; 49:7–10.

Iizuka M, Wakamatsu E, Tsuboi H, Nakamura Y, Hayashi T, Matsui M, Goto D, Ito S, Matsumoto I & Sumida T. Pathogenic role of immune response to M3 muscarinic acetylcholine receptor in Sjögren's syndrome-like sialoadenitis. J Autoimmun 2010; 35:383-389.

Inal V, Kitapcioglu G, Karabulut G, Keser G & Kabasakal Y. Evaluation of quality of life in relation to anxiety and depression in primary Sjogren's syndrome. Mod Rheumatol 2010; 20:588-597.

Ishimaru N, Saegusa K, Yanagi K, Haneji N, Saito I & Hayashi Y. Estrogen deficiency accelerates autoimmune exocrinopathy in murine Sjögren's syndrome through fas-mediated apoptosis. Am J Pathol 1999; 155:173-181.

Ishimaru N, Arakaki R, Yoshida S, Yamada A, Noji S & Hayashi Y. Expression of the retinoblastoma protein RbAp48 in exocrine glands leads to Sjögren's syndrome-like autoimmune exocrinopathy. J Exp Med 2008; 205:2915–2927.

Ittah M, Gottenberg JE, Proust A, Hachulla E, Puechal X, Loiseau P, Mariette X & Miceli-Richard C. No evidence for association between 1858 C/T single-nucleotide polymorphism of PTPN22 gene and primary Sjogren's syndrome. Genes Immun 2005; 6: 457-458.

Ittah M, Miceli-Richard C, Eric Gottenberg J, Lavie F, Lazure T, Ba N, Sellam J, Lepajolec C & Mariette X. B cell-activating factor of the tumor necrosis factor family (BAFF) is expressed under stimulation by interferon in salivary gland epithelial cells in primary Sjogren's syndrome. Arthritis Res Ther 2006; 8: R51-R59.

Ittah M, Miceli-Richard C, Gottenberg JE, Sellam J, Eid P, Lebon P, Pallier C, Lepajolec C & Mariette X. Viruses induce high expression of BAFF by salivary gland epithelial cells through TLR- and type-I IFN-dependent and-independent pathways. Eur J Immunol 2008; 38:1058–1064.

Ittah M, Miceli-Richard C, Gottenberg JE, Sellam J, Lepajolec C & Mariette X. B-cell-activating factor expressions in salivary epithelial cells after dsRNA virus infection depends on RNA-activated protein kinase activation. Eur J Immunol 2009; 39: 1271-1279.

Iwakiri D, Zhou L, Samanta M, Matsumoto M, Ebihara T, Seya T, Imai S, Fujieda M, Kawa K & Takada K. Epstein–Barr virus (EBV)-encoded small RNA is released from EBV-infected cells and activates signaling from Toll-like receptor 3. J Exp Med 2009; 206:2091–2099.

Jonsson R, Moen K, Vestrheim D & Szodoray P. Current issues in Sjögren's syndrome. Oral Dis 2002; 8:130-140.

Jonsson MV, Szodoray P, Jellestad S, Jonsson R & Skarstein K. Association between circulating levels of the novel TNF family members APRIL and BAFF and lymphoid organization in primary Sjogren's syndrome. J Clin Immunol 2005; 25:189-201.

Jonsson R, Bolstad AI, Brokstad KA & Brun JG. Sjögren's syndrome - a plethora of clinical and immunological phenotypes with a complex genetic background. Ann N Y Acad Sci. 2007; 1108:433-447.

Joraku A, Sullivan CA, Yoo JJ & Atala A. Tissue engineering of functional salivary gland tissue. Laryngoscope 2005; 115:244-248.

Kagami H, Agata H & Tojo A. Bone marrow stromal cells (bone marrow-derived multipotent mesenchymal stromal cells) for bone tissue engineering: basic science to clinical translation. Int J Biochem Cell Biol 2011; 43: 286-289.

Kapsogeorgou EK, Abu-Helu RF, Moutsopoulos HM & Manoussakis MN. Salivary gland epithelial cell exosomes: A source of autoantigenic ribonucleoproteins. Arthritis Rheum 2005; 52: 1517-1521.

Karaiskos D, Mavragani CP, Makaroni S, Zinzaras E, Voulgarelis M, Rabavilas A & Moutsopoulos HM. Stress, coping strategies and social support in patients with primary Sjogren'ssyndrome prior to disease onset: a retrospective case-control study. Ann Rheum Dis 2009; 68:40–46.

Kassan SS & Moutsopoulos HM. Clinical manifestations and early diagnosis of Sjögren syndrome. Arch Intern Med 2004; 164:1275-1284.

Katsifis GE, Rekka S, Moutsopoulos NM, Pillermer S & Wahl SM. Systemic and local interleukin-17 and linked cytokines associated with Sjögren's syndrome immunopathogenesis. Am J Pathol 2009; 175:1167–1177.

Kawakami A, Nakashima K, Tamai M, Nakamura H, Iwanaga N, Fujikawa K, Aramaki T, Arima K, Iwamoto N, Ichinose K, Kamachi M, Ida H, Origuchi T & Eguchi K. Toll-like receptor in salivary glands from patients with Sjo¨gren's syndrome: functional analysis by human salivary gland cell line. J Rheumatol 2007; 34:1019–1026.

Khalili S, Liu Y, Sumita Y, Maria OM, Blank D, Key S, Mezey E & Tran SD. Bone marrow cells are a source of undifferentiated cells to prevent Sjögren's syndrome and to preserve salivary glands function in the non-obese diabetic mice. Int J Biochem Cell Biol 2010; 42:1893-1899.

Kishi T, Takao T, Fujita K & Taniguchi H. Clonal proliferation of multipotent stem/progenitor cells in the neonatal and adult salivary glands. Biochem Biophys Res Commun 2006; 340:544-552.

Kittridge A, Routhouska SB & Korman NJ. Dermatological manifestations of Sjogren's syndrome. J Cutan Med Surg 2011; 15:8-14.

Kok MR, Yamano S, Lodde BM, Wang J, Couwenhoven RI, Yakar S, Voutetakis A, Leroith D, Schmidt M, Afione S, Pillemer SR, Tsutsui MT, Tak PP, Chiorini JA & Baum BJ. Local adeno-associated virus-mediated interleukin 10 gene transfer has disease-modifying effects in a murine model of Sjögren's syndrome. Hum Gene Ther 2003; 14:1605–1618.

Konttinen YT, Tensing EK, Laine M, Porola P, Törnwall J & Hukkanen M. Abnormal distribution of aquaporin-5 in salivary glands in the NOD mouse model for Sjogren's syndrome. J Rheumatol 2005; 32:1071-1075.

Konttinen YT, Porola P, Konttinen L, Laine M & Poduval P. Immunohistopathology of Sjogren's syndrome.Autoimmun Rev 2006; 6:16-20.

Korman BD, Kastner DL, Gregersen PK & Remmers EF. STAT4: genetics, mechanisms, and implications for autoimmunity. Curr Allergy Asthma Rep 2008; 8:398-403.

Kwon YJ, Pérez P, Aguilera S, Molina C, Leyton L, Alliende C, Leyton C, Brito M, Romo R, & González MJ. Involvement of specific laminins and nidogens in the active remodeling of the basal lamina of labial salivary glands from patients with Sjogren's syndrome. Arthritis Rheum 2006; 54:3465-3475.

Laine M, Virtanen I, Salo T & Konttinen YT. Segment-specific but pathologic laminin isoform profiles in human labial salivary glands of patients with Sjogren's syndrome." Arthritis Rheum 2004; 50: 3968-3973.

Laine M, Porola P, Udby L, Kjeldsen L, Cowland JB, Borregaard N, Hietanen J, Ståhle M, Pihakari A & Konttinen YT. Low salivary dehydroepiandrosterone and androgen-regulated cysteine-rich secretory protein 3 levels in Sjo¨gren's syndrome. Arthritis Rheum 2007; 56:2575–2584.

Lafitte C, Amoura Z, Cacoub P, Pradat-Diehl P, Picq C, Salachas F, Léger JM, Piette JC, & Delattre JY. Neurological complications of primary Sjögren's syndrome. J Neurol 2001 ; 248:577-584.

Launay D, Hachull AE, Hatron PY, Jais X, Simonneau G & Humbert M. Pulmonary arterial hypertension: a rare complication of primary Sjögren's syndrome: report of 9 new cases and review of the literature. Medicine 2007; 86: 299-315.

Lavie F, Miceli-Richard C, Quillard J, Roux S, Leclerc P & Mariette X. Expression of BAFF (BLyS) in T cells infiltrating labial salivary glands from patients with Sjögren's syndrome. J Pathol 2004; 202:496-502.

Lavie F, Miceli-Richard C, Ittah M, Sellam J, Gottenberg JE & Mariette X. B-cell activating factor of the tumour necrosis factor family expression in blood monocytes and T cells from patients with primary Sjögren's syndrome. Scand J Immunol 2008; 67:185–192.

Li J, Zheng C, Zhang X, Liu X, Zhang C, Goldsmith CM, Baum BJ & Wang S. Developing a convenient large animal model for gene transfer to salivary glands in vivo. J Gene Med 2004; 6:55-63.

Locht H, Pelck R & Manthorpe R. Diagnostic and prognostic significance of measuring antibodies to alpha-fodrin compared to anti-Ro-52, anti-Ro-60, and anti-La in primary Sjögren's syndrome. J Rheumatol 2008; 35:845-849.

Lodde BM, Mineshiba F, Wang J, Cotrim AP, Afione S, Tak PP & Baum BJ. Effect of human vasoactive intestinal peptide gene transfer in a murine model of Sjogren's syndrome. Ann Rheum Dis 2006; 65:195–200.

Loiseau P, Lepage V, Djelal F, Busson M, Tamouza R, Raffoux C, Menkes CJ, Meyer O, Charron D & Goldberg D. HLA class I and class II are both associated with the genetic predisposition to primary Sjögren syndrome. Hum Immunol 2001; 62:725-731.

Lombaert IM, Brunsting JF, Wierenga PK, Faber H, Stokman MA, Kok T, Visser WH, Kampinga HH, de Haan G & Coppes RP. Rescue of salivary gland function after stem cell transplantation in irradiated glands. PLoS One 2008; 3:e2063.

Lu Q, Renaudineau Y, Cha S, Ilei G, Brooks WH, Selmi C, Tzioufas A, Pers JO, Bombardieri S, Gershwin ME, Gay S & Youinou P. Epigenetics in autoimmune disorders: highlights of the 10th Sjögren's syndrome symposium. Autoimmun Rev 2010; 9:627-630.

Ma T, Song Y, Gillespie A, Carlson EJ, Epstein CJ & Verkman AS. Defective secretion of saliva in transgenic mice lacking aquaporin-5 water channels.J Biol Chem 1999; 274: 20071-20074.

Mackay F & Schneider P. Cracking the BAFF code. Nat Rev Immunol 2009; 9:491–502.

Maiti AK, Kim-Howard X, Viswanathan P, Guillén L, Rojas-Villarraga A, Deshmukh H, Direskeneli H, Saruhan-Direskeneli G, Cañas C, Tobön GJ, Sawalha AH, Cherñavsky AC, Anaya JM & Nath SK. Confirmation of an association between rs6822844 at the Il2-Il21 region and multiple autoimmune diseases: evidence of a general susceptibility locus. Arthritis Rheum 2010; 62: 323-329.

Mamtani M, Anaya JM, He W & Ahuja SK. Association of copy number variation in the FCGR3B gene with risk of autoimmune diseases. Genes Immun 2010; 11:155-160.

Manoussakis MN, Dimitriou ID, Kapsogeorgou EK, Xanthou G, Paikos S, Polihronis M & Moutsopoulos HM. Expression of B7 costimulatory molecules by salivary gland epithelial cells in patients with Sjögren's syndrome. Arthritis Rheum 1999; 42:229-239.

Manoussakis MN & Kapsogeorgou EK. The role of intrinsic epithelial activation in the pathogenesis of Sjögren's syndrome. J Autoimmun 2010; 35:219-224.

Mariette X, Roux S, Zhang J, Bengoufa D, Lavie F, Zhou T & Kimberly R. The level of BLyS (BAFF) correlates with the titre of autoantibodies in human Sjögren's syndrome. Ann Rheum Dis 2003; 62:168–171.

Mariette X. Therapeutic potential for B-cell modulation in Sjögren's syndrome. Rheum Dis Clin North Am 2008; 34:1025-1033.

Martínez A, Varadé J, Márquez A, Cénit MC, Espino L, Perdigones N, Santiago JL, Fernández-Arquero M, de la Calle H, Arroyo R, Mendoza JL, Fernández-Gutiérrez B, de la Concha EG & Urcelay E. Association of the STAT4 gene with increased susceptibility for some immune-mediated diseases. Arthritis Rheum 2008; 58:2598-2602.

Mastrangeli A, O'Connell B, Aladib W, Fox PC, Baum BJ & Crystal RG. Direct in vivo adenovirus-mediated gene transfer to salivary glands. Am J Physiol 1994; 266:G1146-G1155.

Matsumura R, Umemiya K, Goto T, Nakazawa T, Kagami M, Tomioka H, Tanabe E, Sugiyama T & Sueishi M. Glandular and extraglandular expression of costimulatory molecules in patients with Sjogren's syndrome. Ann Rheum Dis 2001; 60:473-482.

Mavragani CP & Moutsopoulos HM. The geoepidemiology of Sjögren's syndrome. Autoimmun Rev 2010; 9:A305-A310.

Mavragani CP & Crow MK.Activation of the type I interferon pathway in primary Sjogren's syndrome. J Autoimmun 2010; 35:225-231.

Meijer JM, Meiners PM, Vissink A, Spijkervet FK, Abdulahad W, Kamminga N, Brouwer E, Kallenberg CG & Bootsma H. Effectiveness of rituximab treatment in primary Sjögren's syndrome: a randomized, double-blind, placebo-controlled trial. Arthritis Rheum 2010; 62:960-968.

Miceli-Richard C, Dieude P, Hachulla E, Puechal X, Cornelis F & Mariette X. Tumour necrosis factor receptor 2(TNFRSF1B) association study in Sjögren's syndrome. Ann Rheum Dis 2007; 6:1684–1685.

Miceli-Richard C, Gestermann N, Ittah M, Comets E, Loiseau P, Puechal X, Hachulla E, Gottenberg JE, Lebon P, Becquemont L & Mariette X. The CGGGG insertion/deletion polymorphism of the IRF5 promoter is a strong risk factor for primary Sjögren's syndrome. Arthritis Rheum 2009; 60:1991–1997.

Nakamura Y, Wakamatsu E, Matsumoto I, Tomiita M, Kohno Y, Mori M, Yokota S, Goto D, Ito S, Tsutsumi A & Sumida T. High prevalence of autoantibodies to muscarinic-3 acetylcholine receptor in patients with juvenile-onset Sjögren syndrome. Ann Rheum Dis 2008; 67:136-137.

Naito Y, Matsumoto I, Wakamatsu E, Goto D, Sugiyama T, Matsumura R, Ito S, Tsutsumi A & Sumida T. Muscarinic acetylcholine receptor autoantibodies in patients with Sjögren's syndrome. Ann Rheum Dis 2005; 64:510-511.

Navara SV, Guzmán RM, Gallacher AE, Hall S, Levy RA, Jimenez RE, Li EK, Thomas M, Kim HY, León MG, Tanasescu C, Nasonov E, Lan JL, Pineda L, Zhong ZJ, Freimuth W & Petri MA. BLISS-52 Study Group. Efficacy and safety of belimumab in patients with active systemic lupus erythematosus: a randomised, placebo-controlled, phase 3 trial. Lancet 2011; 377:721-731.

Nguyen CQ, Hu MH, Li Y, Stewart C & Peck AB. Salivary gland tissue expression of interleukin-23 and interleukin-17 in Sjögren's syndrome: findings in humans and mice. Arthritis Rheum 2008; 58:734–743.

Nguyen CQ, Yin H, Lee BH, Chiorini JA & Peck AB. IL17: potential therapeutic target in Sjogren's syndrome using adenovirus-mediated gene transfer. Lab Invest 2011; 91:54-62.

Nordmark G, Kristjansdottir G, Theander E, Eriksson P, Brun JG, Wang C, Padyukov L, Truedsson L, Alm G, Eloranta ML, Jonsson R, Rönnblom L & Syvänen AC. Additive effects of the major risk alleles of IRF5 and STAT4 in primary Sjögren's syndrome. Genes Immun 2009; 10:68–76.

Nordmark G, Kristjansdottir G, Theander E, Appel S, Eriksson P, Vasaitis L, Kvarnström M, Delaleu N, Lundmark P, Lundmark A, Sjöwall C, Brun JG, Jonsson MV, Harboe E, Gøransson LG, Johnsen SJ, Söderkvist P, Eloranta ML, Alm G, Baecklund E, Wahren-Herlenius M, Omdal R, Rönnblom L, Jonsson R & Syvänen AC. Association of EBF1, FAM167A(C8orf13)-BLK and TNFSF4 gene variants with primary Sjögren's syndrome. Genes Immun 2011; 12:100-109.

O'Connell AC, Baccaglini L, Fox PC, O'Connell BC, Kenshalo D, Oweisy H, Hoque AT, Sun D, Herscher LL, Braddon VR, Delporte C & Baum BJ. Safety and efficacy of adenovirus-mediated transfer of the human aquaporin-1 cDNA to irradiated parotid glands of non-human primates. Cancer Gene Ther 1999; 6:505-513.

Ohashi Y, Tsuzaka K, Takeuchi T, Sasaki Y & Tsubota K. Altered distribution of aquaporin 5 and its C-terminal binding protein in the lachrymal glands of a mouse model for Sjögren's syndrome. Curr Eye Res 2008; 33:621-629.

Okumura K, Nakamura K, Hisatomi Y, Nagano K, Tanaka Y, Terada K, Sugiyama T, Umeyama K, Matsumoto K, Yamamoto T & Endo F. Salivary gland progenitor cells induced by duct ligation differentiate into hepatic and pancreatic lineages. Hepatology 2003; 38:104-113.

Palomino-Morales RJ, Diaz-Gallo LM, Witte T, Anaya JM & Martín J. Influence of STAT4 polymorphism in primary Sjögren's syndrome. J Rheumatol 2010; 37:1016-1019.

Pan Y & Sawalha AH. Epigenetic regulation and the pathogenesis of systemic lupus erythematosus. Transl Res 2009; 153:4-10

Parambil JG, Myers JL, Lindell RM, Matteson EL & Ryu JH. Interstitial lung disease in primary Sjögren's syndrome. Chest 2006; 130:1489-1495.

Parke AL. Pulmonary manifestations of Sjogren's syndrome. Rheum Dis Clin North Am 2008; 34:907-920.

Pers JO, Devauchelle V, Daridon C, Bendaoud B, Le Berre R, Bordron A, Hutin P, Renaudineau Y, Dueymes M, Loisel S, Berthou C, Saraux A & Youinou P. BAFF-modulated repopulation of B lymphocytes in the blood and salivary glands of rituximab-treated patients with Sjögren's syndrome. Arthritis Rheum 2007; 56:1464–1477.

Pertovaara M, Bootorabi F, Kuuslahti M, Pasternack A & Parkkila S. Novel carbonic anhydrase autoantibodies and renal manifestations in patients with primary Sjögren's syndrome. Rheumatology 2011; doi:10.1093/rheumatology/ker118, in press.

Pflugfelder SC, Crouse CA, Monroy D, Yen M, Rowe M & Atherton SS. Epstein-Barr virus and the lachrymal gland pathology of Sjögren's syndrome. Am J Pathol 1993; 143:49–64.

Porola P, Virkki L, Przybyla BD, Laine M, Patterson TA, Pihakari A & Konttinen YT. Androgen deficiency and defective intracrine processing of dehydroepiandrosterone in salivary glands in Sjögren's syndrome. J Rheumatol 2008; 35:2229-2235.

Raizis AM, Ferguson MM, Robinson BA, Atkinson CH & George PM. Identification of a novel PTEN mutation (L139X) in a patient with Cowden disease and Sjögren's syndrome. Mol Pathol 1998; 51:339-341

Ramos-Casals M & Font J. Primary Sjögren's syndrome: current and emergent aetiopathogenic concepts. Rheumatology 2005; 44:1354-1367.

Richardson B. Primer: epigenetics of autoimmunity. Nat Clin Pract Rheumatol 2007; 3:521-527.

Rihl M, Ulbricht K, Schmidt RE & Witte T. Treatment of sicca symptoms with hydroxychloroquine in patients with Sjogren's syndrome. Rheumatology 2009; 48:796–799.

Ring, T., M. Kallenbach, Praetorius J, Nielsen S & Melgaard B. Successful treatment of a patient with primary Sjogren's syndrome with Rituximab. Clin Rheumatol 2006; 25:891-894.

Roberts C, Parker GJ, Rose CJ, Watson Y, O'Connor JP, Stivaros SM, Jackson A & Rushton VE. Glandular function in Sjögren syndrome: assessment with dynamic contrast-enhanced MR imaging and tracer kinetic modeling--initial experience. Radiology 2008; 246:845-853.

Sasaki, Y, Tsubota K, Kawedia JD, Manon AG & Yasui M. The difference of aquaporin 5 distribution in acinar and ductal cells in lachrymal and parotid glands. Curr Eye Res 2007; 32:923-929.

Segal B, Carpenter A & Walk D. Involvement of nervous system pathways in primary Sjögren's syndrome. Rheum Dis Clin North Am 2008; 34:885-906.

Sellam, J., Miceli-Richard C, Gottenberg JE, Ittah M, Lavie F, Lacabaratz C, Gestermann N, Proust A, Lambotte O & Mariette X. Decreased B cell activating factor receptor expression on peripheral lymphocytes associated with increased disease activity in primary Sjogren's syndrome and systemic lupus erythematosus." Ann Rheum Dis 2007; 66:790-797.

Sjögren H. Zur kentniss der keratoconjunctivitis sicca. Acta Opthalmol Suppl 1933; 2: 1-151.

Skopouli FN, Dafni U, Ioannidis JP & Moutsopoulos HM. Clinical evolution, and morbidity and mortality of primary Sjögren's syndrome. Semin Arthritis Rheum 2000; 29:296–304.

Soyfoo MS, De Vriese C, Debaix H, Martin-Martinez MD, Mathieu C, Devuyst O, Steinfeld SD & Delporte C. Modified aquaporin 5 expression and distribution in submandibular glands from NOD mice displaying autoimmune exocrinopathy. Arthritis Rheum 2007; 56: 2566-2574.

Spaan M, Porola P, Laine M, Rozman B, Azuma M & Konttinen YT. Healthy human salivary glands contain a DHEA-sulphate processing intracrine machinery, which is deranged in primary Sjögren's syndrome. J Cell Mol Med 2009; 13:1261-1270.

Spachidou MP, Bourazopoulou E, Maratheftis CI, Kapsogeorgou EK, Moutsopoulos HM, Tzioufas AG & Manoussakis MN. Expression of functional Toll-like receptors by salivary gland epithelial cells: increased mRNA expression in cells derived from patients with primary Sjögren's syndrome. Clin Exp Immunol 2007; 147:497–503.

Steinfeld S, Cogan E, King LS, Agre P, Kiss R & Delporte C. Abnormal distribution of aquaporin-5 water channel protein in salivary glands from Sjogren's syndrome patients. Lab Invest 2001; 81:143-148.

Steinfeld SD, Tant L, Burmester GR, Teoh NK, Wegener WA, Goldenberg DM & Pradier O. Epratuzumab (humanised anti-CD22 antibody) in primary Sjögren's syndrome: an open-label phase I/II study. Arthritis Res Ther 2006; 8:R129.

Strietzel FP, Lafaurie GI, Mendoza GR, Alajbeg I, Pejda S, Vuletić L, Mantilla R, Falcão DP, Leal SC, Bezerra AC, Tran SD, Ménard HA, Kimoto S, Pan S, Martín-Granizo RA, Lozano ML, Zunt SL, Krushinski CA, Melilli D, Campisi G, Paderni C, Dolce S, Yepes JF, Lindh L, Koray M, Mumcu G, Elad S, Zeevi I, Barrios BC, López Sánchez RM, Beiski BZ, Wolff A & Konttinen YT. Efficacy and safety of an intraoral electrostimulation device for xerostomia relief: a multicenter, randomized trial. Arthritis Rheum 2011; 63:180-190.

Sumida T, Tsuboi H, Iizuka M, Nakamura Y & Matsumoto I. Functional role of M3 muscarinic acetylcholine receptor (M3R) reactive T cells and anti-M3R autoantibodies in patients with Sjögren's syndrome. Autoimmun Rev. 2010; 9:615-617.

Sumita Y, Liu Y, Khalili S, Maria OM, Xia D, Key S, Cotrim AP, Mezey E & Tran SD. Bone marrow-derived cells rescue salivary gland function in mice with head and neck irradiation. Int J Biochem Cell Biol 2011; 43:80-87.

Taiym S, Haghighat H & Al-Hashimi I. A comparison of the hormone levels in patients with Sjogren's syndrome and healthy controls. Oral Surg Oral Med Oral Pathol Oral Radiol Endod 2004; 97:579-583.

Takagi Y, Kimura Y, Nakamura H, Sasaki M, Eguchi K & Nakamura T. Salivary gland ultrasonography: can it be an alternative to sialography as an imaging modality for Sjogren's syndrome? Ann Rheum Dis 2010; 69:1321-1324.

Tobón GJ, Saraux A, Pers JO & Youinou P. Emerging biotherapies for Sjogren's syndrome. Expert Opin Emerg Drugs 2010; 15:269-282.

Triantafyllopoulou A, Tapinos N & Moutsopoulos HM. Evidence for coxsackievirus infection in primary Sjögren's syndrome. Arthritis Rheum 2004; 50:2897–2902.

Tran SD, Sugito T, Dipasquale G, Cotrim AP, Bandyopadhyay BC, Riddle K, Mooney D, Kok MR, Chiorini JA & Baum BJ. Re-engineering primary epithelial cells from rhesus monkey parotid glands for use in developing an artificial salivary gland. Tissue Eng 2006; 12:2939-2948.

Tran SD, Redman RS, Barrett AJ, Pavletic SZ, Key S, Liu Y, Carpenter A, Nguyen HM, Sumita Y, Baum BJ, Pillemer SR & Mezey E. Microchimerism in salivary glands after blood- and marrow-derived stem cell transplantation. Biol Blood Marrow Transplant 2011; 17:429-433.

Tsinti M, Kassi E, Korkolopoulou P, Kapsogeorgou E, Moutsatsou P, Patsouris E & Manoussakis MN. Functional estrogen receptors alpha and beta are expressed in normal human salivary gland epithelium and apparently mediate immunomodulatory effects. Eur J Oral Sci 2009; 117:498-505.

Tsubota K, Hirai S, King LS, Agre P & Ishida N. Defective cellular trafficking of lachrymal gland aquaporin-5 in Sjogren's syndrome. Lancet 2001; 357:688-689.

Tsunawaki S, Nakamura S, Ohyama Y, Sasaki M, Ikebe-Hiroki A, Hiraki A, Kadena T, Kawamura E, Kumamaru W, Shinohara M & Shirasuna K. Possible function of salivary gland epithelial cells as nonprofessional antigen-presenting cells in the development of Sjogren's syndrome. J Rheumatol 2002; 29:1884-1896.

Tzioufas AG, Hantoumi I, Polihronis M, Xanthou G & Moutsopoulos HM. Autoantibodies to La/SSB in patients with primary Sjögren's syndrome (pSS) are associated with upregulation of La/SSB mRNA in minor salivary gland biopsies (MSGs). J Autoimmun 1999; 13:429–34.

Valtysdóttir ST, Wide L & Hällgren R. Low serum dehydroepiandrosterone sulfate in women with primary Sjögren's syndrome as an isolated sign of impaired HPA axis function. J Rheumatol 2001; 28:1259-1265.

Van Bijsterveld OP. Diagnostic tests in the Sicca syndrome. Arch Ophthalmol 1969; 82:10-14.

Velozo J, Aguilera S, Alliende C, Ewert P, Molina C, Pérez P, Leyton L, Quest A, Brito M, González S, Leyton C, Hermoso M, Romo R & González MJ. Severe alterations in expression and localisation of {alpha}6{beta}4 integrin in salivary gland acini from patients with Sjogren syndrome. Ann Rheum Dis 2009; 68:991-996.

Vitali C, Bombardieri S, Jonsson R, Moutsopoulos HM, Alexander EL, Carsons SE, Daniels TE, Fox PC, Fox RI, Kassan SS, Pillemer SR, Talal N & Weisman MH. European Study Group on Classification Criteria for Sjögren's Syndrome. Classification criteria for Sjögren's syndrome: a revised version of the European criteria proposed by the American-European Consensus Group. Ann Rheum Dis 2002; 61:554-558.

Voulgarelis M & Moutsopoulos HM. Mucosa-associated lymphoid tissue lymphoma in Sjögren's syndrome: risks, management, and prognosis Rheum Dis Clin North Am 2008; 34:921-933.

Voulgarelis M & Tzioufas AG. Pathogenetic mechanisms in the initiation and perpetuation of Sjögren's syndrome. Nat Rev Rheumatol 2010; 6:529-37.

Waterman SA, Gordon TP & Rischmueller M. Inhibitory effects of muscarinic receptor autoantibodies on parasympathetic neurotransmission in Sjögren's syndrome. Arthritis Rheum 2000; 43:1647–1654.

Whitacre C C. Sex differences in autoimmune disease. Nat Immunol 2001; 2:777-780.

Wildenberg ME, van Helden-Meeuwsen CG, van de Merwe JP, Drexhage HA & Versnel MA. Systemic increase in type I interferon activity in Sjögren's syndrome: a putative role for plasmacytoid dendritic cells. Eur J Immunol 2008; 38:2024–2033.

Willeke P, Gaubitz M, Schotte H, Becker H, Mickholz E, Domschke W & Schlüter B. Clinical and immunological characteristics of patients with Sjögren's syndrome in relation to alpha-fodrin antibodies. Rheumatology 2007; 46:479-483.

Xanthou G, Polihronis M, Tzioufas AG, Paikos S, Sideras P & Moutsopoulos HM. Lymphoid chemokine messenger RNA expression by epithelial cells in the chronic inflammatory lesion of the salivary glands of Sjögren's syndrome patients: possible participation in lymphoid structure formation. Arthritis Rheum 2001; 44:408-418

# 4

# Changing Spectrum of Chronic Immune Thrombocytopenic Purpura: New Face for an Old Disease

Indu Sabnani and Patricia Tsang
*Newark Beth Israel Medical Center New Jersey, United States of America*

## 1. Introduction

Characterized by low platelet counts, immune thrombocytopenic purpura (ITP) has been discovered to be an acquired autoimmune disorder since the mid-1900s (Evans et al., 1951). In the 21st century, the modern generation would shudder at Harrington and Hollingsworth's experiment they performed to search for the pathogenesis of ITP. By injecting themselves with 500 ml of blood from a patient from low platelet counts, they developed the same bleeding disorder and were able to reproduce the disease in themselves (Harrington et al., 1951). Since that experiment, the pathogenesis and the therapeutic options of ITP have evolved by leaps and bounds. The traditional model of ITP is that of pathologic destruction of platelets by antiplatelet antibody. For many decades, this model of autoimmune thrombocytopenic purpura has shaped our understanding of the disorder and our therapeutic management of ITP (Buchanan et al, 1977, Hou et al. 1995, Fujisawa K et al. 1992). Recent studies have broadened our perspective beyond humoral dysregulation to include the cellular immune system and abnormalities of megakaryocytes as well (Olsson, et al., 2003, Ballem et al., 1987, McMillan et al., 2004). These recent findings have opened the door for new treatment possibilities for ITP.

In contrast to a more predictable clinical course of acute ITP, the pathogenesis, natural history and management of chronic ITP are significantly more diverse and rapidly evolving. The established treatment practices for chronic ITP have also undergone a major change. After a long period of standard treatment approach using steroids, splenectomy, and immunosuppressive therapy, a breakthrough came with the use of B-cell depletion therapy (Cines and McMillan, 2005). The availability of monoclonal antibody, rituximab, has led hematologists to reconsider the role of splenectomy in the frontline management of chronic ITP (Arnold et al., 2007). A new era has begun with the development of thrombopoietin-mimetic agents that stimulate megakaryocytes to grow and produce platelets (Nurden et al., 2009).

Since chronic ITP remains a heterogeneous disorder; there is no consensus on the definite diagnostic criteria and management. In 1996, the American Society of Hematology published a landmark paper recommending guidelines to assist clinicians in the management of ITP (George et al., 1996). Since then, there have been tremendous advances in the management of both adult and pediatric ITP. These guidelines were updated by the

American Society of Hematology in 2010 (Neunert et al., 2010). In addition, an International Working Group (IWG) of experts on ITP attempted to bring some uniformity to the diagnosis and management of ITP (Rodeghiero et al., 2009). Despite the serious efforts of scientists and specialty societies, the practicing hematologists are still left with many unanswered questions and dilemmas when it comes to treating this benign but challenging disease.

Until recently, adult ITP was considered a disease of young women. However, two recently published studies have shown otherwise (Schoonen et al. 2009, Abrahamson et al., 2009). In these series, the mean ages at presentation were over 50 years, with a slight female predominance (M:F ratio of 1.7:1). In contrary to acute ITP in children, adult ITP is usually insidious in onset, with platelet counts of > 20 x $10^9$/L. The incidence of chronic ITP is 5.8 to 6.6 per 100,000 in the adult population.

## 2. Definition of chronic ITP

While ITP in children usually pursues an acute and self-limited clinical course that responds well to treatment, ITP in adults tends to present as a chronic relapsing condition. Traditionally, the terms chronic ITP, refractory ITP, and chronic persistent ITP are used interchangeably and are used for chronic phase of the disease. Chronic or refractory ITP was previously defined as immune thrombocytopenia persisting for >3 months, failure to respond to splenectomy, and platelet count of less than 50 x $10^9$/L. The definition has become more confusing since the evolution of splenectomy sparing modalities of treatment.

The International Working Group (IWG) consensus panel of both adult and pediatric experts in ITP recently provided guidance on terminology, definitions and outcome criteria for this disorder (Proven et al., 2010). Primary ITP, as defined by the IWG, is platelet count less than 100 x $10^9$/L in the absence of other causes or disorders that may be associated with thrombocytopenia. IWG used a higher platelet cutoff than the traditional criterion of 50 x $10^9$/L based on the observation that there might be physiological variations among different racial groups and that the chances of developing persistent thrombocytopenia of less than 100 x $10^9$/L over 10 years of follow-up seemed to be less in patients presenting with a platelet count between 100 and 150 x $10^9$/L.

The IWG also categorizes ITP as newly diagnosed (diagnosis to 3 months), persistent (3 to 12 months from diagnosis) or chronic (lasting for more than 12 months). However, these definitions may not apply to patients with secondary forms of ITP and have not been formally validated. Specifically, "persistent ITP" includes patients not achieving spontaneous remission or not maintaining therapeutic response after stopping treatment between 3 and 12 months from initial diagnosis. The category "chronic ITP" is reserved for patients with ITP lasting for more than 12 months.

The IWG standardization does not include the degree of thrombocytopenia in classifying the different phases of the disease. The severity of disease varies in patients. Mild, moderate, and severe thrombocytopenia is used commonly in clinical practice. There are no firm guidelines. However, mild thrombocytopenia typically ranges from 50 to 100 x $10^9$/L, moderate thrombocytopenia from 20 to 50 x $10^9$/L, and severe thrombocytopenia under 20 x $10^9$/L. The severity of thrombocytopenia may or may not correlate well with the risk of bleeding. It is well known that the severity and symptoms of ITP in the same patient can vary from time to time. Table 1 summarizes the different terminologies commonly used to define ITP.

| Category | Definition |
|---|---|
| Primary ITP | Platelet count less than 100 x $10^9$/L in the absence of other causes of thrombocytopenia |
| Newly diagnosed ITP | From initial diagnosis to 3 months |
| Persistent ITP | From 3-12 months of initial diagnosis |
| Chronic ITP | ITP lasting for greater than 12 months |
| Mild Thrombocytopenia | Platelet count between 50-100 x $10^9$/L |
| Moderate Thrombocytopenia | Platelet count between 20-50 x $10^9$/L |
| Severe thrombocytopenia | Platelet count below 20 x $10^9$/L |

Table 1. Commonly used definitions in ITP

## 3. Diagnosis of chronic ITP

Fifty years since the discovery of platelet autoantibodies, there is still no definitive laboratory diagnostic test for ITP. Despite the tremendous advances made in the understanding of the pathophysiology, the diagnosis of ITP remains one of exclusion. An initial complete history and physical examination is essential to identify evidence of bleeding and exclude other etiologies of thrombocytopenia or secondary ITP. Secondary causes of thrombocytopenia include autoimmune disorders as well as exposure to drugs (such as quinine), herbs, foods and other substances. A peripheral smear examination usually helps to exclude other hematological disorders, such as thrombotic thrombocytopenic purpura, leukemia, and pseudothrombocytopenia from platelet aggregation. Testing for hepatitis C and HIV infection is recommended for all patients presenting as ITP (Cines et al., 2005, 2009, 2010).

Glycoprotein-specific assays to detect platelet-associated IgG (PAIgG) autoantibodies lack sufficient sensitivity for them to be of use as a diagnostic tool. Therapeutic response to IVIG is considered by many as confirmatory of ITP, in the absence of identifiable causes of thrombocytopenia. As per American Society of Hematology guidelines, there is insufficient evidence for the utility of routine testing for anti-platelet antiphospholipid and antinuclear antibodies, and thrombopoietin levels. There have been recent reports achieving remission in chronic ITP patients with the eradication of Helicobacter pylori infection. Even though there is insufficient evidence to support routine testing for Helicobacter pylori organisms, patients with gastrointestinal symptoms should be investigated further.

Although 2010 ASH guidelines did not find evidence to support an age threshold for which bone marrow is recommended, most hematologists would favor performing bone marrow examination for patients over 60 years of age to rule out myelodysplasia. This practice is especially useful prior to splenectomy in these older patients who do not show good response to treatment. The diagnosis of ITP should always be reassessed during the course of treatment if any atypical clinical or laboratory abnormalities develop to suggest lupus and other autoimmune or hematological disorder. Table 2 outlines the utility of various diagnostic tests for diagnosing ITP according to current guidelines.

| Diagnostic Evaluation | Recommended | Optional |
|---|---|---|
| Personal & Family History of Autoimmune Disorders | √ | |
| Complete Blood Count and Peripheral Smear Examination | √ | |
| ESR ANA and Anticradiolipin Antibodies | | √ |
| Blood Group & Direct Antiglobulin Test | | √ |
| HCV & HIV Serologies | √ | |
| Antiplatelet Antibodies | x | |
| Bone Marrow Aspiration and Biopsy | x | Prior to splenectomy in patients over 60 years, with poor response to medical therapy |
| Thrombopoietin Level | x | |

Table 2. Diagnostic tools for chronic ITP

## 4. Pathogenesis

Since the 1950s, ITP has been firmly established as an acquired autoimmune disorder characterized by low platelet count (Evans et al., 1951). In recent years, there have been significant new insights into the pathophysiologic mechanisms of ITP. Historically, the thrombocytopenia associated with ITP was attributed solely to autoantibodies causing platelet destruction. More recently, it has become evident that the pathophysiology in ITP is complex and multifaceted. In addition to a humoral-mediated mechanism, cytotoxic T-cells and impaired platelet production by abnormal megakaryocytes have recently been found to be important pathogenetic factors in subsets of patients. Our evolving knowledge of the pathogenesis of ITP has led to new therapeutic targets in the clinical management of ITP.

### 4.1 Autoantibody-mediated platelet destruction

In the mid-1900s, it was observed that when experimental subjects were infused with plasma from ITP patients, these subjects developed dose-dependent thrombocytopenia (Harrington et al., 1953). Subsequently, it was shown that the inciting plasma factor was an antiplatelet antibody and that ITP was autoimmune in nature (Schulman et al., 1965).

Platelet-associated autoantibodies are detectable in 50% to 70% of patients with ITP using currently available laboratory methods. Approximately 75% of the autoantibodies detected are directed against the platelet surface glycoprotein (GP) complexes GPIIb-IIIa and GPIb-IX (Hou, et al., 1995). Antibodies against other glycoproteins (GPIa-IIa, IV, and V) are less commonly found (Chang et al. 2003).

These autoantibodies are primarily of the IgG heavy chain type, but IgM and IgA may also be involved (Schulman, et al., 1965). The antibodies are secreted by autoreactive B-cells which are activated by autoreactive CD4+ helper T-cells. In fact, the pathway that leads to platelet destruction involves a complex interplay of the humoral and cellular immune systems.

The initial trigger for the abnormal autoantibody response is unknown. The cause of this loss of self-tolerance probably varies among patients. However, the common pathway appears to involve CD4+ helper T-cells reacting with a specific platelet-associated antigen on the surface of an antigen-presenting cell (such as macrophage, dendritic cell or B-cell). These activated helper T cells produce cytokines that stimulate B-cells to produce specific antibodies. These cytokines can also lead to expansion of CD8+ cytotoxic T-cells.

The primary site of platelet destruction is the spleen, and to a lesser extent, the liver and bone marrow. In these organs, antibody-sensitized platelets are destroyed by phagocytic cells.

### 4.2 Role of cytotoxic T-cells

In 30% or more of the ITP patients with no detectable anti-platelet antibody (Harrington, et al., 1953), alternative mechanisms of platelet destruction are likely to play a role. Recent studies suggest that platelet lysis by CD8+ cytotoxic T-cells may be an important pathogenetic pathway in some ITP patients. These T-cells show increased expression of cytotoxic genes, including tumor necrosis factor α, perforin, granzyme A and granzyme B. In addition to causing lysis of platelets, cytotoxic T-cells may damage megakaryocytes in the bone marrow (Olsson et al, 2003). Therefore, downregulation of cytotoxic T-cell response serves as a potentially effective therapeutic target, especially in ITP patients who are refractory to conventional treatment regimens (Sabnani & Tsang, 2007).

### 4.3 Impaired platelet production

Besides accelerated platelet destruction, abnormal megakaryocytic growth and development are involved in the pathogenesis of ITP. Bone marrow examination under the microscope characteristically reveals normal to increased numbers of megakaryocytes in ITP patients. There may also be a shift to younger forms of megakaryocytes. Despite an apparently adequate number of megakaryocytes, platelet production is impaired. Studies of platelet production have demonstrated decreased or normal turnover in greater than 70% of ITP patients, suggesting an impaired compensatory response of the megakaryocytes to ongoing platelet destruction (Chang et al., 2003; McMillan, et al., 2004). In fact, bone marrow ultrastructural studies have demonstrated abnormalities in 50% to 75% of megakaryocytes in ITP patients. These megakaryocytes show impaired maturation and platelet release, and are unable to adequately compensate for the peripheral platelet destruction (Houwerzijl, et al, 2004).

Produced primarily in the liver, thrombopoietin (TPO) is the hormone responsible for enhancing megakaryocytic maturation and platelet production (Kuter, 2007). When platelet levels are low, free TPO normally increases in the circulation, which then stimulates megakaryocyte proliferation. However, serum levels of TPO fail to increase appropriately in response to thrombocytopenia in ITP patients (Kogusi, et al., 1996). Since TPO binds to both megakaryocytes and platelets, free TPO becomes less available as TPO binds to an increased number of megakaryocytes in the marrow. Furthermore, as platelets to which TPO binds are cleared from the circulation at an increased rate, TPO in turn becomes limited and platelet production is reduced (Kogusi, et al., 1996). These observations involving impaired megakaryocytic growth and relative deficiency of TPO levels have opened new treatment possibilities that involve targeting TPO to stimulate megakaryocytic proliferation and platelet production in ITP.

## 5. Therapeutic challenges and options

### 5.1 Clinical course of ITP

The clinical spectrum of ITP is as heterogeneous as its pathogenesis. Spontaneous remissions occur very rarely. Although the majority of patients with chronic ITP require some type of therapeutic intervention, most have favorable long-term outcomes. However, mortality and morbidity are substantial in patients with severe disease that is refractory to treatment. Despite undergoing splenectomy after initial steroid trial, approximately one-third of ITP patients fail to sustain platelets above $150 \times 10^9/L$, and 15% to 30% of these patients will require continuous therapy to sustain platelets above $30 \times 10^9/L$. Patients with chronic ITP and persistent platelet counts below $30 \times 10^9/L$ have a 4-fold higher risk of mortality than that of the general population. Mortality attributable to thrombocytopenia is usually caused by severe bleeding and infection. Overall, approximately 10% of all patients with ITP are expected to develop refractory disease, posing significant challenge in clinical management. In general, the chances of remission lessen as the duration of chronic ITP increases.

### 5.2 Decision to treat chronic ITP

The decision to treat a patient is usually based upon the individual patient's risk of bleeding. Treatment of patients with ITP is influenced by multiple factors, such as the age of the patient, severity of the illness, and the anticipated natural history. At the present time, treatment for ITP is considered appropriate for symptomatic patients and for those at risk of bleeding. Other factors influencing the decision to treat include a previous history of bleeding episodes, active lifestyle (such as playing contact sports), as well as other risk factors for bleeding such as hypertension, cerebrovascular disease, antiplatelet therapy, and the need for surgery or other invasive procedures. In such situations, treatment can be intermittent for a limited duration unless symptomatic thrombocytopenia persists.

The main goal for treating chronic ITP should be to achieve hemostatic platelet count. Hemostatic platelet count can be defined as the platelet count safe enough in an individual patient to prevent bleeding. Except for patients with severe thrombocytopenia ($<20{,}000 \times 10^9/L$), platelet count is not a reliable surrogate marker for the risk of serious bleeding. Hemostatic platelet count varies in different patients. Most of the studies have shown that the risk of bleeding increases with platelet counts of less than 20 to $30 \times 10^9/L$. Generally, treatment for adults is recommended when platelets fall below 20 to $30 \times 10^9/L$ to avoid life-threatening bleeding episodes.

Management of patients with platelet counts between 30 to $50 \times 10^9/L$ requires individualization and clinical judgment. Since the natural history of ITP varies in each individual patient, the most important factor in treating such ITP patient is to establish the individual record of symptomatology. While establishing the natural history of ITP, it is advisable to keep the platelet count above $30 \times 10^9$. Patients with platelet count greater than $50 \times 10^9/L$ should be treated in the event of active bleeding or anticipated surgical procedures that carry a high risk of bleeding.

The management of chronic ITP varies from observation to aggressive treatment, including stem cell transplantation (Passabeg & Rabusin, 2008). The most critical player in the management of ITP patient is an educated patient. It is strongly suggested that patients understand the full spectrum of options and uncertainties surrounding treatment of this disorder. The availability of technology and support groups has made patients education better. Therapeutic options for chronic ITP are reflective of our understanding of the various pathogenic mechanisms of ITP.

### 5.3 Therapeutic challenges and dilemmas

Despite recommendations from ASH and IWG, there is no single standard treatment of chronic ITP. Once again, treatment should be highly individualized based on the natural history of ITP in the particular individual. Selection of treatment modality is based on age, co-morbid conditions, anticipated efficacy and adverse effects, as well as physician and patient preferences. Overall, the outcome of ITP has improved significantly in the last two decades with the advent of better mapping of the pathophysiology and the availability of new therapeutic agents. Since no single agent is effective in all patients, selecting a treatment regimen that is effective with tolerable toxicity is a challenging task.

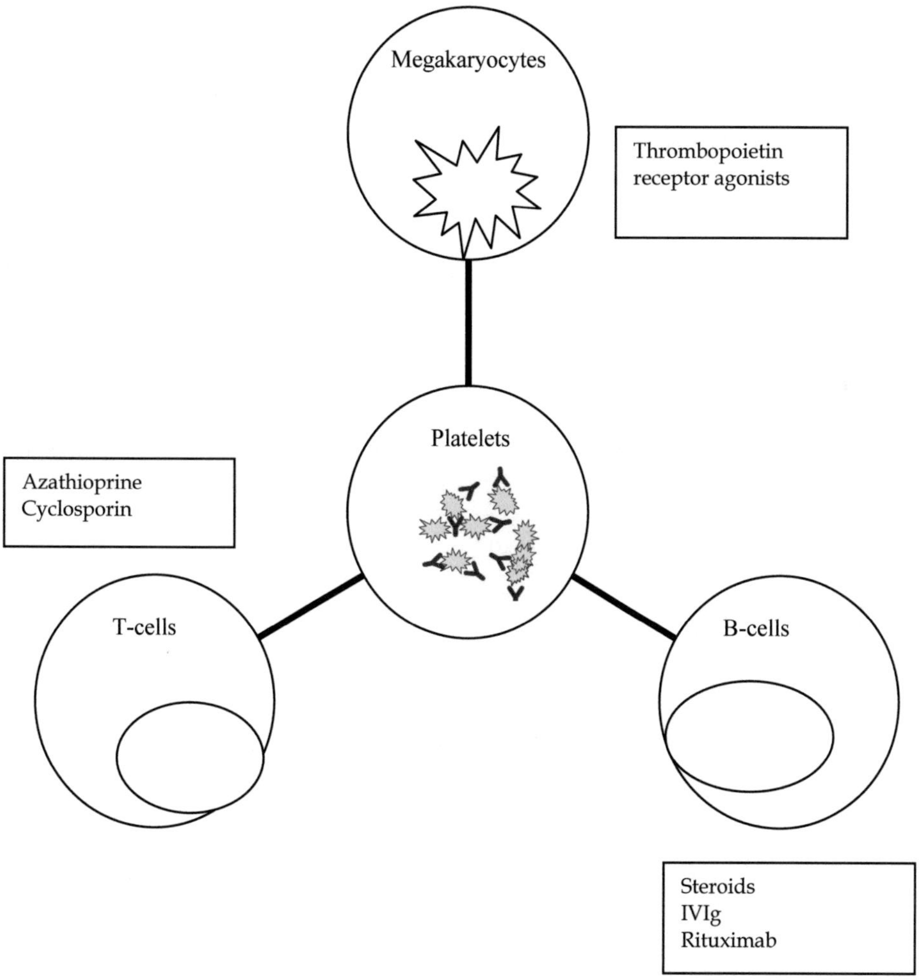


Fig. 1. Treatment modalities targeting various pathophysiologic mechanisms in chronic ITP

### 5.4 Initial treatment of chronic ITP:

Once the diagnosis of persistent or chronic ITP is established and the need for the treatment is determined, underlying infection must be ruled out. Traditional modalities, such as steroids and immunosuppression, could be detrimental in the presence of infection. Intermittent courses of steroids and IVIG are used along with other immunosuppressive modalities. The most commonly used regimens are prednisone at a dose of 1 mg/kg per day orally. The popularity of pulse dosing of high-dose dexamethasone is rising (40 mg/day for 4 days) due to the convenience of short duration of treatment (Cheng et al., 2003). The reported success rate with pulse dexamethasone in chronic ITP is conflicting, and long-lasting durable responses are generally not expected. Intravenous immunoglobulins (dose 1-2gm/kg) can also be used if there is a need to increase platelet count rapidly. Other alternative option is anti-D therapy. It is only recommended in Rh-positive and non-splenectomized patients. Intermittent anti-D therapy can be used on a long-term basis but the potential risk of severe hemolysis should be taken into consideration.

### 5.5 Second line treatment

Until recently, splenectomy was the most common second line option for the treatment of refractory chronic ITP. The use of the anti-CD20 monoclonal antibody, rituximab, as a B-cell depletion therapy has gained tremendous popularity as a spleen saving treatment modality. Rituximab can be used alone or in combination with dexamethasone. However, the complete durable response rate is not as high as splenectomy( Schweizer et al. 2007). Relapsed patients can benefit from re-treatment with rituximab. Long-term immunosuppression and progressive multifocal encephalopathy remains potential serious complications with rituximab use.

### 5.6 The role of splenectomy:

Splenectomy still remains the most effective second line option and offers the highest rate of durable complete remissions. Splenectomy has been shown to lead to durable response in 60% to 70% of patients (Kumar et al. 2002). However, with the introduction of a number of novel treatments, some clinicians recommend delaying splenectomy until later in the course of the illness. Despite the reduced morbidity and mortality with laparoscopic splenectomy in the hands of experienced surgeons, prophylactic appropriate vaccination, and use of antibiotics promptly in the event of febrile illness in post-splenectomy patients; still fewer patients are opting for splenectomy.

### 5.7 Therapeutic options after splenectomy failure

Treatment of patients with refractory ITP following splenectomy is challenging. While many drugs are available, no one treatment is widely accepted (McMillan & Durette, 2004). Intensive treatment should be reserved for patients with persistently low platelet counts in the presence of bleeding. Figure 2 shows an algorithm for managing ITP patients at different severities of disease. Other important considerations in the management of chronic ITP include the time to onset of efficacy, duration of benefit, and whether patients are able to maintain a response off therapy or if continued, the drug dosage necessary to maintain safe platelet counts.

Several immunosuppressive agents alone or in combination have shown some efficacy, including azathioprine (Quiquandon et al 1990), danazol, cyclophosphamide, mycophenylate mofetil (Hou et al. 2003), cyclosporine (Emilia et al. 2001), and vinca alkaloids. Another factor to consider when choosing an agent is patient preference for an oral agent administered daily, or an intravenous agent administered intermittently in an infusion clinic. Hematopoietic stem cell transplantation is used very rarely to treat ITP that has proven to be very refractory to treatment.

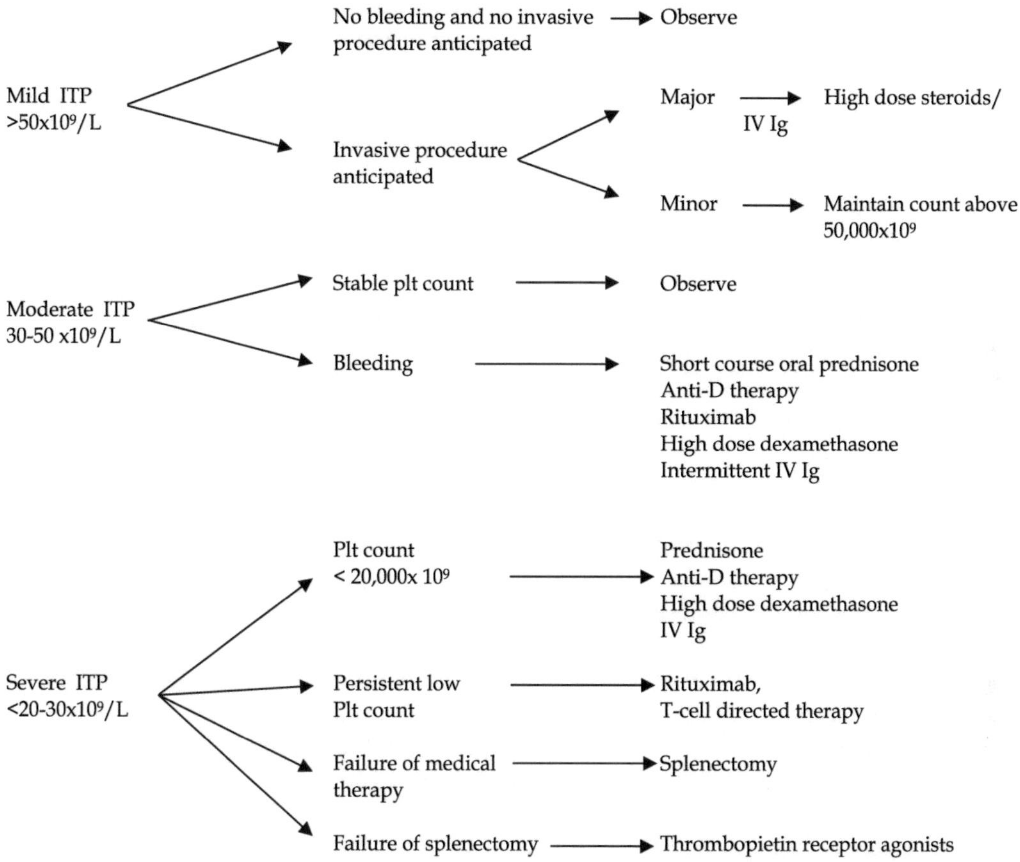


Fig. 2. Algorithm For the Management of Chronic ITP: "Individualize, individualize, and individualize"

Our better understanding of the immunopathogenesis has lead to the development of many novel therapies in the management of chronic ITP. Thrombopoietin receptor agonists (TRAs), which bind and activate the thrombopoietin (TPO) receptor to stimulate platelet production, have opened a new door in the management of chronic refractory ITP. Romiplastin (TPO peptide mimetic) and eltrombopag (nonpeptide TPO mimetic) are two recently approved agents for the treatment of refractory ITP (Burzynski, 2009). These agents have the advantage compared to recombinant TPO agonists of not causing the development of antibodies. The response rate of these agents ranges somewhere between 37% and 50%. To date, the clinical experience with these novel agents for a relatively benign disease is limited. Despite showing a favorable safety profile to date, these agents may have potential long-term side effects, such as thrombosis and myelofibrosis.

## 6. Conclusion

In summary, the diagnosis and management of chronic ITP require a highly individualized approach that is often based on the natural history of the disease in the particular patient as well as the experience of the physician. Published guidelines can certainly provide some guidance to the physicians but the decision of when and how to treat the thrombocytopenia will still depend upon the hematologists. Although ITP is an old disease, our recent understanding of the pathogenesis has caused a marked paradigm shift. For decades, steroids and IVIg have remained frontline treatment. Recently, the developments of newer therapies, such as rituximab and thrombopoietic agonists, have had a major impact on the management of ITP. A combination of different agents may be a useful approach in the future but a single uniform set of guidelines is difficult to establish. To date, optimizing the curative effects of the different therapies available remains a challenge.

## 7. References

Abrahamson, P., Hall, S., Feudjo-Tepie, M., Mitrani-Gold, F. & Logie, J. (2009). The incidence of idiopathic thrombocytopenic purpura among adults: a population-based study and literature review. *European Journal of Haematology,* Vol.83, No.2, (August 2009), pp. 83-89, ISSN 0902-4441

Arnold, D., Dentali, F., Crowther, M., Meyer, R., Cook, R., Sigouin, C., Fraser, G., Lim, W. & Kelton, J. (2007). Systematic review: efficacy and safety of rituximab for adults with idiopathic thrombocytopenic purpura. *Annals of Internal Medicine,* Vol.146, No.1, (January 2007), pp. 25-33, ISSN 0003-4819

Ballem, P., Segal, G., Stratton, J., Gernsheimer, T., Adamson, J. & Slichter, S. (1987). Mechanisms of thrombocytopenia in chronic autoimmune thrombocytopenic purpura. Evidence of both impaired platelet production and increased platelet clearance. *The Journal of Clinical Investigation,* Vol.80, No.1, (July 1987), pp. 33-40, ISSN 0021-9738

Buchanan, G., Scher, C., Button, L. & Nathan, D. (1977) Use of homologous platelet survival in differential diagnoses of chronic thrombocytopenia in childhood. *Pediatrics,* Vol.59, No.1, (January 1977), pp. 45–54, ISSN 0031-4005

Burzynski, J (2009) New options after first-line therapy for chronic immune thrombocytopenic purpura *Am J Health Syst-Pharm* —Vol 66 (Jan 15, 2009) suupl 2 pp. s11-s21

Chang, M., Nakagawa, P., Williams, S., Schwartz, M., Imfeld, K., Buzby, J. & Nugent, D. (2003). Immune thrombocytopenic purpura (ITP) plasma and purified ITP monoclonal autoantibodies inhibit megakaryocytopoiesis in vitro. *Blood,* Vol.102, No.3, (August 2003), pp. 887-895, ISSN 0006-4971

Cheng, Y., Wong, R., Soo, Y., Chui, C., Lau, F., Chan, N., Wong, W. & Cheng, G. (2003). Initial treatment of immune thrombocytopenic purpura with high-dose dexamethasone. *New England Journal of Medicine,* Vol.349, No.9, (August 2003), pp. 831-836, ISSN 0028-4793

Cines, D. & Blanchette, V. (2002). Immune thrombocytopenic purpura. *New England Journal of Medicine,* Vol.346, No.13, (March 2002), pp. 995-1008, ISSN 0028-4793

Cines, D. & Bussell, J. (2005). How I treat idiopathic thrombocytopenic purpura (ITP). *Blood,* Vol.106. No.7, (October 2005), pp. 2244-2251, ISSN 0006-4971

Cines, D. & McMillan, R. (2005). Management of adult idiopathic thrombocytopenic purpura. *Annual Review of Medicine*, Vol.56, (2005), pp. 425-442, ISSN 0066-4219

Evans, R., Takahashi, R., Duane, R., Payne, R. & Liu, C. (1951). Primary thrombocytopenic purpura and acquired hemolytic anemia : evidence for a common etiology. *Archives of Internal Medicine*, Vol.87, No.1, (January 1951), pp. 48-65, ISSN 0003-9926

Emilia, G., Morselli, M., Luppi, M., Longo, G., Marasca, R., Gandini, G., Ferrara, L., D'Apollo, N., Potenza, L., Bertesi, M., & Torelli, G. (2002). Long-term salvage therapy with cyclosporin A in refractory idiopathic thrombocytopenic purpura. *Blood*, Vol.99, No.4, (February 2001), pp. 1482-1485, ISSN 0006-4971

Fujisawa, K., Tani, P., O'Toole, T., Ginsberg, M. & McMillan R. (1992). Different specificities of platelet-associated and plasma autoantibodies to platelet GPIIb-IIIa in patients with chronic immune thrombocytopenic purpura. *Blood*, Vol.79, No.6, (March 1992), pp. 1441-1446, ISSN 0006-4971

George, J., Woolf, S., Raskob, G., Wasser, J., Aledort, L., Ballem, P., Blanchette, V., Bussel, J., Cines, D., Kelton, J., Lichtin, A., McMillan, R., Okerbloom, J., Regan, D. & Warrier, I. (1996). Idiopathic thrombocytopenic purpura: a practice guideline developed by explicit methods for the American Society of Hematology. *Blood*, Vol.88, No.1, (July 1996), pp. 3-40, ISSN 0006-4971

Harrington, W., Minnich, V., Hollingsworth, J., & Moore, C. (1951). Demonstration of a thrombocytopenic factor in the blood of patients with thrombocytopenic purpura. *Journal of Laboratory and Clinical Medicine*, Vol.38, No.1, (July 1951), pp. 1-10, ISSN 0022-2143

Harrington, W., Sprague, C., Minnich, V., Moore, C., Aulvin, R. & Dubach, R. (1953). Immunologic mechanisms in idiopathic and neonatal thrombocytopenic purpura. *Annals of Internal Medicine*, Vol. 38, No.3, (March 1953), pp. 433-469, ISSN 0003-4819

Hou, M., Peng, J., Shi, Y., Zhang, C., Qin, P., Zhao, C., Ji, X., Wang, X., & Zhang, M. (2003). Mycophenolate mofetil (MMF) for the treatment of steroid resistant idiopathicthrombocytopenic purpura. *European Journal of Haematology*, Vol.70, No.6, (June 2003), pp. 353-357, ISSN 0902-4441

Hou, M., Stockelberg, D., Kutti, J. & Wadenvik, H. (1995). Antibodies against GPIb/IX, GPIIb/IIIa, and other platelet antigens in chronic idiopathic thrombocytopenic purpura. *European Journal of Haematology*, Vol.55, No.5, (November 2005), pp. 307–314, ISSN 0902-4441

Houwerzijl, EJ., Blom, NR., van der Want, JJ., Esselink, MT., Koornstra, JJ., Smit, JW., Louwes, H., Vellenga, E. & Wolf, JT. (2004). Ultrastructural study shows morphologic features of apoptosis and para-apoptosis in megakaryocytes from patients with idiopathic thrombocytopenic purpura. *Blood*, Vol.103, (January 2004), pp. 500-506, ISSN 0006-4971

Kosugi, S., Kurata Y., Tomiyama, T., et al. (1996). Circulating thrombopoietin level in chronic immune thrombocytopenic purpura. *British Journal of Hematology*, Vol 93, No.3, (June 1996), pp. 704-706, ISSN 0007-1048

Kumar, S., Diehn, F., Gertz, M. & Tefferi, A. (2002). Splenectomy for immune thrombocytopenic purpura: long-term results and treatment of postsplenectomy relapses. *Annals of Hematology*, Vol.81, No.6, (June 2002), pp. 312–319, ISSN 0939-5555

Kuter, DJ. New thrombopoietic growth factors. (2007). *Blood,* Vol.109, No. 11, (June 2007), pp. 4607-4616, ISSN 1557-9190

McMillan, R. & Durette, C. (2004). Long-term outcomes in adults with chronic ITP after splenectomy failure. *Blood,* Vol.104, No.4, (August 2004), pp. 956–960, ISSN 0006-4971

McMillan, R., Wang, L., Tomer, A., Nichol, J., & Pistillo, J. (2004). Suppression of in vitro megakaryocyte production by antiplatelet autoantibodies from adult patients with chronic ITP. *Blood,* Vol.103, No.4, (February 2004), pp. 1364–1369, ISSN 0006-4971

Nurden, A., Villard, J. & Nurden, P. (2009). New-generation drugs that stimulate platelet production in chronic immune thrombocytopenic purpura. *Lancet,* Vol.373, No.9674, (May 2009), pp. 1562-1569, ISSN 0140-6736

Nunert, C., Lim, W., Crowther, M., Cohen, A., Solberg, L. & Crowther, MA ( 2011). The American Society of Hematology evidence-basedpractice guideline for immune thrombocytopenia. *Blood,* prepublished online, March 16, print ISSN 0006-4971, online ISSN 1528-0020),

Olsson, B., Andersson, P., Jernas, M., Jacobsson, S., Carlsson, B., Carlsson, L. & Wadenvik, H. (2003). T-cell mediated cytotoxicity toward platelets in chronic idiopathic thrombocytopenic purpura. *Nature Medicine,* Vol.9, No.9, (September 2003), pp. 1123-1124, ISSN 1061-4036

Passweg, J. & Rabusin, M. (2008). Hematopoietic stem cell transplantation for immune thrombocytopenia and other refractory autoimmune cytopenias. *Autoimmunity,* Vol.41, No.8, (December 2008), pp. 660–665, ISSN 0891-6934

Quiquandon, I., Fenaux, P., Caulier, M., Pagniez, D., Huart, J. & Bauters, F. (1990). Re-evaluation of the role of azathioprine in the treatment of adult chronic idiopathic thrombocytopenic purpura: a report on 53 cases. *British Journal of Haematology,* Vol.74, No.2, (February 1990), pp. 223-228, ISSN 0007-1048

Rodeghiero, F., Stasi, R., Gernsheimer, T., Michel, M., Provan, D., Arnold, D., Bussel, J., Cines, D., Chong, B., Cooper, N., Godeau, B., Lechner, K., Mazzucconi, M., McMillan, R. Sanz, M., Imbach, P., Blanchette, V., Kühne, T., Ruggeri, M. & George, J. Standardization of terminology, definitions and outcome criteria in immune Thrombocytopenic purpura of adults and children: report from an international working group. *Blood,* Vol.113, No.11, (March 2009), pp. 2386-2393, ISSN 0006-4971

Sabnani, I. & Tsang, P. (2006). Are clonal T-cell large granular lymphocytes to blame for unexplained haematological abnormalities? *British Journal of Haematology,* Vol.136, No.1, (January 2007), pp. 30-37, ISSN 0007-1048

Schoonen, W., Kucera, G., Coalson, J., Li, L., Rutstein, M., Mowat, F., Fryzek, J., & Kaye, J. (2009). Epidemiology of immune thrombocytopenic purpura in the General Practice Research Database. *British Journal of Haematology,* Vol.145, No.2, (April 2009), pp. 235–244, ISSN 0007-1048

Schweizer, C., Reu, F., Ho, A. & Hensel, M. (2007). Low rate of long-lasting remissions after successful treatment of immune thrombocytopenic purpura with rituximub. *Annals of Hematology,* Vol.86, No.10, (October 2007), pp. 711–717, ISSN 0939-5555

Shulman, N., Marder, V. & Weinrach, R. (1965). Similarities between known antiplatelet antibodies and the factor responsible for thrombocytopenia in idiopathic purpura. Physiologic, serologic and isotopic studies. *Annals of the New York Academy of Sciences,* Vol.124, No.2, (June 1965), pp. 499-542, ISSN 0077-8923

# 5

# Autoimmune-Associated Hemophagocytic Syndrome/Macrophage Activation Syndrome

Maciej Machaczka[1], Wojciech Sydor[2], Małgorzata Rucińska[3], Marta Szostek[3] and Jacek Musiał[2]
[1]*Hematology Center, Karolinska University Hospital Huddinge, Stockholm*
[2]*The Second Chair and Department of Internal Medicine, Collegium Medicum, Jagiellonian University, Kraków*
[3]*Chair and Department of Hematology, Collegium Medicum, Jagiellonian University, Kraków*
[1]*Sweden*
[2,3] *Poland*

## 1. Introduction

Hemophagocytic syndrome (HPS), also known as hemophagocytic lymphohistiocytosis (HLH) encompasses an infrequent group of non-malignant, yet potentially life-threatening disorders caused by massive cytokine release from activated lymphocytes and macrophages (Filipovich, 2009; Henter et al., 1998, 2007; Janka et al., 1998; Janka, 2009). This multisystem inflammatory syndrome is associated with a range of genetic and acquired factors. Hectic and persistent fever, cytopenias, hepatitis, jaundice, edema, splenomegaly, neurological symptoms and hemophagocytosis in bone marrow (BM), liver or lymph nodes are common clinicopathological features of HLH.

## 2. Historical background and terminology of HLH

The first published report on HLH is presumably an observation of hemophagocytosis in malignancy (Tschistowitsch & Bykova, 1928). In 1939, Scott and Robb-Smith reported four similar cases of adults with an HLH-like picture and proposed to call this condition histiocytic medullary reticulosis (HMR) (Scott & Robb-Smith, 1939). The term HMR was later succeeded by the disease entity known as malignant histiocytosis (MH) (Rappaport, 1966). The familial form of HLH (named FHL or FHLH) was first described in a family with two affected siblings (Farquhar & Claireaux, 1952). Risdall et al. later reported a series of 19 patients with active viral infection, whose bone marrow smears disclosed histiocytic hyperplasia with prominent hemophagocytosis (Risdall et al., 1979). Of note, 14 of 19 patients in this study were immunosuppressed and active infection with herpes group viruses was documented in 74% (14/19) of patients. They proposed to term this condition virus-associated hemophagocytic syndrome (VAHS). Some authors argue that this paper by Risdall and colleagues is the first well documented report of acquired (or secondary) HLH (sHLH) (Kumakura, 2005). Five years later, Risdall et al. also reported HPS in three patients with bacterial sepsis (Risdall et al., 1984). This condition was named bacteria-associated hemophagocytic syndrome (BAHS). To date, sHLH is known to be associated not only with viral or bacterial infections, but also with different types of other disseminated infections, including fungal or parasitic infections (Janka et al., 1998). Therefore, HLH associated with any infection type is collectively called infection-associated hemophagocytic syndrome (IAHS) or infection-associated hemophagocytic lymphohistiocytosis (I-HLH) (Kumakura et al., 2004).

The origin of the proliferating cells in MH has been thought to be the precursors of histiocytes, but then it has been clarified that the proliferating cells are lymphoma cells (Kumakura, 2005). In 1981, a case of T-cell lymphoma resembling MH was reported (Kadin, 1981). Following this report, many lymphoma cases associated with HPS have been reported worldwide (Han et al., 2007; Hasselblom et al., 2004; Ishii et al., 2007; Janka et al., 1998; Reiner & Spivak, 1988; Tong et al., 2008). In most of these cases it was proven that the proliferating cells were not of histiocytic origin, but that they were lymphoma cells. Therefore, the 'true MH', which is recognized as a neoplastic disease of immature histiocytes, is thought to be very infrequent, and secondary HLH associated with lymphoma is called lymphoma-associated hemophagocytic syndrome (LAHS) (Kumakura, 2004). Later, it has become clear that other hematological malignancies (e.g. myelodysplastic syndromes, acute and chronic leukemias, multiple myeloma) and solid cancers (e.g. thymoma, carcinoma, germ cell tumor, hepatocellular carcinoma) can be associated with HLH as well (Gupta et al., 2009; Ishii et al., 2007; Janka et al., 1998; Lackner et al., 2008; Machaczka et al., 2010; Reiner & Spivak, 1988; Shabbir et al., 2010). Thus, HLH associated with any malignancy should be collectively called malignancy-associated hemophagocytic syndrome (MAHS) or malignancy-associated hemophagocytic lymphohistiocytosis (M-HLH).

In 1991, Wong reported six patients with active systemic lupus erythematosus (SLE) who demonstrated reactive bone marrow hemophagocytosis (Wong et al., 1991). Since there was no evidence of an underlying infection, hemophagocytosis was thought to be solely associated with the activity of SLE, and the authors proposed to name this condition acute lupus hemophagocytic syndrome (ALHS). Shortly thereafter, Kumakura et al. reported cases of secondary HLH associated with autoimmune diseases other than SLE, and postulated to consider a new disease entity autoimmune-associated hemophagocytic syndrome (AAHS) (Kumakura et al., 1995, 1997). Albert et al. were the first to use the term 'macrophage activation syndrome' (MAS) in a description of the disorder (Albert et al., 1992). Shortly after, Stephan et al. used the term MAS in their description of 4 children suffering from chronic rheumatic disease characterized by a pro-inflammatory milieu (Stephan et al., 1993). MAS has been often reported in cases of systemic juvenile idiopathic arthritis (sJIA), but is also a known complication of adult onset Still's disease (AOSD), systemic lupus erythematosus (SLE), rheumatoid arthritis, Sjögren's syndrome, dermatomyositis, Kawasaki disease, mixed connective tissue disease and systemic sclerosis (Carvalheiras et al., 2010; Davi et al., 2011; Fukaya et al., 2008; Grom & Mellins, 2010; Hendricks et al., 2010; Kumakura et al., 2004; Parodi et al., 2009; Sawhney et al., 2001; Simonini et al., 2010; Titze et al., 2009; Tristano, 2008).

Recognition in recent years that MAS belongs to the class of sHLH has led to a proposal to rename it according to the contemporary classification of histiocytic disorders (Ramanan & Baildam, 2002). Some authors have suggested that the term MAS be dropped in favor of reactive HLH to reflect this similarity and to better familiarize pediatric rheumatologists with treatment options, particularly in patients not responding to frontline therapy (Grom 2003). Nevertheless, use of the term MAS still remains prevalent in the rheumatology literature, whereas syndromes described in the hematology and infectious disease literature often describe a similar phenomenon as secondary HLH (Deane et al., 2010). Some authors suggest that the terms MAS and HLH are interchangeable (Behrens, 2008; Behrens et al., 2008; Emmenegger et al., 2005; Ramanan & Baildam, 2002), whereas others describe MAS as a distinct subset of sHLH (Arceci, 2008; Janka, 2007, 2009), and still others highlight the heterogeneity of disorders described by both terms and call for revised terminology based more precisely on pathophysiology (Grom et al., 2003; Grom & Mellins, 2010).

## 3. Classification of HLH

According to the aforementioned historical background and current progress in understanding of its pathophysiology, HLH is generally divided into two distinct forms: an inherited, familial form and an acquired, secondary form (Arceci 2008; Janka, 2009; Henter et al., 2007). FHL has an autosomal recessive inheritance pattern, and usually arises in infants (80% cases), however in rare cases it can also occur in adults (Gupta & Weitzman, 2010; Henter et al., 1991b, 1998, 2007; Nagafuji et al., 2007). Acquired HLH can develop at any age, from childhood to the elderly, as a result of intensive immunological activation due to severe infections, autoimmune inflammatory disorders or malignancies (Janka, 2009; Henter et al., 2007). HLH as a serious complication of autoimmune diseases is commonly called macrophage activation syndrome or autoimmune-associated hemophagocytic syndrome. Macrophage activation syndrome as a severe complication of the systemic form of juvenile idiopathic arthritis (sJIA) is a prototype of AAHS. Nowadays MAS is considered a special form of acquired HLH by most rheumatologists. However, it should be emphasized that in the literature dealing with HLH in adults, MAS is sometimes used synonymously with acquired HLH regardless of its cause (Janka, 2009). The contemporary classification of HLH is presented in Table 1.

## 4. Epidemiology of HLH

Until recently, it was widely believed that FHL because of genetic causes arose during infancy and early childhood. In a retrospective Swedish study the incidence of FHL was estimated to be 0.12/100,000 children per year (Henter et al., 1991b). With the more widespread availability of genetic testing, it is apparent that the first significant episode of HLH can occur throughout life from prenatal presentations through to the seventh decade.
There is no exact data on the incidence of any form of the acquired HLH. In 2007, a retrospective study was published analyzing HLH cases diagnosed in Japan between 2001 and 2005 (Ishii et al., 2007). The most frequent form of HLH in all age groups in Japan was EBV-associated HLH (35%; 163/469 pts), followed by other infection-associated HLH (29%; 138/469 pts), lymphoma-associated HLH (18%; 84/469 pts), autoimmune-associated HLH (11%; 53/496), FHL (4.5%; 20/469 pts) and post-HSCT (hematopoietic stem cell transplantation) HLH (2.5%; 11/469 pts). The authors estimated that the annual incidence of all types of HLH and in all age groups of Japanese patients was 1 case in 800,000 individuals per year (Ishii et al., 2007). However, this number is probably underestimated, due to the retrospective nature of the study, certain diagnostic difficulties and overlooking or misdiagnosing of some HLH cases. In the same study, the reported 5-year overall survival was highest in EBV- or other infection-associated HLH (> 80%) and in autoimmune-associated HLH (almost 90%), intermediate in FHL or B-cell lymphoma-associated HLH

(50%), and lowest in T/NK-cell lymphoma-associated HLH (< 15%) (Ishii et al., 2007). A recent retrospective population-based study revealed the annual incidence of M-HLH in adults to be 1:280,000 per year or 0.36/100,000 individuals per year (Machaczka et al., 2011a). The results of this study were limited by the small population of the Swedish region of northern Halland, but the long observation period of over 14 years strengthened these findings.

<table>
<tr><th colspan="3">Genetic HLH</th><th colspan="3">Acquired HLH</th></tr>
<tr><td rowspan="5">Familial HLH</td><td rowspan="4"><u>Known gene defects:</u><br><br>?(FHL1)<br>PFR1(FHL2)<br>UNC13D (FHL3)<br>STX11 (FHL4)<br>STXBP2 (FHL5)</td><td rowspan="4"><u>Mutation's location:</u><br><br>9q21.3–22<br>10q21–22<br>17q25<br>6q24<br>19p13</td><td rowspan="4">Infection-associated</td><td>Virus-associated</td><td>EBV, CMV, HSV, adenovirus, influenza</td></tr>
<tr><td>Bacteria-associated</td><td>different species</td></tr>
<tr><td>Fungus-associated</td><td>Aspergillus spp., Candida spp., etc.</td></tr>
<tr><td>Other organisms</td><td>Pneumocystis jiroveci, Malaria, Leishmania</td></tr>
<tr><td>Unknown gene defects</td><td>ND</td><td>Autoimmune-associated</td><td colspan="2">sJIA, adult onset Still's disease, Kawasaki disease, rheumatoid arthritis, vasculitis, polymyositis/dermatomyositis, systemic sclerosis, systemic lupus erythematosus</td></tr>
<tr><td rowspan="4">Immune deficiency syndromes</td><td rowspan="2">Chédiak-Higashi syndrome (LYST)</td><td rowspan="2">1q42.1–q42.2</td><td rowspan="2">Malignancy-associated</td><td>Lymphoma-associated</td><td>T/NK-cell leukemia and lymphoma, B-cell lymphoma, Hodgkin lymphoma</td></tr>
<tr><td>Other malignancies</td><td><u>Hematological:</u><br>MDS, AML, ALL, MM<br><u>Solid tumors:</u><br>melanoma, thymoma, hepatocellular carcinoma, germ cell tumor</td></tr>
<tr><td>Griscelli syndrome 2 (RAB27A)</td><td>15q21</td><td colspan="3">Immune supression/post-transplantation<br>immune suppressive therapy<br>post-autologous SCT HLH and post-allogeneic SCT HLH</td></tr>
<tr><td>X-linked lymphoproli-pherative syndrome:<br><br>(SH2D1A)<br><br>(XIAP)</td><td><br><br><br><br>xq25<br><br>xq25</td><td colspan="3">Drug-associated<br>Anticonvulsants<br>(e.g., phenytoin, carbamazepine)</td></tr>
</table>

HLH - hemophagocytic lymphohistiocytosis; EBV - Epstein-Barr virus; CMV - cytomegalovirus; HSV - herpes simplex virus; ND - not determined; sJIA - systemic onset juvenile idiopathic arthritis; NHL - non-Hodgkin lymphoma; MDS - myelodysplastic syndromes; AML - acute myeloid leukemia; ALL - acute lymphoblastic leukemia; MM - multiple myeloma; SCT - stem cell transplantation.

Table 1. The contemporary classification of different HLH forms

The reported incidence of juvenile idiopathic arthritis (JIA) varies from 1 to 22 cases per 100,000 children, with a prevalence of 8 to 150 cases per 100,000 children (Cassidy & Petty, 2005; Weiss & Ilowite, 2007). Of these, approximately 10% of patients have the systemic form of the disease (i.e., sJIA). It is estimated that approximately 7-10% of patients with sJIA develop life-threatening MAS (Janka, 2009; Sawhney et al., 2001), which may occur at any time during the course of the disease, with a mortality between 10-20%. Moreover, two studies suggested that a mild, subclinical form of MAS may be present in as many as 25-30% patients with sJIA (Bleesing et al., 2007, Behrens et al., 2007). Although there are also numerous reports of MAS in adult onset Still's disease, SLE, and Kawasaki disease, the incidence of MAS in these entities is unknown. However, in considering MAS in general, the mortality rate is presumably about 8-22% (Gupta & Weitzman, 2010).

## 5. Clinical and laboratory features of HLH and AAHS/MAS

The most typical signs of HLH are fever (duration ≥7 days, with peaks ≥38.5°C) and splenomegaly associated with pancytopenia (affecting ≥2 cell lineages in peripheral blood), cerebromeningeal symptoms, skin rash, lymph node enlargement, jaundice and edema (Henter et al., 1991b; Kumakura, 2005; Öst et al., 1998; Reiner & Spivak, 1988). Laboratory findings include hyperferritinemia, hypertriglyceridemia, hypofibrinogenemia, coagulopathy, liver function abnormalities (i.e., elevated transaminases and bilirubin), hypoproteinemia, and hyponatremia (Henter et al., 1991b, 1998, 2007; Janka et al., 1998). Histopathological examination reveals accumulation of lymphocytes and histiocytes (macrophages), sometimes with hemophagocytic activity, observed in the spleen, bone marrow, liver, lymph nodes and cerebrospinal fluid (Henter & Nennesmo, 1997; Henter et al., 2007; Janka, 2009; Öst et al., 1998). The histological picture of liver biopsy resembles chronic persistent hepatitis (Henter et al., 2007). In the brain the leptomeninges and perivascular spaces are involved (Akima & Sumi, 1984; Henter & Nennesmo, 1997). Other typical findings in HLH are low natural killer (NK) cell activity and high levels of the alpha chain of the soluble interleukin-2 receptor (sIL-2R, also named sCD25) in serum and CSF (Henter et al., 2007; Janka, 2009). Soluble IL-2R (together with an elevated level of ferritin) is a marker of generalized inflammation, but very high levels of sIL-2R are almost never seen outside of HLH (Filipovich, 2009). Normal ranges of sIL-2R vary with age being highest in infants, and lower in teenagers and adults. All the key clinical and laboratory features of HLH can be explained by hypercytokinemia and organ infiltration as shown in Table 2 (Janka, 2009).

Another important marker of HLH is soluble CD163 (sCD163). The macrophage hemoglobin scavenger receptor CD163 is restricted in its expression exclusively to cells of the monocyte-macrophage lineage (Schaer et al., 2005). The extracellular part of the protein is shed into plasma (sCD163), because of proteolytic cleavage upon macrophage activation. Thus, sCD163 is a reliable clinical marker of disorders associated with overwhelming macrophage activity (Filipovich, 2009; Grom & Mellins, 2010; Schaer et al., 2005). Because sIL-2R and sCD163 are soluble molecules shed from the surfaces of activated T cells and macrophages, respectively, their levels are likely to increase in the serum regardless of the tissue localization of these cells (Grom & Mellins, 2010).

AAHS/MAS may exhibit all of the characteristic features of HLH. Coagulopathy and cardiac impairment are common (Janka, 2009). Neurological symptoms in MAS may progress to a severe encephalopathy and coma. Of note, not all patients with

| HLH symptom/sign | Causative factors |
|---|---|
| Fever | IL-1; IL-6, TNF-α |
| Cytopenia in peripheral blood | suppressive acitivity of TNF-α, INF-γ, and the heavy unit of ferritin on hematopoiesis; hemophagocytosis |
| High concentration of triglycerides in blood | supressive action of increased levels of TNF-α on lipoprotein lipase |
| Low concentration of fibrinogen in blood | high levels of plasminogen activator secreted by macrophages stimulate plasmine and in consequence lead to hiperfibrynolisis |
| High concentration of ferritin in serum | released by activated histiocytes/macrophages |
| High concentration of the α chain of the sIL-2R in blood | secreted by activated T lymphocytes |
| Hepatosplenomegaly | organ infiltrations with activated lymphocytes and histiocytes/macrophages |
| Increased liver transaminases and bilirubin in blood | |
| Neurological abnormalities | |

HLH - hemophagocytic lymphohistiocytosis; IL - interleukin; TNF - tumor necrosis factor; sIL-2R - soluble IL-2 receptor (also named sCD25).

Table 2. Signs and symptoms of HLH and their causes

autoimmune/autoinflamatory diseases and MAS fulfill at the beginning diagnostic criteria for HLH (Janka, 2009). In patients, who already have signs of inflammation such as high leukocytosis, elevated platelet count, and elevated levels of fibrinogen, a decline in these parameters, without reaching pathological values, may herald MAS (Ravelli et al., 2005). MAS as a first symptom of sJIA may be indistinguishable from other cases of HLH when arthritis is missing. A high interleukin-1β concentration in blood may also suggest MAS rather than classic HLH (Janka, 2009; Henter et al., 1996). Although mild elevation of sIL-2R has been reported in many rheumatic diseases including JIA and SLE, a several-fold increase in the levels of sIL-2R in these diseases is highly suggestive of MAS (Grom & Mellins, 2010). Importantly, other clinical entities associated with high levels of sIL-2R include malignancies and some viral infections, such as viral hepatitis, and so these conditions should be considered in the differential diagnosis. Nevertheless, sIL-2R receptor and sCD163 are now increasingly recognized as important biomarkers of AAHS/MAS (Filipovich, 2009; Grom & Mellins, 2010).

## 6. Diagnosis of HLH and AAHS/MAS

In 1991 the HLH Study Group of the Histiocyte Society published the first diagnostic guidelines for HLH which were later updated in 2004 (Henter et al., 1991c, 2007). According to the current guidelines (HLH-2004), five of the following eight criteria must be fulfilled for the diagnosis of HLH: (1) fever, (2) splenomegaly, (3) cytopenias affecting two or three lineages (Hb <90 g/l; PLT <100 × $10^9$/l; neutrophils <1.0 × $10^9$/l), (4) hypertriglyceridemia (fasting triglycerides >3.0 mmol/l) and/or hypofibrinogenemia (<1.5 g/l), (5) hemophagocytosis in bone marrow, spleen, or lymph nodes, (6) hyperferritinemia (>500 µg/l), (7) low or absent NK-cell activity, (8) elevated level of sIL-2R (sCD25) >2400 U/ml. The last three HLH criteria were introduced in the revised diagnostic guidelines for HLH in 2004 (Henter et al., 2007).

There are no validated diagnostic criteria addressed exclusively for AAHS/MAS, and early diagnosis is often difficult (Filipovich et al., 2010; Fukaya et al., 2008; Grom & Mellins, 2010). In general, in a patient with persistently active underlying rheumatologic disease, a fall in the ESR and platelet count, particularly in combination with persistently high CRP and increasing levels of serum D-dimer and ferritin, should raise a suspicion of impeding MAS (Grom & Mellins, 2010). According to Janka, a C-reactive protein >100 mg/l, increased granulopoiesis with left shift in the bone marrow and peripheral blood, and s-ferritin concentration >10,000 µg/L (if EBV infection has been excluded) are features strongly suggestive of MAS (Janka, 2009). The diagnosis of MAS is usually confirmed by demonstration of hemophagocytosis in the bone marrow, liver, lymph nodes, etc. However, false negative results may occur owing to sampling errors, particularly at the early stages of the syndrome (Grom & Mellins, 2010; Janka 2009). In some patients, subsequent biopsies may reveal hemophagocytic macrophages. In patients with negative bone marrow biopsies, assessment of the levels of sIL-2R and sCD163 in serum may help with the timely diagnosis of MAS (Grom & Mellins, 2010; Komp et al., 1989; Schaer et al., 2005).

In particular, application of the HLH diagnostic criteria to sJIA patients with suspected MAS is problematic. Some of the HLH markers such as lymphadenopathy, splenomegaly, and hyperferritinemia are common features of active sJIA itself and therefore do not distinguish MAS from a conventional systemic JIA flare (Davi et al., 2011; Grom & Mellins, 2010). Other HLH criteria, such as cytopenias and hypofibrinogenemia, become evident only at the late stages. This is related to the fact that sJIA patients often have increased white blood cell and platelet counts and elevated s-fibrinogen as a part of the inflammatory response in sJIA. Therefore, when they develop MAS, they demonstrate cytopenias and hypofibrinogenemia to the extent seen in HLH only at the later stage of MAS, when its management becomes challenging (Davi et al., 2011; Grom & Mellins, 2010). Diagnosis of MAS is even more problematic in SLE patients with autoimmune cytopenias, which are difficult to distinguish from cytopenias caused by MAS (Carvalheiras et al., 2010; Grom & Mellins, 2010; Parodi et al., 2009). In these patients, the presence of extreme hyperferritinemia and elevated LDH should raise suspicion of MAS (Parodi et al., 2009). Attempts to modify the HLH criteria to increase their sensitivity and specificity for the diagnosis of MAS in rheumatic conditions have been initiated and continue today (Ravelli et al., 2005; Davi et al., 2011).

## 7. Case presentations

Here we present three illustrative cases of patients with different autoimmune diseases developing severe AAHS/MAS in the course of their autoimmune disorder.

### 7.1 MAS complicating juvenile arthritis and ankylosing spondylitis

A 31-year-old male was referred from community hospital to the University Hospital (The Second Chair of Internal Medicine, Collegium Medicum, Jagiellonian University, Krakow,

Poland) because of persistent fever and progressive haemostatic abnormalities (skin bruises, undetectable fibrinogen level, prolonged aPTT and INR, markedly elevated FDP and D-dimer levels). The patient was admitted to a community hospital 3 weeks earlier with signs of a possible upper respiratory tract infection (fever, dry cough, sore throat) accompanied by herpes labialis. Broad spectrum antibiotic and acyclovir treatment were both ineffective. Because of a progressing bi-cytopenia (thrombocytopenia with neutropenia; Fig. 1) a fine needle bone marrow biopsy was performed showing no signs of significant primary bone marrow suppression.

Past medical history revealed that the patient suffered from a polyarticular seropositive juvenile arthritis since the age of 8 years. In the following years the patient was hospitalized several times because of disease exacerbations. Non-steroidal inflammatory drugs, gold salts, azathioprine, methotrexate and systemic corticosteroids together with physiotherapy were administered at various time periods; synoviectomy was performed twice. At the age of 29 a diagnosis of ankylosing spondylitis was established (sacroilitis, presence of HLA-B27). Approximately 5 months before admission to our Center the patient's immunosuppressive treatment was modified because of poor disease control, and he received a TNF-α inhibitor (adalimumab) with good clinical response.

On admission the patient complained of pain localized to the right subcostal region and persistent fever. On physical examination body temperature was 39.2°C, and slight hepatomegaly and skin ecchymoses with mucosal bleeding were present. Selected laboratory results and hematologic parameters at admission are shown in Table 3.

Differential diagnosis included DIC with sepsis (blood cultures later showed negative results), neutropenic fever (neutrophils $0.29 \times 10^9/l$), and opportunistic infections (HBV, HCV, EBV, CMV, and HIV infection were excluded). Adalimumab side effects were also taken into consideration. Filgrastim, ganciclovir and intravenous gammaglobulins were instituted with no improvement. Concomitant medications included ceftazidime, vancomycin, amikacin, sulfamethoxazole/trimethoprim, linezolide, tranexamic acid, fresh frozen plasma and cryoprecipitate.

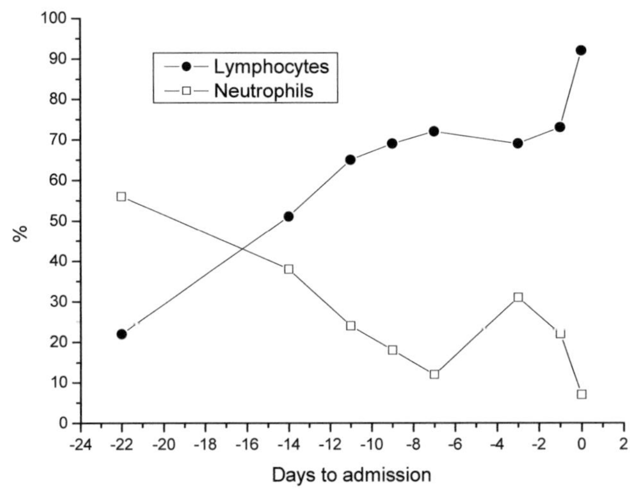


Fig. 1. Changes in neutrophils and lymphocyte counts before the admission

| Hematological parameters | | Reference range | Patient's result |
|---|---|---|---|
| Hemoglobin | g/l | 120–170 | 99 |
| White blood cells | × $10^9$/l | 4.0–10 | 1.0 |
| Lymphocytes | % | 20–40 | 64 |
| Neutrophils | % | 58–66 | 29 |
| Platelets | × $10^9$/l | 150–400 | 90 |
| Reticulocytes | ‰ | 3–15 | 2 |
| **Biochemistry** | | | |
| AspAT | U/l | 17–59 | 263 |
| AlAT | U/l | 21–72 | 116 |
| LDH | U/l | 313–618 | 7,700 |
| CRP | mg/l | <5 | 56.1 |
| **Coagulation tests** | | | |
| INR | | 0.85–1.15 | 1.30 |
| aPTT | sec | 25–31.5 | 55.60 |
| Fibrinogen | g/l | 1.8–3.5 | undetectable |
| Fibrinogen (nephelometry) | g/l | 1.8–3.5 | 0.7 |
| Trombin time | sec | 14–21 | 60.1 |
| D-dimer | ng/ml | <500 | >10,000 |
| Factor II | % | 70–120 | 45.9 |
| Factor V | % | 70–120 | 106.5 |
| Factor VII | % | 70–120 | 109.7 |
| Factor VIII | % | 50–120 | 39.8 |
| Factor IX | % | 70–120 | 94.6 |
| Factor X | % | 70–120 | 76.2 |
| Factor XI | % | 70–120 | 110.9 |
| Factor XII | % | 70–120 | 81.5 |

Table 3. The patient's laboratory results on admission

Because of a rapidly progressive thrombocytopenia and neutropenia, bone marrow biopsy was reinterpreted towards a diagnosis of hemophagocytic syndrome. Multiple macrophages (10–15% of nucleated bone marrow cells) together with several hemophagocytes were found (Fig. 2).

A diagnosis of macrophage activation syndrome complicating recent adalimumab treatment was established. Six days after the patient's admission, treatment with etoposide, dexamethasone, and cyclosporine A was instituted as recommended by the modified HLH-2004 protocol (Fig. 3). Body temperature normalized at day 3 of therapy. Etoposide-related nadir occurred at day 20 (platelets 14 × $10^9$/l; leukocytes 0.42 × $10^9$/l) (Table 4). One dose of etoposide was omitted and filgrastim (G-CSF) was administered (48 mln units b.i.d) with a beneficial effect. Etoposide was then continued for the next 9 months.

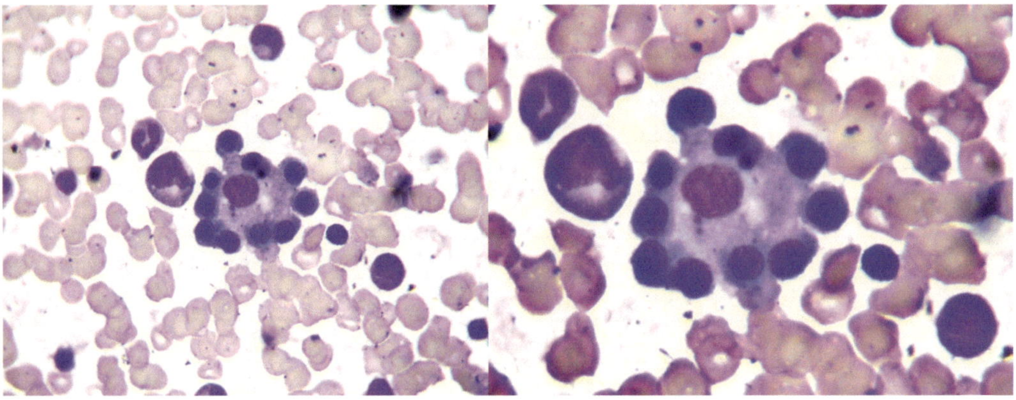

Fig. 2. Bone marrow aspirate smears showing the centrally placed macrophage laden with erythroblasts. Normally developed myeloid cells are present nearby. Wright's stain, lower (× 400) and higher (× 1000) magnification

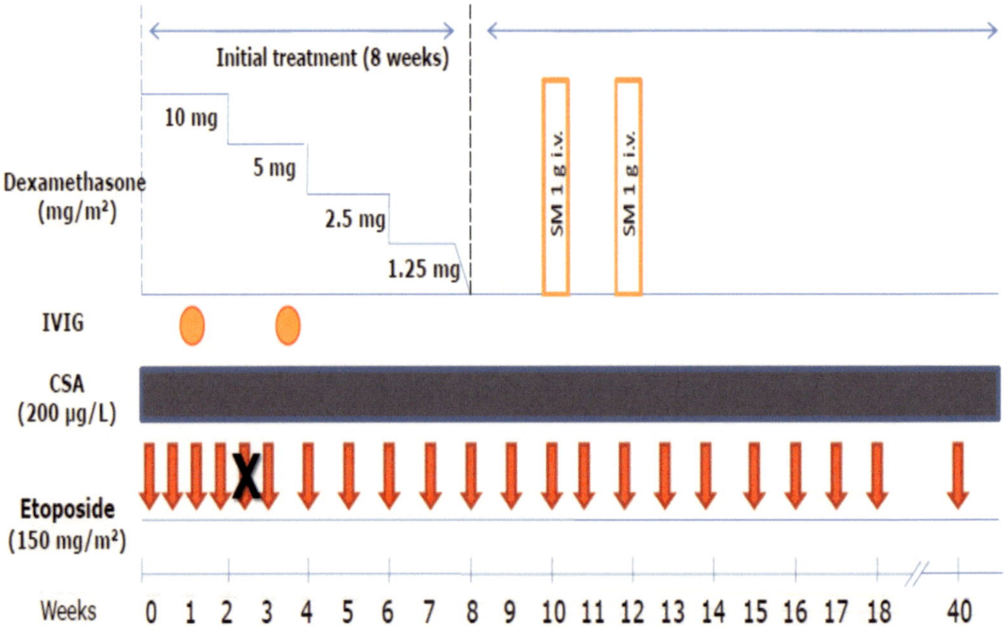


Fig. 3. The patient's treatment scheme with a HLH-2004 protocol

Control examination of bone marrow with a fine needle biopsy performed at week 40 of treatment confirmed the disappearance of activated macrophages. The patient felt well and continues treatment with cyclosporine and low-dose corticosteroids.

| Parameter (units) | Baseline (nadir/zenith) | After treatment |
|---|---|---|
| Fever (°C) | 39.2 | 35.8 |
| Splenomegaly | slight | - |
| Hepatomegaly | + | - |
| Hemoglobin (g/l) | 85 | 137 |
| Platelets (× $10^9$/l) | 14 | 260 |
| Neutrophils (× $10^9$/l) | 0.29 | 5.3 |
| Triglycerides (mmol/l) | 6.5 | 2.84 |
| Fibrinogen (g/l) | undetectable | 4.8 |
| Ferritin (µg/l) | >20,000 | 233.2 |
| AlAT (U/l) | 116 | 25 |
| Bilirubin (µmol/l) | 19 | 15 |
| LDH (U/l) | 7,687 | 624 |
| Hemophagocytosis | + | - |

Table 4. Changes in selected laboratory and clinical parameters characteristic for MAS during the applied therapy (HLH-2004)

### 7.2 MAS complicating rheumatoid arthritis

A 58-years-old patient, suffering from rheumatoid arthritis for 12 years, about 13 months after a course of TNF-α inhibitor (etanercept) treatment was admitted to hospital in another country due to progressive weakness, weight loss, intensive ankle joint pain and fever reaching 40°C. RA flare and infection were excluded and etanercept-related bone marrow dysfunction was suspected due to agranulocytosis, leukopenia, and thrombocytopenia. The patient had decided to leave the hospital and sought consultation in our University Hospital (The Second Chair of Internal Medicine, Collegium Medicum of the Jagiellonian University, Krakow, Poland). On admission his general condition was satisfactory; physical examination having revealed *livedo reticularis* on the lower limbs, swelling and redness of the left ankle joint, slight splenomegaly and caries of teeth 11 and 24. The most important laboratory abnormalities are shown in Table 5. Rheumatoid arthritis with Felty syndrome was diagnosed 12 years ago based on the presence of 5 ACR criteria, positive rheumatoid factor (RF) and elevated anti-cyclic citrullinated peptide antibodies (anti-CCP). About a year ago etanercept was started due to the ineffectiveness of corticosteroids and methotrexate.

After admission the patient received three injections of filgrastim (48 mln. units each) and antimicrobial treatment was implemented (ceftazidim, amikacin, fluconazole). Teeth 11 and 24 were extracted. The patient was seen by a hematologist and a fine needle bone marrow biopsy was performed showing numerous, typical hemophagocytes (Figure 4).

A macrophage activation syndrome associated with rheumatic disease (RA) was diagnosed. On day 8 of hospitalization, dexamethasone (20 mg qd) and cyclosporine A (dose adjusted to trough blood levels) were initiated. Treatment led to a quick decrease in body temperature and little later to normalization of the peripheral blood picture (Table 6).

| Hematological parameters | | Reference range | Patient's result |
|---|---|---|---|
| Hemoglobin | g/l | 120–170 | 108 |
| White blood cells | × $10^9$/l | 4.0–10 | 0.62 |
| Lymphocytes | % | 20–40 | 80 |
| Neutrophils | % | 58–66 | 13 |
| Platelets | × $10^9$/l | 150–400 | 56 |
| Reticulocytes | ‰ | 3–15 | 43 |
| **Biochemistry** | | | |
| AspAT | U/l | 21–72 | 16 |
| AlAT | U/l | 21–72 | 11 |
| Bilirubin | μmol/l | 3–22 | 12 |
| LDH | U/l | 313–618 | 420 |
| CRP | mg/l | <5 | 54.3 |
| **Coagulation tests** | | | |
| INR | | 0.85–1.15 | 1.08 |
| aPTT | sec | 25–31.5 | 31 |
| Fibrinogen | g/l | 1.8–3.5 | 1.5 |

Table 5. The patient's laboratory results on admission to the University Hospital

| Parameter (units) | Baseline (nadir/zenith) | After treatment |
|---|---|---|
| Fever (°C) | 37.2 | 36.6 |
| Splenomegaly | + | - |
| Hepatomegaly | - | - |
| Hemoglobin (g/l) | 108 | 133 |
| Platelets (× $10^9$/l) | 25.2 | 173 |
| Neutrophils (× $10^9$/l) | 0.6 | 3.43 |
| Triglycerides (mmol/l) | 2.83 | 2.7 |
| Fibrinogen (g/l) | 1.40 | 5.2 |
| Ferritin (μg/l) | 1,855 | 717.5 |
| AlAT (U/l) | 16 | 52 |
| Bilirubin (μmol/l) | 12 | not determined |
| LDH (U/l) | 420 | not determined |
| Hemophagocytosis | + | not determined |

Table 6. Changes of selected laboratory and clinical parameters of MAS during the treatment with modified HLH-2004 protocol

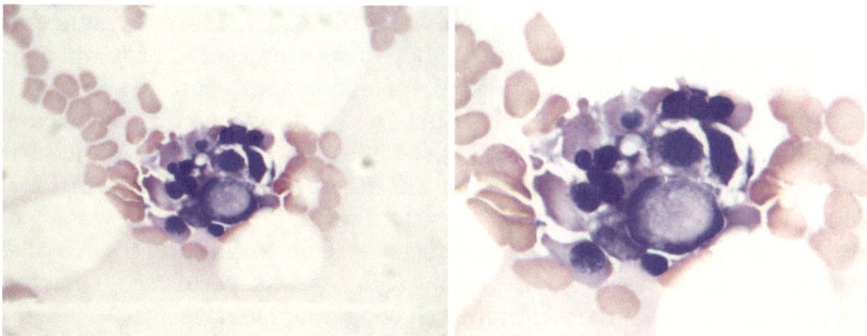

Fig. 4. Bone marrow aspirate smears. The centrally located macrophage shows phagocytosis of erythrocytes, erythroblasts and myeloid cells. Wright's stain, lower (× 400) and higher (× 1000) magnification

### 7.3 MAS complicating systemic lupus erythematosus

A 46-year-old man was admitted to the University Hospital (The Second Chair of Internal Medicine, Collegium Medicum of the Jagiellonian University, Krakow, Poland) in 2010 because of persistent fever and pulmonary nodules and consolidations. He has been treated for the last 10 years for systemic lupus erythematosus (SLE) with renal involvement. His SLE was diagnosed in 1991 based on the presence of several ARA criteria (fever, arthralgias, pleuritis and pericarditis, proteinuria, anemia, and the presence of ANA in high titer as well as ds-DNA antibodies) and typical results of renal biopsy. His medical history revealed arterial hypertension, peripherial artery occlusive disease and deep vein thrombosis of both lower limbs. Initially SLE was treated with corticosteroids and oral cyclophosphamide, then treatment was frequently modified according to the disease activity (azathioprine, cyclosporine A, mycophenolate mofetil and plasmapheresis).

| Hematological parameters | | Reference range | Patient's result |
|---|---|---|---|
| Hemoglobin | g/l | 120-150 | 134 |
| White blood cells | × $10^9$/l | 4.0-10 | 9.0 |
| Lymphocytes | % | 20-40 | 12.2 |
| Neutrophils | % | 58-66 | 83.0 |
| Platelets | × $10^9$/l | 150-400 | 57 |
| Reticulocytes | ‰ | 3-15 | 10 |
| **Biochemistry** | | | |
| AspAT | U/l | 21-72 | 38 |
| AlAT | U/L | 21-72 | 50 |
| Bilirubin | μmol/l | 3-22 | 11 |
| LDH | U/l | 313-618 | 1,114 |
| CRP | mg/l | <5 | 75.7 |
| **Coagulation tests** | | | |
| INR | | 0.85-1.15 | 0.94 |
| aPTT | sec | 25-31.5 | 25.9 |
| Fibrinogen | g/l | 1.8-3.5 | 5.0 |

Table 7. The patient's laboratory results on admission to the University Hospital

The patient's general condition on admission was satisfactory. His body temperature was 38.4°C, physical examination revealed neither hepatosplenomegaly nor lymphadenopathy. Selected laboratory results and hematologic parameters on admission are shown in Table 7. Microbial analysis of bronchoalveolar lavage obtained at bronchoscopy revealed a group I Mycobacteria-other-than-tuberculosis (MOTT). Targeted therapy was instituted (rifampicin 450 mg qd, isoniazide 250 mg qd, ethambutol 750 mg qd and clarithromycin 1000 mg bid) with no effect on the fever. Because of the persistent fever, bronchoscopy was repeated one month later, but MOTT's were no longer detectable. Due to the progressive anemia and thrombocytopenia a fine needle bone marrow biopsy was performed showing typical hemophagocytes, with some of these forming cell conglomerates (Fig. 5).

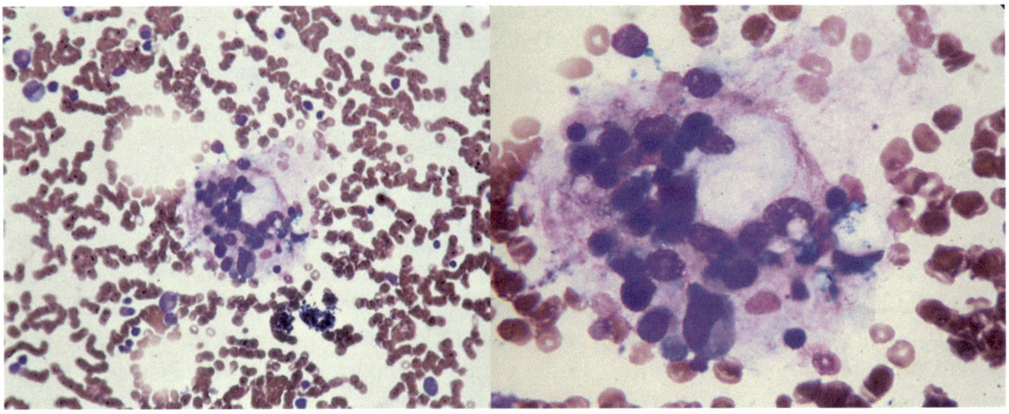

Fig. 5. Wright's stain of bone marrow aspirate smears. The centrally placed large cell conglomerate consists of activated macrophages presenting hemophagocytosis of erythroblasts and myeloid cells. Lower (× 200) and higher (× 400) magnification

| Parameter (units) | Reference range | Baseline (nadir/zenith) | After treatment |
|---|---|---|---|
| Fever (°C) | | 40.0 | 36.5 |
| Splenomegaly | | - | - |
| Hepatomegaly | | - | - |
| Hemoglobin (g/l) | 120-170 | 85 | 153 |
| Platelets (× $10^9$/l) | 150-400 | 42.2 | 118.2 |
| Neutrophils (× $10^9$/l ) | | 6,100 | 3,500 |
| Triglycerides (mmol/l) | 0.3-2.26 | 2.63 | 1.07 |
| Fibrinogen (g/l) | 1.8-3.5 | 3.60 | 3.1 |
| Ferritin (µg/l) | 13-400 | 1,387 | 105 |
| AlAT (U/L) | 21-72 | 142 | 57 |
| Bilirubin (µmol/l) | 3-22 | 12 | 11 |
| LDH (U/L) | 313-618 | 804 | 452 |
| Hemophagocytosis | | ++ | single cells |

Table 8. Changes of selected laboratory and clinical parameters typical for MAS during treatment (HLH-2004)

Macrophage activation syndrome was diagnosed and one month after the patient's admission treatment with dexamethasone, cyclosporine A, and etoposide was started resulting in the normalization of body temperature and peripherial blood morphology. Etoposide-related nadir occurred at day 14 (platelets $18 \times 10^9/l$, leukocytes $1.0 \times 10^9/l$). Two etoposide doses were omitted and filgrastim was administered twice (48 mln units qd). Intravenous pulses of etoposide were given for the next 2 months, followed by oral administration. A control bone marrow examination performed on week 40 of treatment showed disappearance of activated macrophages. The patient has continued treatment with cyclosporine A in combination with low-dose corticosteroids with continuous improvement of his clinical and laboratory parameters (Table 8).

## 8. Pathophysiologic and molecular mechanism of HLH

Although significant progress in understanding the genetics and pathophysiology of primary HLH has been achieved during recent years, the pathogenesis of acquired forms of HLH is still not fully understood. An exaggerated immune response is the final common pathway of HLH, however, there are multiple roads leading to it (Arceci, 2008; Janka, 2009). The immune response is often triggered by different stimulants (e.g., infection) and the underlying inherited or acquired immune defect. It has been proposed that the clinical presentation of HLH is due to uncontrolled activation of immune cells, macrophages and $CD8^+$ T lymphocytes (cytotoxic), leading to a massive release of various mediators of inflammation such as TNF-α (tumor necrosis factor α), interleukin(IL)-6, IL-8, IL-10, IL-12, IL-18, interferon γ, macrophage inflammatory protein (MIP 1-α), and hematopoietic growth factors (e.g., GM-CSF) (Filipovich, 2009; Henter et al., 1991a, 1996, 2007; Janka & Schneider, 2004; Osugi et al., 1997). IL-10 with its anti-inflammatory properties plays many important roles in the regulation of autoimmune inflammatory responses, particularly of systemic autoimmune disorders such as HLH/MAS. The role of IL-10 as part of an important regulatory mechanism involved in HLH has long been proposed (Behrens et al., 2011; Benveniste et al., 2000; Osugi et al., 1997). Recently, the roles of T regulatory cells in HLH have also been discussed (Verbsky & Grossman, 2006). Low or absent NK-cell function is present in many HLH patients and results in difficulties in termination of the exaggerated immune response (Filipovich, 2009; Henter et al., 2007).

There are two major subtypes of genetic causes of HLH. First are those genetic defects, grouped under the term FHL, that present with HLH as the primary and only manifestation of disease (Gupta & Weitzman, 2010; Henter et al., 2007). A second group of genetic disorders include HLH as only one, although often fatal, manifestation of the disease (Gupta & Weitzman, 2010; Janka, 2009). All known genetic abnormalities causing FHL involve genes that regulate proteins important in the secretory cytolytic pathway of NK-cells and $CD8^+$ T lymphocytes. In 1999, the first FHL-inked locus was discovered on chromosome 9q21.3–22 in several Pakistani families and was later defined as the FHL1 subtype (Ohadi et al., 1999). Shortly thereafter, mutations in the perforin gene *PRF1* were discovered on chromosome 10q21 in a group of patients with FHL (FHL2 subtype) (Stepp et al., 1999). Furthermore, mutations in genes *UNC13D* (located on chromosome 17q25; FHL3 subtype), *STX11* (located on chromosome 6q24; FHL4 subtype), and most recently *STXBP2* (located on chromosome 19p13; FHL5 subtype) were described (Feldmann 2003; zur Stadt et al., 2005, 2009). In view of the remarkable progress since the discovery of the first genetic defect in

FHL in 1999, it is expected that many new mutations in the known genes will be identified, as well as some novel gene mutations (Gupta & Weitzman, 2010).
Viruses, non-steroidal anti-inflammatory drugs, methotrexate, gold salts, and even TNF-α inhibitors have been reported as triggers for AAHS/MAS (Gupta & Weitzman, 2010). Interestingly, distinctions between genetically determined and acquired HLH become increasingly blurred as brand new genetic causes are identified, and patients who develop HLH beyond early childhood or in the contexts of EBV infection or autoimmune disease are being found to share some of the same genetic etiologies (Arceci, 2008; Hazen et al., 2008; Nagafuji et al., 2007; Zhang et al., 2008). Patients who develop sHLH may also have a genetic predisposition, but the molecular basis of the defects in sHLH has yet to be discovered (Arceci, 2008). This supposition has recently been strengthened by recent studies showing decreased NK cell function or reduced perforin expression in children with sJIA complicated by MAS, similarly to patients with FHL (Grom et al., 2003; Wulffraat et al., 2003). Of note, mutations in *UNC13D* gene, mutated in FHL type 3, were also described in patients with sJIA (Hazen et al., 2008; Zhang et al., 2008).

## 9. Treatment of HLH and AAHS/MAS

Early diagnosis and the prompt introduction of adequate therapy to produce a rapid response are crucial for a positive outcome in HLH. The treatment of any HLH type should focus on: (1) suppression of the hyperinflammatory state by destruction of activated $CD8^+$ T lymphocytes and macrophages, and (2) treatment of any existing triggers (Gupta & Weitzman, 2010; Henter et al., 2007). In cases of FHL, an additional aim is the correction of the underlying immune defect (Filipovich, 2009; Henter et al., 2007; Janka, 2009). HLH treatment categories include: (1) proapoptotic chemotherapy with etoposide (100–150 $mg/m^2$/dose i.v.), and (2) immunosuppressive drugs, targeting the hyperactivated macrophages (e.g., etoposide, corticosteroids, intravenous immunoglobulin), and T lymphocytes (e.g., corticosteroids, cyclosporine A [CyA]) (Henter et al., 2007). In 1994 the first prospective international treatment protocol (HLH-94) was introduced (Henetr et al., 1997). The experience from the HLH-94 protocol (including etoposide and dexamethasone [DXM]) and other studies have led to the development of a new treatment protocol, HLH-2004 (including etoposide, DXM, CyA) (Henter et al., 2007). However, immunochemotherapy (i.e., HLH-94 and HLH-2004 protocols) is only temporarily effective in the control of FHL, and the outcome is uniformly fatal unless the patient undergoes allogeneic stem cell transplantation (alloSCT) (Jordan & Filipovich, 2008; Henter et al., 2007). Last but not least, since patients with HLH represent a unique population with high morbidity/mortality and disease-specific complications, consideration should be given to referring these patients to centers with significant experience in the treatment and care of HLH.

### 9.1 Immunochemotherapy

Initially mild cases of HLH can deteriorate rapidly within a short period of time. Therefore, prompt administration of effective HLH therapy may prevent development of the full-blown syndrome. So far, treatment of AAHS/MAS is not standardized and remains highly variable across clinical centers (Deane et al., 2010). Nevertheless, a frontline treatment of AAHS/MAS (particularly of milder grades) usually involves corticosteroids with or without

intravenous immunoglobulin (IVIG), which may be sufficient to control hyperinflammation (Janka, 2009). In order to achieve rapid reversal of the coagulation abnormalities and cytopenias, most clinicians prefer starting with intraveneous methylprednisolone pulse therapy (30 mg/kg for 3 consecutive days) followed by 2 to 3 mg/kg/day divided by 4 doses (Filipovich et al., 2010). After improvement of the complete blood count and resolution of the coagulopathy, steroids are tapered slowly to avoid relapses of MAS (Janka, 2009; Filipovich et al., 2010). High-dose corticosteroids alone have been reported to induce remission in approximately half of MAS patients (Sawhney et al., 2001 Stephan et al., 2001).
Administration of IVIG might be effective in AAHS/MAS. High dose IVIG infusions are immunosuppressive, in part engaging Fc-receptors, which can play an important role in same patients with autoimmune/autoinflammatory diseases (Arceci, 2008; Kumakura et al., 2004). IVIG may also provide an anti-pathogen effect, which is particularly important if MAS is triggered by a viral infection.
Even when treatment is introduced in a timely manner, MAS can be fatal and deaths have been reported among patients treated with massive doses of steroids (Filipovich et al., 2010). However, corticosteroid resistant non-responders may benefit from second-line therapies, such as CyA or etoposide. Parenteral administration of CyA has been shown to be effective in patients with corticosteroid-resistant MAS (Mouy et al., 1996; Ravelli et al., 1996). Of note, in author's experience, some patients with MAS have not responded until etoposide was added to the HLH therapy. The similar conclusion has recently been postulated by other authors (Gupta & Weitzman, 2010). Thus, if there is no response to the aforementioned drugs (corticosteroids, IVIG, CyA), use of the HLH-2004 protocol including etoposide is recommended (Table 9). In summary, patients with suspected AAHS/MAS could be started on therapy without etoposide, as long as treatment adjustments are made rapidly in refractory cases (Gupta & Weitzman, 2010).
The utility of biological response modifiers in MAS treatment remains unclear, and at the present there is no consensus on recommendations in respect to this group of drugs. The use of TNF-α inhibitors (etanercept, infliximab) in MAS has produced conflicting results, being the effective therapy in some patients (Makay et al., 2008; Sellmer et al., 2011), while triggering MAS in others (Sandhu et al., 2007). Biological agents that neutralize IL-1 (anakinra) and IL-6 (tocilizumab) have been reported to be effective in occasional MAS patients (Filipovich et al., 2010; Kelly & Ramanan, 2008), but the clinical experience is as yet limited. In the case of patients with a form of sHLH other than AAHS/MAS, which proved refractory to frontline HLH therapy, anecdotal reports on the beneficial use of plasma exchange, hemofiltration, antithrombin III, anti-CD52 antibodies (alemtuzumab), and anti-CD25 antibodies (daclizumab) have been published previously, but the role of these therapies is not yet validated for any type of HLH (Gupta & Weitzman, 2010). Lastly, if MAS is driven by EBV infection, monoclonal anti-CD20 antibodies (rituximab) which deplete B lymphocytes, the main type of cells harboring EBV virus, should be used (Balamuth et al., 2007).

### 9.2 Stem cell transplantation

The first successful allogeneic bone marrow transplantation in a case of HLH was reported in 1986 (Fischer et al., 1986). Since then, information regarding the role of alloSCT in the treatment of HLH has mostly concerned FHL (Janka, 2009; Marsh et al., 2010). In FHL, alloSCT is the only available curative treatment option with the reported 5-year overall

<table>
<tr><th></th><th>Children</th><th>Adults*</th></tr>
<tr><td rowspan="14">Initial therapy (weeks 1–8) aiming remission of HLH</td><td colspan="2">Etoposide</td></tr>
<tr><td>150 mg/m² i.v.<br>twice weekly in 2 weeks followed by once weekly administration (week 3–8)</td><td>50–120 mg/m² i.v.<br>twice weekly in 2 weeks followed by once weekly administration (week 3–8)</td></tr>
<tr><td colspan="2">Caution! Adults usually do not tolerate as high etoposide doses as children, therefore dose reduction is indicated as proposed above</td></tr>
<tr><td colspan="2">Dexamethasone</td></tr>
<tr><td colspan="2">10 mg/m² p.o. daily in 2 weeks (week 1–2)<br>5 mg/m² p.o. daily in 2 weeks (week 3–4)<br>2.5 mg/m² p.o. daily in 2 weeks (week 5–6)<br>1.25 mg/m² p.o. daily in 1 week (week 7)<br>tapering and discontinuation during week 8</td></tr>
<tr><td colspan="2">Cyclosporine A</td></tr>
<tr><td colspan="2">3 mg/kg p.o. twice daily during the first week of therapy, followed by dose aiming CyA concentration at trough of 200 μg/l (week 2–8)</td></tr>
<tr><td colspan="2">Caution! Adults usually do not tolerate as high CyA concentrations as children, and CyA concentrations of 100–200 μg/l may be acceptable</td></tr>
<tr><td colspan="2">General remarks:</td></tr>
<tr><td colspan="2">1. Maximal initial supportive care is suggested, inclusive: appropriate broad-spectrum antibiotics (until culture results); prophylactic co-trimoxazole (equivalent to 5 mg/kg of trimethoprim 3 times weekly); an oral antimycotic therapy; antiviral therapy in patients with ongoing viral infection; and IVIG (0.5 g/kg) once every 4 weeks</td></tr>
<tr><td colspan="2">2. Gastroprotection due to the high steroids doses is recommended (e.g., PPIs)</td></tr>
<tr><td colspan="2">3. If after 2 weeks there is clinical evidence of progressive neurological symptoms or if abnormal CSF (pleocytosis and elevated proteins) has not improved, 4 weekly intrathecal Methotrexate injections are recommended</td></tr>
<tr><td rowspan="6">Continuation therapy (≥ week 9) after achieved HLH remission until alloSCT or therapy discontinuation</td><td colspan="2">Etoposide</td></tr>
<tr><td>150 mg/m² i.v.<br>once weekly every alternating (with Dexamethasone) second week</td><td>50–100 mg/m² i.v.<br>once weekly every alternating (with Dexamethasone) second week</td></tr>
<tr><td colspan="2">Dexamethasone</td></tr>
<tr><td colspan="2">pulses of 10 mg/m² p.o. for 3 consecutive days, given every alternating (with etoposide) second week</td></tr>
<tr><td colspan="2">Cyclosporine A</td></tr>
<tr><td colspan="2">dose aiming CyA concentration at trough of 200 μg/l (adults 100–200 μg/l)</td></tr>
</table>

* – etoposide dose recommendations for adults are not validated proposal, but based on clinical experience (personal communication with Jan-Inge Henter)
HLH - hemophagocytic lymphohistiocytosis; CSF – cerebrospinal fluid; CyA – cyclosporine A; IVIG - intravenous immunoglobulin; PPI – proton pump inhibitor.

Table 9. The HLH-2004 immunochemotherapy protocol for management of hemophagocytic lymphohistiocytosis

survival rate of 50–70% with myeloablative conditioning (MAC) (Baker et al., 1997; Cesaro et al., 2008; Dürken et al., 1999; Horne et al., 2005; Imashuku et al., 1999; Jabado et al., 1997; Ouachèe-Chardin et al., 2006), and 75–92% with reduced-intensity conditioning (RIC) (Cooper et al., 2006; Marsh et al., 2010).

So far, alloSCT has been performed only occasionally in cases of acquired HLH and its role in the treatment of sHLH is not yet established. Sporadic case reports have previously been published on refractory EBV-HLH successfully treated by means of alloSCT (Minegishi et al., 2001; Sovinz et al., 2010; Toubo et al., 2004). A recent Japanese survey revealed a curative effect of alloSCT on sHLH in 7 out of 11 patients (64%) with refractory EBV-HLH (Ogha et al., 2010). Similarly, Yoon et al. reported that alloSCT could be a curative treatment not only for FHL, but also for relapsed/refractory sHLH (Yoon et al., 2010). Anecdotal reports have also shown the efficacy of alloSCT in M-HLH therapy (Chang et al., 2009; Goi et al., 1999; Kelly et al., 2011; Machaczka et al., 2011b).

No concerted effort to apply alloSCT for the definitive treatment of MAS has yet been made. Given the high mortality associated with the current management of AAHS/MAS, the option of alloSCT using less intensive conditioning protocols, is reasonable to consider, especially in cases of severe or recurrent MAS episodes (Filipovich et al., 2010). Of note, sometimes fatal MAS was observed as a complication of prolonged T lymphocyte immunodeficiency in early trials of autologous stem cell transplantation for severe progressive systemic or polyarticular juvenile idiopathic arthritis (Filipovich et al., 2010). These observations suggested a failure to control the underlying disease given the patient's genetically predisposed hematopoietic stem cells (Bleesing et al., 2007).

## 10. Conclusions

Autoimmune-associated hemophagocytic syndrome/macrophage activation syndrome is a life-threatening hyperinflammatory syndrome which remains a major cause of morbidity and mortality in patients with autoimmune/autoinflammatory diseases. Awareness of AAHS/MAS, its symptoms and diagnostic criteria should be made mandatory among all physicians, especially those providing care to patients with autoimmune/autoinflammatory diseases. There are no validated diagnostic criteria making early MAS diagnosis difficult in part owing to strong similarities between MAS and sepsis. The treatment of MAS remains highly variable across clinical centers. Nevertheless, the frontline treatment of AAHS/MAS usually involves corticosteroids with or without intravenous immunoglobulin. In some patients with corticosteroid-refractory MAS, administration of cyclosporine A circumvents refractoriness. If there is no response to the aforementioned treatments a use of etoposide is recommended. The progress in understanding the pathophysiology behind MAS and identification of the pathways associated with the early stages of this syndrome bring hope to the idea of developing new biomarkers and treatments for clinical practice.

## 11. Acknowledgments

This work was supported by ALF resources (the agreement on clinical research between the Stockholm County Council and Karolinska Institutet). The authors thank Mr. J. Hubert and Mr. F. Kasina for linguistic assistance.

## 12. References


Albert, A., Azgui, Z., Buisine, J., Ciaudo, M., Fenneteau, O., Fillola, G., et al. (1992). Macrophage activation syndromes. *Nouv. Rev. Fr. Hematol.* Vol. 34 (No. 6): 435–441.

Akima, M. & Sumi, S.M. (1984). Neuropathology of familial erythrophagocytic lymphohistiocytosis: six cases and review of the literature. *Hum. Pathol.* Vol. 15 (No. 2): 161–168.

Arceci, R.J. (2008). When T cells and macrophages do not talk: the hemophagocytic syndromes. *Curr. Opin. Hematol.* Vol. 15 (No. 4): 359–367.

Baker, K.S., DeLaat, C.A., Steinbuch, M., Gross, T.G., Shapiro, R.S., Loechelt, B., et al. (1997). Successful correction of HLH with related or unrelated bone marrow transplantation. *Blood* Vol. 89 (No. 10): 3857–3863.

Balamuth, N.J., Nichols, K.E., Paessler, M. & Taechey, D.T. (2007). Use of rituximab in conjunction with immunosuppressive chemotherapy as a novel therapy for Epstein-Barr virus-associated hemophagocytic lymphohistiocytosis. *J. Pediatr. Hematol. Oncol.* Vol. 29 (No. 8): 569–573.

Behrens, E.M. (2008). Macrophage activation syndrome in rheumatic disease: what is the role of the antigen presenting cell? *Autoimmun. Rev.* Vol. 7 (No. 4): 305–308.

Behrens, E.M., Beukelman, T., Gallo, L., Spangler, J., Rosenkranz, M., Arkachaisri, T., et al. (2008). Evaluation of the presentation of systemic onset juvenile rheumatoid arthritis: data from the Pennsylvania Systemic Onset Juvenile Arthritis Registry (PASOJAR). *J. Rheumatol.* Vol. 35 (No. 2): 343–348.

Behrens, E.M., Beukelman, T., Paessler, M. & Cron, R.Q. (2007). Occult macrophage activation syndrome in patients with systemic juvenile idiopathic arthritis. *J. Rheumatol.* Vol. 34 (No. 5): 1133–1138.

Behrens, E.M., Canna S.W., Slade, K., Rao, S., Kreiger, P.A., Paessler, M., et al. (2011). Repeated TLR9 stimulation results in macrophage activation syndrome-like disease in mice. *J. Clin. Invest.* Vol. 121 (No. 6): 2264–2277.

Benveniste, O., Dereuddre-Bosquet, N., Clayette, P., Leport, C., Vildé, J.L. & Dormont, D. (2000). High levels of IL-10 and determination of other cytokines and chemokines in HIV-associated haemophagocytic syndrome. Clin. Exp. Immunol. Vol 121 (No. 2): 320-323.

Bleesing, J., Prada, A., Siegel, D.M., Villanueva, J., Olson, J., Ilowite, N.T., et al. (2007). The diagnostic significance of soluble CD163 and soluble interleukin-2 receptor alpha-chain in MAS and untreated new-onset systemic juvenile idiopathic arthritis. *Arthritis Rheum.* Vol. 56 (No. 3): 965–971.

Carvalheiras, G., Anjo, D., Mendonca, T., Vasconcelos, C. & Farinha, F. (2010). Hemophagocytic syndrome as one of the main primary manifestations in acute SLE - case report and literature review. *Lupus* Vol. 19 (No. 6): 756–761.

Cassidy, J.T. & Petty, R.E. (2005). Chronic arthritis in childhood, *in* Cassidy, J.T., Petty, R.E., Laxer, R.M. & Lindsley C.B. (eds.), *Textbook of Pediatric Rheumatology* (5th edition), Elsevier Saunders, Philadelphia, pp. 206–260.

Cesaro, S., Locatelli, F., Lanino, E., Porta, F., Di Maio, L., Messina, C., et al. (2008). Hematopoietic stem cell transplantation for hemophagocitic lymphohistiocytosis: a retrospective analysis of data from the Italian Association of Pediatric Hematology Oncology (AIEOP). *Haematologica* Vol. 93 (No. 11): 1694–1701.

Chang, Y.H., Lu, P.J., Lu, M.Y., Wang, J.S., Tung, C.L. & Shaw, C.F. (2009). Sequential transplants for respective relapse of Hodgkin disease and HLH: a treatment dilemma. *J. Pediatr. Hematol. Oncol.* Vol. 31 (No. 10): 778–781.

Cooper, N., Rao, K., Gilmour, K., Hadad, L., Adams, S., Cale, C., et al. (2006). Stem cell transplantation with RIC for hemophagocytic lymphohistiocytosis. *Blood* Vol. 107 (No. 3): 1233–1236.

Davi, S., Consolaro, A., Guseinova, D., Pistorio, A., Ruperto, N., Martini, A., et al.; MAS Study Group. (2011). An international consensus survey of diagnostic criteria for macrophage activation syndrome in systemic juvenile idiopathic arthritis. *J. Rheumatol.* Vol. 38 (No. 4): 764–768.

Deane, S., Selmi, C., Teuber, S.S. & Gershwin M.E. (2010). Macrophage activation syndrome in autoimmune disease. *Int. Arch. Allergy Immunol.* Vol. 153 (No. 2): 109–120.

Dürken, M., Horstmann, M., Bieling, P., Erttmann, R., Kabisch, H., Löliger, C., et al. (1999). Improved outcome in HLH after BMT from related and unrelated donors: a single-centre experience of 12 patients. *Br. J. Haematol.* Vol. 106 (No. 4): 1052–1058.

Emmenegger, U., Schaer, D.J., Larroche, C. & Neftel, K.A. (2005). Haemophagocytic syndromes in adults: current concepts and challenges ahead. *Swiss Med. Wkly.* Vol. 135 (No. 21-22): 299–314.

Farquhar, J.W. & Claireaux, A.E. (1952). Familial haemophagocytic reticulosis. *Arch. Dis. Child.* Vol. 27 (No. 136): 519–525.

Feldmann, J., Callebaut, I., Raposo, G., Certain, S., Bacq, D., Dumont, C., et al. (2003). Munc13-4 is essential for cytolytic granules fusion and is mutated in a form of familial hemophagocytic lymphohistiocytosis (FHL3). *Cell* 2003 Vol. 115 (No. 4): 461–473.

Filipovich, A.H. (2009). Hemophagocytic lymphohistiocytosis (HLH) and related disorders. *Hematology Am. Soc. Hematol. Educ. Program*: 127–131.

Filipovich, A., McClain, K. & Grom, A. (2010). Histiocytic disorders: recent insights into pathophysiology and practical guidelines. *Biol. Blood Marrow Transplant.* Vol. 16 (1 Suppl): S82–S89.

Fischer, A., Cerf-Bensussan, N., Blanche, S., Le Deist, F., Bremard-Oury, C., Leverger, G., et al. (1986). Allogeneic BMT for erythrophagocytic lymphohistiocytosis. *J. Pediatr.* Vol. 108 (No. 2): 267–270.

Fukaya, S., Yasuda, S., Hashimoto, T., Oku, K., Kataoka, H., Horita, T., et al. (2008). Clinical features of haemophagocytis syndrome in patients with systemic autoimmune diseases: analysis of 30 cases. *Rheumatology (Oxford)* Vol. 47 (No. 11): 1686–1691.

Goi, K., Sugita, K., Nakamura, M., Miyamoto, N., Karakida, N., Iijima, K., et al. (1999). Development of acute lymphoblastic leukemia with t(4;11) in a girl with familial pericentric inv 12. *Cancer Genet. Cytogenet.* Vol. 110 (No. 2): 124–127.

Grom, A.A. (2003). Macrophage activation syndrome and reactive HLH: the same entities? *Curr. Opin. Rheumatol.* Vol. 15 (No. 5): 587–590.

Grom, A.A., Villanueva, J., Lee, S., Goldmuntz, E.A., Passo, M.H. & Filipovich, A. (2003). Natural killer cell dysfunction in patients with systemic-onset juvenile rheumatoid arthritis and macrophage activation syndrome. *J. Pediatr.* Vol. 142 (No. 3): 292–296.

Grom, A.A. & Mellins, E.D. (2010). Macrophage activation syndrome: advances towards understanding pathogenesis. *Curr. Opin. Rheumatol.* Vol. 22 (No. 5): 561-566.

Gupta, A.A., Tyrrell, P., Valani, R., Benseler, S., Abdelhaleem, M. & Weitzman, S. (2009). Experience with hemophagocytic lymphohistiocytosis/macrophage activation syndrome at a single institution. *J. Pediatr. Hematol. Oncol.* Vol. 31 (No. 2): 81–84.

Gupta, S. & Weitzman, S. (2010). Primary and secondary hemophagocytic lymphohistiocytosis: clinical features, pathogenesis and therapy. *Expert Rev. Clin. Immunol.* Vol. 6 (No. 1): 137–154.

Han, A.R., Lee, H.R., Park, B.B., Hwang, I.G., Park, S., Lee, S.C., et al. (2007). Lymphoma-associated hemophagocytic syndrom: clinical features and treatment outcome. *Ann. Hematol.* Vol. 86 (No. 7): 493-498.

Hasselblom, S., Linde, A. & Ridell, B. (2004). Hodgkin's lymphoma, EBV reactivation and fatal haemophagocytic syndrome. *J. Intern. Med.* Vol. 255 (No. 2): 289-295.

Hazen, M.M., Woodward, A.L., Hofmann, I., Degar, B.A., Grom, A., Filipovich, A.H., et al. (2008). Mutations of the hemophagocytic lymphohistiocytosis-associated gene UNC13D in a patient with systemic juvenile idiopathic arthritis. *Arthritis Rheum.* Vol. 58 (No. 2): 567–570.

Hendricks, M., Pillay, S., Davidson, A., De Decker, R. & Lawrenson, J. (2010). Kawasaki disease preceding haemophagocytic lymphohistiocytosis: challenges for developing world practitioners. *Pediatr. Blood Cancer* Vol. 54 (No. 7): 1023–1025.

Henter, J.-I., Andersson, B., Elinder, G., Jakobson, A., Lübeck, P.O. & Söder, O. (1996). Elevated circulating levels of interleukin-1 receptor antagonist but not IL-1 agonist in hemophagocytic lymphohistiocytosis. *Med. Pediatr. Oncol.* Vol. 27 (No. 1): 21–25.

Henter, J.-I., Arico, M., Egeler, R.M., Elinder, G., Favara, B.E., Filipovich, A.H., et al. (1997). HLH-94: a treatment protocol for hemophagocytic lymphohistiocytosis. *Med. Pediatr. Oncol.* Vol. 28 (No. 5): 342–347.

Henter, J.-I., Arico, M., Elinder, G., Imashuku, S. & Janka, G. (1998). Familial hemophagocytic lymphohistiocytosis (primary HLH). *Hematol. Oncol. Clin. North Am.* Vol. 12 (No. 2): 417–433.

Henter, J.-I., Elinder, G., Söder, O., Hansson, M., Andersson, B. & Andersson, U. (1991a). Hypercytokinemia in familial hemophagocytic lymphohistiocytosis. *Blood* Vol. 78 (No. 11): 2918–2922.

Henter, J.-I., Elinder, G., Söder, O. & Öst Å. (1991b). Incidence in Sweden and clinical features of familial hemophagocytic lymphohistiocytosis. *Acta Paediatr. Scand.* Vol. 80 (No. 4): 428-435.

Henter, J.-I., Elinder, G. & Öst, Å. (1991c). Diagnostic guidelines for hemophagocytic lymphohistiocytosis. The FHL Study Group of the Histiocyte Society. *Semin. Oncol.* Vol. 18 (No. 1): 29–33.

Henter, J.-I., Horne, A.C., Arico, M., Egeler, R.M., Filipovich, A.H., Imashuku, S., et al. for the Histiocyte Society. (2007). HLH-2004: Diagnostic and therapeutic guidelines for hemophagocytic lymphohistiocytosis. *Pediatr. Blood Cancer* Vol. 48 (No. 2): 124–131.

Henter, J.-I. & Nennesmo, I. (1997). Neuropathologic findings and neurologic symptoms in twenty-three children with hemophagocytic lymphohistiocytosis. *J. Pediatr.* Vol. 130 (No. 3): 358–365.

Horne, A., Janka, G., Maarten Egeler, R., Gadner, H., Imashuku, S., Ladisch, S., et al.; Histiocyte Society. (2005). Haematopoietic stem cell transplantation in haemophagocytic lymphohistiocytosis. *Br. J. Haematol.* Vol. 129 (No. 5): 622–630.

Imashuku, S., Hibi, S., Todo, S., Sako, M., Inoue, M., Kawa, K., et al. (1999). Allogenic hematopoietic SCT for patients with hemophagocytic syndrome (HPS) in Japan. *Bone Marrow Transplant.* Vol. 23 (No. 6): 569–572.

Ishii, E., Ohga, S., Imashuku, S., Yasukawa, M., Tsuda, H., Miura, .I, et al. (2007). Nationwide survey of hemophagocytic lymphohistiocytosis in Japan. *Int. J. Hematol.* Vol. 86 (No. 1): 58–65.

Jabado, N., de Graeff-Meeder, E.R., Cavazzana-Calvo, M., Haddad, E., Le Deist, F., Benkerrou, M., et al. (1997). Treatment of familial hemophagocytic lymphohistiocytosis with bone marrow transplantation from HLA genetically nonidentical donors. *Blood* Vol. 90 (No. 12): 4743–4748.

Janka, G., Imashuku, S., Elinder, G., Schneider, M. & Henter, J.-I. (1998). Infection- and malignancy-associated hemophagocytic syndromes. Secondary hemophagocytic lymphohistiocytosis. *Hematol. Oncol. Clin. North Am.* Vol. 12 (No. 2): 435–444.

Janka, G.E. & Schneider, E.M. (2004). Modern management of children with haemophagocytic lymphohistiocytosis. *Br. J. Haematol.* Vol. 124 (No. 1): 4–14.

Janka, G.E. (2007). Familial and acquired hemophagocytic lymphohistiocytosis. Eur. J. Pediatr. Vol. 166 (No. 2): 95–109.

Janka, G. (2009). Hemophagocytic lymphohistiocytosis: When the immune system runs amok. *Klin. Padiatr.* Vol. 221 (No. 5): 278–285.

Jordan, M.B. & Filipovich, A.H. (2008). Hematopoietic cell transplantation for hemophagocytic lymphohistiocytosis: a journey of a thousand miles begins with a single (big) step. *Bone Marrow Transplant.* Vol. 42 (No. 7): 433–437.

Kadin, M.E., Kamoun, M. & Lamberg, J. (1981). Erythrophagocytic T gamma lymphoma: a clinicopathologic entity resembling malignant histiocytosis. *N. Engl. J. Med.* Vol. 304 (No. 11): 648–653.

Kelly, C., Salvi, S., McClain, K. & Hayani, A. (2011). HLH associated with precursor B acute lymphoblastic leukemia. *Pediatr. Blood Cancer* Vol. 56 (No. 4): 658–660.

Kelly, A. & Ramanan, A.V. (2008). A case of macrophage activation syndrome successfully treated with anakinra. *Nat. Clin. Pract. Rheumatol.* Vol. 4 (No. 11): 615–620.

Komp, D.M., McNamara, J. & Buckley, P. (1989). Elevated soluble interleukin-2 receptor in childhood hemophagocytic histiocytic syndromes. *Blood* Vol. 73 (No. 8): 2128–2132.

Kumakura, S., Ishikura, H., Endo, J. & Kobayashi, S. (1995). Autoimmune-associated hemophagocytosis. *Am. J. Hematol.* Vol. 50 (No. 2): 148–149.

Kumakura, S., Ishikura, H., Umegae, N., Yamagata, S. & Kobayashi, S. (1997). Autoimmune-associated hemophagocytic syndrome. *Am. J. Med.* Vol. 102 (No. 1): 113–115.

Kumakura, S., Ishikura, H., Kondo, M., Murakawa, Y., Masuda, J. & Kobayashi, S. (2004). Autoimmune-associated hemophagocytic syndrome. *Mod. Rheumatol.* Vol. 14 (No. 3): 205–215.

Kumakura, S. (2005). Hemophagocytic syndrome. *Intern. Med.* Vol. 44 (No. 4): 278–280.

Lackner, H., Urban, C., Sovinz, P., Benesch, M., Moser, A. & Schwinger, W. (2008). Hemophagocytic lymphohistiocytosis as severe adverse event of antineoplastic treatment in children. *Haematologica* Vol. 93 (No. 2): 291–294.

Machaczka, M., Vaktnäs, J., Klimkowska, M., Nahi, H. & Hägglund, H. (2010). Acquired HLH associated with multiple myeloma. *Med. Oncol.* Apr 1. [Epub]

Machaczka, M., Vaktnäs, J., Klimkowska, M. & Hägglund, H. (2011a). Malignancy-associated HLH in adults: a retrospective population-based analysis from a single center. *Leuk. Lymphoma* Vol. 52 (No. 4): 613–619.

Machaczka, M., Nahi, H., Karbach, H., Klimkowska, M. & Hägglund, H. (2011b). Successful treatment of recurrent malignancy-associated HLH with a modified HLH-94 immunochemotherapy and allogeneic SCT. *Med. Oncol.* Apr 29. [Epub]

Makay, B., Yilmaz, S., Türkyilmaz, Z., Unal, N., Oren, H. & Unsal, E. (2008). Etanercept for therapy-resistant macrophage activation syndrome. *Pediatr. Blood Cancer* Vol. 50 (No. 2): 419–421.

Marsh, R.A., Vaughn, G., Kim, M.O., Li, D., Jodele, S., Joshi, S., et al. (2010). Reduced-intensity conditioning significantly improves survival of patients with hemophagocytic lymphohistiocytosis undergoing allogeneic hematopoietic cell transplantation. *Blood* Vol. 116 (No. 26): 5824–5831.

Minegishi, M., Ohashi, Y., Kumaki, S., Sasahara, Y., Hayashi, T., Asada, H., et al. (2001). Successful umbilical cord blood transplantation from an unrelated donor for a patient with Epstein-Barr virus-associated hemophagocytic lymphohistiocytosis. *Bone Marrow Transplant.* Vol. 27 (No. 8): 883–886.

Mouy, R., Stephan, J.L., Pillet, P., Haddad, E., Hubert, P. & Prieur, A.M. (1996). Efficacy of cyclosporine A in the treatment of macrophage activation syndrome in juvenile arthritis: report of five cases. *J. Pediatr.* Vol. 129 (No. 5): 750-754.

Nagafuji, K., Nonami, A., Kumano, T., Kikushige, Y., Yoshimoto, G., Takenaka, K., et al. (2007). Perforin gene mutations in adult-onset hemophagocytic lymphohistiocytosis. *Haematologica* Vol. 92 (No. 7): 978–981.

Ohga, S., Kudo, K., Ishii, E., Honjo, S., Morimoto, A., Osugi, Y., et al. (2010). Hematopoietic SCT for familial hemophagocytic lymphohistiocytosis and EBV-associated HLH in Japan. *Pediatr. Blood Cancer* Vol. 54 (No. 2): 299–306.

Ohadi, M., Lalloz, M.R., Sham, P., Zhao, J., Dearlove, A.M., Shiach, C., et al. (1999). Localization of a gene for familial hemophagocytic lymphohistiocytosis at chromosome 9q21.3–22 by homozygosity mapping. *Am. J. Hum. Genet.* Vol. 64 (No. 1): 165–171.

Ouachèe-Chardin, M., Elie, C., de Saint Basile, G., Le Deist, F., Mahlaoui, N., Picard, C., et al. (2006). Hematopoietic stem cell transplantation in HLH: a single-center report of 48 patients. *Pediatrics* Vol. 117 (No. 4): e743–750.

Öst, Å., Nilsson-Ardnor, S., Henter, J.-I. (1998). Autopsy findings in 27 children with haemophagocytic lymphohistiocytosis. *Histopathology* Vol. 32 (No. 4): 310–316.

Osugi, Y., Hara, J., Tagawa, S., Takai, K., Hosoi, G., Matsuda, Y., et al. (1997). Cytokine production regulating Th1 and Th2 cytokines in hemophagocytic lymphohistiocytosis. *Blood.* Vol. 89 (No. 11): 4100–4103.

Parodi, A., Davì, S., Pringe, A.B., Pistorio, A., Ruperto, N., Magni-Manzoni, S., et al. Lupus Working Group of the Paediatric Rheumatology European Society. (2009). Macrophage activation syndrome in juvenile systemic lupus erythematosus: a multinational multicenter study of 38 patients. *Arthritis Rheum.* Vol. 60 (No. 11): 3388–3399.

Ramanan, A.V. & Baildam, E.M. (2002). Macrophage activation syndrome is hemophagocytic lymphohistiocytosis - need for the right terminology. *J. Rheumatol.* Vol. 29 (No. 5): 1105.

Rappaport, H. (1966). Tumors of the hematopoietic systems, *in Atlas of tumor pathology*, Armed Forces Institutes of Pathology, Washington DC, pp. 49-63.

Ravelli, A., De Benedetti, F., Viola, S. & Martini, A. (1996). Macrophage activation syndrome in systemic juvenile rheumatoid arthritis successfully treated with cyclosporine. *J. Pediatr.* Vol. 128 (No. 2): 275–278.

Ravelli, A., Magni-Manzoni, S., Pistorio, A., Besana, C., Foti, T., Ruperto, N., et al. (2005). Preliminary diagnostic guidelines for macrophage activation syndrome complicating systemic juvenile idiopathic arthritis. *J. Pediatr.* Vol. 146 (No. 5): 598–604.

Reiner, A.P. & Spivak, J.L. (1988). Hematophagic histiocytos. A report of 23 new patients and a review of the literature. *Medicine (Baltimore)* Vol. 67 (No. 6): 369–388.

Risdall, R.J., McKenna, R.W., Nesbit, M.E., Krivit, W., Balfour, H.H. Jr, Simmons, R.L., et al. (1979). Virus-associated hemophagocytic syndrome: a benign histiocytic proliferation distinct from malignant histiocytosis. *Cancer* Vol. 44 (No. 3): 993–1002.

Risdall, R.J., Brunning, R.D., Hernandez, J.I. & Gordon, D.H. (1984). Bacteria-associated hemophagocytic syndrome. *Cancer* Vol. 54 (No. 12): 2968–2972.

Sandhu, C., Chesney, A., Piliotis, E., Buckstein, R. & Koren, S. (2007). Macrophage activation syndrome after etanercept treatment. *J. Rheumatol.* Vol. 34 (No. 1): 241–242.

Sawhney, S., Woo, P. & Murray, K.J. (2001). Macrophage activation syndrome: a potentially fatal complication of rheumatic disorders. *Arch. Dis. Child.* Vol. 85 (No. 5): 421–426.

Schaer, D.J., Schleiffenbaum, B., Kurrer, M., Imhof, A., Bächli, E., Fehr, J., et al. (2005). Soluble hemoglobin-haptoglobin scavenger receptor CD163 as a lineage-specific marker in the reactive hemophagocytic syndrome. *Eur. J. Haematol.* Vol. 74 (No. 1): 6–10.

Scott, R.B. & Robb-Smith, A.H.T. (1939). Histiocytic medullary reticulosis. *Lancet* Vol. 234 (No. 6047): 194–198.

Sellmer, A., Stausbøl-Grøn, B., Krag-Olsen, B. & Herlin, T. (2010). Successful use of infliximab in macrophage activation syndrome with severe CNS involvement. *Scand. J. Rheumatol.* Vol. 40 (No. 2): 156–157.

Shabbir, M., Lucas, J., Lazarchick, J. & Shirai, K. (2010). Secondary hemophagocytic syndrome in adults: a case series of 18 patients in a single institution and a review of literature. *Hematol. Oncol.* Aug 30. [Epub]

Simonini, G., Pagnini, I., Innocenti, L., Calabri, G.B., De Martino, M. & Cimaz, R. (2010). Macrophage activation syndrome/hemophagocytic lymphohistiocytosis and Kawasaki disease. *Pediatr. Blood Cancer* Vol. 55 (No. 3): 592.

Sovinz, P., Schwinger, W., Lackner, H., Benesch, M., Moser, A., Raicht, A., et al. (2010). Severe Epstein-Barr virus encephalitis with hemophagocytic syndrome. Rapid clearance of virus following allogeneic stem cell transplantation from a seropositive donor. *Pediatr. Infect. Dis. J.* Vol. 29 (No. 6): 553–556.

Stephan, J.L., Kone-Paut, I., Galambrun, C., Mouy, R., Bader-Meunier, B. & Prieur, A.M. (2001). Reactive haemophagocytic syndrome in children with inflammatory disorders. A study of 24 patients. *Rheumatology (Oxford)* Vol. 40 (No. 11): 1285–1292.

Stephan, J.L., Zeller, J., Hubert, P., Herbelin, C., Dayer, J.M. & Prieur, A.M. (1993). Macrophage activation syndrome and rheumatic disease in childhood: a report of four new cases. *Clin. Exp. Rheumatol.* Vol. 11 (No. 4): 451–456.

Stepp, S.E., Dufourcq-Lagelouse, R., Le Deist, F., Bhawan, S., Certain, S., Mathew, P.A., et al. (1999). Perforin gene defects in familial hemophagocytic lymphohistiocytosis. *Science* Vol. 286 (No. 5446): 1957–1959.

Titze, U., Janka, G., Schneider, E.M., Prall, F., Haffner, D. & Classen, C.F. (2009). HLH and Kawasaki disease: combined manifestation and differential diagnosis. *Pediatr. Blood Cancer* Vol. 53 (No. 3): 493–495.

Tong, H., Ren, Y., Liu, H., Xiao, F., Mai, W., Meng, H., et al. (2008). Clinical characteristics of T-cell lymphoma associated with hemophagocytic syndrome: comparison of T-cell lymphoma with and without hemophagocytic syndrome. *Leuk. Lymphoma* Vol. 49 (No. 1): 81–87.

Toubo, T., Suga, N., Ohga, S., Nomura, A., Onoe, Y., Takada, H., et al. (2004). Successful unrelated cord blood transplant for EBV-associated lymphoproliferative disease with hemophagocytic syndrome. *Int. J. Hematol.* Vol. 80 (No. 5): 458–462.

Tristano, A.G. (2008). MAS: a frequent but under-diagnosed complication associated with rheumatic diseases. *Med. Sci. Monit.* Vol. 14 (No. 3): RA27–36.

Tschistowitsch, T. & Bykova, O. (1928). Retikulose als eine systemerkrankung der blutbildenden organe. *Virchovs Arch.* Vol. 267 (No. 1): 91–105.

Verbsky, J.W. & Grossman, W.J. (2006). Hemophagocytic lymphohistiocytosis: diagnosis, pathophysiology, treatment, and future perspectives. *Ann. Med.* Vol. 38 (No. 1): 20–31.

Weiss, J.E. & Ilowite, N.T. (2007). Juvenile idiopathic arthritis. *Rheum. Dis. Clin. North Am.* Vol. 33 (No. 3): 441-470, vi.

Wong, K.F., Hui, P.K., Chan, J.K., Chan, Y.W. & Ha, S.Y. (1991). The acute lupus hemophagocytic syndrome. *Ann. Intern. Med.* Vol. 114 (No. 5): 387–390.

Wulffraat, N.M., Rijkers, G.T., Elst, E., Brooimans, R. & Kuis, W. (2003). Reduced perforin expression in systemic juvenile idiopathic arthritis is restored by autologous stem cell transplantation. *Rheumatology (Oxford)* Vol. 42 (No. 2): 375–379.

Yoon, H.S., Im, H.J., Moon, H.N., Lee, J.H., Kim, H.J., Yoo, K.H., et al. (2010). The outcome of hematopoietic stem cell transplantation in Korean children with hemophagocytic lymphohistiocytosis. *Pediatr. Transplant.* Vol. 14 (No. 6): 735–740.

Zhang, K., Biroschak, J., Glass, D.N., Thompson, S.D., Finkel, T., Passo, M.H., et al. (2008). Macrophage activation syndrome in patients with systemic juvenile idiopathic arthritis is associated with *MUNC13-4* polymorphism. *Arthritis Rheum.* Vol. 58 (No. 9): 2892–2896.

zur Stadt, U., Schmidt, S., Kasper, B., Beutel, K., Diler, A.S., Henter, J.-I., et al. (2005). Linkage of familial HLH (FHL) type-4 to chromosome 6q24 and identification of mutations in syntaxin 11. *Hum. Mol. Genet.* Vol. 14 (No. 6): 827–834.

zur Stadt, U., Rohr, J., Seifert, W., Koch, F., Grieve, S., Pagel, J., et al. (2009). Familial hemophagocytic lymphohistiocytosis type 5 (FHL-5) is caused by mutations in Munc18-2 and impaired binding to syntaxin 11. *Am. J. Hum. Genet.* Vol. 85 (No. 4): 482–492.

# 6

# Ocular Myasthenia Analysis of Diagnostic and Treatment Options

Austin Hake and Henry J. Kaminski
*Department of Neurology & Psychiatry, Saint Louis University, St. Louis, MO USA*

## 1. Introduction

Myasthenia gravis (MG) is an autoimmune disease of the neuromuscular junction caused by antibodies directed towards the skeletal muscle nicotinic acetylcholine receptor (AChR), the muscle specific kinase (MuSK), and perhaps as yet undefined antigens, which compromise neuromuscular transmission (Figure 1) (Vincent et al. 2001; Conti-Fine et al. 2006). The disorder has a distinct predilection for the ocular muscles - the extraocular muscles (EOM), which move the globe, and the levator palpebrae that elevates the eyelid (Kusner et al. 2006). MG may produce weakness of any skeletal muscle to varying degrees with the potential for a broad range of clinical presentations (Seybold 1999; Kuks and Oosterhuis 2003); however, almost all patients will have ocular manifestations during the disease course, and a large subset will have manifestations restricted to the ocular muscles, so-called ocular myasthenia (OM) (Kusner et al. 2006). Diagnostic tests for OM include clinical evaluations, serum autoantibodies, and electrophysiological evaluation, all of which differ in their diagnostic predictive value depending on whether a patient has generalized MG or OM (Roh et al. 2011). Treatment for OM includes well-studied modalities; however, none that are supported by rigorous, controlled trials. This analysis will discuss the ocular manifestations, diagnostic testing, and treament of OM, with a focus on the current evidence to support clinical decision-making (Luchanok and Kaminski 2008).

## 2. Epidemiology

MG has a prevalence of 20-400 per million based on large population studies, and OM comprises approximately 20% of all cases (Somnier et al. 1991; Phillips et al. 1992; Christensen et al. 1993; Phillips and Torner 1996; MacDonald et al. 2000; Casetta et al. 2010). The classic statement of the disease being of old men and young woman is true with an age distribution being bimodal with incidence peaks in the 20's for women and 40's for men (Phillips and Torner 1996; Grob 1999; Mantegazza et al. 2003; Vincent et al. 2003; Matsuda et al. 2005). OM is more likely to present at a later age and is more often seen in men (Gilbert and Savino 2007). In Asian populations, OM is more common and has a distinct predilection for a juvenile onset, quite different from that observed in European and American populations (Chiu et al. 1987; Hawkins et al. 1989; Wong et al. 1992). One study from South Africa found that OM in the black population was more likely to be treatment resistant than in the white (Heckmann et al. 2007).

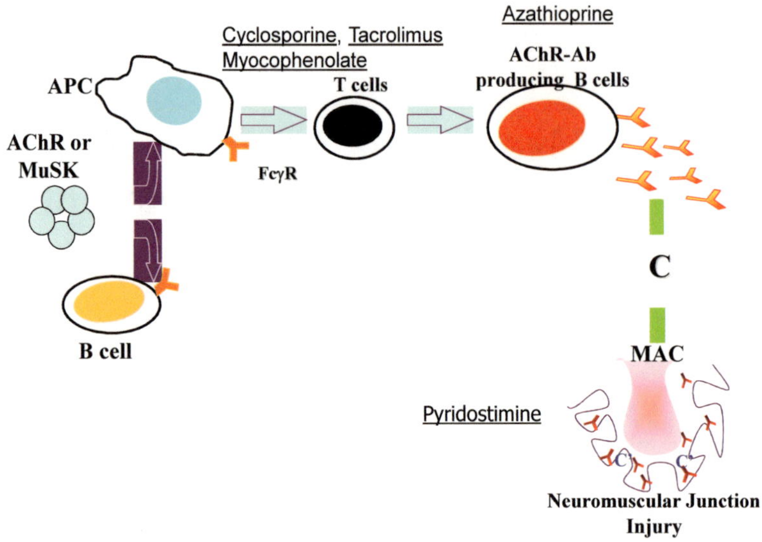


Fig. 1. Summary of Myasthenia Gravis Pathogenesis. Antibodies directed at neuromuscular junction proteins are produced by B cells under T cell regulation. Antibodies compromise the AChR density at the neuromuscular junction and thereby impair neuromuscular transmission producing weakness. Treatments used for ocular myasthenia are indicated. APC-antigen presenting cell.

## 3. Ocular manifestations of myasthenia gravis

Over seventy-five percent of MG patients initially present with ptosis or diplopia and almost all MG patients experience ocular manifestations sometime during the course of the disease (Beekman et al. 1997; Barton and Fouladvand 2000; Daroff and Benatar 2009). About half of patients who present with isolated ocular manifestations develop generalized weakness within six months and up to eighty percent will generalize within 2 years (Bever et al. 1983; Oosterhuis 1989; Kupersmith et al. 2003). It is likely that symptoms will remain restricted to the ocular muscles once a patient has had restricted ocular manifestations for over two years (Evoli et al. 1988; Oosterhuis 1989; Grob 1999; Verschuuren et al. 2010). The natural history of the disease impacts therapeutic decision-making.

The hallmark of MG manifestations is their variable nature, which may range in severity over a day, over weeks to months, and include periods of complete resolution. The variations in severity assist in diagnostic recognition of MG but may complicate clinical recognition, if a patient is examined at a time of relative good strength. Ptosis may be unilateral or bilateral, and usually differs in severity between lids. OM is the only diagnostic consideration in a patient with a history of alternating or recurrent painless ptosis (Daroff and Benatar 2009). Some patients do not immediately appreciate lid droop and complain primarily of blurred vision secondary to the lid's obstruction of the pupil. Due Hering's law of equal innervation, central compensation for unilateral ptosis may lead to hyper-retraction of a less affected lid leading to ocular irritation from exposure. When the ptotic lid is manually elevated, the retracted lid droops, a sign commonly considered specific for MG. The presence of Cogan's sign also strongly supports the diagnosis of MG. Cogan's sign is elicited by instructing the patient to look down and then rapidly return the eyes to primary gaze. During the refixation, the eyelid overshoots and appears retracted momentarily and then becomes ptotic again (Cogan 1965).

Other causes of ptosis may rarely be confused with OM. Senile ptosis and levator dehiscence are readily differentiated by absence of significant fluctuation. Chronic progressive external ophthalmoplegia produces symmetric ptosis and ophthalmoparesis, but with slow saccades which should distinguish it from OM (Barton et al. 1995; Leigh and Zee 1999; Hirano and DiMauro 2001). Brainstem disorders of the third nerve nuclear complex will usually have associated central nervous system pathology. Horner's syndrome is identified by miosis and elevation of the lower lid, while the ptosis in complete third nerve palsy is associated with pupillary dilatation. Clinically evident pupillary abnormalities *never* occur in MG, although subclinical alterations in pupillary constriction are reported (Tsiptsios et al. 2008).

Ophthalmoparesis is the second most common manifestation of OM. Most MG patients complain of frank double vision; however, complaints may include dizziness, gait instability, or visual blurring without significant complaints of diplopia. Symptoms may improve with closure of one eye. Nearly 90% of patients who present with diplopia have associated ptosis, and the combination should immediately lead to the consideration of MG as a diagnosis (Barton and Fouladvand 2000; Elrod and Weinberg 2004; Fouladvand et al. 2005; Daroff and Benatar 2009). The eye movement abnormalities of MG mimic any peripheral or central nervous system ocular motility abnormality, and the degree of impairment varies from paralysis to subtle weakness with isolated nystagmus. Dissociated gaze-evoked nystagmus contralateral to a paretic eye may be observed in OM, which represents adaptive increases in innervational pulse. On dynamic testing, saccadic velocity may be preserved or increased in a limited range of movement (highly suggestive of MG) or intrasaccadic fatigue may be identified when a fast eye movement suddenly slows and becomes disconjugate in mid-flight (Khanna et al. 2007). Graves ophthalmopathy can mimic OM by presence of a restrictive deficit but ptosis is absent and if the patient is thyrotoxic, lid retraction may be present. Ptosis in a patient with Graves disease suggests the coexistence MG.

Orbicularis oculi weakness in combination with ptosis or ophthalmoparesis is a strong indicator of MG (Barton and Fouladvand 2000; Fouladvand et al. 2005). OM may mimic any pupil-sparing ocular motility disorder including fourth, sixth, and partial third nerve palsies, and central gaze disorders, such as internuclear ophthalmoplegia, the one and a half syndrome, and chronic progressive external ophthalmoplegia (Leigh and Zee 1999; Fouladvand et al. 2005; Daroff and Benatar 2009). Other neuromuscular junction disorders may mimic OM such as Lambert-Eaton myasthenic syndrome, botulism, or organophosphate poisoning, but purely ocular presentations of these disorders are rare. Appropriate history, physical examination, and ancillary testing should distinguish these conditions from MG.

## 4. Diagnostic testing

The diagnosis of OM may be made based on clinical grounds when no other conditions are consistent with a patient's examination and history. However, at times the clinical manifestations are difficult to detect by routine examination or may be absent at time of an examination leading to the need for additional evaluation. In addition, therapy for MG is not benign, and most clinicians and patients desire definitive confirmation of the diagnosis. However, the clinician must appreciate the limitations of tests used for diagnosis.

### 4.1 Edrophonium test

The edrophonium test involves intravenous infusion of edrophonium chloride, which inhibits the action of acetylcholinesterase (AChE). Procedures for edrophonium administration are not standardized, but in general, an initial 1 mg dose is given to assure patient tolerance followed by slow infusion over a few minutes until improvement in strength of a muscle is observed or a maximum of 10 mg is administered, although 7 mg is usually the maximum required to achieve a positive response (Kupersmith et al. 2003). Because of the objective nature of the response, unequivocal improvement in strength of a ocular muscle is the best endpoint to judge a test as positive (Daroff 1986).

Improvement of ptosis in response to edrophonium may be as high as 95% and the specificity has been reported at 97%; however EOM weakness does not respond as well to an edrophonium challenge (Nicholson GA 1983; Evoli et al. 1988; Kupersmith et al. 2003; Pascuzzi 2003). However, these high response rates have been determined in the controlled environments of academic institutions and not in standard clinical practices. The specificity of the edrophonium is likely to be high as long as the evaluation is performed by experienced clinicians. The potential for false positives exists, in the busy office practice, especially when the examiner rarely performs such evaluations. Other neuromuscular transmission disorders, such as Lambert-Eaton syndrome and botulism, can also cause a positive response to edrophonium (Oh SJ 1990), and false positive tests are reported with Guillain-Barre syndrome, compressive cranial neuropathies, and brain stem pathology (Pascuzzi 2003; Daroff and Benatar 2009).

There has been concern raised regarding the safety of edrophonium testing, which has led to some institutions requiring cardiac monitoring during the procedure. However, serious complications of bradycardia and syncope are rare (Ing et al. 2000), and it is the authors' opinion that cardiac monitoring is not necessary for most patients. Cardiac dysrhythmias and bronchial asthma are relative contraindications for edrophonium administration. Beyond muscarinic effects of tearing, salivation, sweating, abdominal cramps, and nausea, the test has limited morbidity (Pascuzzi 2003; Daroff and Benatar 2009).

### 4.2 Other clinical evaluations

The ice pack, rest, and sleep tests are non-pharmacological evaluations, which have been developed in order to avoid the need for edrophonium infusion and have close to no morbidity. However, the limitation of all these evaluations is that sensitivity and specificity assessments have been performed (Benatar 2006). All studies have small sample sizes. Inter-observer reliability is also not known.

The ice pack test is performed by placement of an ice pack across the eyes for two to five minutes followed by the examiner's assessment for improvement of ptosis or ocular motility deficit (Golnik et al. 1999; Ellis et al. 2000). Some patients may have difficulty tolerating the ice pack. The rest test requests the patient close their eyelids for up to 5 minutes, and then improvement in ptosis is assessed. For the sleep test, the patient lies with eyes closed in a quiet, dark room for 30 minutes and then ptosis and ophthalmoparesis are assessed for improvement. For the ice test, sensitivity of 80-97 percent and specificity of 97-100 percent are reported (Golnik 1997; Golnik et al. 1999; Benatar 2006). In a study of edrophonium-positive patients all had positive sleep tests as well (Odell et al. 1991). A small, randomized trial compared the ice test to the rest test and found that the median improvement of ptosis with the rest test was 2 mm and with the ice test 4.5 mm, but no improvement found among patients without MG (Kubis et al. 2000). One value of these tests is that they may be performed in patients in whom edrophonium infusion is contraindicated.

### 4.3 Serum autoantibody evaluation

Serum AChR antibody examinations are performed concurrently, or instead of the clinical tests described (Howard et al. 1987). The sensitivity of AChR antibodies testing for OM ranges between 39 and 71 percent. The specificity achieved is 95-100 percent (Benatar 2006). The detection of AChR antibodies may increase the risk of progression to generalized MG, but studies are inconsistent (Seybold 1999; Kupersmith et al. 2003) AChR antibodies have been detected without evidence of MG among patients with autoimmune liver disease, systemic lupus erythematosus, rheumatoid arthritis, Lambert Eaton syndrome, inflammatory neuropathies, amyotrophic lateral sclerosis, thyroid ophthalmopathy, thymoma patients, in patients taking D-penicillamine, and first degree relatives of patients with MG (Lennon 1997). Therefore, their detection is not absolutely specific for the diagnosis.

The binding AChR antibody is the most sensitive test and the studies described above dealt with the binding assay. The modulating AChR antibody may increase the diagnostic yield slightly for generalized MG patients but has not been assessed for OM. The modulating AChR antibody suffers from higher rates of false positives. The third AChR antibody evaluation is the blocking antibody, but it may only slightly increase sensitivity of the binding assay. Therefore, the authors generally only order the binding AChR antibody examination.

About a three percent of patients with generalized MG have antibodies against MuSK, a neuromuscular junction protein that provides the clustering signal for AChR (Hoch et al. 2001; Liyanage et al. 2002; Evoli et al. 2003; Vincent et al. 2003; Zhou et al. 2004). Rare cases of pure OM in association with MuSK antibodies are described (Caress et al. 2005; Bennett et al. 2006; Chan and Orrison 2007); however, large case series of MuSK antibody positive patients have not identified OM patients, but patients may present with ocular manifestions (Evoli et al. 2003; Zhou et al. 2004). MuSK examinations are about 16 times the cost of the binding AChR antibody test and therefore, should not be routinely requested unless clinically indicated.

Patients with clinical symptoms of MG with electrophysiological evidence of neuromuscular junction impairment, but no evidence of serum autoantibodies are deemed to have seronegative MG (Argov 2010; Roh et al. 2011). Up to half of OM patients do not have detectable antibodies to the AChR. A small percentage (15%) of initially seronegative patients may become seropositive for AChR antibodies later in the disease course (Chan et al. 2007). With specialized testing two-thirds of patients with generalized MG without traditional antibodies for AChR or MuSK are positive for low-affinity IgG autoantibodies to AChR (Leite et al. 2008). Therefore, even in OM patients pathogenic antibodies may be directed against the AChR but be undetected by standard testing.

### 4.4 Electrodiagnosis

A significant proportion of OM patients will have negative AChR antibody evaluations and have non-definitive clinical assessments. Electrodiagnostic testing needs then to be performed to objectively confirm a diagnosis of OM. Repetitive nerve stimulation measures the action potential amplitude produced by repetitive low frequency stimulation. A decrement of 10% or more is considered positive for MG (Oh SJ 1992). The sensitivity of repetitive nerve stimulation for OM is poor (11-54 percent), but specificity is high (89-98 percent) (Roh et al. 2011). Evaluation of the orbicularis oculi (especially the lower orbicularis oculi), orbicularis oris, or nasalis will increase the percentage of patients identified, but such evaluations are much more difficult to tolerate for patients than extremity evaluations (Mercelis and Merckaert 2011). Although identification of decremental responses in non-ocular muscles indicates subclinical disease in other muscles, the finding does not indicate the presence or predict progression to generalized MG.

Single fiber electromyography (SFEMG) involves repetitive measures of the time between action potentials of two fibers in a muscle during a slight contraction. Abnormalities occur because of a fiber's slowed transmission of an action potential because of a compromised endplate potential that does not reach threshold. A fiber may not be activated which produces a neuromuscular block. If the mean jitter - time between activation of all fiber pairs (or endplates) - exceeds the upper limit of normal for that muscle, or if more than 10% of pairs have jitter that exceeds the upper limit of jitter during voluntary activation, then the study is considered abnormal. SFEMG is 62 to 99 percent sensitive for detection of MG, and its specificity is reported to be from 66 to 98 percent (Ukachoke et al. 1994; de Entrambasaguas et al. 2007; Mercelis and Merckaert 2011); however, it implementation is limited due to the requirements of specially-trained, experienced examiners. Although it is labor-intensive, SFEMG should be considered in patients with a strong clinical suspicion for OM in which repetitive nerve stimulation is negative, due to its higher sensitivity (Srivastava et al. 2007). The SFEMG is also useful in ruling out myasthenic weakness. If the SFEMG is normal in a clinically weak muscle, then the weakness is not due to a neuromuscular transmission disorder (Sanders and Stalberg 1996; Katirji and Kaminski 2002; Meriggioli and Sanders 2004; Sanders 2004).

### 4.5 Other evaluations

When the clinician thinks the OM diagnosis is likely additional testing is necessary. Thyroid dysfunction is a common co-morbidity and therefore, it is appropriate to screen all OM patients for hypo- or hyperthyroidism. Identification of concurrent thyroid dysfunction may improve MG related weakness. If clinically indicated the co-existence of other autoimmune disorders should be evaluated, in particular pernicious anemia, Chest imaging should be performed to exclude thymoma although thymoma is rare in OM patients. In anticipation of immunosuppressive treatments, screening for tuberculosis is appropriate.

## 5. Treatment

The treatment goal for patients with OM is to produce normal vision with a minimum of adverse effects. Unfortunately, treatment of OM has not been subject to rigorous evaluation and longitudinal studies of the risks of chronic treatment do not exist. Also, the individual tolerance of patients needs to be considered in making treatment recommendations. Some patients with OM respond well to non-pharmacologic therapies that are often overlooked by neurologists. If non- pharmacologic therapies cannot provide adequate relief, acetylcholesterase are typically administered, but the majority of patients do not respond well, and immunosuppressive treatments are required (Table).

| Drug | Cost in USA | Mechanism of action |
|---|---|---|
| Pyridostigmine 60 mg tablets<br><br>Pyridostigmine 180 mg controlled release (time span) | $17.99 (30 tabs)<br><br>$137.99 (30) | Inhibits acetylcholinesterase at neuromuscular junction but also at muscarinic synapses |
| Prednisone<br>20 mg tablet | $11.99 (30) | Anti-inflammatory effects related to: a) redistribution of lymphocytes and reduction of production and differentiation, b) alterations of function of TNF, IL-1 and IL-2, c) inhibition of antigen processing and presentation by macrophage. |
| Immuran® 50 mg tablet<br>Azathioprine 50 mg tablet | $159.99 (30)<br><br>$27.99 (30) | Inhibits T- and B-cell proliferation |
| CellCept® 500 mg tablet<br>Mycophenolate mofetil 500 mg | $951.33 (100)<br><br>$129.99 (100) | Inhibits T- and B-cell proliferation through inhibition of guanosine nucleotide synthesis. Also produces: a) apoptosis of activated T-lymphocytes, b) decrease in cell adhesion molecules thus reducing lymphocyte recruitment, c) reduction of inducible NOS activity. |
| Prograf® 1 mg capsule<br>Tacrolimus 1 mg capsule | $409.94 (100)<br><br>$345.97 (100) | Calcineurin mediated pathway inhibition of T-cell and IL-2 production. Modulates the activity of T-cells, increases their apoptosis and may enhance T regulatory cells. |

* From Epocrates® online Searched April 2011.

Table 1. Ocular Myasthenia Treatment Options

### 5.1 Non-pharmaceutical treatment options

Ptosis may be improved by eyelid tape or crutches; however, patients often are intolerant of these approaches finding them uncomfortable. Also, scleral irritation may occur by exposure and lead to drying or abrasion. Visual occlusive devices, such as eye patches or opaque contact lenses, eliminate diplopia but reduce the visual field. Custom corrective lenses with prisms may correct diplopia temporarily, but because patients with OM have fluctuation of their visual axes, they require frequent correction of their prism. Prism therapy may be considered in patients with stable strabismus for six months to a year. Eye muscle surgery may be beneficial in rare patients when a fixed strabismus occurs and non-variable ptosis (Ohtsuki et al. 1996; Bentley et al. 2001). Botulinum toxin may also be considered to correct ocular alignment by chemodenervation of the involved extraocular muscles, but it must be used cautiously given the potential for systemic neuromuscular transmission blockade. Although there are challenges associated with the treatments, non-pharmacological options may be favored by some patients and be the only options for patients with disease resistant to pharmacological treatments.

Thymectomy is not generally indicated of OM, but case series do support its use (Schumm et al. 1985; Roberts et al. 2001). Of course, OM patients with a thymoma should undergo tumor removal and co-incident removal of the remainder of the thymus.

### 5.2 Acetylcholesterase inhibition

AChE inhibitors are the first line of medical treatment for OM, and pyridostigmine is the most commonly used drug in the class. While AChE inhibitors are effective for ptosis, diplopia is of often resistant to treatment (Sommer et al. 1993; Sommer et al. 1997; Mehndiratta et al. 2011). In some patients, unilateral ptosis "unmasks" ocular misalignment producing the symptom of diplopia which may be more troublesome for the patient (Daroff and Benatar 2009). Patients presenting with both ptosis and diplopia tend to have an inferior response to pyridostigmine (Chirapapaisan N 2007), and many OM patients move on to corticosteroid treatment(Kupersmith and Ying 2005).

Pyridostigmine 30-60 mg three to four times per day are typical starting doses and may be increased to 90 to 120 mg every 3-4 hours per day, if symptoms respond and adverse effects are kept to a minimum. Complications are primarily related to muscarinic effects, in particular abdominal cramps, nausea, vomiting and diarrhea, which occur in at least a third of patients (Beekman et al. 1997). Atropine or glycopyrrolate may be used to limit muscarinic activity. AChE inhibitor treatment should be used with caution in patients with bradycardia and prostatic hypertrophy. Patients with MG treated with AChR inhibitors, who have reactive airway disease, may have worsening of respiratory function secondary increased respiratory secretions leading to a false conclusion that respiratory insufficiency is caused by myasthenic weakness. An open label prospective trial demonstrated improved quality of life with the sustained-release form of pyridostigmine, which requires less frequent administration (Sieb and Kohler 2010). However, in the author's experience, more reliable improvements in strength occur with the standard preparation. Cholinergic weakness is often discussed but probably does not occur in this era that patients move to immunotherapy and do not rely on extremely high doses of AChE inhibitors. However, if a clinician is concerned that cholinergic weakness is a cause of worse OM symptoms, the AChE inhibitor may be reduced.

### 5.3 Corticosteroid treatment

Most patients will not receive significant benefit from the non-pharmacological and AChE inhibitor treatments and will choose to proceed to immunosuppressive treatment (Kupersmith and Ying 2005). Prednisone is the most frequently used immunosuppressive treatment for OM, and unless corticosteroids are contraindicated due to comorbities, it is the first-line immunosuppressive for OM. Although this is based on retrospective analysis(Benatar and Kaminski 2007, Bhanushali et al. 2008).

Dosing regimens vary but typically, 10-20 mg once a day is started and increased by 5-10 mg every 3 days until visual symptoms are improved significantly, which usually occurs in the first few weeks of therapy (Kupersmith et al. 2003; Mee et al. 2003; Papapetropoulos et al. 2003). 60-80 mg per day is a maximum dose. At times mild double vision that does not impair function may persist and need to be tolerated. After symptom resolution is maintained for a month, a slow taper is instituted at a rate of 5-10 mg per day every 2 weeks until a dose of 20 mg every day is achieved and the dose reductions slowed further. Rapid tapers often lead to recurrence of symptoms, but even with gradual dose reductions a large percentage of patients will have symptom recurrence. Patients will need an increase in dose when symptoms recur. Most patients require maintenance doses for years, which should be the lowest possible to prevent recurrence of visual complaints. More than three-quarters of patients experience significant improvement (Evoli et al. 1988; Sommer et al. 1997; Tackenberg et al. 2001; Kupersmith and Ying 2005). To reduce corticosteroid complications every other day dosing of prednisone may be used. Patients should be instructed to take a single morning dose, which mimics the diurnal peak of endogenous corticosteroid. Patients need to be educated about steroid side effects, which include weight gain, glucose tolerance, hypertension, osteoporosis, insomnia, anxiety, depression, and the numerous other complications of prednisone. The neurologist or ophthalmologist should work with the patient's primary care physician to monitor for complications.

Based on retrospective analysis, corticosteroids may delay or prevent the progression of OM to generalized MG (Agius 2000; Kaminski and Daroff 2000; Kupersmith 2004). However, there has not been a randomized, controlled trial to assess whether steroids have a disease modifying effect (Gilbert et al. 2007; Gilbert and Savino 2007). Future studies should consider visual outcome and quality of life to determine whether the benefits of corticosteriods outweigh the complications of chronic corticosteroid use.

### 5.4 Immunotherapy

Some patients will not respond to corticosteroids, have contraindications to their use, or have intolerable adverse effects necessitating use of other immunotherapies (Tackenberg et al. 2001). Assessment of efficacy for immunosuppressives specific to treatment for OM is extremely limited and is entirely based on retrospective investigation. Support for their use also derives from administration for the generalized disease, but these studies are also not robust. Azathioprine was demonstrated to reduce corticosteroid requirements in a randomized, placebo-controlled trial of generalized MG patients (Palace et al. 1998), and retrospective analyses support its efficacy in OM patients (Mertens et al. 1981; Matell 1987; Hohlfeld et al. 1988; Mantegazza et al. 1988). The clinician and the patient then need to consider immunosuppressant therapy, and here the evidence base relies on data from the generalized disease and expert opinion. For generalized MG, cyclosporine, tacrolimus, and mycophenolate mofetil have steroid sparing effects demonstrated in double-blind, placebo-controlled or retrospective studies (Sanders and Evoli 2010).

## 6. Conclusion

The analysis provides a focused review of clinical manifestations, diagnosis, and treatment of OM and highlights the significant limitations of the literature. Diagnosis of OM is generally straightforward, when the clinician thinks of the disorder. Confirmation of clinical diagnosis is challenging for OM. Serum AChR antibodies are found in only half of patients, and while the MuSK antibody is detected in about three percent of the generalized MG population, it is found only rarely among patients with isolated OM. Therefore the majority of patients lack detectable autoantibodies and confirmation of a neuromuscular transmission disorder relies on specialized, electrophysiological testing. Although expert opinion suggests that treatment is highly effective, significant knowledge gaps exist as to severity of treatment complications and over-all quality of life of patients with OM. Only through prospective trials or multi-center, rigorously constructed outcome databases will improvements in treatment be achieved.

## 7. References

Agius, M. A. (2000). Treatment of ocular myasthenia with corticosteroids: yes. *Arch Neurol* 57(5): pp. 750-751.

Argov, Z. (2010). Current approach to seronegative myasthenia. *Journal of Neurology* 258(1): pp. 14-18.

Barton, J. J. and Fouladvand, M. (2000). Ocular aspects of myasthenia gravis. *Semin Neurol* 20(1): pp. 7-20.

Barton, J. J., Jama, A. and Sharpe, J. A. (1995). Saccadic duration and intrasaccadic fatigue in myasthenic and nonmyasthenic ocular palsies. *Neurology* 45(11): pp. 2065-2072.

Beekman, R., Kuks, J. B. and Oosterhuis, H. J. (1997). Myasthenia gravis: diagnosis and follow-up of 100 consecutive patients. *J Neurol* 244(2): pp. 112-118.

Benatar, M. (2006). A systematic review of diagnostic studies in myasthenia gravis. *Neuromuscul Disord* 16(7): pp. 459-467.

Benatar, M. and Kaminski, H. J. (2007). Evidence report: the medical treatment of ocular myasthenia (an evidence-based review): report of the Quality Standards Subcommittee of the American Academy of Neurology. *Neurology* 68(24): pp. 2144-2149.

Bennett, D. L., Mills, K. R., Riordan-Eva, P., Barnes, P. R. and Rose, M. R. (2006). Anti-MuSK antibodies in a case of ocular myasthenia gravis. *J Neurol Neurosurg Psychiatry* 77(4): pp. 564-565.

Bentley, C. R., Dawson, E. and Lee, J. P. (2001). Active management in patients with ocular manifestations of myasthenia gravis. *Eye* 15(Pt 1): pp. 18-22.

Bever, C. T., Aquino, A. V., Penn, A. S., Lovelace, R. E. and Rowland, L. P. (1983). Prognosis of ocular myasthenia. *Ann Neurol* 14: pp. 516-519.

Bhanushali, M. J., Wuu, J. and Benatar, M. (2008). Treatment of ocular symptoms in myasthenia gravis. *Neurology* 71(17): pp. 1335-1341.

Caress, J. B., Hunt, C. H. and Batish, S. D. (2005). Anti-MuSK myasthenia gravis presenting with purely ocular findings. *Arch Neurol* 62(6): pp. 1002-1003.

Casetta, I., Groppo, E., Gennaro, R., Cesnik, E., Piccolo, L., Volpato, S. and Granieri, E. (2010). Myasthenia gravis: a changing pattern of incidence. *Journal of Neurology* 257(12): pp. 2015-2019.

Chan, J. W. and Orrison, W. W. (2007). Ocular myasthenia: a rare presentation with MuSK antibody and bilateral extraocular muscle atrophy. *Br J Ophthalmol* 91(6): pp. 842-843.

Chan, K. H., Lachance, D. H., Harper, C. M. and Lennon, V. A. (2007). Frequency of seronegativity in adult-acquired generalized myasthenia gravis. *Muscle & Nerve* 36(5): pp. 651-658.

Chirapapaisan N, T. S., Chuenkongkaew W (2007). Factors associated with insensitivity to pyridostigmine therapy in Thai patients with ocular myasthenia gravis. *Asian Pac J Allergy Immunol* 25(1): pp. 13-16.

Chiu, H.-C., Vincent, A., Nemsom-Davis, J., Hsieh, K.-H. and Hung, T.-p. (1987). Myasthenia gravis: population differences in disease expression and acetylcholine receptor antibody titers between Chinese and Caucasians. *Neurology* 37: pp. 1854-1857.

Christensen, P., Jensen, T., Tsiropoulos, I., Sorensen, T., Kjaer, M., Hojer-Pedersen, E., Rasmussen, M., Lehfeldt, E. and de Fine Olivarius, B. (1993). Incidence and prevalence of myasthenia gravis in western Denmark 1975 to 1989. *Neurology* 43: pp. 1779-1783.

Cogan, D. (1965). Myasthenia gravis: a review of the disease and a description of lid twitch as a characteristic sign. *Arch Ophthalmol*(74): pp. 217–221.

Conti-Fine, B. M., Milani, M. and Kaminski, H. J. (2006). Myasthenia gravis: past, present, and future. *J Clin Invest* 116(11): pp. 2843-2854.

Daroff, R. and Benatar, M. (2009). Ocular Myasthenia. Myasthenia Gravis and Related Disorders. H. J. Kaminski. Totowa, NJ, Humana Press: 95-104.

Daroff, R. B. (1986). The office tensilon test for ocular myasthenia gravis. *Arch Neurol* 43: pp. 843-844.

de Entrambasaguas, M., Lopez-Bernabe, R. and Lopez-Alemany, M. (2007). [Ocular myasthenia gravis: diagnostic aspects and evolution]. *Rev Neurol* 44(7): pp. 397-403.

Ellis, F. D., Hoyt, C. S., Ellis, F. J., Jeffery, A. R. and Sondhi, N. (2000). Extraocular muscle responses to orbital cooling (ice test) for ocular myasthenia gravis diagnosis. *J Aapos* 4(5): pp. 271-281.

Elrod, R. D. and Weinberg, D. A. (2004). Ocular myasthenia gravis. *Ophthalmol Clin North Am* 17(3): pp. 275-309; v.

Evoli, A., Tonali, P., Bartoccioni, E. and LoMonaco, M. (1988). Ocular myasthenia: Diagnostic and therapeutic problems. *Acta Neurol Scand* 77: pp. 31-35.

Evoli, A., Tonali, P. A., Padua, L., Monaco, M. L., Scuderi, F., Batocchi, A. P., Marino, M. and Bartoccioni, E. (2003). Clinical correlates with anti-MuSK antibodies in generalized seronegative myasthenia gravis. *Brain* 126(Pt 10): pp. 2304-2311.

Fouladvand, M., Ledoux, D. and Barton, J. S. (2005). Ocular Myasthenia Gravis. *Comprehensive Opthalmology Update* 6: pp. 25-36.

Gilbert, M. E., De Sousa, E. A. and Savino, P. J. (2007). Ocular Myasthenia Gravis treatment: the case against prednisone therapy and thymectomy. *Arch Neurol* 64(12): pp. 1790-1792.

Gilbert, M. E. and Savino, P. J. (2007). Ocular myasthenia gravis. *Int Ophthalmol Clin* 47(4): pp. 93-103, ix.

Golnik, K. (1997). An ice test for the diagnosis of myasthenia gravis. *Ophthalmology* 106(7): pp. 1282-1286.

Golnik, K. C., Pena, R., Lee, A. G. and Eggenberger, E. R. (1999). An ice test for the diagnosis of myasthenia gravis. *Ophthalmology* 106(7): pp. 1282-1286.

Grob, D. (1999). Natural History of Myasthenia Gravis. Myasthenia Gravis and Myasthenic Disorders. A. G. Engel. New York, Oxford University Press: 131-154.

Hawkins, B. R., Yu, Y. L., Wong, V., Woo, E., Ip, M. S. and Dawkins, R. L. (1989). Possible evidence of a variant of myasthenia gravis based on HLA and acetylcholine receptor antibody in Chinese patients. *Quart J Med* 70: pp. 235-241.

Heckmann, J. M., Owen, E. P. and Little, F. (2007). Myasthenia gravis in South Africans: Racial differences in clinical manifestations. *Neuromuscul Disord.*

Hirano, M. and DiMauro, S. (2001). ANT1, Twinkle, POLG, and TP: New genes open our eyes to ophthalmoplegia. *Neurology* 57(12): pp. 2163-2165.

Hoch, W., McConville, J., Helms, S., Newsom-Davis, J., Melms, A. and Vincent, A. (2001). Auto-antibodies to the receptor tyrosine kinase MuSK in patients with myasthenia gravis without acetylcholine receptor antibodies. *Nat Med* 7(3): pp. 365-368.

Hohlfeld, R., Michels, M., Heininger, K., Besinger, U. and Toyka, K. V. (1988). Azathioprine toxicity during long-term immunosuppression of generalized myasthenia gravis. *Neurology* 38: pp. 258-261.

Howard, F. J., Lennon, V., Finley, J., Matsumoto, J. and Elveback, L. (1987). Clinical correlations of antibodies that bind, block, or modulate human acetylcholine receptors in myasthenia gravis. *Ann NY Acad Sci* 505: pp. 526-538.

Ing, E. B., Ing, S. Y., Ing, T. and Ramocki, J. A. (2000). The complication rate of edrophonium testing for suspected myasthenia gravis. *Can J Ophthalmol* 35(3): pp. 141-144; discussion 145.

Kaminski, H. J. and Daroff, R. B. (2000). Controversies in Neurology. Treatment of ocular myasthenia: steroids only when compelled. *Arch Neurol* 57: pp. 752-753.

Katirji, B. and Kaminski, H. J. (2002). An electrodiagnostic approach to the patient with neuromuscular junction disorder. *Neur Clin* 20: pp. 557-586.

Khanna, S., Liao, K., Kaminski, H. J., Tomsak, R. L., Joshi, A. and Leigh, R. J. (2007). Ocular myasthenia revisited: Insights from pseudo-internuclear ophthalmoplegia. *Journal of Neurology* 254(11): pp. 1569-1574.

Kubis, K. C., Danesh-Meyer, H. V., Savino, P. J. and Sergott, R. C. (2000). The ice test versus the rest test in myasthenia gravis. *Ophthalmology* 107(11): pp. 1995-1998.

Kuks, J. and Oosterhuis, H. J. G. H. (2003). Clinical Presentation and Epidemiology of Myasthenia Gravis. Myasthenia Gravis and Related Disorders. H. J. Kaminski. Totowa, NJ, Humana Press: 93-114.

Kupersmith, M. J. (2004). Does early treatment of ocular myasthenia gravis with prednisone reduce progression to generalized disease? *J Neurol Sci* 217(2): pp. 123-124.

Kupersmith, M. J., Latkany, R. and Homel, P. (2003). Development of generalized disease at 2 years in patients with ocular myasthenia gravis. *Arch Neurol* 60(2): pp. 243-248.

Kupersmith, M. J. and Ying, G. (2005). Ocular motor dysfunction and ptosis in ocular myasthenia gravis: effects of treatment. *Br J Ophthalmol* 89(10): pp. 1330-1334.

Kusner, L. L., Puwanant, A. and Kaminski, H. J. (2006). Ocular myasthenia: diagnosis, treatment, and pathogenesis. *Neurologist* 12(5): pp. 231-239.

Leigh, R. J. and Zee, D. S. (1999). The Neurology of Eye Movements. Philadelphia, F.A. Davis.

Leite, M. I., Jacob, S., Viegas, S., Cossins, J., Clover, L., Morgan, B. P., Beeson, D., Willcox, N. and Vincent, A. (2008). IgG1 antibodies to acetylcholine receptors in 'seronegative' myasthenia gravis. *Brain* 131(7): pp. 1940-1952.

Lennon, V. (1997). Serologic profile of myasthenia gravis and distinction from Lambert-Eaton myasthenic syndrome. *Neurology* 48 (Suppl 5): pp. S23-27.

Liyanage, Y., Hoch, W., Beeson, D. and Vincent, A. (2002). The agrin/muscle-specific kinase pathway: new targets for autoimmune and genetic disorders at the neuromuscular junction. *Muscle Nerve* 25(1): pp. 4-16.

Luchanok, U. and Kaminski, H. J. (2008). Ocular myasthenia: diagnostic and treatment recommendations and the evidence base. *Curr Opin Neurol* 21(1): pp. 8-15.

MacDonald, B. K., Cockerell, O. C., Sander, J. W. and Shorvon, S. D. (2000). The incidence and lifetime prevalence of neurological disorders in a prospective community-based study in the UK. *Brain* 123(Pt 4): pp. 665-676.

Mantegazza, R., Antozzi, C., Peluchetti, D., Sghirlanzoni, A. and Cornelio, F. (1988). Azathioprine as a single drug or in combination with steroids in the treatment of myasthenia gravis. *J Neurol* 235: pp. 449-453.

Mantegazza, R., Baggi, F., Antozzi, C., Confalonieri, P., Morandi, L., Bernasconi, P., Andreetta, F., Simoncini, O., Campanella, A., Beghi, E. and Cornelio, F. (2003). Myasthenia gravis (MG): epidemiological data and prognostic factors. *Ann N Y Acad Sci* 998: pp. 413-423.

Matell, G. (1987). Immunosuppressive drugs: azathioprine in the treatment of myasthenia gravis. *Ann N Y Acad Sci* 505: pp. 589-594.

Matsuda, M., Dohi-Iijima, N., Nakamura, A., Sekijima, Y., Morita, H., Matsuzawa, S., Sato, S., Yahikozawa, H., Tabata, K., Yanagawa, S. and Ikeda, S. (2005). Increase in incidence of elderly-onset patients with myasthenia gravis in Nagano Prefecture, Japan. *Intern Med* 44(6): pp. 572-577.

Mee, J., Paine, M., Byrne, E., King, J., Reardon, K. and O'Day, J. (2003). Immunotherapy of ocular myasthenia gravis reduces conversion to generalized myasthenia gravis. *J Neuroophthalmol* 23(4): pp. 251-255.

Mehndiratta, M. M., Pandey, S. and Kuntzer, T. (2011). Acetylcholinesterase inhibitor treatment for myasthenia gravis. *Cochrane Database Syst Rev* 2: pp. CD006986.

Mercelis, R. and Merckaert, V. (2011). Diagnostic utility of stimulated single-fiber electromyography of the orbicularis oculi muscle in patients with suspected ocular myasthenia. *Muscle & Nerve* 43(2): pp. 168-170.

Meriggioli, M. N. and Sanders, D. B. (2004). Myasthenia gravis: diagnosis. *Semin Neurol* 24(1): pp. 31-39.

Mertens, H. G., Hertel, G., Reuther, P. and Ricker, K. (1981). Effect of immunosuppressive drugs (azathioprine). *Ann N Y Acad Sci* 377: pp. 691-699.

Nicholson GA, M. J., Griffiths LR (1983). Comparison of diagnostic tests in myasthenia gravis. *Clin Exp Neurol*(19): pp. 45-49.

Odell, J. G., Winterkorn, J. M. S. and Behrens, M. M. (1991). The sleep test for myasthenia gravis. Safe alternative to Tensilon. *J Clin Neuro Opthalmol* 11: pp. 288-292.

Oh SJ, C. H. (1990). Edrophonium responsiveness not necessarily diagnostic of myasthenia gravis. *Muscle Nerve*(13): pp. 187-191.

Oh SJ, K. D., Kuruoglu R, et al (1992). Diagnostic sensitivity of the laboratory tests in myasthenia gravis. *Muscle Nerve*(15): pp. 720–724. indentation

Ohtsuki, H., Hasebe, S., Okano, M. and Furuse, T. (1996). Strabismus surgery in ocular myasthenia gravis. *Ophthalmologica* 210(2): pp. 95-100.

Oosterhuis, H. (1989). The natural course of myasthenia gravis. *J Neurol Neurosurg Psychiatry* 52: pp. 1121-1127.

Palace, J., Newsom-Davis, J. and Lecky, B. (1998). A randomized double-blind trial of prednisolone alone or with azathioprine in myasthenia gravis. Myasthenia Gravis Study Group. *Neurology* 50(6): pp. 1778-1783.

Papapetropoulos, T. H., Ellul, J. and Tsibri, E. (2003). Development of generalized myasthenia gravis in patients with ocular myasthenia gravis. *Arch Neurol* 60(10): pp. 1491-1492.

Pascuzzi, R. M. (2003). The edrophonium test. *Semin Neurol* 23(1): pp. 83-88.

Phillips, L., Torner, J., Anderson, M. and Cox, G. (1992). The epidemiology of myasthenia gravis in central and western Virginia. *Neurology* 42: pp. 1888-1893.

Phillips, L. H. and Torner, J. C. (1996). Epidemiologic evidence for a changing natural history of myasthenia gravis. *Neurology* 47: pp. 1233-1238.

Roberts, P. F., Venuta, F., Rendina, E., De Giacomo, T., Coloni, G. F., Follette, D. M., Richman, D. P. and Benfield, J. R. (2001). Thymectomy in the treatment of ocular myasthenia gravis. *J Thorac Cardiovasc Surg* 122(3): pp. 562-568.

Roh, H. S., Lee, S. Y. and Yoon, J. S. (2011). Comparison of clinical manifestations between patients with ocular myasthenia gravis and generalized myasthenia gravis. *Korean J Ophthalmol* 25(1): pp. 1-7.

Sanders, D. B. (2004). Electrophysiologic tests of neuromuscular transmission. *Suppl Clin Neurophysiol* 57: pp. 167-169.

Sanders, D. B. and Evoli, A. (2010). Immunosuppressive therapies in myasthenia gravis. *Autoimmunity* 43(5-6): pp. 428-435.

Sanders, D. B. and Stalberg, E. V. (1996). AAEM minimonograph #25: single-fiber electromyography. *Muscle Nerve* 19(9): pp. 1069-1083.

Schumm, F., Wiethölter, H., Fateh-Moghadam, A. and Dichgans, J. (1985). Thymectomy in myasthenia with pure ocular symptoms. *J Neurol Neurosurg Psychiatry* 48: pp. 332-337.

Seybold, M. E. (1999). Diagnosis of myasthenia gravis. Myasthenia gravis and myasthenic disorders. A. G. Engel. New York, Oxford University Press: 146-166.

Sieb, J. P. and Kohler, W. (2010). Benefits from sustained-release pyridostigmine bromide in myasthenia gravis: results of a prospective multicenter open-label trial. *Clin Neurol Neurosurg* 112(9): pp. 781-784.

Sommer, N., Melms, A., Weller, M. and Dichgans, J. (1993). Ocular myasthenia gravis, a critical review of clinical and pathophysiological aspects. *Doc Ophthalmol* 84: pp. 309-333.

Sommer, N., Sigg, B., Melms, A., Weller, M., Schepelmann, K., Herzau, V. and Dichgans, J. (1997). Ocular myasthenia gravis: response to long term immunosuppressive treatment. *J Neurol Neurosurg Psychiatry* 62: pp. 156-162.

Somnier, F., Keiding, N. and Paulson, O. (1991). Epidemiology of myasthenia gravis in Denmark: a longitudinal and comprehensive study. *Arch Neurol* 48: pp. 733-739.

Srivastava, A., Kalita, J. and Misra, U. K. (2007). A comparative study of single fiber electromyography and repetitive nerve stimulation in consecutive patients with myasthenia gravis. *Electromyogr Clin Neurophysiol* 47(2): pp. 93-96.

Tackenberg, B., Hemmer, B., Oertel, W. H. and Sommer, N. (2001). Immunosuppressive treatment of ocular myasthenia gravis.

Tsiptsios, D., Fotiou, D. F., Haidich, A. B., Brozou, G. C., Nakou, M., Giantselidis, C., Karlovasitou, A. and Fotiou, F. (2008). Evaluation of pupil mobility in patients with myasthenia gravis. *Electromyogr Clin Neurophysiol* 48(5): pp. 209-218.

Ukachoke, C., Ashby, P., Basinski, A. and Sharpe, J. A. (1994). Usefulness of single fiber EMG for distinguishing neuromuscular from other causes of ocular muscle weakness. *Can J Neurol Sci* 21(2): pp. 125-128.

Verschuuren, J. J., Palace, J. and Gilhus, N. E. (2010). Clinical aspects of myasthenia explained. *Autoimmunity* 43(5-6): pp. 344-352.

Vincent, A., Bowen, J., Newsom-Davis, J. and McConville, J. (2003). Seronegative generalised myasthenia gravis: clinical features, antibodies, and their targets. *Lancet Neurol* 2(2): pp. 99-106.

Vincent, A., Clover, L., Buckley, C., Grimley Evans, J. and Rothwell, P. M. (2003). Evidence of underdiagnosis of myasthenia gravis in older people. *J Neurol Neurosurg Psychiatry* 74(8): pp. 1105-1108.

Vincent, A., Palace, J. and Hilton-Jones, D. (2001). Myasthenia gravis. *Lancet* 357(9274): pp. 2122-2128.

Wong, V., Hawkins, B. R. and Yu, Y. L. (1992). Myasthenia gravis in Hong Kong Chinese. *Acta Neurol Scand* 86: pp. 68-72.

Zhou, L., McConville, J., Chaudhry, V., Adams, R. N., Skolasky, R. L., Vincent, A. and Drachman, D. B. (2004). Clinical comparison of muscle-specific tyrosine kinase (MuSK) antibody-positive and -negative myasthenic patients. *Muscle Nerve* 30(1): pp. 55-60.

# 7

# Sweet Syndrome

Manuel Ginarte and Jaime Toribio
*Department of Dermatology. Complejo Hospitalario Universitario de Santiago. Faculty of Medicine. Santiago de Compostela, Spain*

## 1. Introduction

Sweet syndrome (SS) was first described by Robert Sweet in 1964 as acute febrile neutrophilic dermatosis (Sweet, 1966). Despite of the descriptive value of this denomination and the advice of Robert Sweet to keep it, the eponymous became prevalent on the time. SS was the first neutrofilic dermatosis (ND) described and it represents the paradigm of them. There are three key points of SS that are of interest not only for the dermatologists but also for the general practitioners: a) its marked clinical manifestations, b) the potential systemic repercussion of neutrophilic reaction, and c) its association with extracutaneos diseases, especially with malignancies.

## 2. Definition and classification

SS is a neutrophilic dermatosis characterized by specific clinical and histopathological manifestations. In fact, the best way of defining SS is based on its diagnostic criteria. Typically, SS appears abruptly with multiple, edematous, tender red plaques that are distributed bilaterally but asymmetrically in a febrile patient. The dermatopathological image shows a neutrophilic diffuse infiltrate without vasculitis located in upper dermis. Besides this typical picture, several clinical and histopathological variants have been described (table 1). The current classification of SS is based on the associated or trigger conditions and has clinical value for the management of these patients (table 2).

| |
|---|
| Transitional forms with other neutrophlic dermatosis |
| Located forms: dorsal hands and facial |
| Chronic recurrent neutrophilic dermatosis |
| Histiocytoid Sweet syndrome |

Table 1. Main clinical and histopathological subtypes of Sweet syndrome

| |
|---|
| Idiopatic |
| Parainflammatory |
| Paraneoplastic |
| Drug-induced |
| Associated to pregnancy |

Table 2. Classification of Sweet syndrome

## 3. Epidemiology

There is not reliable data regarding the incidence and prevalence of SS in general population. This relies on the fact that SS is an infrequent condition and the available data are based on series´ reports of and patient´s records from hospitals and dermatology departments. Moreover, it is necessary to take into account that the incidence of SS is determined by the incidence of infectious causes in general population (Hommel et al, 1993). With all these limitations, it has been reported that the incidence of SS in Scotland is 2.7 cases per million inhabitants and year (Kemmett & Hunter, 1990).
Gender distribution of SS is conditioned by the underlying or trigger disorder. There is a female predominance in parainflammatory and idiopathic cases which disappears in the infantile and paraneoplastic ones. There is no racial predilection.

## 4. Pathogenesis

The pathogenesis of SS remains to be definitively determined. Three possible pathogenical mechanisms have been considered, but none of them have been consistently demostrated (Requena, 2007): a) a type III hypersensitivity reaction, b) an activation of T cells by antigens or superantigens, and c) a disturbance of neutrophils´ function. It seems that genetic factors play a role since SS has been associated to several HLA, especially to Bw54 (Mizoguchi, 1988). Because of female predominace in parainflammatory and idiopathic cases and both pregnancy and contraconceptive pills implication in some cases of SS, hormonal background can also be involved in the development of SS.
Numerous cytokines are involved in the pathogenesis of this condition, including interleukins 1, 2, 3, 6, and 8 and gamma interferon, but the key substance is the granulocyte-colony stimulating factor (G-CSF). The administration of G-CSF can result in an outbreak of SS and this substance is elevated in serum of patients with SS and its levels are directly related with the disease activity (Kawakami et al, 2004; Ginarte & Toribio, 2010).

## 5. Clinical manifestations

### 5.1 Skin

SS begins as an alarming feature for the patient because of its abrupt onset, the presence of general malaise, and the pain or tenderness of the multiple erythematoedematous plaques (Gunawardena et al 1975; Kemmett & Hunter, 1990; Zamora et al 1990; Sitjas et al, 1993; von den Driesch 1994; Chan et al, 1994; Ginarte et al, 1997). The appearance of each individual lesion may be variable: the colour goes from vivid red to violaceus, sometimes with central paleness due to dermal edema. This edema can also be represented by pseudovesicular or true bullous lesions (figure 1). It is relatively frequent to oberve dome like lesions, especially on tenar and hypotenar eminences (in "mountain range") (figure 2). Individual lesions can also be pustular. Up to a third of the lesions have an annular appearance. Plaque´s size is variable but the majority range between 1 and 10 cm. The lesions are distributed bilaterally but asymmetrically. Common locations are face, neck, upper trunk, shoulders, and hands. On pretibial aspect of the legs, the lesions may exhibit a nodular morphology, which may be the clinical manifestation of a typical SS, a subcutaneous Sweet or an erythema nodosum (see forward). Pathergy may be present in up to 8% of the patients.

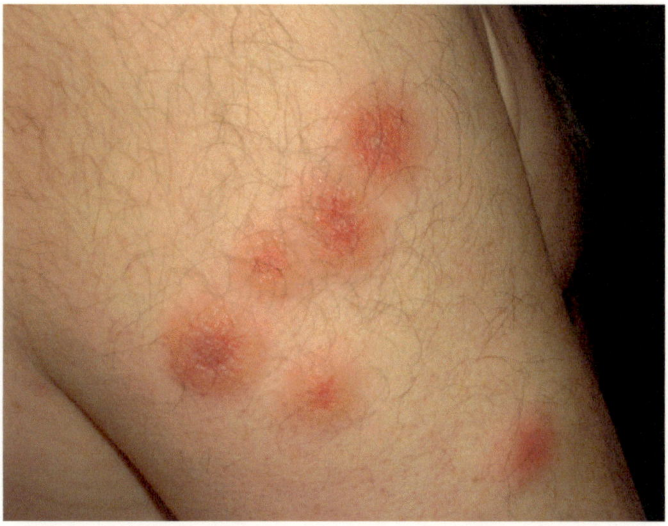

Fig. 1. Erythematous plaques with vesicular and bullous appearance due to a intense dermal edema.

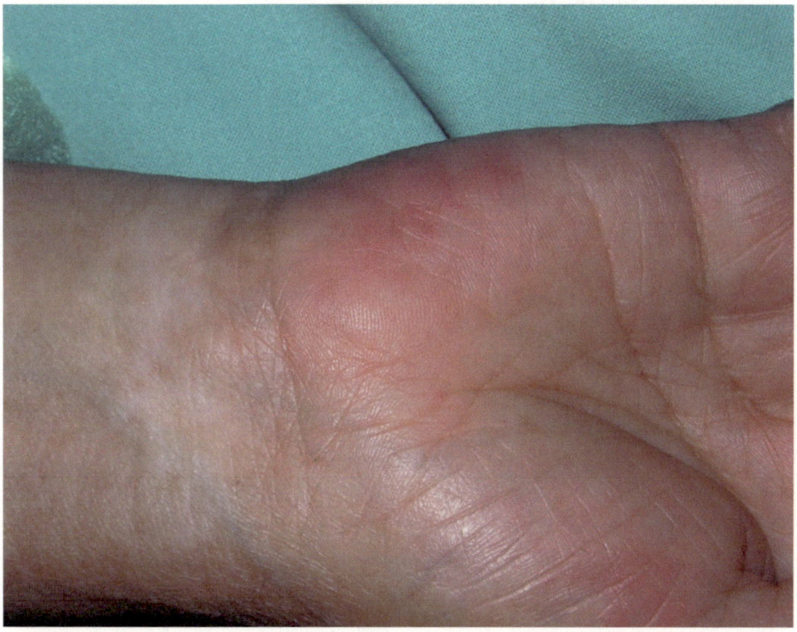

Fig. 2. The plaques on tenar and hypotenar skin have frequently a characteristic appearance of "montain range"

### 5.2 Mucous membranes

The mucous membranes are frequently involved, especially the ocular as conjunctivitis or epiescleritis (Gottlieb et al, 2008) (figure 3). Less frequent is the affectation of the oral mucosa, usually as aphtous ulcers.

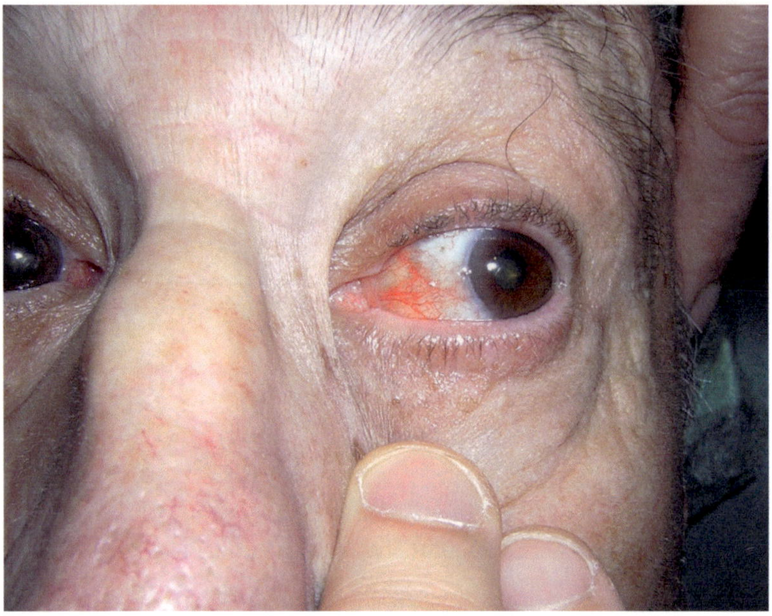

Fig. 3. Epiescleritis in a patient with Sweet syndrome

### 5.3 Laboratory findings

Analytic alterations are very frequent and they can have diagnostic significance. The most typical but not constant alteration is leukocytosis with neutrophilia that only in the 50% of the patients exceed by 10.0 x$10^3$ cells/$mm^3$. The majority of patients have the acute reactants (erythrocyte sedimentation rate and C-reactive protein) elevated and a third have mild alterations in urinary tests (haematuria, leukocyturia, and/or proteinuria) without affectation of renal function (Ginarte et al, 1997). It is necessary to distinguish the laboratory findings related to SS from the analytic changes due to trigger or associated diseases. For example, the presence of anemia, trombocytosis and/or massive leukocytosis should force us to rule out an haematologic malignancy (Cohen & Kurzrock, 1993).

### 5.4 Extracutaneous manifestations

Frequently patients with SS have extracutaneous manifestations that can be caused by two different mechanisms: a) a systemic neutrophilic reaction that affects not only the skin but also internal organs, and b) a disease or trigger condition causing the SS. These two different possibilities make more difficult the management of the patients because it is hard to distinguish by means the clinical and routine complementary tests if an internal disorder is the cause or the consequence of the SS. For example, the existence of respiratory manifestations, pulmonary infiltrates in X-ray chest, fever and leukocytosis with neutrophilia in a patient with SS set the doubt between an infectious pneumonia or a neutrophilic pneumonitis (which has important practical consequences since their treatment is quite different, i.e., antibiotics versus glucocorticoids). Despite of its original denomination as acute febrile neutrophilic dermatosis, the fever is only present in 50 to 72% of the cases (Ginarte et al, 1997). Joint involvement appear in 37 to 51% of the patients, usually as arthralgias or, more rarely, as true arthritis, which is commonly located on knees and ankles. Neutrophilic infiltration of internal organs is less frequent. Although the infiltration of the majority of the organs has been reported, the most frequently affected are the lungs (up to 6% of the patient in a serie) (Sitjas et al, 1993). Pulmonary involvement expresses as neutrophilic alveolitis. In the literature there are abundant references about the neutrophilic affectation of internal organs, which may induce to think that it is a frequent event even though it is actually an uncommon fact. This situation is secondary to a bias in reporting the more extreme cases of SS. Nevertheless, the possibility of internal organ involvement in SS patients should always be taken in consideration and it is important distinguish it from other diseases or trigger factors (especially the infectious ones) since their clinical management is quite different. As neutrophilic internal organ involvement is relatively more frequent in paraneoplastic SS than in other subtypes of SS, its presence obligates us to rule out a malignancy (Cohen & Kurzrock, 1993). Table 3 shows the main extracutaneous manifestations of SS.

| ORGAN | CLINICAL MANIFESTATIONS | REFERENCES |
|---|---|---|
| Bones | Chronic recurrent osteomyelitis (in children) | Majeed et al, 1989; Marie et al, 1998 |
| Bowel | Neutrophilic bowel infiltration, pancolitis | McDermott et al, 2001; Fain et al, 1996 |
| Central nervous system | Neuro-Sweet | Hisanaga et al, 1999; Nobeyama & Kamide, 2003; Ramos et al, 2003; Hisanaga et al, 2005; Sobol et al, 2009; Watanabe et al, 2009 |
| Heart | Aortitis, myocarditis, cardiac insuficiency, isquemic cardiopathy | Muster et al, 1983; Shimizu, 1998; Guia et al, 1999; Dorenkamp et al, 2003 |
| Kindney | Glomerulonephritis, alterations of urinalysis | Christ et al, 1996 |
| Liver | Neutrophilic hepatitis, changes in liver function tests and analysis | Kemmett & Hunter, 1990; Zamora et al, 1990; Fett et al, 1995; Ginarte et al, 1997 |
| Lung | Neutrophilic alveolitis, pleural effusion; radiologic sterile infiltrates | Cohen & Kurzrock, 1992; Sitjas et al, 1993; Fett et al, 1995; Peters et al, 1998; Astudillo et al, 2006 |
| Muscle | Tendosinovitis, myositis, myalgias | Attias et al, 1995; Brown et al, 2002 |

Table 3. Systemic involvement in Sweet syndrome

## 6. Characteristics of the subsets of SS

### 6.1 Idiopatic

Clasically it is the most frequent subset of SS and it represents up to 70% of the cases in old series (Requena, 2007). It predominates in women, especially in patients aged under 45 years. Most recently, this subset has become less prevalent possibly due to the better study of the patients (Corazza et al, 2008).

### 6.2 Parainflammatory

This group encompasses the SS associated or triggered by inflammatory and infectious conditions. There is a broad number of entities related with SS, some of them only based on isolated or few case reports, which makes difficult to assess the true power of the association (reviewed by Requena, 2007; von den Driesch, 1994; Cohen, 2007). The best documented inflammatory diseases associated with SS are Beçhet disease, bowel inflammatory disease, rheumatoid arthritis, lupus erythematous, and other autoimmune collagenosis. The infectious conditions more related with SS are oropharingeal infection (especially due to streptococcus pyogenes) and intestinal infections by *Salmonella* and *Yersinia*. Less constantly SS has been linked to other bacterial infections, tuberculosis, lepra, histoplasmosis, toxoplasmosis, HIV, and viral hepatitis. Recent reports suggest that the patients with previous oropharingeal infection have a less severe form of this syndrome (Borges Da Costa et al, 2009).

### 6.3 Paraneoplastic SS

It is a well established subset of SS with an obvious interest. Up to 20% of SS are paraneoplastic (Cohen & Kurzrock, 1993). The SS may precede (sometime in years) or follow the malignancy. It also may arise in relation with the recurrence of previous malignancy. There are some characteristics more related to paraneoplastic than to non-paraneoplastic SS: a) lack of female predominance; b) advanced age; c) presence of anemia and/or other hematological disturbances; d) extracutaneous involvement; e) atypical, pustular, or necrotic skin lesions (Cohen & Kurzrock, 1993; Watanabe et al, 2009). The majority of paraneoplastic SS are associated with hematologic malignancies, especially with acute myelogenous leukemia and myelodysplastic syndromes (Buck et al, 2008). About 15% of paraneoplastic SS are related with solid cancers, predominating breast, gastrointestinal, and genitourinary origin.

### 6.4 Drug-induced SS

More than 25 drugs have been related to the flare of SS, but the most frequently implicated is the granulocyte-colony stimulating factor (G-CSF). Other drugs that are commonly associated with the development of SS are trimethoprim-sulphamethoxazole, oral contraceptive pills, retinoids, minocicline, hydralazine, carbamacepine, bortezomib, and imatinib. As it is usual in other skin eruptions induced by drugs, the disease fades with the withdrawal of the drug and flares up if it is re-administrated.

### 6.5 SS associated with pregnancy

It is not unanimously considered as a subgroup of SS, but its existence should be taken into account due to its relative frequency.

## 7. Clinical variations and associations with other dermatoses

The typical cases of SS present very characteristics clinicopathological manifestations so that their diagnosis usually does not represent particular difficulty. Nevertheless, the SS may occasionally show a different clinical picture or it may be associated with other cutaneous signs making difficult to set the diagnosis and/or imply a change in the patient´s management. There is controversy about the need of describing such cases as "atypical" SS or as individualizing them as different entities.

### 7.1 Overlap and relationship with other ND

The group of ND represents a *continuum* of diseases that share clinical, histopathological, and causal features. The individualization of each entity is mainly based on clinical criteria. This fact explains that SS occasionally shares clinical characteristics with other ND (overlap), especially with generalized vesiculobullous forms of pyoderma gangrenosum. Other ND such as Behçet disese, bowel bypass syndrome, and neutrophilic eccrine hidradenitis may clinically resemble SS (Mizuashi et al, 2010). Sometimes patients with these features can only be diagnosed generically as suffering a ND, without a more specific denomination. In the same way, there have been reported patients suffering both SS and other ND (either simultaneously or sequentially) (Callen, 1985; Sherertz, 1987; Villanueva et al, 1989; Ginarte et al, 1997).

### 7.2 Chronic recurrent annular neutrophilic dermatosis

As its denomination indicates, it is a subtype of SS characterized by erythematoedematous plaques with a chronic and recurrent evolution. It has neither extracutaneous signs, nor fever or neutrophilia (Christensen et al, 1989; Romero et al, 1994; Cabanillas et al, 2008).

### 7.3 Subcutaneous fat involvement

Frequently, patients with SS have nodular lesions, especially on anterior aspects of the legs. These nodules are the clinical manifestation of the alteration of the subcutaneous fat, which can be originated by two different mechanisms. The first one called subcutaneous SS is characterized by a neutrophilic inflammatory infiltrate located on subcutaneous fat (either exclusively or accompanied by dermal affectation). Such infiltrate is usually located in fat lobules, but occasionally it may be septal or mixed (Cohen & Kurzrock, 2003). In a recent study, subcutaneous SS was shown by 16% of the patients (Abbas et al, 2010). The second possibility of subcutaneous fat involvement in SS is the association between this syndrome and erythema nodosum. This association is relatively frequent (up to 30% of the cases) and can be explained because both entities share several common features: essentially both are reactive dermatoses triggered by similar stimuli and pathogenically mediated by neutrophils. They are also treated with similar treatments (Ginarte et al, 1997; Ginarte & Toribio, 2000; Ginarte & Toribio, 2007). Due to the different significance of subcutaneous SS and erythema nodosum, it is necessary to make a deep biopsy from one of the nodules.

### 7.4 Sweet syndrome in infancy

About 16% of SS appears in children (Abbas et al, 2010). Pediatric SS is similar to that in adult population, with only three differences: a) it is associated with immunodeficiency

(HIV infection and other immune disorders), b) it is less associated with malignancy (although it is necessary to investigate this condition), and c) it is particularly susceptible to recurrences (Mohr et al, 2010).

### 7.5 Located forms

It has been described as located subtypes of SS cases with clinical lesions limited to a particular body´s area. The neutrophilic dermatosis of the dorsal hands shows characteristics as much SS as pyoderma gangrenosum exclusively located in this area. There is a controversy about if this entity is a subtype of SS or it is an independient disease (Walling et al, 2006; Laguna et al, 2007; Takahama & Kanbe, 2010). The same consideration is discussed about the located form in facial region (Whittle et al, 1968).

## 8. Histopathology

It is very characteristic and one of the diagnostic criteria of SS: a diffuse infiltrate of neutrophils located in the upper half of the dermis accompanied by intense edema. This edema causes the clinical appearance of pseudovesicular or bullous plaques. Leukocytoclasia is frequently present and may be prominent, but obvious vasculitis (neutrophils and fibrin deposits into blood vessel walls) must be absent in order to set the diagnosis. Ocasionally swollen endothelial cells, scattered eosinophils (more typical of drug-induced SS), and epidermal exocytosis of neutrophils (even with formation of subcorneal pustules) can be observed. In older lesions the neutrophilic infiltrate is substituted by linfohistiocytic infiltrate (Jordaan, 1989). Requena et al (Requena et al, 2005; Requena, 2007) have described the called *histiocytoid Sweet syndrome*, characterized by a dermal infiltrate constituted by immature neutrophilic granulocytes that have an appearance indistinguishable from histiocytoid cells on optic microscopy with routine stains. The majority of this histiocytoid SS is associated with hematological malignancies, although it has recently been reported an histiocytoid SS induced by trimethoprim-sulfamethoxazole therapy with bone marrow granulocytic maturation arrest (Wu et al, 2008) and two patients with inflammatory bowel disease (Requena et al, 2005; Spencer et al, 2008). Immunohistochemical analysis is necessary when histyocites are present in SS in order to distinguish histiocytoid SS (immature neutrophils) from true histiocytes that can be present in the typical neutrophilic infiltrate, sometimes in a moderate or predominant amount (specially in older lesions) (Corazza et al, 2008).

## 9. Diagnosis

Typical forms of SS are easily diagnosed by means of criteria of Su and Liu published in 1986 (Su & Liu, 1986) (table 4). Von den Driesch provided a more evolved modification of these criteria in 1994 (von den Driesch, 1994) (table 5), but it has had less acceptation. As we previously indicated, there are patients with "atypical" SS, transitional forms of SS and other ND, as well as cases in which it is only possible to set a generic diagnosis of ND.

## 10. Differential diagnosis

As typical forms of SS exhibit a very characteristic clinicopathological picture they rarely cause problems with differential diagnosis. The disease that clinically more resembles SS is the erythema multiforme. Other clinical differential diagnosis are drug eruptions and Behçet disease. All of these entities can be ruled out by means of a skin biopsy. Other ND (atypical pyoderma gangrenosum, bowel bypass syndrome, neutrophilic eccrine hidradenitis), vasculitis (specially erythema elevatum diutinum), and erythema nodosum may occasionally set problems with differential diagnosis both from the histopathological and clinical points of view.

**Major criteria**

- Clinic criterium: abrupt onset of tender or painful erythematous or violaceus plaques or nodules
- Histopathological criterium: predominantly neutrophilic infiltration in the dermis without leukocytoclastic vasculitis

**Minor criteria**

- Preceded by fever or infections
- Accompanied by fever, arthralgia, conjunctivitis, or underlying malignancy
- Leukocitosis
- Good response to systemic steroids and not to antibiotics

The definite diagnosis of SS demands the fulfillment of both major criteria and at least two of the minor criteria

Table 4. Diagnostic criteria by Su y Liu (1986)

**Major criteria**

1. Clinical criterium: abrupt onset of tender or painful erythematous plaques or nodules occasionally with vesicles, pustules or bullae
2. Histopathological criterium: predominantly neutrophilic infiltration in the dermis without leukocytoclastic vasculitis

**Minor criteria**

1. Preceded by a nonspecific respiratory or gastrointestinal tract infection or vaccination or associated with:
   a. Inflammatory diseases such as chronic autoimmune disorders, infections
   b. Hemoproliferative disorders or solid malignant tumors
   c. Pregnancy
2. Accompanied by periods of general malaise and fever (>38°C)
3. Three of four of the following laboratory values during onset:
   a. ESR > 20 mm
   b. C-reactive protein positive
   c. Segmented-nuclear neutrophils and stabs > 70% in peripheral blood smear
   d. Leukocytosis > 8000
4. Excellent response to treatment with systemic corticosteroids or potassium iodide

Table 5. Diagnostic criteria by von den Driesch (1992)

1. Non-steroidal anti-inflammatory drugs: indometacin, naproxen
2. Tetracyclines: doxicycline, minocycline
3. Dapsone
4. Clofazimine
5. Cyclosporine

Table 6. Second-line therapies of Sweet syndrome.

## 11. Treatment

Nowadays, the first line therapies for SS are systemic corticosteroids, potassium iodide, and colchicine (Cohen, 2009). Systemic corticosteroids are the most widely used: the clinical response is so fast and brilliant that it is considered a diagnostic criterion (Su & Liu, 1986). The general malaise fades into hours and skin lesions into days (less than 10 days) (von den Driesch, 1994). Oral prednisone is given at a dosage of 0.5-1 mg/kg/day (in a single dose or divided in two doses). The dosage is progressively lowered during 3-6 weeks. Such brilliant response to prednisone is darken by the frequent recurrences: 20-30% of the patients will suffer recurrences after treatment withdrawal and up to 10% of the cases will have a chronic and recurrent evolution for more than 1 year (Kemmett & Hunter, 1990; Sitjas et al, 1993, von den Driesch, 1994; Ginarte et al, 1997). The recurrences respond well to a new cycle of systemic corticosteroids (Ginarte et al, 1997), but their use is limited by their long-term side effects. Another limitation of systemic corticosteroids is the potential existence of an active infection that may trigger the SS. It is important to ruled out such possiblity.

Potassium iodide is a therapy as fast and effective as systemic corticosteroids. In fact, the response to this agent was included in the diagnostic criteria by von den Driesch (von den Driesch, 1994). Systemic symptoms disappear within 24 to 48 hours and cutaneous plaques in as much as 1 week. The dosage of potassium iodide is 300 mg administrated orally, three times daily (or if it is used the Lugol saturated solution, 3 drops three times each day and then increasing progressively the dose to a maximum of 15 drops three times each day). The main adverse effects are gastrointestinal intolerance (nausea and/or diarrhea), hypotiroidism, and vasculitis (Horio et al, 1983).

The other first-line therapy for SS is colchicine. This drug is administered at a dosage of 0.5 mg, two or three times per day. It can be maintained from 2 to 4 weeks. About 90% of the patients respond favorably within a few days and its main limitation are the gastrointestinal side effects (nausea and/or diarrhea) (Maillard et al, 1999).

There have been reported favorable responses to a wide and heterogeneous group of drugs. The response to several of these drugs is only based in isolated case reports, so it must be considered with caution. Table 6 summarized the drugs most repeatedly pointed out in the literature (isolated case reports are not included). These drugs are considered second-line treatments, but it is important to keep them in mind because they may be an effective therapy in patients with frequent recurrences, intolerance or adverse effects to the first-line treatments. This fact is especially applicable to elderly or polymedicated patients.

Obviously, although it was not mentioned, it is also important to treat the underlying process when possible.

## 12. References

Abbas O, Kibbi A-G, Rubeiz N. (2010). Sweet's syndrome: Retrospective study of clinical and histologic features of 44 cases from a tertiary care center. *Int J Dermatol* 2010; 49: 1244-9. ISSN 0011-9059.

Astudillo L, Sailler L, Launay F, Josse AG, Lamant L, Couret B, Arlet-Suau E. (2006). Pulmonary involvement in Sweet's syndrome: a case report and review of the literature. *Int J Dermatol* 2006; 45: 677-680. ISSN 0011-9059.

Attias D, Laor R, Zuckermann E, Naschitz JE, Luria M, Misselevitch I,Boss JH. (1995). Acute neutrophilic myositis in Sweet's syndrome: late phase transformation into fibrosing myositis and panniculitis. *Hum Pathol* 1995; 26: 688-690. ISSN 0046-8177.

Borges Da Costa J, Silva R, Soares De Almeida L, Filipe P, Marques Gomes M. Sweet's syndrome: A retrospective study of 42 admitted patients in a Portuguese hospital. (2009). *Int J Dermatol* 2009; 48: 953-5. ISSN 0011-9059.

Brown AM, Davies MG, Hickling P. (2002). Recurrent tenosynovitis in Sweet's syndrome. *Rheumatology (Oxford)* 2002; 41: 1067-1069. ISSN 1462-0324.

Buck T, Gonzalez LM, Lambert WC, Schwartz RA. (2008). Sweet's syndrome with hematologic disorders: a review and reappraisal. *Int J Dermatol* 2008; 47: 775-82. ISSN 0011-9059.

Cabanillas M, Suárez-Amor O, Sánchez-Aguilar D, Pereiro MªM, Toribio J. (2008). Dermatosis neutrofílica crónica recurrente: una posible variante en el espectro de las dermatosis neutrofílicas. *Actas Dermosifiliogr* 2008; 99: 61-3. ISSN 0001-7310.

Callen JP. (1985). Acute febrile neutrophilic dermatosis (Sweet's syndrome) and the related conditions of "bowel bypass" syndrome and bullous pyoderma gangrenosum. *Dermatol Clin* 1985; 3: 153-63. ISSN 0733-8635.

Chan H-L, Lee Y-S, Kuo T-T. (1994). Sweet's syndrome: clinicopathologic study of eleven cases. *Int J Dermatol* 1994; 33: 425-432. ISSN 0011-9059.

Christ E, Linka A, Jacky E, Speich R, Marincek B, Schaffner A. (1996). Sweet's syndrome involving the musculoskeletal system during treatment of promyelocytic leukemia with all-trans retinoic acid. *Leukemia* 1996; 10: 731-734. ISSN 0887-6924.

Christensen OB, Holst R, Svensson A. (1989). Chronic recurrent annular neutrophilic dermatosis. An entity? *Acta Derm Venereol (Stockh)* 1989; 69: 415-8. ISSN 0001-5555.

Cohen PR, Kurzrock R. (1992). Extracutaneous manifestations of Sweet's syndrome: steroid-responsive culture-negative pulmonary lesions. *Am Rev Respir Dis* 1992, 146:269. ISSN 0003-0805.

Cohen PR, Kurzrock R. (1993). Sweet's syndrome and cancer. *Clin Dermatol* 1993; 11: 149-157. ISSN 0738-081X.

Cohen PR, Kurzrock R. (2003). Sweet's syndrome revisited: a review of disease concepts. *Int J Dermatol* 2003; 42: 761-78. ISSN 0011-9059.

Cohen PR. (2007). Sweet's syndrome - a comprehensive review of an acute febrile neutrophilic dermatosis. *Orphanet J Rare Dis* 2007; 2: 34. ISSN: 1750-1172.

Cohen PR. (2009). Neutrophilic dermatoses: a review of current treatment options. *Am J Clin Dermatol* 2009; 10: 301-12. ISSN: 1175-0561.

Corazza M, Lauriola MM, Broghi A, Marzola A, Virgili A. (2008). Sweet's syndrome: a retrospective clinical, histopathological and immunohistochemical analysis of 11 cases. *Acta Derm Venereol (Stockh)* 2008; 88: 601-6. ISSN 0001-5555.

Dorenkamp M, Weikert U, Meyer R, Schwimmbeck PL, Morguet AJ. (2003). Heart failure in acute febrile neutrophilic dermatosis. *Lancet* 2003; 362: 1374. ISSN 0140-6736.

Fain O, Mathieu E, Feton N, Sibony M, Sitbon M, Lejeune F, Thomas M. (1996). Intestinal involvement in Sweet's syndrome. *J Am Acad Dermatol* 1996; 35: 989-990. ISSN 0190-9622.

Fett DL, Gibson LE, Su WPD. (1995). Sweet's syndrome: systemic signs and symptoms and associated disorders. *Mayo Clin Proc* 1995; 70: 234-240. ISSN 0025-6196.

Ginarte M, Garcia-Doval I, Toribio J. (1997). Síndrome de Sweet: studio de 16 casos. *Med Clin (Barc)* 1997, 109:588-591. ISSN 0025-7753.

Ginarte M, Toribio J. (2000). Association of Sweet´s syndrome and erythema nodosum. *Arch Dermatol* 2000; 136: 673-674. ISSN 0003-987X.

Ginarte M, Toribio J. (2007). Sweet syndrome and erythema nodosum: two neutrophilic dermatoses? *Clin Rheumatol* 2007; 26: 1215-1216. ISSN 0770-3198 .

Ginarte M, Toribio J. (2010). Sobre la patogenia del síndrome de Sweet. *Med Clin (Barc)* 2010; 134: 424. ISSN 0025-7753.

Gottlieb CC, Mishra A, Belliveau D, Green P, Heathcote JG. (2008). Ocular involvement in acute febrile neutrophilic dermatosis (Sweet syndrome): new cases and review of the literature. *Surv Ophthalmol* 2008; 53: 219-26. ISSN 0039-6257.

Guia JM, Frias J, Castro FJ, Gracian M. (1999). Cardiovascular involvement in a boy with Sweet's syndrome. *Pediatr Cardiol* 1999; 20: 295-297. ISSN 0172-0643.

Gunawardena DA, Gunawardena KA, Ratnayaka RM, Vasanthanathan NS. (1975). The clinical spectrum of Sweet's syndrome (acute febrile neutrophilic dermatosis)-a report of eighteen cases. *Br J Dermatol* 1975; 92: 363-73. ISSN 0007-0963.

Hisanaga K, Hosokawa M, Sato N, Mochizuki H, Itoyama Y, Iwasaki Y. (1999). "Neuro-Sweet disease": benign recurrent encephalitis with neutrophilic dermatosis. *Arch Neurol* 1999; 56: 1010-1013. ISSN 0003-9942.

Hisanaga K, Iwasaki Y, Itoyama Y, Neuro-Sweet Disease Study Group. (2005). Neuro-Sweet disease: clinical manifestations and criteria for diagnosis. *Neurology* 2005; 64: 1756-1761. ISSN 0028-3878.

Hommel L, Harms M, Saurat JH. (1993). The incidence of Sweet's syndrome in Geneva. A retrospective study of 29 cases. *Dermatology* 1993; 187: 303-305. ISSN 1018-8665.

Horio T, Danno K, Okamoto H, Miyachi Y, Imamura S. (1983). Potassium iodide in erythema nodosum and other erythematous dermatoses. *J Am Acad Dermatol* 1983; 9: 77-81. ISSN 0190-9622.

Jordaan HF. (1989). Acute febrile neutrophilic dermatosis. A histopathological study of 37 patients and a review of the literature. *Am J Dermatopathol* 1989, 11:99-111. ISSN 0193-1091.

Kawakami T, Ohashi S, Kawa Y, Takahama H, Ito M, Soma Y, Mizoguchi M. (2004). Elevated serum granulocyte colony-stimulating factor levels in patients with active phase of Sweet syndrome and patients with active Behçet disease: implication in neutrophil apoptosis dysfunction. *Arch Dermatol* 2004; 140: 570-4. ISSN 0003-987X.

Kemmett D, Hunter JAA. (1990). Sweet's syndrome: a clinicopathologic review of twenty-nine cases. *J Am Acad Dermatol* 1990; 23: 503-507. ISSN 0190-9622.

Laguna C, Vilata JJ, Martín B. (2007). Dermatosis neutrofílica del dorso de manos. *Actas Dermosifiliogr* 2007; 98: 102-4. ISSN 0001-7310.

Maillard H, Leclech C, Peria P, Avenel-Audran M, Verret JL (1999). Colchicine for Sweet's syndrome. A study of 20 cases. *Br J Dermatol* 1999; 140: 565-566. ISSN 0007-0963 .

Majeed HA, Kalaawi M, Mohanty D, Teebi AS, Tunjekar MF, Al-Gharbawy F, Majeed SA, Al-Gazzar AH. (1989). Congenital dyserythropoietic anemia and chronic recurrent multifocal osteomyelitis in three related children and the association with Sweet's syndrome in two siblings. *J Pediatr* 1989; 115: 730-734. ISSN 0022-3476.

Marie I, Boyer A, Heron F, Joly P, Levesque H, Thomine E, Courtois H. (1998). Focal aseptic osteitis underlying neutrophilic dermatosis. *Br J Dermatol* 1998; 139: 744-745. ISSN 0007-0963

McDermott MB, Corbally MT, O'Marcaigh AS. Extracutaneous Sweet syndrome involving the gastrointestinal tract in a patient with Fanconi's anemia. (2001). *J Pediatr Hematol Oncol* 2001; 23: 59-62. ISSN 1077-4114.

Mizoguchi M, Matsuki K, Mochizuki M, Watanabe R, Ogawa K, Harada S, Hino H, Amagai M, Juji T. (1998). Human leukocyte antigen in Sweet's syndrome and its relationship to Behçet's disease. *Arch Dermatol* 1988; 124: 1069-73. ISSN 0003-987X.

Mizuashi M, Sugawara M, Tanita M, Aiba S. (2010). A case of pustular vasculopathy. An atypical variant of Sweet's syndrome? *Int J Dermatol* 2010; 49:1461-3. ISSN 0011-9059.

Mohr MR, Torosky CM, Hood AF, Cunnion KM, Fisher RG, Williams JV. (2010). Sweet syndrome in infancy. *Pediatr Dermatol* 2010; 27: 208-9. ISSN 0736-8046.

Muster AJ, Bharati S, Herman JJ, Esterly NB, Gonzales-Crussi F, Holbrook KA. (1983). Fatal cardiovascular disease and cutis laxa following acute febrile neutrophilic dermatosis. *J Pediatr* 1983; 102: 243-248. ISSN 0022-3476.

Nobeyama Y, Kamide R. (2003). Sweet's syndrome with neurologic manifestation: case report and literature review. *Int J Dermatol* 2003; 42: 438-443. ISSN 0011-9059.

Peters FPJ, Drent M, Verhaegh M, van Pampus ECM, Schouten HC. (1998). Myelodysplasia presenting with pulmonary manifestations associated with neutrophilic dermatosis. *Ann Hematol* 1998; 77:135-138. ISSN *0939-5555.*

Ramos JC, Sanz J, Oliveira E, Garcia M. (2003). Meningitis aséptica y síndrome de Sweet. *Med Clin (Barc)* 2003; 121: 437. ISSN 0025-7753.

Requena L, Kutzner H, Palmedo G, Pascual M, Fernández-Herrera J, Fraga J,García-Díez A, Yus ES. (2005). Histiocytoid Sweet syndrome: a dermal infiltration of immature neutrophilic granulocytes. *Arch Dermatol* 2005; 141: 834-42. ISSN 0003-987X.

Requena L. Síndrome de Sweet histiocitoide. (2007). En Agustín España. Fisiopatología de las enfermedades cutáneas V. Aula Médica. Madrid, 2007. Pág 61-108. ISBN 978-84-7885-444-8.

Romero G, López-Estebaranz JL, De PabloP, Ortiz JL, Vanaclocha F, Iglesias L. (1994). Dermatosis neutrofílica afebril crónica recurrente. *Actas Dermosifiliogr* 1994; 85: 305-308. ISSN 0001-7310.

Sherertz EF. (1987). Pyoderma gangrenosum versus acute febrile neutrophilic dermatosis (Sweet's síndrome). *Am J Med* 1987; 83: 1011-2. ISSN 0002-9343.

Shimizu K. (1998). Neutrophilic infiltration of the myocardium in a patient with myelodysplastic syndrome. *Am J Hematol* 1998; 58: 337-338. ISSN 0361-8609.

Sitjas D, Cuatrecasas M, De Moragas JM. (1993). Acute febrile neutrophilic dermatosis (Sweet's syndrome). *Int J Dermatol* 1993; 32: 261-268. ISSN 0011-9059.

Sobol UA, Sherman KL, Smith J, Nagda SN, Micetich K, Nickoloff BJ, Shoup MC. (2009).Sweet's syndrome with neurologic manifestations in a patient with esophageal adenocarcinoma: case report and review of the literature. *Int J Dermatol* 2009; 48: 1062-5. ISSN 0011-9059.

Spencer B, Nanavati A, Greene J, Butler DF. (2008).Dapsone-responsive histiocytoid Sweet's syndrome associated with Crohn's disease. *J Am Acad Dermatol* 2008; 59 (2 SUPPL.): S58-S60. ISSN 0190-9622.

Su WPD, Liu HNH. (1986). Diagnostic criteria for Sweet's syndrome. *Cutis* 1986, 37:167-174. ISSN 0011-4162.

Sweet RD. (1964). An acute febrile neutrophilic dermatosis. *Br J Dermatol* 1964; 76: 349-356. ISSN 0007-0963.

Takahama H, Kanbe T. (2010). Neutrophilic dermatosis of the dorsal hands: a case showing HLA B54, the marker of Sweet's syndrome. *Int J Dermatol* 2010; 49: 1079-80. ISSN 0011-9059.

Villanueva C, Monés J, Pujol R, Puig L, Such J, Sancho FJ. (1989). Erupción vesículopustulosa y síndrome de Sweet asociado a 2 exacerbaciones de colitis ulcerosa en una mujer de 76 años. *Med Clin (Barc)* 1989; 93: 298-300. ISSN 0025-7753.

von den Driesch P. (1994). Sweet's syndrome (acute febrile neutrophilic dermatosis). *J Am Acad Dermatol* 1994; 31: 535-556. ISSN 0190-9622.

Walling HW, Snipes CJ, Gerami P, Piette WW. (2006). The relationship between neutrophilic dermatosis of the dorsal hands and Sweet syndrome. *Arch Dermatol* 2006; 142: 57-63. ISSN 0003-987X.

Watanabe T, Nakashima K, Shindo M, Yoshida Y, Yamamoto O. (2009).Multiorgan involvement in Sweet's syndrome. *Clin Exp Dermatol* 2009; 34: e343-4. ISSN 0307-6938.

Whittle CH, Beck GA, Champion RH. (1968). Recurrent neutrophilic dermatisis of face: a variant of Sweet´s syndrome. *Br J Dermatol* 1968; 80: 806-810. ISSN 0007-0963.

Wu AJ, Rodgers T, Fullen DR. (2008). Drug-associated histiocytoid Sweet's syndrome: A true neutrophilic maturation arrest variant. *J Cutan Pathol* 2008; 35: 220-4. ISSN 0303-6987.

Zamora E, Martin L, de Castro A, Barat A. (1990). Síndrome de Sweet. Estudio de 10 casos y revisión de la literatura. *Rev Clin Esp* 1990, 186:264-269. ISSN 0014-2565.

# Part 2

## Diagnostics & Prognostics

# 8

# Validation of Protein Biomarkers to Advance the Management of Autoimmune Disorders

David S. Gibson[1,2], Sorcha Finnegan[1], Stephen Pennington[3], Ji Qiu[4], Joshua LaBaer[4], Madeleine E. Rooney[1] and Mark W. Duncan[2,5]
[1]*Centre of Infection and Immunity, Queen's University of Belfast,*
[2]*Division of Endocrinology, Metabolism and Diabetes, University of Colorado, Denver,*
[3]*Proteome Research Center, Conway Institute, University College Dublin, Dublin,*
[4]*Center for Personalized Diagnostics, Arizona State University, Tempe,*
[5]*Obesity Research Center, King Saud University,*
[1]*United Kingdom*
[2,4]*United States of America*
[3]*Ireland*
[5]*Saudi Arabia*

## 1. Introduction

Despite the anticipated boom stemming from proteomic investigations, the rate at which novel protein biomarkers are introduced into clinical practice has remained static over the past 20 years. The reality is that approaches to both discover and validate protein biomarkers remain inadequate, and consequently, many areas of medicine, including the broad field of autoimmune disorders, remain deprived of the tools essential for the optimal management of patients. Most importantly, there is a huge backlog of candidate biomarkers that are yet to undergo thorough investigation and validation to assess their clinical utility. A recent assessment of the situation has estimated that although many tens of thousands of publications claim biomarker discoveries, there are roughly only 100 routinely used in clinical practice (Poste, 2011).

This chapter reviews the potential applications of protein biomarkers to manage autoimmune diseases with a special focus on the transition from the biomarker discovery through to validation phases using proteomic strategies. We emphasize the importance of careful review of the discovery data, the critical roles of protein isoform verification, and the essential features of targeted and thorough validation. Ultimately, when these factors are appropriately considered and implemented, we are optimistic that autoimmune disorders can be transformed by omics technologies and personalized practice can become a reality.

### 1.1 Biochemical markers and their potential role in autoimmune disease

Biological markers are widely used in medicine and can provide an objective measure of normal and pathogenic processes or pharmacologic responses to a therapeutic intervention. By the term '*biological markers*' (or biomarkers) we mean an objective molecular indicator or surrogate of pathological processes which possess diagnostic, prognostic or predictive utility. These are distinct from *'clinical markers'* which rely on physical variables or symptoms such as joint count, pain assessment or radiological findings. Biomarker examples include: cardiovascular risk assessment through cholesterol checks; pituitary and target gland hormone determinations to assess endocrine function and dysfunction; hemoglobin A1c (HbA1c) evaluations to monitor blood glucose levels in diabetic patients; liver function tests (LFT) in liver disease; and, prostate-specific antigen (PSA) determinations to assess prostate cancer risk. Not surprisingly, there is considerable interest in developing additional clinical biomarkers in medicine; however, the path from their discovery to routine adoption is painstakingly complex and slow.

### 1.2 Why target protein biomarkers

Although genomic and transcriptomic methods are powerful, they cannot predict downstream events. Specifically, they can't predict what protein forms will be expressed in a particular tissue or biofluid, nor can they reliably estimate expressed protein levels. Because it is the gene products that contribute directly to physiological or pathological change, they alone provide the best clues to function in health and dysfunction in disease. Just as importantly, protein modifications including a plethora of post-translational changes are not evident upstream. As discussed later, proteins may require cleavage of a specific sequence to become biologically active, additional sidegroups may be added at specific amino acids including phosphorylation to propagate signal transduction or glycosylation to transport the molecule to a specific site. The analysis of hundreds if not thousands of proteins - proteomics - is therefore potentially the most illuminating of all multiplexed strategies.

Proteomics, however, is an imperfect science, and although its methods are rapidly evolving, it is important to acknowledge that all existing approaches have serious limitations. Notably, the available discovery tools offer poor precision, sensitivity, specificity and low throughput. An example of a low throughput proteomic platform is classic liquid chromatography separation of a single complex biological sample, coupled with electrospray ionization to generate of mass spectra. These limitations place severe constrains on study design (*e.g.*, small sample numbers) and they can lead investigators to place a disproportionate confidence in the data generated in a discovery setting. Regardless of these shortcomings, proteomic methods have been widely adopted and have generated many potential candidate markers. As we will illustrate, candidates identified using these techniques should be considered a set of ideas or leads from which the investigator can generate testable hypotheses. The study design and process of testing or validating these candidates is especially important if the test is to be applied in a clinical setting.

This chapter focuses on several key areas of the biomarker development process and uses rheumatoid arthritis as a case model of autoimmune disease for discussion. We first discuss the issue of clinical need, *i.e.,* how biomarkers *are currently* used in the practice of rheumatology what biomarkers might offer in *the future* in a clinical setting, then highlight some clinical scenarios describing considerations for study design. Because discovery methods have been reviewed elsewhere (Gibson & Rooney, 2007; Hu et al., 2006; Tilleman et al., 2005) our emphasis here is on describing and evaluating the targeted proteomic methods that are essential to candidate validation. It is the authors' belief that the task of validation has not received adequate attention. We are overwhelmed with discovery studies and data arising from them; validation approaches are infrequently reviewed and relatively little validation data have been reported. The significance of major barriers to their widespread clinical adoption is also briefly discussed. These challenges to new marker development and commercialization include factors such as study design, pre-analytical variables, data interpretation, bioinformatics, validation, ethics and commerce. While our focus is on protein biomarkers and proteomic methods in rheumatology, the principles we discuss are generally applicable to other analytes and areas.

### 1.3 Biomarkers currently used in the practice of rheumatology

The biomarkers currently used in the practice of rheumatology can be subdivided into three distinct molecular classes: nucleic acid, proteins, and metabolites. Some of these tests and their applications are included in Table 1. This is not an exhaustive list and while an invaluable armamentarium, it is limited in number, clinical utility and performance. With the exception of anti-CCP autoantibody and S100 proteins, the list has remained essentially static for the last 5-10 years. Additional potential biomarkers have been reported, but few, if any, have been adopted in routine practice. There is, however, no dispute that better tools are urgently required for both objective diagnosis and optimal management of rheumatoid arthritis.

### 1.4 The future: additional markers & rheumatology practice

Several areas of medicine lack objective, quantitative measures of a disease and its response to therapy and the inflammatory forms of arthritis are no exception. Below, we define three distinct stages in the clinical progression to chronic inflammatory disease exemplified by some autoimmune disorders and outline where and how biomarkers could aid in managing the RA patient.

i. *The pre-symptomatic stage*: Here asymptomatic individuals, especially those who are genetically susceptible to rheumatoid arthritis (RA), need to be screened for early indications of disease onset. Biochemical markers could remove uncertainty in detecting the disease in its early stages and would allow early and appropriate intervention. Such early detection could help clinicians minimize or even halt disease progression, reduce morbidity and mortality, and markedly lower the costs of health care delivery in rheumatology.

ii. *The early clinical stage*: In the early stages of rheumatic diseases patients may be symptomatic but there are insufficient clinical or laboratory findings to confirm the diagnosis. A few biomarkers exist which are helpful in predicting outcome at a population level, such as rheumatoid factor and, more recently, anti-cyclic citrullinated peptide antibodies (anti-CCP) for the diagnosis of rheumatoid arthritis (See Table 1). Clinicians believe that early diagnosis and treatment are essential for the best outcome. In the past, the presence of the biomarker, IgM rheumatoid factor (RF), has helped to identify patients likely to have more aggressive disease (Vocovsky et al., 2003). In the last decade, anti-CCP antibodies have been shown to predict a more aggressive disease course in very early disease (van Venrooij, et al., 2008). However, the relatively low sensitivity and specificity of their assay offers relatively low diagnostic sensitivity and this means that a significant minority of patients with aggressive disease cannot be identified (Kastbom et al., 2004; Lindqvist et al., 2005). Furthermore, neither RF nor anti-CCP antibodies are of any use in the other inflammatory arthritides of adulthood, such as psoriatic arthritis and ankylosing spondylitis, or for the vast majority of children with juvenile idiopathic arthritis.

| Marker | Molecular Class | Example Application |
|---|---|---|
| *Creatinine* | Metabolite | *Creatinine* is used together with liver enzyme determinations (AST and ATL) as an index of drug toxicity and kidney function (Anders et al., 2002). |
| *C-reactive protein (CRP)* | Protein | A plasma protein routinely measured as a non-specific index of acute inflammation. CRP levels are typically integrated into clinical response scores, such as DAS28, which help to titer drug dosage (Pepys & Hiirschfield, 2003). |
| *S100 proteins* | Protein | Phagocyte derived proteins found in a variety of inflammatory diseases , with the ability to discriminate between diseases (Wittkowski et al., 2008). |
| *Anti-nuclear antibody (ANA)* | Protein- Auto-antibody | Used along with other tests, ANA helps with the diagnosis of arthritides. ANA titers and nuclear stain patterns can vary between patients depending on the condition (≈ 95% of systemic lupus erythrematosis (SLE)) (Wilk, 2005). Specific subsets of ANA's can be used to distinguish the type of autoimmune disease, *e.g.*, Sjögren's syndrome. ANA positivity increases the risk of eye disease in juvenile idiopathic arthritis patients. |
| *Rheumatoid Factor (RF)* | Protein- Auto-antibody | RF antibodies target the Fc region of IgG and are detected in 60-80% of RA patients, though are present in other inflammatory and connective tissue diseases (Chen et al. , 1987).The presence of RF early in the course of RA is associated with more active disease (Nakamura, 2000). |
| *Anti-cyclic citrullinated peptide (CCP)* | Protein- Auto-antibody | Anti-CCP antibody positivity predicts the development of RA and may occur long before the onset of symptoms (Nielen, 2004). Anti-CCP is associated with severe erosive disease and can predict disease progression in RA patients (Meyer et al., 2003). |
| *Anti-Ds DNA antibodies* | Protein-Auto-antibody | Anti dsDNA antibodies are highly specific for the diagnosis of SLE with a specificity of 95% but with a low sensitivity of <60% (Kavanaugh et al., 2002). |
| *HLA-DR4 or HLA-DRB* | Nucleic acid-Gene | Human leukocyte antigen genes have been found to be associated with RA. This association is particularly strong for HLA-DRB-1 alleles which share a similar amino acid sequence known as the shared epitope (van der Horst-Bruinsma et al., 1999). The presence of these alleles both increases the risk of RA and associate with more severe disease (Wagner et al., 1997). |
| *PTPN22* | Nucleic acid-Gene | The protein tyrosine phosphatase, non-receptor 22 (PTPN22) allele is a major risk factor for several autoimmune diseases. The protein product increases the tyrosine dephosphorylation of T-cell receptor resulting in decreased signaling via this pathway (Vang et al., 2005). |
| *TRAF1/C5* | Nucleic acid-Gene | TNF-receptor-associated factor-1 is one of many single nucleotide polymorphisms involved in the pathway of tumour necrosis factor alpha. The protein encoded by TRAF1 mediates signal transduction from the family of TNF receptors (Kurreeman et al., 2007). Increased susceptibility to and severity of RA is associated with this SNP, by influencing TRAF1/C5 function. |
| *TLR/ TNFR/ NF-κB* | Nucleic Acid-Transcript | Pharmacogenomic tests which use cellular transcript measurements to predict drug response are yet to be implemented in the clinic. Interesting data has emerged on the association between anti-TNF antagonist response and genetic variation (Bowes et al., 2009; Potter et al., 2010). |

Table 1. Biomarkers routinely used in the diagnosis & treatment of arthritides and some potential future markers-arthritides.

iii. *The disease management stage*: Early commencement of effective therapy is essential if joint damage and other complications are to be avoided. Historically, monitoring response to treatment is a composite of clinical findings and laboratory markers such as erythrocyte sedimentation rate (ESR), C-reactive protein (CRP) and disease activity score (e.g. DAS28) . Treatment is modified according to these parameters. However disease response can take many months, indeed years. Thus by the time the patients disease is deemed unresponsive substantial joint damage can have occurred. The identification of biomarkers that would predict disease response would have an enormous impact on outcome. Treatment may also be discontinued due poor tolerability. Identifying such patients in advance would improve patient care and reduce stress. Biologic drugs, as third line therapy such as anti-TNF have revolutionised the treatment of rheumatic diseases and systematic reviews have confirmed their efficacy and relative safety (Alonso-Ruiz et al. 2008). However these drugs are extremely expensive. Months of treatment can be required before the clinician knows whether they are effective. This is both costly and inefficient. The identification of biomarkers that would predict the response of individual patients to these expensive agents would help patients, clinicians and funding agencies alike. Finally there are concerns associated with the use of such targeted therapy i.e. the risk of life threatening infections using and more worryingly the long term risk of malignancy (Bongartz et al. 2006). The ability to identify such patients in advance would protect them from such serious adverse reactions.

## 2. The proteomics biomarkers development pipeline

### 2.1 Overview

There is no dispute that new biomarkers would advance the diagnosis and management of autoimmune disorders. The ongoing challenge, however, is how to discover candidate markers and how to validate them, *i.e.*, define their performance characteristics when adopted in a routine clinical setting.

A major impetus for increased interest in biomarkers has been the introduction of the omics technologies. In a single study these allow interrogation of hundreds (or thousands) of independent variables, such as genes, mRNA, metabolites or proteins and given the volume of information generated from such studies, many have anticipated candidate biomarkers would flow quickly from each new investigation. The reality, however, is otherwise. Comparing the levels of hundreds (or thousands) of data points in several distinct groups, especially when the sample numbers are small, gives rise to many apparent differences, only some of which are related to biology. Chance alone gives rise to many apparent "distinguishing features" - the trick is identifying the biologically relevant differences and ignoring the others.

For example, consider a proteomics experiment in which 200 proteins are measured simultaneously in a control and a test sample. At $P < 0.05$, 10 proteins will appear to be different by chance alone and unrelated to the treatment or condition. This consideration is not presented to undermine the value or utility of omics research, but rather, to underscore the importance of verifying any observed differences in follow-up studies. In more conventional scientific studies it is typical to examine a single dependent variable, run replicates, and to use standard statistical approaches to analyze the outcomes.

Omics studies are very different. Data sets are typically of high dimensionality, but the sample size is small. There are typically very few if any replicates and any interesting trends are hidden within the combination the variables. Under these circumstances the probability of finding associations by random chance is high. Although multivariant statistics can help with the analysis of these complex data sets, there is no easy way out. Any single omics study is best considered as an observational investigation that aids in generating novel hypotheses that can direct their future studies. Contrary to what was hoped, the omics methods do not provide a fast-track to biomarkers or shortcut the scientific process. They do, however, allow an investigator to operate independent of existing knowledge and to be less dependent on insight, instinct or experience. A single omics study can provide data from which dozens of testable hypotheses can be formulated or, put another way, it can identify dozens of biomarker *candidates*. Accordingly, the validation of each candidate biomarker is analogous to hypothesis testing where the investigator sets out to falsify (or disprove) the claim that candidate "x" is a valid biomarker in defined clinical scenario "y".

In the sections that follow some of the other important components of the biomarker development pipeline are discussed and we highlight the primary concerns that are necessary to optimize the success of biomarker development.

### 2.2 The clinical objective and study design considerations

Several types of biomarkers can be developed, but in each instance the process requires a different study design and unique sample sets. Biomarker development in autoimmune disease must incorporate a cross-section of patients representing the full spectrum of the specific disorder, and given its complex and heterogeneous nature, a panel of markers, not a single marker, will likely be necessary to reflect all relevant clinical parameters. Depending on the groups incorporated into the study and the comparisons made, integrated panels of individual biomarkers may be identified that provide valuable screening/diagnostic, predictive or prognostic information.

*Screening biomarkers:* Biomarkers that can be used to screen and identify disease before the onset of any symptoms are the Holy Grail of autoimmune disease; however, their discovery and validation presents substantial challenges. While some of the biomarkers evident in symptomatic disease *may* be present early on in asymptomatic individuals, it is more likely that these will be low abundance and masked by more abundant, non-specific biomarkers of inflammatory and secondary processes related to the disease. Therefore, reliable identification of the biochemical events that earmark early stage, asymptomatic disease requires access to biobanks with adequate numbers of samples to give statistical power collected from affected individuals well before disease onset. (In the case of juvenile RA these samples should ideally be collected from birth onwards.) When samples are available from the same individual both before and after disease onset, patients can serve as their own controls and therefore changes characteristic of the disease can be measured against a relatively constant biochemical background. Sample sets for these studies are, however, difficult to come by and require substantial long-term logistical and financial investment. Consequently, a compromised study design incorporating a relevant control group and early stage (symptomatic) subjects is more commonly adopted to meet this objective.

*Diagnostic biomarkers:* Typically, a case-control approach is used in this setting, such that a cohort of disease-free controls is compared to a similarly-sized cohort of diseased subjects. Comparisons of this type require careful design and implementation because observed differences may be non-specific and associated with the consequences of end-stage disease, rather than related to RA itself. Although widely used, for this reason alone the case-control study design is frequently problematic. Case and control samples need to be age- and lifestyle-matched, detailed clinical histories must be available on both cohorts, and strict inclusion/exclusion criteria are required. The value of any markers identified by this approach, and especially those that are not specific to autoimmune disorders alone, can only be assessed through large-scale hypothesis-driven studies performed in a defined clinical setting.

*Prognostic or predictive biomarkers:* For a prognostic or predictive biomarker study, suitable samples must be available both before and after the measured outcome from each subject. Often these studies use samples collected from completed studies that addressed a different clinical question, but are then used to identify and track a molecular signature (biomarker profile) that may have predictive/prognostic value. (*i.e.,* They employ retrospective samples.) However, in all instances, prospective (purpose-driven) sample collection is preferred. Although logistically difficult, this approach affords greater control over pre-analytical variables including storage time, storage conditions and use of additives. With foresight and planning, a randomized controlled trial with longitudinal sample collection can incorporate multiple nested outcome studies relating, for example, to therapeutic response, disease progression or disease recurrence.

### 2.3 Samples and sampling considerations

It is important to state the obvious: a biomarker study can only be as good as the clinical samples and their associated records. If there are errors with annotation, if patient details are inaccurate, or if the samples themselves have not been collected and stored properly, the exercise of biomarker development may be futile (Poste, 2011). Although there are limited numbers of biobanks available at this time, thankfully, more and more investigators, research centers and commercial entities are committing to establishing and maintaining high-quality sample repositories linked to accurate clinical records.

With respect to samples, factors such as the timing from sample collection to freezer, the complexity and reproducibility of any sample handling steps, length of storage time, storage temperature and freeze-thaw cycles, may affect the stability of some analytes. For example, samples sourced from different cohorts at different locations may 'carry forward' pre-analytical background signals with discriminating features unrelated to the biology of the disease (Addona et al., 2009; Davis et al., 2010; Ransohoff, 2010). Ideally, samples should be processed immediately, then aliquoted into airtight tubes and frozen in liquid nitrogen or -70°C freezers. Similarly, multiple freeze-thaw cycles can affect the stability of potential biomarkers (Flower et al., 2000; Rai et al., 2005). Protease inhibition may help preserve sample integrity, but this approach is not without its complications. For example, irreversibly-binding to sample components can have undesirable downstream consequences.

Fluids or tissues proximal to the sites of pathology can act as biomarker sinks. As a result, these should also be considered, when available, alongside plasma or serum as a means of focusing the search on pathologically-relevant candidates. For example, in the case of arthritis, synovial fluid, cartilage and synovium are potential sources for biomarker discovery. Here protein variants unique to the site and pathology can be measured before they escape into plasma (Gibson et al., 2009).

Studies indicate that plasma is likely a better substrate for proteome analysis than serum due to the obfuscation of results associated with the high proportion (>40%) of clot-related proteins and peptides in serum (Haab et al., 2005; Rai et al., 2005; Tammen, 2005). Less invasive samples also amenable to protein biomarker discovery include urine, saliva and tear fluid. Although putative biomarkers can come from discovery work, candidates can also come from literature searches and genomic or transcriptomic mining. All candidates, however, must undergo subsequent verification and validation (Pepe et al., 2008).

### 2.4 Discovery strategies

Discovery strategies allow many analytes to be measured simultaneously (*i.e.,* multiplexed analysis). The objective is to identify qualitative and/or quantitative differences across distinct clinical phenotypes that are reproducible and can then be adopted in a clinical setting. As discussed previously, however, what is observed in a discovery setting could be an artifact of statistical chance or experimental bias, and any findings must be rigorously validated. Discovery is typically costly, slow (low-throughput) and labor-intensive. Further, because the methods are not optimized for any single analyte, their performance characteristics are compromised (*i.e.,* limited sensitivity, selectivity and precision). The methods are therefore only suitable to survey - they are not suited to efficient, precise and accurate quantification. When proteins are the targets of the discovery process then there are two orthogonal strategies that are adopted: peptide-centric and protein-centric.

*Peptide-centric (bottom-up or shotgun) strategies*: This approach begins with proteolytic digestion of proteins to peptides and the 'digest' is then subjected to fractionation (HPLC) and tandem mass spectrometry (Duncan et al., 2010; Aebersold & Mann, 2003; Chait, 2006). The tandem mass spectra are then converted to peptide sequences and their precursor proteins are "assumed" by computational approaches. Refinements of this approach sometimes incorporate fractionation prior to digestion and/or multiple stages of fractionation post digestion (Washburn et al., 2001; Wolters et al. 2001). The principal assumption of a bottom-up strategy is that the identity of intact proteins can be ascertained from their constituent peptide fragments. As discussed elsewhere, this assumption is frequently invalid (Duncan et al., 2010).

*Protein-centric (top-down) strategies*: With protein-centric approaches intact proteins are first separated, typically by 2D gel electrophoresis, then the proteins are isolated and identified by mass spectrometry. Typically identification involves enzymatic cleavage of each individual protein to peptides and then either: (a) the masses of the peptide products of each pure protein are determined (*via* single stage mass spectrometry); or (b) the tandem mass spectrum (fragmentation pattern) of one (or more) of the peptides is determined (*via* tandem mass spectrometry). One or both these data sets is/are then used to interrogate a database and identify the protein. Relative protein amounts can be determined from the gel by staining. Because a top-down approach retains the protein integrity, modifications and sequence variations can be investigated.

As we will illustrate, the discovery findings should be considered a set of leads that require meticulous validation, especially with respect to the utility of the biomarker(s) in a routine clinical setting.

### 2.5 Biostatistical considerations

Because proteomic studies of clinical samples can generate cumbersome data sets, bioinformaticians are frequently involved in study design (*e.g.,* patient selection and study size calculation) and the hunt for significant and reproducible patterns in the data. Their objective is to find reproducible differences which correlate with a defined clinical outcome and that are independent of the influence of experimental bias, over-fitting and statistical chance.

The incorporation of a randomization strategy in sample analysis reduces bias by accounting for the day-to-day variations in the analytical technique. Similarly, it is prudent to calibrate and record the performance characteristics of the instruments used in the analyses. Calibration in proteomic analyses entails, for example in mass spectrometry, initialising the mass accuracy to a standard mixture of purified proteins or peptides of known mass. Routine calibration of sensitive instruments subject to 'drift' in measurement over a period of time should become part of good laboratory practice. Further, in the discovery phase, the objective is to have sufficient sample numbers to provide confidence that the list of protein candidates is worthy of follow-up during the validation phase. Typically in this phase of biomarker development, the sample size is small due to the cost and time of analysis, and sometimes because of the difficulty associated with obtaining samples. However, the number of proteins (independent variables) measured in each sample is typically very large. This ratio of samples to variable size is contrary to the traditional application of multivariate statistics and leads to some unique considerations that have been discussed by others (Dowsey et al., 2009; Karp & Lilley, 2007). Conversely in the validation phase this relationship is inverted so that patient cohorts are much larger (typically 100's -1000's) and the number of biomarker candidates carried over from discovery are reduced depending on the strength of their relationship to the clinical outcome or measure being assessed. The costs incurred by the validation phase therefore sit in a multi-million dollar range far exceeding the costs of discovery. The financial implications alone may account for the relative dearth of publications on this phase as the main players, large pharmaceutical or diagnostic corporations, having invested large amounts of time and money likely strive to protect the resultant intellectual property prior to further clinical testing and pre-market approval.

Bias, or any discrimination occurring due to a non-biological signal, can potentially confound discovery. For example, spurious results may arise because of differences in how patient samples are collected, *e.g.*, type of blood collection tube, time taken to freeze sample, or the order in which the samples are analyzed. Over-fitting can occur when regression analysis tools are used to 'fit' (too) many variables to a limited set of outcomes. The discriminating 'pattern' or 'signature' then becomes an artifact of the patient cohorts. To resolve issues of bias, statistical analyses must consider the biology of the system being analyzed and take into account the assumptions and limitations of the methods (Ransohoff, 2009). Statistical tests capable of gauging the level of false positives across multiple comparisons include the student's unpaired t-test (for two group comparisons), ANOVA (for three or more group comparisons) and linear regression (for quantitative or correlative studies) (Dowsey et al., 2009). Alternatively, if the data are not normally distributed, non-parametric Mann Whitney and Kruskal-Wallis tests should be substituted (Karp & Lilley, 2007). These methods can be used to analyze the features one-at-a-time and then to compile a ranked list of them based on a combination of p values and effect size. As noted earlier, a longitudinal design can minimize the potential for bias relative to a typical case-control study. Nevertheless, false biomarker leads are common and therefore rigorous validation essential.

The false discovery rate (FDR) can also be calculated (Benjamini et al., 2003; Storey, 2003; Strimmer, 2008). By setting the FDR level, it is possible to diminish the risk of a false positive identification for a differentially-expressed protein, i.e., at $P \leq 0.05$, we expect only 5% false positives. However, by doing so, the process of discovery may be compromised by overly stringent criteria. Although proteins displaying the most dramatic changes may appear to be useful biomarkers, it is important to attempt to rationalize their changes to the pathology. For example, acute phase proteins are frequently identified in plasma or serum-based studies as 'specific' biomarkers of a wide range of chronic disorders, including arthritis and cancer but clearly they are not specific to any one disease (Addona et al., 2009).

Cross-validation procedures can be used to reduce false positives. In this instance one data set is used to build the model (called training) and a second data set generated from an independent patient cohort is used to assess the predictive accuracy of the model (called testing). Another commonly-used validation strategy is known as K-fold cross-validation where the analysis is repeated over many random splits of the data. For each analysis, a subset of the data is used to build K number of predictive models, with the remaining subset available for a test of predictive accuracy. Although useful initially after discovery, validation based on splitting a single data set is of limited use because confounding factors can introduce systematic biases into both training and test splits.

Given the issues noted above, it advisable to validate intial 'discoveries' on independent sample sets, perhaps incorporating analysis by orthogonal methods which are more amenable to the requirements of clinical throughput and precision (Dupuy & Simon, 2007). Re-analysis or meta-analysis using raw data coming from other research groups is another possibility, although data standards, such as the 'minimum information about a proteomics experiment' (MIAPE) (Taylor et al., 2007), often do not extend into the initial design of clinical studies. Consequently, detailed clinical data may not be captured and reported consistently for clinical proteomics experiments, limiting the ability of investigators to independently verify, combine or correlate data from multiple experiments.

For thorough validation, the number of patient samples required should be determined through the use of statistical tools that take into account the imprecision of the analytical method, inter-patient variability and the acceptable threshold of difference that is deemed significant for a given biomarker application (Ye et al., 2009). Patient numbers (biological replicates) and other statistical considerations of power have also been discussed in detail elsewhere (Cairns et al., 2009).

### 2.6 Feature selection and classifier assessment

Several multivariate analysis tools are available for the analysis of large multidimensional data sets and some of these have been arranged into commercial software packages. Visual tools, including principle component analysis, hierarchical cluster analysis and heat maps which display variance, relatedness and patterns in data (respectively), are also available and are useful preliminary aids in data analysis. These analyses stive to represent variance in a graphical fashion and give for example an overall view protein expression prevalence within outcome groups in the case of heat maps or 'relatedness' of expression levels between different proteins with hierarchical trees (Marengo et al. 2006; Marengo et al. 2008). Emphasis however, should be placed on using supervised or semi-supervised methods such as distribution free learning (kernel- based or Bayesian analysis) or support vector machine (SVM) which allow for advanced categorization and classification of multidimensional proteomic data with respect to clinical data. This process known as 'feature selection' and leads ultimately to the creation of a 'classifier' or biomarker driven algorithm specific to the disease and outcome being measured (Liu et al., 2009; Zhu et al., 2009). Since most protein expression profiles will likely not be correlated to a specific outcome, supervised methods screen out uninformative proteins and select protein combinations to develop a 'classifier'. A recent application of the SVM principle has been used to guide feature selection of exhaled peptides as potential biomarkers of asthma (Bloemen et al., 2011).

Depending on whether proteome studies are focused on biomarkers for (i) diagnosis (class discovery), (ii) prognosis (outcome-related) or (iii) prediction (supervised prediction), various rationales should be employed to generate and assess the reliability a classifier. Class discovery methods are best suited for grouping proteins into subsets that elucidate pathways with similar expression profiles across patient subgroups. In outcome-related studies, the goal is to identify which proteins have expression levels that correlate with outcomes grouped into discrete classes: for example, in arthritis patients with a good versus a bad prognosis. When prediction of patient outcome is the aim, supervised prediction methods that use a selected proteome profile are used to generate an algorithm based on individual profiles. In supervised class prediction studies, a totally independent cohort should be used for cross-validation purposes when rigorous testing of a predictive model is desired (Dupuy & Simon, 2007).

The statistical significance of a selected proteome 'classifier' gives an incomplete estimate of its predictive ability and potential clinical utility. The number of true and false positives or negatives should be presented allowing the calculation of sensitivity and specificity. This reveals clinically-relevant information on how the classifier performs in each outcome category. List of statistical tools and recommendations for their application have been reported (Dupuy & Simon, 2007; Karp & Lilley, 2007; Marengo et al. 2006). Depending on the clinical question there may however be multiple outcome measures that are not amenable to a simple binary classification system. Statistical evidence of prevalence and analytical limits of detection of a specific group of isoforms can then direct the study towards validation of candidate biomarkers in a much larger group of multi-center patient populations.

## 3. The biomarker development process

Three distinct phases can be delineated within a typical development pipeline: discovery, verification and validation. These can be further subdivided so there is a reduced number of candidates at each stage, each with an increased probability of utility [51]. In the subsequent sections we aim to clearly segregate these phases in the biomarker 'pipeline' and further expand on the vastly different requirements of each (Figure 1). This process is prefaced by a brief overview of pre-analytical factors which can introduce unwanted bias or variation.

### 3.1 The discovery phase

In the discovery phase, proteomic platforms are unsupervised and are used to highlight qualitative and/or quantitative differences in multiple proteins across distinct clinical phenotypes. The process of discovery is focused on assessing many candidates, while minimizing the probability of false positives and negatives.

Discovery by definition requires an analytical approach which does not preempt the identity of the biomarker candidates. Generally speaking as most discovery methods prioritise the measurement of as many proteins as possible they have inherently low throughput, are labor intensive and offer a low dynamic range. These characteristics preclude their use in later phases of the biomarker pipeline. It is also important to realize that as yet there is no single method available for looking at the complete complexity of the proteome within a given clinical sample. Because we are working with a relatively blunt set of tools in discovery we need to transition to more precise methods for validation.

A two-step approach to the discovery phase, though widely used, is not well defined in the literature. In the initial pilot exploration of a low number of individuals the aim is to gain a grasp of the variability of whole proteome being measured across the cohort, selecting a suitable sample type, optimizing the separation and quantification platform and ultimately calculating appropriate patient numbers to power a second (discovery) round with greater statistical confidence.

| Phase | Aim | Platform | Precision/ Accuracy | Sample Turnover |
|---|---|---|---|---|
| Candidate Discovery | Relative, Unsupervised | 2DE DIGE LC-MS | Low | Low |
| Specificity Verification | Qualititative, PTM Isoform Targeted | MS/MS | High | Low |
| Sensitivity Qualification | Quantitative, Prevalence, Classifier Test | ELISA MRM | High | Medium |
| Clinical Validation | Classifier Validated, Standardized, FDA Approved IVDMIA | MRM High Content Array MALDI profiling | High | High |

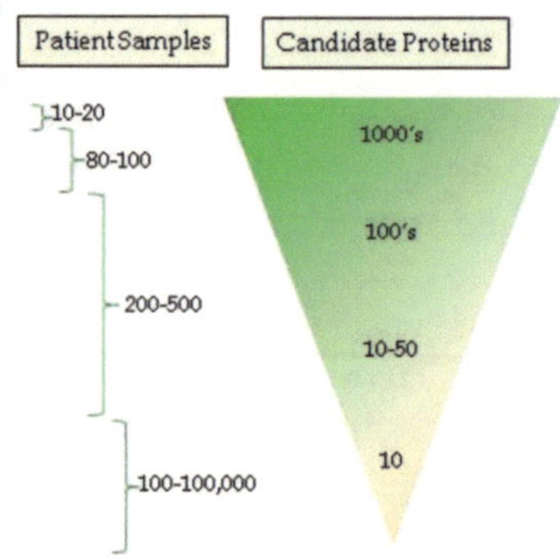


Fig. 1. Biomarker pipeline

Table describes the aim, the likely analytical platform and associated characteristics of each phase in an ideal biomarker discovery pipeline through verification to validation and final pre-market approval. The schema represents the increase in patient sample and decrease in candidate protein numbers as a biomarker study moves from discovery (two-step) through to validation phases; 2DE- 2-dimensional gel electrophoresis, DIGE- difference in-gel electrophoresis, LC-MS- liquid chromatography associated with mass spectrometry, ELISA- enzyme linked immuno-adsorbant assay, MRM- multiple reaction monitoring mass spectrometry, IVDMIA-in vitro diagnostic multivariate index assay.

### 3.2 Verification of protein modifications

Protein modifications are common but are frequently overlooked, especially during the discovery phase. Amongst the most significant modifications are covalent alternations to amino acids (*e.g.*, phosphorylation, nitration or redox changes) and covalent addition of large groups (*e.g.*, glycosylation). These modifications can have dramatic effects on protein function and may play a significant role in a range of arthritides and autoimmune disorders. Because most biomarker candidate identification strategies rely on peptide surrogate based mass spectrometry, there is added potential to characterize low abundance PTM variants. MALDI-TOF is an example mode of mass spectrometry can scrutinize multiple variants of a given protein in a concurrent, swift and relatively sensitive fashion. Several criteria determine accurate structural assignment and the quantification of specific modifications via a peptide-centric approach (Duncan et al., 2010), including spectra search criteria, sequence coverage and database completeness.

Accordingly, changing levels of a modified protein may represent a better biomarker than changes in the total expression levels of a given protein. For example, alterations in the levels of naturally-occurring glycosylation motifs can serve as a marker of inflammation, lymphocyte tolerance and senescence in arthritis (Garcia et al., 2005), *viz.* increased branching of sugar moieties on alpha-1 acid glycoprotein can act as biomarkers of inflammation, whereas decreased branching of T-cell receptor affects the development of Th1/Th2 cells increasing susceptibility to autoimmunity (Havenaar et al., 1998; Morgan et al., 2004).

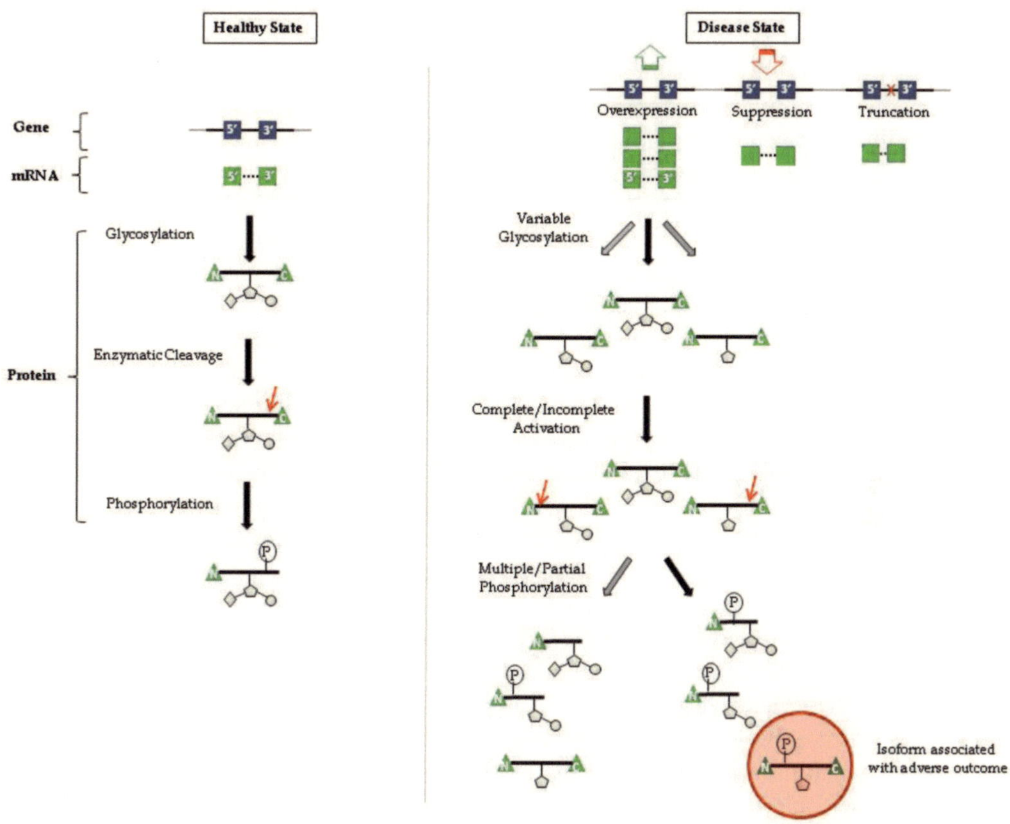


Fig. 2. Protein isoform verification

A depiction of possible qualitative and quantitative changes in protein isoforms between health and a disease state. The illustration of an isoform of a given protein associated with a specific adverse outcome demonstrates that it can only be detected by high 'resolution' proteomic strategies which can detect variance in post translational modifications. Conventional genomic and antibody based methods will only pick up on a change in expression of recognized transcripts or epitopes, giving a high likely hood of missing the significance of the isoform prevalent in a particular disease outcome.

Recent evidence suggests that oxidative modifications to the proteins S100A8 and S100A9 shifts function from macrophage and neutrophil activation in inflammatory arthritis towards a protective role (Lim et al., 2009). In this case, the modification appears to serve as a regulatory switch. Citrulination of arginine side chains has the potential to alter structure, antigenicity and protein function (Wegner et al., 2010). In fact, synthetic peptides modified to mimic possible neo-antigens which trigger an autoimmune response have been used to identify novel diagnostic/prognostic autoantibodies (McLaren et al., 2005; Papini et al., 2009).

Before disease becomes apparent, it is likely that a particular disease pathology 'specific' protein isoform combination has been expressed for some time, impacting normal physiological pathways. These disease 'specific' proteins may also be expressed in a benign or developing state of the disease devoid of clinical symptoms and may contain a sub pool of surrogate markers of chronic inflammation. An example from the world of autoimmune disease is presented by a study of systemic lupus erythematosus patients in whom autoantibodies were detected prior to clinical symptoms (Eriksson et al., 2011). Susceptibility to develop several other auoimmune diseases including diabetes and rheumatoid arthritis can be predicted by long periods of pre-clinical autoantibody expression (Bastra et al., 2001; Rantapaa-Dahlquist et al, 2003). Another recent study indicates that galactosylation of IgG precedes disease onset, correlates with disease activity, and is prevalent in autoantibodies in rheumatoid arthritis patients (Ercan et al., 2010).

Evidently these preclinical biomarker 'screening' studies are unique in that they rely heavily on concerted biobanking of samples in a prospective fashion, generally have focused on more easily retrieved antibodies and may incur long 'wait times' until a specific disorder may occur. They do however offer a fascinating glimpse of what could be occurring at the protein level prior to disease onset, which arguably could offer a window of opportunity to diagnose earlier, manage the pathology before it becomes clinically symptomatic and possibly prevent aberrant processes all together. Alterations in protein isoforms therefore may also comprise part of the milieu of pathological changes and thereby serve as biomarkers. Studies aimed at full length characterization of proteins indicate that preliminary discovery stages may therefore not reflect the full extent of protein variants due to the low cohort sizes (and low throughput techniques) typical of this stage. For example, a study of diabetes patients revealed that, within a cohort of 96 individuals, an average of 3 variants of each protein were observed; a further 8 variants were observed across 1000 individuals (Borges et al., 2010). This highlights the importance of accounting for protein micro-heterogeneity across patient populations and correlation of prevalence with specific disease outcome sub-groups (Figure 2). Statistical evidence of prevalence and analytical limits of detection of a specific group of isoforms should then direct the study towards validation of candidates in a much larger group of multi-center patient populations.

## 4. Emerging tools for targeted biomarker validation

The biggest challenge in proteomics remains independent validation of changes 'discovered' in observational investigations. Traditionally, validation has been undertaken by antibody-based approaches, including Western blotting, ELISA and immunohistochemistry (IHC). However, despite major efforts to generate proteome-scale panels of suitable antibodies (most notably the impressive Human Protein Atlas initiative [http:// www. proteinatlas.

org/ index.php]), this remains a slow process. It requires antibody generation and characterization to establish specificity and utility in different assay formats.

### 4.1 Multiple reaction monitoring

Antibody-independent strategies are highly desirable. The most popular of these is based on peptide-centric, multiple reaction monitoring (MRM). MRM is a technology that has unique potential for reliable quantification of analytes of low abundance in complex mixtures. In an MRM assay, a predefined precursor ion and one of its fragments are selected by the two mass filters of a triple quadrupole instrument and monitored over time for precise quantification. A series of transitions (precursor/fragment ion pairs) in combination with the retention time of the targeted peptide can constitute a definitive assay (Lange et al., 2008). The combination of MRM, chemistry and software to aid with the selection of suitable proteotypic peptides, has provided the opportunity to rapidly develop quantitative multiplexed assays of protein expression and post-translational modification that are both highly specific and sensitive (Scheiss et al., 2009). In recent years, significant advances have been made in the measurement of protein expression using MRM on triple quadrupole (QQQ) mass spectrometers (Pan et al., 2009). In this system, one or more peptide ions of unique and known mass are preselected in the first quadrupole (Q1), induced to fragment in the second quadrupole (Q2), and some of the resulting 'product ions' (or fragments) are selected for transmission to the detector in the third quadrupole (Q3) (Figure 3A). MRM supports the simultaneous measurement of multiple proteotypic peptides and synthetic mass variants of them (usually spiked into samples in known amounts). The strategy enables the absolute quantification of multiple proteins (Keshishan et al., 2007; Kuzyk et al., 2009). When MRM is combined with immunoaffinity purification and internal peptide standards, for example SISCAPA, detection is in the sub-femtomolar range (Whiteaker et al., 2010).

In a relatively early demonstration of peptide MRM, assays were developed to simultaneously quantify the expression of sixteen cytochrome P450 enzymes - proteins important in determining susceptibility to adverse drug reactions (Jenkins et al., 2006). Previously, a method was described for the MRM assay of C-reactive protein (CRP) as a means of differentiating erosive from non-erosive RA patients (Kuhn et al., 2004). The same research team then applied the same MRM technique to measure elevated levels in synovial fluid of six additional members of the S100 calcium-binding proteins associated with an erosive subtype of RA (Liao et al., 2004).

### 4.2 Nucleic acid programmable protein arrays

The production of antibodies against self-antigens (autoantibodies) is a characteristic feature of many autoimmune diseases. At a clinical level, tests for specific autoantibodies, such as ANA positivity, are routinely employed to aid the diagnosis and track the progress of these diseases. Traditionally, autoantibodies have been identified with a one-antigen-at-a-time, hypothesis-driven approach using methods such as immunofluorescence and ELISA.

Microarrays provide a particularly effective platform for the systematic study of thousands of proteins in parallel because they are sensitive and require low sample volumes (MacBeath & Schreiber, 2000; Zhu et al., 2001). Protein microarrays involve the display of thousands of different proteins with high spatial density on a microscopic surface. Protein microarrays have been applied to autoimmune biomarker studies focused on pre-symptomatic screening and diagnosis, clinical outcome prognosis and therapeutic response prediction (Hueber et al., 2005; Quitana et al., 2004) With particular relevance to the remit of this chapter, conventional printed arrays have been used to study rheumatoid arthritis, systemic lupus erythematosus, multiple sclerosis, hepatitis and encephalomyelitis (Fattal et al., 2010; Hueber et al. 2009; Li et al., 2005; Somers et al., 2009; Song et al., 2010).

**A** In protein multiple reaction monitoring (MRM), one or more peptides of unique and known mass (proteotypic peptides) are preselected in the first quadrupole (Q1), induced to fragment in Q2 by collisional excitation with a neutral gas in a pressurized cell and some of the resulting 'product ions' (fragments) are selected for transition to the detector in the third quadrupole (Q3). **B1** Nucleic acid programmable protein array (NAPPA) spotted with genes of interest; All proteins are tagged at the c-terminus to ensure only full length translated proteins can be captured in situ by co-spotted anti-tag antibodies. NAPPA has consistent protein amounts displayed at each spot; most are within two fold of the average (Ramachandaran et al., 2008). Proteins are expressed "just-in-time" for assay, which eliminates concern of protein stability. **B2** Image of NAPPA with randomly selected 768 genes probed with a synovial fluid sample from a patient with juvenile arthritis. Antibodies in patient samples bind to their antigen targets on the array and are detected by Alexa647-conjugated goat anti-human IgG. **B3** Scatterplot of reactivity on NAPPA between paired plasma and synovial fluid samples from arthritis patients. Median correlation is 0.982. **C1** Matrix assisted laser desorption ionization- time of flight (MALDI-TOF) mass spectrometry whereby proteins or peptides imbedded in a crystallized matrices are ionized by a high frequency laser beam and accelerated through a flight tube by electrical field; ions 'fly' and reach the detector plate with respect to their mass:charge ratio. **C2** A spectra is generated which reflects the energy of a given ion vs the mass:charge ratio (m/z). **C3** A birds eye view representation of the spectra reveals distinguishing peaks (*) from the six samples analysed.

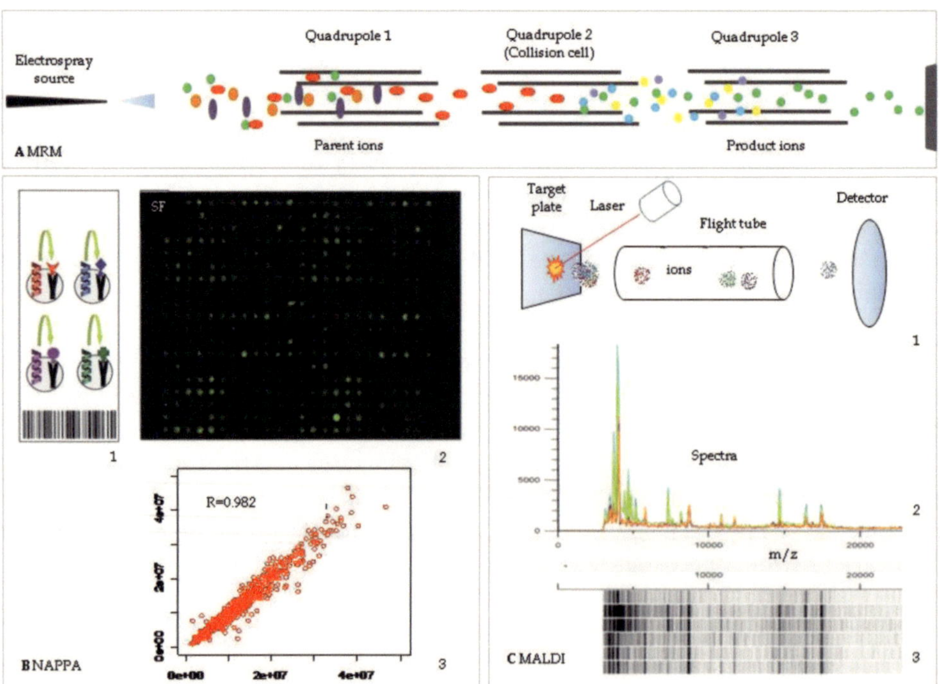


Fig. 3. Targeted identification methods

Nucleic Acid Programmable Protein Array (NAPPA) is an innovative method to produce protein microarrays, where cDNAs encoding proteins of interest are spotted onto activated surfaces and proteins are produced *in situ* using mammalian *in vitro* expression systems (Ramachandran et al., 2004; Ramachandran et al., 2008). The freshly made protein is captured by co-spotted antibodies specific for a 'tag' encoded at the end of the amino acid sequence. This approach circumvents the labor and cost considerations associated with conventional spotting of labile recombinant proteins into arrays. NAPPA technology recently revealed that ankylosing spondylitis patients' autoantibody responses were targeted towards connective, skeletal and muscular tissue, unlike those of RA patients (Wright et al., 2010). In a recent pilot study, a strong correlation was observed between 768 autoantibodies in paired plasma and synovial fluid samples from patients with juvenile arthritis (Figure 3B).

### 4.3 Proteomic profiling methods

Intact protein profiling across clinical cohorts gives a glimpse into the degree of variation evident in a single gene product (Borges et al., 2008a). The same approach may be useful in the study of arthritis. Mass spectrometry-based techniques can potentially distinguish these physical and structural variations and allow the relative abundance of one isoform to be determined (Duncan et al., 2010). By contrast, these variants would be overlooked by conventional ELISA methods (Figure 2). A brief description and recent application of such techniques follows.

*MALDI / SELDI Profiling (Immuno-MALDI):* Matrix assisted laser desorption ionisation (MALDI) mode of mass spectrometry allows the 'soft' ionization of complete proteins which are liable to fragment under conventional ionization methods. The type of a mass spectrometer most widely used with MALDI is the time-of-flight (TOF), mainly due to its large mass range (Figure 3C). Purifying a protein from a clinical sample by immunoprecipitation can greatly reduce the complexity of the proteome being analysed. In one approach, purified polyclonal antibodies that capture the target protein isoforms can be immobilized onto sepharose beads packed within a pipette tip or 'fret' (Borges et al., 2008b). Eluted proteins can then be spotted on a MALDI target plate and spectra obtained. For example, some recent MALDI profiling applications have demonstrated the ability to diagnose early RA and hypertension and distinguish active SLE (Dai et al., 2010; Long et al., 2010; Reid et al., 2010). Glycosylation heterogeneity of selected inflammation associated molecules such as serum amyloid and vitamin D binding protein have been investigated in cancer and diabetic patients (Rehder et al., 2009; Weiss et al., 2011).

As a modification of MALDI, surface-enhanced laser desorption ionization (SELDI) methods can be used to target lower molecular weight proteins (<20 KDa) to differentiate arthritides and therapeutic response (de Seny et al., 2008; Miyame et al. 2005). The technology is currently being developed to affinity capture the protein of interest directly to the mass spectrometry target plate (Brauer et al., 2010).

### 4.4 Biomarker research and grant funding

Although proteomics has been full of promise, few validated biomarkers have made their way into the public domain and even fewer influence clinical practice. There is little doubt that validation is a serious bottleneck in the biomarker development process. While there is abundant discussion of approaches to discovery, the tools for validation and their applications have received little attention. It is very often difficult to receive funding from traditional grant programs to validate markers: funding agencies balk at the prospect of funding a 're-measurement' of the same entity in larger independent cohorts. Additionally, the continuum from discovery through to validation is tedious and extends well beyond the time-frame of a typical research grant. In fact, the time from initial discovery to routine use can take up to a decade (Anderson, 2010; Wilson et al., 2007). A recent example illustrates the seven year journey from discovery to FDA approval for the multivariate diagnostic test OVA1, used to screen ovarian cancer patients (Fung, 2010).

Similarly, when validation fails it is difficult for academic investigators to publish these 'negative' results; when validation succeeds, the emphasis frequently shifts to commercialization rather than publication.

## 5. Conclusions

While there is widespread recognition of the value of biomarkers, scientific progress is slow. Over the years, biomarkers have sometimes been the center of excessive "hype", prompting excessive or unreasonable expectations. In addition, the use of biomarkers as surrogate endpoints have led to some public failures when they were felt to be falsely reassuring, creating general skepticism amongst scientists and clinicians alike (e.g. Petricoin et al., 2002). In addition to limited validation, resistance still hindering biomarker acceptance includes:

- Resistance to sharing data across independent efforts - Organizations may work on similar research or discover keystone advances yet resist sharing knowledge because they feel that doing so will jeopardize their competitive advantage. However, sharing information could help companies achieve greater overall progress and reduce costs.
- Need for new R&D models with greater precision and flexibility - The industry needs an R&D model with greater precision to improve pipelines, leveraging active clinical knowledge to offset the declining success in new drug development. Some research and development leaders are concerned that using an approach that targets treatment for only a subset of patients decreases profits and increases research costs. Others recognize that this direction has already created value beyond costs and are building these capabilities into their business strategy. For example, Herceptin® is considered an effective targeted treatment for breast cancer. Targeted treatments could actually increase both the medical and economic success of a therapeutic.
- Insufficient interoperability - Traditional data resides in disparate places that often do not easily connect. Factor in imaging biomarkers constituted by terabytes of data and you have a complex mix of data from which it is difficult to extract new insights (Poste, 2011). The path forward - interoperability - is a design and intent to have systems share information that relies on data standards, and more importantly, semantics. Semantics use common vocabularies and business rules to relate clinical terms reported across different sources to find common meaning.

Tools to support development, medical care, health policy such as the FDA's critical path, and BioPharma investment decisions. The biomarker development and validation process is necessary but costly for one company. Innovation takes place in many organizations and, as such, stakeholders work redundantly on the same effort. Many collaborative forums exist but these usually involve sharing "safe" information that really does not hasten overall progress. Consequently, most existing biomarkers have taken decades to become part of medical practice.

Currently there are few FDA-approved proteomic tests for autoimmune disease. Although there is little doubt that such tests could help the diagnosis and treatment of arthritis, it is a major clinical and financial challenge to develop, validate and market them. Robust validation data including evidence of sensitivity, specificity and correlation to the existing limited set of clinical or laboratory criteria are necessary to support clinical utility. Disease activity scores (DAS-CRP and DAS28), for example, combine inflamed joint count and ESR/CRP to document levels of disease activity at a static time point. The measurement of specific proteins that flag a particular patient's status add objectivity in circumstances where the clinician currently relies on clinical judgment alone.

From a clinician's perspective, it is important to address several questions in a timely fashion for a given patient presenting with autoimmune disease. In each instance, the clinician is attempting to minimize underlying disease and adverse outcomes, such as joint damage in arthritis. Key questions that can currently only be partially answered by clinical observation and patient history include: (a) is this true autoimmune-driven arthritis (i.e., diagnosis), (b) how severe or at what stage is the disease process, (c) what is this patient's likely outcome (i.e., prognosis) and (d) which drugs could abrogate that outcome (i.e., prediction)? Decision-making also extends to selection of therapy: (e) what is the patient-specific titer, (f) which disease subgroups will benefit from a specific therapeutic strategy and (g) when should treatment be terminated?

This chapter has addressed and discussed three key areas for consideration, which if addressed after initial discovery work could provide solid evidence of their clinical utility and commercial viability: (i) limiting bias in study design, (ii) thorough protein isoform verification and (iii) modes of orthogonal and targeted validation.

## 6. Glossary- the language of biomarker and proteomic research

*Bias-* In statistics, bias is systematic favoritism present in data collection, analysis or reporting of quantitative research

*Biomarker-* or *biological marker,* is a molecular characteristic that is objectively measured and evaluated as an indicator of normal biological processes, pathogenic processes, or pharmacologic responses to a therapeutic intervention.

*Classifier-* in statistics is the formula or criteria for identifying a sub-population based on quantitative information on one or more measurements, traits or characteristics.

*Development pipeline-* represents the process from candidate discovery, through verification, validation and final pre-market approval.

*Diagnostic-* in the context of medicine is any test performed or criteria applied to aid to determine and/or identity a possible disease or disorder.

*Discovery-* in the context of biomarkers, describes the initial process of observation, identification and quantification of one or more biological molecules which may act as a classifier.

*Isoform-* describes the biological phenomenon of several different structural forms of the same protein which may arise by alternate gene splicing and single-nucleotide polymorphisms before messenger RNA translation and chemical modifications e.g. phosphorylation or glycosylation which occur post-translation of proteins.

*Multiplex-* in the context of protein assay is a method or platform which permits the simultaneously measururement of multiple analytes (dozens or more) in a single test.

*Omics*- this suffix, often used in modern biological research, refers to the lofty aim of observing, identifying and quantifying the totality of a particular class of molecules i.e. genomics, proteomics.
*Orthogonal method*- describes the ideal of using alternate types of analyses to corroborate the original findings by independent means.
*Peptide-centric*- or *bottom-up,* proteomics is a common method used to identify proteins by proteolytic digestion of proteins prior to analysis by mass spectrometry.
*Protein-centric*- or *top-down,* proteomics is a method of intact protein identification e.g. an ion trapping mass spectrometer used to store an isolated protein ion for mass measurement and tandem mass spectrometry analysis.
*Power analysis*- to calculate the number of samples required for a study to reach statistically sound conclusions.
*Predictive model*- in the context of medicine, is created or chosen to try to predict the probability of a clinical outcome by use of one or more *classifiers.*
*Prognostic*- is a clinical test which can forecast the likely course or outcome of an illness.
*Sensitivity*- measures the proportion of true positives which are correctly identified as such (e.g. the percentage of sick people who are correctly identified as having the condition).
*Specificity*- measures the proportion of true negatives which are correctly identified (e.g. the percentage of healthy people who are correctly identified as not having the condition).
*Throughput*- refers to the rate of analysis of samples by a particular method e.g. analysis of a single protein by Western blotting is relatively low throughput compared to ELISA.
*Validation*- later stage in the biomarker pipeline is defined as the documented act of demonstrating that putative biomarker classifiers will consistently lead to the expected results i.e establish *sensitivity* and *specificity* performance in large populations and begin to optimize the assay for commercial use.
*Verification*- intermediate phase in biomarker pipeline bridging *discovery* and *validation,* which typically reduces the number of candidates, confirms specific protein isoforms within a *classifier* and begins to assess the sensitivity in expanded populations.

## 7. Acknowledgement

DSG would like to acknowledge continued support from Arthritis Research UK in the form of a Travelling Fellowship (No. 19250). The UCD Conway Institute and the Proteome Research Centre are funded by the Programme for Research in Third Level Institutions, as administered by the Higher Education Authority of Ireland. SRP acknowledges support for equipment from Science Foundation Ireland. DSG and MR would like to acknowledge the funding of this research by Arthritis Research UK in the form of a Project Grant (No. 18748).

## 8. References

Alonso-Ruiz A., Pijoan J.I., Ansuategui E., Urkaregi A., Calabozo M. & Quintana A. Tumor necrosis factor alpha drugs in rheumatoid arthritis: systematic review and metaanalysis of efficacy and safety. *BMC Musculoskelet. Disord.,* 9, (2008), pp 52.

Anders H.J., Rihl M., Vielhauer V. & Schattenkirchner M. Assessment of renal function in rheumatoid arthritis: validity of a new prediction method. *J. Clin. Rheumatol.,* 8(3), (2002), pp 130-3.

Addona T.A. Abbatiello S.E., Schilling B., Skates S.J., Mani D.R., Bunk D.M., Spiegelman C.H., Zimmerman L.J., Ham A.J., Keshishian H., Hall S.C., Allen S., Blackman R.K., Borchers C.H., Buck C., Cardasis H.L., Cusack M.P., Dodder N.G., Gibson B.W., Held J.M., Hiltke T., Jackson A., Johansen E.B., Kinsinger C.R., Li J., Mesri M., Neubert T.A., Niles R.K., Pulsipher T.C., Ransohoff D., Rodriguez H., Rudnick P.A., Smith D., Tabb D.L., Tegeler T.J., Variyath A.M., Vega-Montoto L.J., Wahlander A., Waldemarson S., Wang M., Whiteaker J.R., Zhao L., Anderson N.L., Fisher S.J., Liebler D.C., Paulovich A.G., Regnier F.E., Tempst P. & Carr S.A.. Multi-site assessment of the precision and reproducibility of multiple reaction monitoring-based measurements of proteins in plasma. *Nat. Biotechnol.*, 27, (2009), pp 633-641.

Aebersold R. & Mann M. Mass spectrometry-based proteomics. *Nature*, 422, (2003), pp 198-207.

Anderson N.L. The clinical plasma proteome: a survey of clinical assays for proteins in plasma and serum. *Clin. Chem.*, 56(2), (2010), pp 177-85.

Batstra M.R., Aanstoot H.J. & Herbrink P. Prediction and diagnosis of type 1 diabetes using beta-cell autoantibodies. *Clin. Lab.*, 47(9-10), (2001), pp 497-507.

Bloemen K., Van Den Heuvel R., Govarts E., Hooyberghs J., Nelen V., Witters E., Desager K. & Schoeters G. A new approach to study exhaled proteins as potential biomarkers for asthma. *Clin. Exp. Allergy*, 41(3), (2011), pp 346-56.

Bongartz T., Sutton A.J., Sweeting M.J., Buchan I., Matteson E.L. & Montori V. Anti-TNF antibody therapy in rheumatoid arthritis and the risk of serious infections and malignancies: systematic review and meta-analysis of rare harmful effects in randomized controlled trials. *JAMA*, 295(19), (2006), pp 2275-85.

Borges C.R., Jarvis J.W., Oran P.E. & Nelson R.W. Population studies of Vitamin D Binding Protein microheterogeneity by mass spectrometry lead to characterization of its genotype-dependent O-glycosylation patterns. *J. Proteome Res.*, 7(9), (2008), pp 4143-53.

Borges C.R., Jarvis J.W., Oran P.E., Rogers S.P. & Nelson R.W. Population studies of intact vitamin D binding protein by affinity capture ESI-TOF-MS. *J. Biomol. Tech.*, 19(3), (2008), pp 167-76.

Borges C.R., Rehder D.S., Jarvis J.W., Schaab M.R., Oran P.E. & Nelson R.W. Full-length characterization of proteins in human populations. *Clin. Chem.*, 56(2), (2010), pp 202-11.

Bowes J.D., Potter C., Gibbons L.J., Hyrich K., Plant D., Morgan A.W., Wilson A.G., Isaacs J.D.,Worthington J. & Barton A. Investigation of genetic variants within candidate genes of the TNFRSF1B signalling pathway on the response to anti-TNF agents in a UK cohort of rheumatoid arthritis patients. *Pharmacogenet. Genomics*, 19(4), (2009), pp 319-23.

Brauer H.A., Lampe P.D., Yasui Y.Y., Hamajima N. & Stolowitz M.L. Biochips that sequentially capture and focus antigens for immunoaffinity MALDI-TOF MS: a new tool for biomarker verification. *Proteomics*, 10(21), (2010), pp 3922-7. Cairns D.A., Barrett J.H., Billingham L.J., Stanley A.J., Xinarianos G., Field J.K., Johnson P.J., Selby P.J. & Banks R.E. Sample size determination in clinical proteomic profiling experiments using mass spectrometry for class comparison. *Proteomics*, 9(1), (2009), pp 74-86.

Chait, B. T. Chemistry. Mass spectrometry: bottom-up or top-down? *Science*, 314, (2006), pp 65-66.

Chen P.P., Robbins D.L., Jirik F.R., Kipps T.J. & Carson D.A. Isolation and characterization of a light chain variable region gene for human rheumatoid factors. *J. Exp. Med.*, 166(6), (1987), pp 1900-1905.

Dai Y., Hu C., Wang L., Huang Y., Zhang L., Xiao X. & Tan Y. Serum peptidome patterns of human systemic lupus erythematosus based on magnetic bead separation and MALDI-TOF mass spectrometry analysis. *Scand. J. Rheumatol.*, 39(3), (2010), pp 240-246.

Davis M.T., Auger P.L. & Patterson S.D. Cancer biomarker discovery via low molecular weight serum profiling--are we following circular paths? *Clin. Chem.*, 2010, 56(2), pp 244-247.

de Seny D., Fillet M., Ribbens C., Marée R., Meuwis M.A., Lutteri L., Chapelle J.P., Wehenkel L., Louis E., Merville M.P. & Malaise M. Monomeric calgranulins measured by SELDI-TOF mass spectrometry and calprotectin measured by ELISA as biomarkers in arthritis. *Clin. Chem.*, 54(6), (2008), pp 1066-1075.

Dowsey, A.W., Morris, J.S., Gutstein, H.B. & Yang, G.Z. in Proteome Bioinformatics (eds Hubbard, S. J. & Jones, A. R.) 239 (Humana Press, New York, 2009).

Duncan M.W., Aebersold R. & Caprioli R.M. The pros and cons of peptide-centric proteomics. *Nat. Biotechnol.*, 28(7), (2010), pp 659-64.

Dupuy A. & Simon R.M. Critical review of published microarray studies for cancer outcome and guidelines on statistical analysis and reporting. *J. Natl. Cancer Inst.*, 99(2), (2007), pp 147-157.

Ercan, A. Cui J., Chatterton D.E., Deane K.D., Hazen M.M., Brintnell W., O'Donnell C.I., Derber L.A., Weinblatt M.E., Shadick N.A., Bell D.A., Cairns E., Solomon D.H., Holers V.M., Rudd P.M. & Lee D.M. Aberrant IgG galactosylation precedes disease onset, correlates with disease activity, and is prevalent in autoantibodies in rheumatoid arthritis. *Arthritis Rheum.*, 62, (2010), pp 2239-2248.

Eriksson C., Kokkonen H., Johansson M., Hallmans G., Wadell G. & Rantapaa-Dahlqvist S. Autoantibodies predate the onset of Systemic Lupus Erythematosus in northern Sweden. *Arthritis Res. Ther.,*. 13(1), (2011), pp R30.

Fattal I., Shental N., Mevorach D., Anaya J.M., Livneh A., Langevitz P., Zandman-Goddard G., Pauzner R., Lerner M., Blank M., Hincapie M.E., Gafter U., Naparstek Y., Shoenfeld Y., Domany E. & Cohen I.R. An antibody profile of systemic lupus erythematosus detected by antigen microarray. *Immunology*, 130(3), (2010), pp 337-343.

Flower L., Ahuja R.H., Humphries S.E. & Mohamed-Ali V. Effects of sample handling on the stability of interleukin 6, tumour necrosis factor-alpha and leptin. *Cytokine*. 12(11), (2000), pp 1712-1716.

Fung E.T. A recipe for proteomics diagnostic test development: the OVA1 test, from biomarker discovery to FDA clearance. *Clin. Chem.*, 56(2), (2010), pp 327-329.

Garcia G.G., Berger S.B., Sadighi Akha A.A. & Miller R.A.. Age-associated changes in glycosylation of CD43 and CD45 on mouse CD4 T cells. *Eur. J. Immunol.*, 35(2), (2005), pp 622-31.

Gibson D.S. & Rooney M.E. The human synovial fluid proteome: A key factor in the pathology of joint disease. *PROTEOMICS - CLINICAL APPLICATIONS*, 1, (2007), pp 889-899.

Gibson, D.S. Blelock S., Curry J., Finnegan S., Healy A., Scaife C., McAllister C., Pennington S., Dunn M. & Rooney M.. Comparative analysis of synovial fluid and plasma proteomes in juvenile arthritis--proteomic patterns of joint inflammation in early stage disease. *J. Proteomics*, 72, (2009), pp 656-676.

Haab B.B, Geierstanger B.H., Michailidis G., Vitzthum F., Forrester S., Okon R., Saviranta P., Brinker A., Sorette M., Perlee L., Suresh S., Drwal G., Adkins J.N., Omenn G.S. Immunoassay and antibody microarray analysis of the HUPO Plasma Proteome Project reference specimens: systematic variation between sample types and calibration of mass spectrometry data. *Proteomics*, 5(13), (2005), pp 3278-3291.

Havenaar E.C., Axford J.S., Brinkman-van der Linden E.C., Alavi A., Van Ommen E.C., van het Hof B., Spector T., Mackiewicz A. & Van Dijk W.. Severe rheumatoid arthritis prohibits the pregnancy-induced decrease in alpha3-fucosylation of alpha1-acid glycoprotein. *Glycoconj. J.*, 15(7), (1998), pp 723-729.

Hu, S., Loo, J.A. & Wong, D.T. Human body fluid proteome analysis. *Proteomics*, 6, (2006), pp 6326-6353.

Hueber W., Kidd B.A., Tomooka B.H., Lee B.J., Bruce B., Fries J.F., Sønderstrup G., Monach P., Drijfhout J.W., van Venrooij W.J., Utz P.J., Genovese M.C. & Robinson W.H. Antigen microarray profiling of autoantibodies in rheumatoid arthritis. *Arthritis Rheum.*, 52(9), (2005), pp 2645-2655.

Hueber W., Tomooka B.H., Batliwalla F., Li W., Monach P.A., Tibshirani R.J., Van Vollenhoven R.F., Lampa J., Saito K., Tanaka Y., Genovese M.C., Klareskog L., Gregersen P.K. & Robinson W.H. Blood autoantibody and cytokine profiles predict response to anti-tumor necrosis factor therapy in rheumatoid arthritis. *Arthritis Res. Ther.*, 11(3), (2009), pp R76.

Jenkins R.E., Kitteringham N.R., Hunter C.L., Webb S., Hunt T.J., Elsby R., Watson R.B.,Williams D., Pennington S.R., Park B.K. Relative and absolute quantitative expression profiling of cytochromes P450 using isotope-coded affinity tags. Proteomics, 6(6), (2006), pp 1934-1947.

Karp N.A. & Lilley K.S. Design and analysis issues in quantitative proteomics studies. *Proteomics*, 7 Suppl 1, (2007), pp 42-50.

Kastbom A., Strandberg G., Lindroos A. & Skogh T. Anti-CCP antibody test predicts the disease course during 3 years in early rheumatoid arthritis (the Swedish TIRA project). *Ann. Rheum. Dis.*, 63(9), (2004), pp 1085-1089.

Kavanaugh A.F., Solomon D.H. & American College of Rheumatology Ad Hoc Committee on Immunologic Testing Guidelines. Guidelines for immunologic laboratory testing in the rheumatic diseases: anti-DNA antibody tests. *Arthritis Rheum.*, 47(5), (2002), pp 546-555.

Keshishian H., Addona T., Burgess M., Kuhn E. & Carr S.A. Quantitative, multiplexed assays for low abundance proteins in plasma by targeted mass spectrometry and stable isotope dilution. *Mol. Cell. Proteomics*, 6(12), (2007), pp 2212-2229.

Kuhn E., Wu J., Karl J., Liao H., Zolg W. & Guild B. Quantification of C-reactive protein in the serum of patients with rheumatoid arthritis using multiple reaction monitoring mass spectrometry and 13C-labeled peptide standards. *Proteomics*, 4(4), (2004), pp 1175-86.

Kurreeman F.A., Padyukov L., Marques R.B., Schrodi S.J., Seddighzadeh M., Stoeken-Rijsbergen G., van der Helm-van Mil A.H., Allaart C.F., Verduyn W., Houwing-Duistermaat J., Alfredsson L., Begovich A.B., Klareskog L., Huizinga T.W. & Toes R.E. A candidate gene approach identifies the TRAF1/C5 region as a risk factor for rheumatoid arthritis. *PLoS Med.*, 4(9), (2007), pp e278.

Kuzyk M.A., Smith D., Yang J., Cross T.J., Jackson A.M., Hardie D.B., Anderson N.L. & Borchers C.H. Multiple reaction monitoring-based, multiplexed, absolute quantitation of 45 proteins in human plasma. *Mol. Cell. Proteomics*, 8(8), (2009), pp 1860-1877.

Lange V., Picotti P., Domon B.& Aebersold R. Selected reaction monitoring for quantitative proteomics: a tutorial. *Mol .Syst. Biol.*, 4, (2008), pp 222.

Li Q.Z., Xie C., Wu T., Mackay M., Aranow C., Putterman C. & Mohan C. Identification of autoantibody clusters that best predict lupus disease activity using glomerular proteome arrays. *J. Clin. Invest.*, 115(12), (2005), pp 3428-39.

Liao H., Wu J., Kuhn E., Chin W., Chang B., Jones M.D., O'Neil S., Clauser K.R., Karl J., Hasler F., Roubenoff R., Zolg W. & Guild B.C. Use of mass spectrometry to identify protein biomarkers of disease severity in the synovial fluid and serum of patients with rheumatoid arthritis. *Arthritis Rheum.*, 50(12), (2004), pp 3792-803.

Lim S.Y., Raftery M.J., Goyette J., Hsu K. & Geczy C.L. Oxidative modifications of S100 proteins: functional regulation by redox. *J. Leukoc. Biol.*, 86(3), 2009, pp 577-587.

Lindqvist E., Eberhardt K., Bendtzen K., Heinegard D. & Saxne T. Prognostic laboratory markers of joint damage in rheumatoid arthritis. *Ann. Rheum. Dis.*, 64(2), (2005), pp 196-201.

Liu Q., Sung A.H., Chen Z., Liu J., Huang X. & Deng Y. Feature selection and classification of MAQC-II breast cancer and multiple myeloma microarray gene expression data. *PLoS One*, 4(12), (2009), pp e8250.

Long L., Li R., Li Y., Hu C. & Li Z. Pattern-based diagnosis and screening of differentially expressed serum proteins for rheumatoid arthritis by proteomic fingerprinting. *Rheumatol. Int.*, (2010).

MacBeath G. & Schreiber S.L. Printing proteins as microarrays for high-throughput function determination. *Science*, 289(5485), (2000), pp 1760-1763.

Marengo E., Robotti E., Bobba M., Liparota M.C., Rustichelli C., Zamò A., Chilosi M. & Righetti P.G. Multivariate statistical tools applied to the characterization of the proteomic profiles of two human lymphoma cell lines by two-dimensional gel electrophoresis. *Electrophoresis*, 27(2), (2006), pp 484-494.

McLaren M,. Waring A., Galarraga B., Rudd A., Morley K. & Belch J.J. Investigation of platelet glycoprotein IIIa polymorphism using flow cytometry in patients with rheumatoid arthritis. *Scand. J. Rheumatol.*, 34, (2005), pp 437-440.

Meyer O., Labarre C., Dougados M., Goupille P., Cantagrel A., Dubois A., Nicaise-Roland P., Sibilia J. & Combe B.Anticitrullinated protein/peptide antibody assays in early rheumatoid arthritis for predicting five year radiographic damage. *Ann. Rheum. Dis.*, 62(2), (2003), pp 120-126.

Miyamae T., Malehorn D.E., Lemster B., Mori M., Imagawa T., Yokota S., Bigbee W.L.,Welsh M., Klarskov K., Nishomoto N., Vallejo A.N. & Hirsch R. Serum protein profile in systemic-onset juvenile idiopathic arthritis differentiates response versus nonresponse to therapy. Arthritis Res. Ther., 7(4), (2005), pp R746-755.

Morgan R., Gao G., Pawling J., Dennis J.W., Demetriou M. & Li B. N-acetylglucosaminyltransferase V (Mgat5)-mediated N-glycosylation negatively regulates Th1 cytokine production by T cells. *J. Immunol.*, 173(12), (2004), pp 7200-7208.

Nakamura RM. Progress in the use of biochemical and biological markers for evaluation of rheumatoid arthritis. *J. Clin. Lab. Anal.*, 14(6), (2000), pp 305-313.

Nielen M.M., van Schaardenburg D., Reesink H.W., van de Stadt R.J., van der Horst-Bruinsma I.E., de Koning M.H., Habibuw M.R., Vandenbroucke J.P. & Dijkmans B.A. Specific autoantibodies precede the symptoms of rheumatoid arthritis: a study of serial measurements in blood donors. *Arthritis Rheum.*, 50(2), (2004), pp 380-6.

Pan S., Aebersold R., Chen R., Rush J., Goodlett D.R., McIntosh M.W., Zhang J., Brentnall T.A. Mass spectrometry based targeted protein quantification: methods and applications. *J. Proteome Res.*, 8(2), (2009), pp 787-797.

Papini, A.M. The use of post-translationally modified peptides for detection of biomarkers of immune-mediated diseases. *J. Pept. Sci.*, 15, (2009), pp 621-628.

Pepe M.S., Feng Z., Janes H., Bossuyt P.M. & Potter J.D. Pivotal evaluation of the accuracy of a biomarker used for classification or prediction: standards for study design. *J. Natl. Cancer Inst.*, 100(20), (2008), pp 1432-1438.

Pepys M.B. & Hirschfield G.M. C-reactive protein: a critical update. *J. Clin. Invest.*, 111(12), (2003), pp 1805-1812.

Petricoin, E.F. Ardekani A.M., Hitt B.A., Levine P.J., Fusaro V.A., Steinberg S.M., Mills G.B., Simone C., Fishman D.A., Kohn E.C. & Liotta L.A. Use of proteomic patterns in serum to identify ovarian cancer. *Lancet*, 359, (2002), pp 572-577. Potter C., Cordell H.J., Barton A., Daly A.K., Hyrich K.L., Mann D.A., Morgan A.W., Wilson A.G., the Biologics in Rheumatoid Arthritis Genetics and Genomics Study Syndicate (BRAGGSS) & Isaacs J.D.. Association between anti-tumour necrosis factor treatment response and genetic variants within the TLR and NF{kappa}B signalling pathways. *Ann. Rheum. Dis.*, 69(7), (2010), pp 1315-1320.

Poste G. Bring on the Biomarkers. *Nature*, 469, (2011), pp 156-157.

Quintana F.J., Farez M.F., Viglietta V., Iglesias A.H., Merbl Y., Izquierdo G., Lucas M., Basso A.S., Khoury S.J., Lucchinetti C.F., Cohen I.R. & Weiner H.L. Antigen microarrays identify unique serum autoantibody signatures in clinical and pathologic subtypes of multiple sclerosis. *Proc. Natl. Acad. Sci. USA*, 105(48), (2008), pp 18889-18894.

Quintana F.J., Hagedorn P.H., Elizur G., Merbl Y., Domany E. & Cohen I.R. Functional immunomics: microarray analysis of IgG autoantibody repertoires predicts the future response of mice to induced diabetes. *Proc. Natl. Acad. Sci. USA*, 101 Suppl. 2, (2004), pp 14615-14621.

Rai A.J., Gelfand C.A., Haywood B.C., Warunek D.J., Yi J., Schuchard M.D., Mehigh R.J., Cockrill S.L., Scott G.B., Tammen H., Schulz-Knappe P., Speicher D.W., Vitzthum F., Haab B.B., Siest G. & Chan D.W. HUPO Plasma Proteome Project specimen collection and handling: towards the standardization of parameters for plasma proteome samples. *Proteomics*, 5(13), (2005), pp 3262-3277.

Ramachandran N., Hainsworth E., Bhullar B., Eisenstein S., Rosen B., Lau A.Y., Walter J.C. & LaBaer J. Self-assembling protein microarrays. *Science*, 305(5680), (2004), pp 86-90.

Ramachandran N., Raphael J.V., Hainsworth E., Demirkan G., Fuentes M.G., Rolfs A., Hu Y. & LaBaer J. Next-generation high-density self-assembling functional protein arrays. Nat. Methods, 5(6), (2008), pp 535-538.

Ransohoff D.F. & Gourlay M.L. Sources of bias in specimens for research about molecular markers for cancer. *J. Clin. Oncol.*, 28(4), (2010), pp 698-704.

Ransohoff D.F. Promises and limitations of biomarkers. *Recent Results Cancer Res.* 181, (2009), pp 55-59.

Ransohoff D.F. Proteomics research to discover markers: what can we learn from Netflix? *Clin. Chem.* 56, (2010), pp 172-176.

Rantapää-Dahlqvist S., de Jong B.A., Berglin E., Hallmans G., Wadell G., Stenlund H., Sundin U. & van Venrooij WJ. Antibodies against cyclic citrullinated peptide and IgA rheumatoid factor predict the development of rheumatoid arthritis. *Arthritis Rheum.*, 48(10), (2003), pp 2741-2749.

Rehder D.S., Nelson R.W. & Borges C.R. Glycosylation status of vitamin D binding protein in cancer patients. *Protein. Sci.*, 18(10), 2009, pp 2036-2042.

Reid J.D., Holmes D.T., Mason D.R., Shah B. & Borchers C.H. Towards the development of an immuno MALDI (iMALDI) mass spectrometry assay for the diagnosis of hypertension. *J. Am. Soc. Mass Spectrom.*, 21(10), (2010), pp 1680-6.

Reiner A., Yekutieli D. & Benjamini Y. Identifying differentially expressed genes using false discovery rate controlling procedures. *Bioinformatics*, 19(3), (2003), pp 368-375.

Robinson W.H., DiGennaro C., Hueber W., Haab B.B., Kamachi M., Dean E.J., Fournel S., Fong D., Genovese M.C., de Vegvar H.E., Skriner K., Hirschberg D.L., Morris R.I., Muller S., Pruijn G.J., van Venrooij W.J., Smolen J.S., Brown P.O., Steinman L. & Utz P.J. Autoantigen microarrays for multiplex characterization of autoantibody responses. Nat. Med., 8(3), (2002), pp 295-301.

Robinson W.H., Fontoura P., Lee B.J,. de Vegvar H.E., Tom J., Pedotti R., DiGennaro C.D., Mitchell D.J., Fong D., Ho P.P., Ruiz P.J., Maverakis E., Stevens D.B., Bernard C.C., Martin R., Kuchroo V.K., van Noort J.M., Genain C.P., Amor S., Olsson T., Utz P.J., Garren H. & Steinman L. Protein microarrays guide tolerizing DNA vaccine treatment of autoimmune encephalomyelitis. *Nat. Biotechnol.*, 21(9), (2003), pp 1033-9.

Schiess R., Wollscheid B. & Aebersold R. Targeted proteomic strategy for clinical biomarker discovery. *Mol. Oncol.*, 3(1), (2009), pp 33-44.

Smith M.P., Banks R.E., Wood S.L., Lewington A.J. & Selby P.J. Application of proteomic analysis to the study of renal diseases. *Nat. Rev. Nephrol.*, 5(12), (2009), pp 701-712.

Somers K., Govarts C., Stinissen P. & Somers V. Multiplexing approaches for autoantibody profiling in multiple sclerosis. *Autoimmun. Rev.*, 8(7), (2009), pp 573-579.

Song Q., Liu G., Hu S., Zhang Y., Tao Y., Han Y., Zeng H., Huang W., Li F., Chen P., Zhu J., Hu C., Zhang S., Li Y., Zhu H. & Wu L. Novel autoimmune hepatitis-specific autoantigens identified using protein microarray technology. *J. Proteome Res.*, 9(1), (2010), pp 30-39.

Storey J.D. & Tibshirani R. Statistical significance for genomewide studies. *Proc. Natl. Acad. Sci. USA*, 100(16), (2003), pp 9440-9445.

Strimmer K. A unified approach to false discovery rate estimation. *BMC Bioinformatics*, 9, (2008), pp 303.

Tammen H., Schulte I., Hess R., Menzel C., Kellmann M. & Schulz-Knappe P. Prerequisites for peptidomic analysis of blood samples: I. Evaluation of blood specimen qualities and determination of technical performance characteristics. *Comb. Chem. High Throughput Screen.*, 8(8), (2005), pp 725-733.

Taylor C.F., Paton N.W., Lilley K.S., Binz P.A., Julian R.K. Jr, Jones A.R., Zhu W., Apweiler R., Aebersold R., Deutsch E.W., Dunn M.J., Heck A.J., Leitner A., Macht M., Mann M., Martens L., Neubert T.A., Patterson S.D., Ping P., Seymour S.L., Souda P., Tsugita A.,Vandekerckhove J., Vondriska T.M., Whitelegge J.P., Wilkins M.R., Xenarios I., Yates J.R. 3rd & Hermjakob H. The minimum information about a proteomics experiment (MIAPE). *Nat. Biotechnol.*, 25(8), (2007), pp 887-93.

Tilleman K., Deforce D. & Elewaut D. Rheumatology: a close encounter with proteomics. *Rheumatology (Oxford)*, 44, (2005), pp 1217-1226.

van der Horst-Bruinsma I.E., Visser H., Hazes J.M., Breedveld F.C., Verduyn W., Schreuder G.M., de Vries R.R., Zanelli E. HLA-DQ-associated predisposition to and dominant HLA-DR-associated protection against rheumatoid arthritis. Hum. Immunol., 60(2), (1999), pp 152-158.

van Venrooij W.J., van Beers J.J. & Pruijn G.J. Anti-CCP Antibody, a Marker for the Early Detection of Rheumatoid Arthritis. *Ann. N. Y. Acad. Sci.*, 1143, (2008), pp 268-285.

Vang T., Congia M., Macis M.D., Musumeci L., Orrú V., Zavattari P., Nika K., Tautz L., Taskén K., Cucca F., Mustelin T. & Bottini N. Autoimmune-associated lymphoid tyrosine phosphatase is a gain-of-function variant. Nat. Genet., 37(12), (2005), pp 1317-1319.

Vencovsky J., Machacek S., Sedova L., Kafková J., Gatterová J., Pesáková V. & Růzicková S. Autoantibodies can be prognostic markers of an erosive disease in early rheumatoid arthritis. *Ann. Rheum. Dis.*, 62(5), (2003), pp 427-30.

Wagner U, Kaltenhauser S, Sauer H, Arnold S, Seidel W, Häntzschel H, Kalden JR, Wassmuth R. HLA markers and prediction of clinical course and outcome in rheumatoid arthritis. Arthritis Rheum., 40(2), (1997), pp 341-351.

Washburn M.P., Wolters D. & Yates J.R.,3rd. Large-scale analysis of the yeast proteome by multidimensional protein identification technology. *Nat. Biotechnol.* 19, (2001), pp 242-247.

Wegner N., Lundberg K., Kinloch A., Fisher B., Malmström V., Feldmann M. & Venables P.J. Autoimmunity to specific citrullinated proteins gives the first clues to the etiology of rheumatoid arthritis. *Immunol. Rev.*, 233, (2010), pp 34-54.

Weiss N.G., Jarvis J.W., Nelson R.W. & Hayes M.A. Examining serum amyloid P component microheterogeneity using capillary isoelectric focusing and MALDI-MS. *Proteomics*, 11(1), (2011), pp 106-113.

Whiteaker J.R., Zhao L., Anderson L. & Paulovich A.G. An automated and multiplexed method for high throughput peptide immunoaffinity enrichment and multiple reaction monitoring mass spectrometry-based quantification of protein biomarkers. *Mol. Cell. Proteomics*, 9(1), (2010), pp 184-196.

Wiik A.S. Anti-nuclear autoantibodies: clinical utility for diagnosis, prognosis, monitoring, and planning of treatment strategy in systemic immunoinflammatory diseases. Scand. *J. Rheumatol.*, 34(4), (2005), pp 260-268.

Wilson C., Schulz S. & Waldman S.A. Biomarker development, commercialization, and regulation: individualization of medicine lost in translation. *Clin. Pharmacol. Ther.*, 81(2), (2007), pp 153-155.

Wittkowski H., Frosch M., Wulffraat N., Goldbach-Mansky R., Kallinich T.,Kuemmerle-Deschner J., Frühwald M.C., Dassmann S., Pham T.H., Roth J. & Foell D. S100A12 is a novel molecular marker differentiating systemic-onset juvenile idiopathic arthritis from other causes of fever of unknown origin. *Arthritis Rheum.*, 58(12), (2008), pp 3924-3931.

Wolters D.A., Washburn M.P. & Yates J.R.,3rd. An automated multidimensional protein identification technology for shotgun proteomics. *Anal. Chem.* 73, (2001), pp 5683-5690.

Wright C., Sibani S., Trudgian D., Fischer R., Kessler B., Labaer J. & Bowness P. Detection of multiple autoantibodies in patients with ankylosing spondylitis using nucleic acid programmable protein arrays. *Mol. Cell. Proteomics*, (2010).

Ye X., Blonder J. & Veenstra T.D. Targeted proteomics for validation of biomarkers in clinical samples. *Brief. Funct .Genomic Proteomic*, 8(2), (2009), pp 126-135.

Zhu H., Bilgin M., Bangham R., Hall D., Casamayor A., Bertone P., Lan N., Jansen R., Bidlingmaier S., Houfek T., Mitchell T., Miller P., Dean R.A., Gerstein M. & Snyder M. Global analysis of protein activities using proteome chips. Science, 293(5537), (2001), pp 2101-2105.

Zhu Y., Shen X. & Pan W. Network-based support vector machine for classification of microarray samples. *BMC Bioinformatics*, 10 Suppl 1, (2009), pp S21.

9

# Relevance of Autoantibodies for the Classification and Pathogenesis of Neurological Diseases

Simone Mader[1], Benjamin Obholzer[2] and Markus Reindl[1]
[1]*Clinical Department of Neurology, Innsbruck Medical University*
[2]*University of Innsbruck*
*Austria*

## 1. Introduction

In the last decade research on autoantibodies in neurological diseases of the central nervous system (CNS) has been very successful. An increasing number of autoantibodies and their target antigens have been detected, supporting stratification of patients and enabling specific treatment. The detection of autoantibodies depends on the assay used, as antibody binding requires the native conformation of the antigen. Although cumulative data is suggesting an important role of B cells and antibodies in Multiple Sclerosis (MS), numerous studies failed to identify specific biomarkers for MS (Figure 1). Even though several clinical, immunological and radiological studies tried to discover risk factors for disease progression, it remains an open issue to predict the individual disease course. However, recently autoantibodies have been discovered in some rare CNS demyelinating disease closely resembling MS (Table 1). Particularly Neuromyelitis Optica (NMO) gained enormous interest due to the discovery of autoantibodies targeting the water channel protein aquaporin-4 (AQP4) (Lennon et al., 2004; Lennon et al., 2005), which is expressed on astrocytic endfeet at the blood brain barrier (Nicchia et al., 2004) (Figure 1). This inflammatory demyelinating disease represents itself with optic neuritis and longitudinally extensive transverse myelitis (Wingerchuk et al., 1999) and was long considered as a severe variant of MS. Due to the detection and validation of this highly sensitive and specific biomarker, NMO is now regarded as a separate disease entity to MS. Consequently, the anti-AQP4 antibody serostatus was included into the diagnostic criteria of NMO (Jarius et al., 2007; Wingerchuk et al., 2007). Compared to MS, patients with NMO have a worse prognosis and require different treatment strategies according to the dominant humoral immunopathogenesis. With the advent of anti-AQP4 antibodies as biomarkers in NMO spectrum disorders (NMOSD), different NMO antibody assays have been developed, whereby cell based assays using the M23 isoform of AQP4 yield highest sensitivity (Takahashi et al., 2007; Waters & Vincent, 2008; Mader et al., 2010). Despite the high percentage of anti-AQP4 IgG positive NMO patients, various studies described a lack of these autoantibodies in a cohort of NMO patients, which we will critically discuss in this chapter. It remains an open question whether these patients form their own subgroup of NMO patients or if the antibodies are not detected due to a sensitivity problem of the applied assays. Moreover, we will address the relevance of autoantibodies for the classification of neurological diseases and discuss novel findings of a potential involvement of T cells in NMO.

| | MS | NMO | ADEM |
|---|---|---|---|
| Prevalence | 100 / 100,000 | 1 / 100,000 | 1 / 100,000 |
| Female : Male ratio | 3 : 1 | 9 : 1 | 1 : 2 |
| Disease onset | 20-30 years | 40 years | Childhood |
| Disease course | Relapsing-remitting progressive | Relapsing-remitting | Monophasic, recurrent |
| Clinical symptoms | Variable | Optic neuritis, myelitis | Encephalopathy, multifocal |
| Brain MRI | Multiple white matter lesions | Normal or atypical for MS | Multifocal large bilateral lesions |
| Spinal MRI | Short-segment (<3) lesions | Long-segment (>3) lesions | Confluent |
| CSF IgG OCB + | Frequent (>90%) | Rarely | Rarely |
| Relapse treatment | Intravenous high-dose methylprednisolone, plasma exchange | | |
| Interval treatment | IFN-ß, GA, Tysabri, Fingolimod, AZT | AZT + steroids, Rituximab | None |
| Environmental triggers | Infections, Vitamin-D, smoking | Unknown | Infection, vaccination |
| Diagnostic marker | | AQP4-IgG | MOG-IgG |

Table 1. Important human inflammatory demyelinating diseases. IFN-ß = interferon-beta, GA = glatiramer acetate, AZT = azathioprine, MRI = Magnetic resonance imaging, OCB = oligoclonal bands.

Controversial results regarding the detection of autoantibodies to myelin oligodendrocyte glycoprotein (MOG) in patients with MS have confused researchers for several years. Latest findings showed increased anti-MOG antibody titers in a subgroup of patients with acute disseminated encephalomyelitis (ADEM) and childhood MS, but not in adult MS (O'Connor et al., 2007; Brilot et al., 2009; Di Pauli et al., 2011; Lalive et al., 2011). The target antigen MOG is expressed on the outer surface of the myelin sheath (Figure 1) and can only be detected using cell based assays expressing MOG on their surface. Early stratification from MS is of great relevance as ADEM is usually a self-limiting disease. However, due to the high number of anti-MOG antibody negative ADEM patients, early diagnosis remains challenging in some cases.

An early detection of autoantibodies to the NMDA (*N*-methyl *D*-aspartate) receptor is crucial in anti-NMDA-receptor encephalitis, an acute form of encephalitis, which can have a neuropsychiatric presentation, seizures, dyskinesias or autonomic instability (Dalmau et al., 2007). This disease is potentially reversible if it is recognized and treated as early as possible. In paraneoplastic courses a removal of the tumour is mandatory, but NMDA-receptor encephalitis can also be non-paraneoplastic and affect both genders. Detection of antibodies to the neuronal cell surface antigen NMDA-receptor (NMDA-R, Figure 1) in serum of patients supported a better understanding of the disease pathomechanism. In this chapter we will report on the latest findings of autoantibodies in CNS diseases, primarily focusing on anti-AQP4 antibodies in NMO, the relevance of anti-MOG antibodies in ADEM and MS and antibodies to NMDA-R in anti-NMDA-receptor encephalitis.

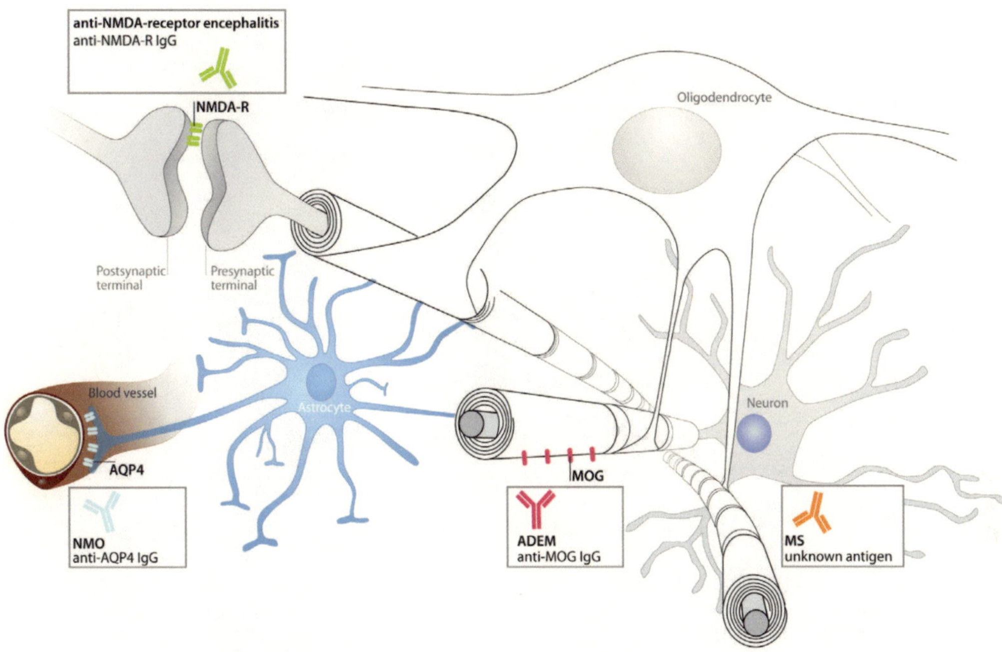


Fig. 1. Discovery of autoantibodies and their target antigens in different CNS diseases.

## 2. B cells and antibodies in MS

MS is the most frequent inflammatory demyelinating disease in young adults with a high risk of future disability and a heterogeneous clinical presentation (Noseworthy et al., 2000). Approximately 2.5 million people are affected, experiencing different disease courses. In the majority of patients (85-90%), the disease follows a relapsing-remitting course (RR-MS), characterized by acute relapses and subsequent complete or incomplete remission (Sospedra & Martin, 2005). RR-MS patients often convert into a secondary progressive disease course (SP-MS) (Sospedra & Martin, 2005). In contrast, a minority of patients suffer from the primary-progressive disease course (PP-MS, 10-15%) with a steady disease progression (Sospedra & Martin, 2005). Although the etiology of MS remains unresolved, currently it is believed that components of the myelin sheath are attacked by autoreactive T cells involving the cellular and humoral immune system (Sospedra & Martin, 2005). This infiltration of inflammatory cells within the CNS results in inflammation, thus leading to demyelination of the myelin sheaths, which cover the nerve fibers. Brain MRI shows typically multiple white matter lesions, with frequent development of new lesions. In the last decade, increasing research is focusing on the relevance of B cells and antibodies in MS, investigating their role and contribution in the initiation and propagation of inflammatory demyelinating processes at different disease stages (Figure 2).

In at least a subset of MS patients, pathogenic antibodies are believed to cause demyelination and axonal loss. This resulted in an extensive research in order to identify the still unknown target antigen. The detection of intrathecal IgG synthesis and the occurrence of oligoclonal bands (OCB) in the CSF of more than 90% of MS patients supports the impact

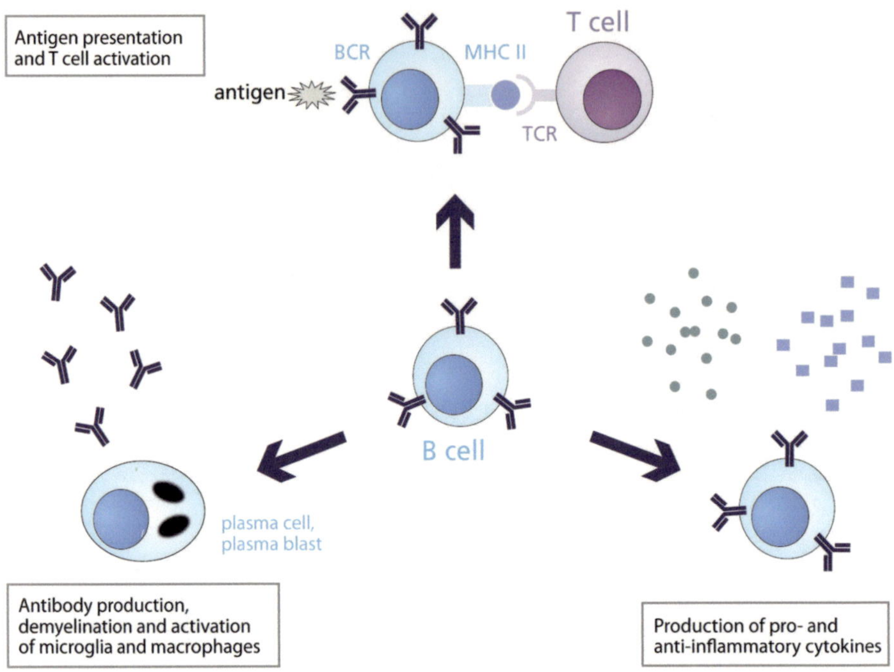


Fig. 2. Increasing evidence suggests an important role of B cells in MS. Currently, research is focusing on their relevance for antigen presentation and T cell activation, production of cytokines and antibodies.

of humoral immune responses in the pathogenesis of MS (Kabat et al., 1948). This seminal finding in 1948 is still an immunological hallmark for the disease, with the incorporation of OCB as diagnostic marker for MS (Freedman et al., 2005). However, OCBs are not unique for MS, as they are commonly detected in infectious diseases (Freedman et al., 2005), underlining the urgent need for specific biomarkers. A central role for B cells in the disease pathology can be attributed to studies showing a deposition of antibodies and complement in acute MS lesions (Lucchinetti et al., 2000) and histopathological studies confirming an antibody mediated demyelination (Lucchinetti et al., 1996; Storch et al., 1998) . Furthermore, clonally expanded B lymphocytes were discovered in chronic MS plaques and in the CSF of MS patients (Qin et al., 1998; Colombo et al., 2000; Owens et al., 2003). Latest studies highlight the role of B cells in the disease pathogenesis, as B cell depletion with the chimeric anti-CD20 monoclonal antibody rituximab had an impact on reduced inflammatory brain lesions in MS patients (Hauser et al., 2008). Nevertheless, there is a lack of unique biomarkers for MS, although numerous studies have focused on the presence of autoantibodies against potential antigens of the myelin sheath (Figure 3) and infectious agents in serum and CSF of patients (Reindl et al., 2006).

### 2.1 Anti-MOG antibodies and MS

One promising potential candidate as target antigen for MS is the myelin oligodendrocyte glycoprotein (MOG), a CNS specific antigen, which has been studied for several decades now. This transmembrane protein is localized on the outer membrane of myelin sheaths and oligodendrocytes (Figure 3) (Brunner et al., 1989).

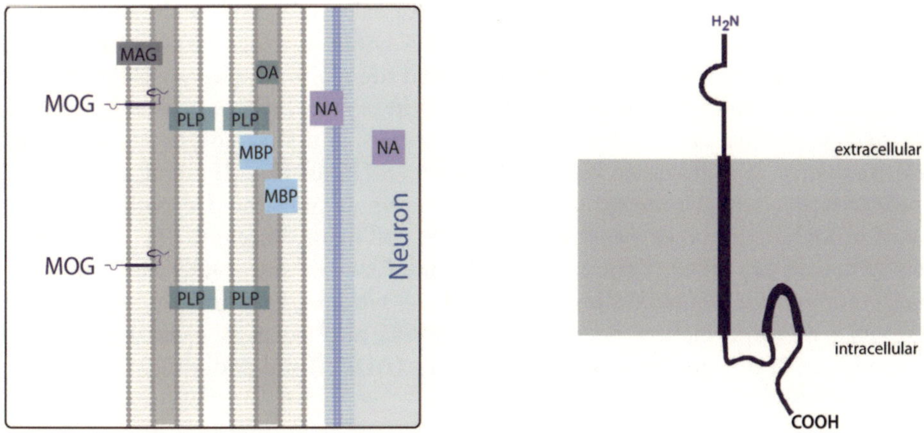


Fig. 3. MOG is expressed on the outer myelin surface.

Anti-MOG antibodies are pathogenic *in vitro* (Kerlero de Rosbo et al., 1990) and *in vivo*, as immunization with the MOG protein induces severe experimental autoimmune encephalomyelitis (EAE), which is commonly used as animal model for MS (Linington et al., 1993; Amor et al., 1994; Adelmann et al., 1995; Genain et al., 1995; Weissert et al., 1998). Immunization of MOG in adjuvant or adoptive transfer of activated myelin-specific T cells results in a MS like pathology in EAE (Goverman, 2009). Anti-MOG antibodies are proposed to augment disease severity by enhancing T cell and macrophage initiated demyelination (Zhou et al., 2006). In addition to their relevance in animal models, anti-MOG autoantibodies were discovered in active MS brain lesions (Genain et al., 1999), yet their presence in the CSF and serum of MS patients remains controversial and there are ongoing studies trying to solve these conflicting outcomes (Reindl et al., 2006). Following a publication of our group showing that increased serum anti-MOG and anti-MBP IgM antibodies in patients with clinically isolated syndrome (CIS), the most common first manifestation of MS, predict early conversion to clinically definite MS (Berger et al., 2003), numerous other studies were performed with correlations ranging from highly significant (Greeve et al., 2007; Tomassini et al., 2007), significant in a subanalysis (Rauer et al., 2006; Kuhle et al., 2007a) or not significant at all (Rauer et al., 2006; Kuhle et al., 2007a; Kuhle et al., 2007b). Possible explanations for this controversy could be linked to discrepancies in antibody assays, study designs and the investigated populations (Bar-Or & Antel, 2008). Former studies used mainly Western Blot, ELISA and liquid phase assays for the analysis of anti-MOG antibodies, which detect primarily linear epitopes of the MOG protein or partially refolded MOG. These assays were performed using bacterially expressed fragments of the MOG protein ($MOG^{1\text{-}125}$). However, binding of pathogenic serum anti-MOG antibodies might require native MOG with its posttranslational modifications. As the commonly used Western Blot and ELISA techniques led to inconsistent results, new assays were developed detecting conformational epitopes of MOG. Therefore, cell-based assays were used reflecting the correct formation and glycosylation of native MOG in the human CNS. Increased levels of autoantibodies to native MOG were observed in MS patients during relapse and in SP-MS, compared to patients in remission and controls when performing an ELISA coated with native MOG expressed by eukaryotic cells (Gaertner et al., 2004). A higher frequency of antibodies to native MOG was detected using cell lines expressing full length human MOG (Lalive et al., 2006; Zhou et al., 2006). Although both studies used cell based assays, the frequency of anti-MOG antibodies within the MS disease course varied in both studies. Lalive and colleges reported increased titers of serum anti-MOG antibodies in patients with CIS, RR-MS and to a smaller extend in SP-MS, but not in healthy controls or PP-MS patients (Lalive et al., 2006). This is in contrast to a study of Zhou, observing the highest frequency of pathogenic autoantibodies to MOG in PP-MS patients using a flow cytometry-based assay. Moreover, Zhou and colleges demonstrated a pathogenic role of human anti-MOG antibodies *in vitro* and *in vivo* following injection into susceptible rat models (Zhou et al., 2006). Summarizing, the relevance of anti-MOG antibodies in MS remains controversial. Latest findings using a novel tetramer radioimmunoassay indicated the presence of conformation dependent anti-MOG antibodies is a subset of pediatric patients with acute disseminated encephalomyelitis (ADEM) and pediatric MS, but rarely in adult onset MS (O'Connor et al., 2007).

### 2.2 High titer anti-MOG antibodies in ADEM patients

ADEM is a rarely occurring inflammatory demyelinating disease of the CNS, brain and spinal cord, with an unknown relationship to MS. In patients with ADEM, acute or subacute multifocal large bilateral white matter lesions, frequently involving deep grey matter regions are accompanied by the occurrence of encephalopathy (Mikaeloff et al., 2004; Krupp et al., 2007). Although guidelines have been published to support the diagnosis of ADEM, diagnosis can be complicated, as exact diagnostic criteria are missing. Thus, the incidence remains to be investigated. Some publications suggest a prevalence rate of 0.8 per 100,000 affected patients per year (Leake et al., 2004). Whereas some reports describe no gender predisposition (Dale et al., 2000; Leake et al., 2004), most studies indicate a slight male preponderance in ADEM patients (Pavone et al., 2010). Although the majority of patients with ADEM follow a monophasic disease course, recently recurrent or multiphasic forms have been described with a lower incidence rate (Rust, 2000; Hynson et al., 2001). ADEM commonly occurs after a vaccination (post-vaccination encephalomyelitis) or infection (post-infection encephalomyelitis). In a study of Tenembaum, analyzing 84 pediatric ADEM patients, neurological disturbances occurred in 74% of patients following vaccination or infection (Tenembaum et al., 2002). ADEM is more often described in pediatric patients and juveniles (Leake et al., 2004), however, adult cases have also been reported (Schwarz et al., 2001). In contrast to the persistent disease course of MS, 57-89% of ADEM patients show complete recovery (Dale et al., 2000; Tenembaum et al., 2002). Furthermore, acute treatment with corticosteroids, immunoglobulins and plasma exchange often results in amelioration of ADEM patients, for which reason a biomarker is of high relevance in order to stratify MS and ADEM. Primarily at disease onset, ADEM can be misdiagnosed as CIS (Mikaeloff et al., 2007). The International Consensus criteria of 2007 can serve as guidelines for diagnosing CIS or ADEM (Krupp et al., 2007). Recently, a retrospective study was published analyzing the role of MRI in 28 children with MS and 20 ADEM patients (Callen et al., 2009). Herby, Callen et al. demonstrated a lower age of onset for ADEM patients compared to pediatric MS. This study invented new MRI diagnostic criteria to help differentiating RR-MS from monophasic ADEM at disease onset, yielding a high sensitivity (81%) and specificity (95%) (Callen et al., 2009). Contrary to MS which is typically associated with the development of new lesions, ADEM lesions usually resolve or show residual findings (Kesselring et al., 1990). Therefore, a follow-up MRI within a time period not shorter than 6 months is helpful for diagnosis (Kesselring et al., 1990). Analysis of CSF can support the diagnosis, as OCB are infrequently detected in patients with ADEM (Stuve et al., 2005; Franciotta et al., 2008), yet a biomarker with high specificity is warranted. Recently, ADEM has attracted rising interest due to the discovery of anti-MOG autoantibodies in a subset of patients (O'Connor et al., 2007). In their study, O`Connor and colleges used a tetramer radioimmunoassay and detected serum antibodies directed to folded MOG tetramer in patients with ADEM in higher concentrations compared to adult MS cases (O'Connor et al., 2007). This observation was confirmed by several other publications (Brilot et al., 2009; Di Pauli et al., 2011; Lalive et al., 2011). Serum antibodies to native MOG were most commonly reported in pediatric ADEM patients. Although, a recent study of our group detected native MOG autoantibodies predominantly in children, we additionally observed few adult anti-MOG antibody positive ADEM cases (Di Pauli et al., 2011). Furthermore, we performed longitudinal analysis of anti-MOG antibodies and showed that a decrease of anti-MOG antibodies in ADEM patients was associated with a more favorable clinical outcome (Di Pauli et al., 2011). Anti-MOG IgG was detected in the CSF of high titer seropositive patients, suggesting a rather peripheral production of antibodies directed to MOG (Di Pauli et al., 2011). Even though anti-MOG antibodies might support the diagnosis of ADEM in a subset of patients, additional biomarkers are warranted for the remaining large proportion of anti-MOG antibody negative ADEM patients. Furthermore, the relevance of ADEM specific high titer anti-MOG antibodies for disease pathogenesis should be further analyzed.

## 3. Anti-AQP4 autoantibodies in NMO

NMO is a rare devastating inflammatory demyelinating disease of the CNS. In former times it was believed to be a severe variant of MS, the most common neurological disease in young adults. In contrast to MS, it has several unique features (Table 1). NMO is characterized by the occurrence of optic neuritis (ON) and longitudinally extensive transverse myelitis (LETM) extending over three or more vertebral segments (Wingerchuk et al., 1999; Cree, 2008), which can lead to blindness and paraplegia within several years of disease onset (Wingerchuk et al., 1999; Wingerchuk & Weinshenker, 2003). Furthermore, NMO commonly follows a more aggressive disease course compared to MS and has a high rate of morbidity and mortality in patients who receive no special treatment (Wingerchuk & Weinshenker, 2003). Especially at disease onset, the diagnosis can be complicated by a long lasting time interval between the occurrence of LETM and ON. Whereas OCB are detected in the CSF of approximately 90% of MS patients (Kabat et al., 1948), they are rarely or transiently present in patients with NMO (0-37%) (Wingerchuk et al., 1999). In addition, the diagnosis of NMO can be supported by the detection of CSF pleocytosis (>50 $x10^6$ white blood cell count / L) during acute relapses (Zaffaroni, 2004), which is not indicative for MS. Originally, NMO was described in 1894 by Eugene Devic and Gault as acute monophasic disorder with simultaneous occurrence of ON and LETM (Minagar et al., 2002). Due to a tremendous increase in the scientific interest for this disease, many aspects from the original view of NMO have changed. Nowadays, NMO is characterized as a mainly relapsing disease (80-90%), with a minority of patients suffering from a monophasic course (Wingerchuk et al., 2007; Sellner et al., 2010). Whereas NMO was initially described by a lack of brain MRI lesions, MS-atypical brain lesions are found in some NMO patients primarily at sites of high AQP4 expression (Pittock et al., 2006). However, a negative brain MRI at disease onset is not indicative for MS (Jarius et al., 2008b). The explosive rise in the field of NMO research was mainly due to the discovery of NMO-IgG autoantibodies, mostly IgG1, in serum of NMO patients, but not in classical MS or any other controls (Lennon et al., 2004). This marvelous achievement is attributed to Vanda Lennon and her group, discovering one year later the AQP4 water channel protein as target antigen of NMO autoantibodies (Lennon et al., 2004; Lennon et al., 2005). This transmembrane channel protein constitutes an essential part of the blood brain barrier due to its localization in pericapillary endfeet processes and ependymal cells facing the ventricles (Figure 1) (Nielsen et al., 1997; Rash et al., 1998; Nicchia et al., 2004). The discovery and validation of this highly specific biomarker resulted in the incorporation of the anti-AQP4 antibody serostatus in the diagnostic criteria of NMO, achieving high sensitivity (99%) and specificity (90%) (Jarius et al., 2007; Wingerchuk et al., 2007) (Table 2).

| Absolute criteria | Supportive criteria |
|---|---|
| 1. Optic neuritis | 1. Brain MRI atypical for MS |
| 2. Acute myelitis | 2. Spinal cord MRI with contiguous T2-weighted signal abnormality extending over 3 or more vertebral segments |
| | 3. Anti-AQP4 IgG seropositive status |

Table 2. Revised diagnostic criteria of NMO (Wingerchuk et al., 2007). Definite NMO requires fulfillment of both absolute criteria and of two of the 3 supportive criteria.

Since the discovery of anti-AQP4 IgG, NMO is considered as a separate disease entity with an unknown relationship to MS. Thus, the detection of anti-AQP4 antibodies facilitates an early stratification of NMO and MS, which is highly important due to the different treatment recommendations. Compared to MS, NMO patients have a worse prognosis and require distinct treatment strategies due to the dominant humoral immunopathogenesis. Whereas immunomodulatory therapies are frequently applied for treating MS, immunosuppressive treatment is more promising for NMO (Sellner et al., 2010). Interferon beta (IFN-ß) and glatiramer acetate (GA) were shown to be beneficial in MS, whereas in NMO patients these drugs have an ineffective or even deleterious effect (Papeix et al., 2007; Warabi et al., 2007). Acute attacks are commonly treated by a combination of corticosteroids and immunosuppressive agents. Plasma exchange or treatment with rituximab can prevent NMO attacks in patients not responding to corticosteroids (Cree et al., 2005; Watanabe et al., 2007; Jacob et al., 2008; Bonnan et al., 2009).

### 3.1 NMO epidemiology and genetic factors

Limited reports are published concerning the epidemiology of NMO in different ethnic groups (Kira, 2006; Cabrera-Gomez et al., 2009; Collongues et al., 2010), and thus the incidence and prevalence of NMO remains unknown. Some studies indicate a prevalence of one per 100,000 patients (Cabre, 2009; Cabrera-Gomez et al., 2009), however these studies use different antibody assays. Presumably, a proportion of patients remains to be falsely diagnosed as severe variant of MS. Available data suggest a higher incidence in non-Caucasian countries, especially in Latin American, East Asian and African populations compared to Northern European countries (Osuntokun, 1971; Kira et al., 1996; Papais-Alvarenga et al., 2002). NMO occurs up to nine times more often in women than in men

(Wingerchuk et al., 2007), with a median age of onset at around 40 years (Wingerchuk et al., 2007). Female patients were far more likely to develop the recurrent disease course (Wingerchuk, 2009), yet the gender had no impact on the type or severity of initial attacks, recovery from initial attacks, relapse frequency or disease related mortality (Wingerchuk, 2009). A genetic predisposition for NMO was recently indicated by some case reports, which are mainly based on studies of sibling pairs and a parent-child case (Mirsattari et al., 2001; Rivera & Cabrera, 2001; Braley & Mikol, 2007; Cabrera-Gomez et al., 2009). Furthermore, 12 pedigrees of NMO patients with a total number of 25 patients were recently analyzed by Mattiello and his group, resulting in 3% familial NMO cases in patients with clinical definite NMO (Matiello et al., 2010). This number might be larger when also including patients with high risk NMO, as the disease can have a heterogeneous presentation (Pellkofer et al., 2009).

### 3.2 Anti-AQP4 antibodies as biomarkers for NMO-spectrum disorders

With the advent of anti-AQP4 antibodies as biomarkers in NMOSD (Lennon et al., 2004; Lennon et al., 2005), various NMO antibody assays have been developed (Lennon et al., 2004; Lennon et al., 2005; Paul et al., 2007; Takahashi et al., 2007; Marignier et al., 2008; Waters & Vincent, 2008; Mader et al., 2010). The choice of assay is crucial for the identification of NMO IgG autoantibodies in serum and CSF samples of patients. The first assay describing the presence of NMO autoantibodies applied an indirect immunofluorescence (IF) assay with a composite substrate of adult mouse cerebellum sections (Lennon et al., 2004). This assay was described by the group of Vanda Lennon, achieving 58-73% sensitivity and 91-100% specificity for NMO. One year later the AQP4 water channel protein was detected as target antigen using human embryonic kidney cells (HEK) transfected with human AQP4 (Lennon et al., 2005). The establishment of cell based assays using transfected HEK cells resulted in an even higher sensitivity than the tissue based IF assays, resembling most likely the native conformation of the AQP4 protein (Takahashi et al., 2006; Takahashi et al., 2007; Mader et al., 2010). For this purpose, the cells were transfected with the AQP4 protein fused to a green fluorescence protein. After addition of the NMO samples, the bound anti-AQP4 antibodies were detected using a secondary antibody. Positive samples were visualized by a co-staining of NMO IgG (red) with the AQP4 expressing cells (green), as demonstrated in Figure 4 (Takahashi et al., 2006; Mader et al., 2010).

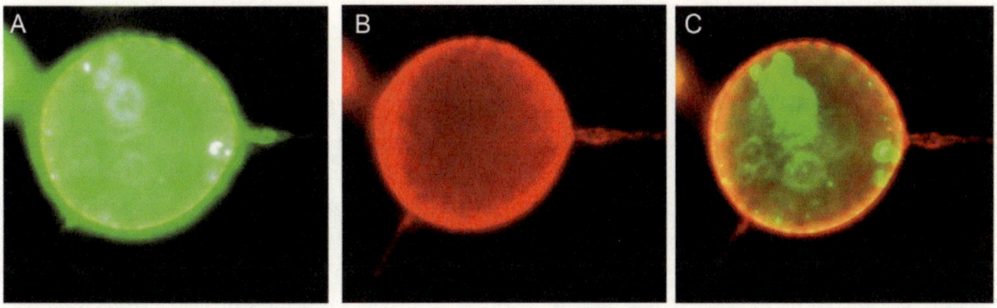


Fig. 4. Detection of an anti-AQP4 IgG seropositive patient with our live cell staining IF assay (Mader et al., 2010). Human anti-AQP4 IgG (red, B) in patient`s serum bind to the AQP4-EmGFP transfected cells (green, A), resulting in co-localisation (merge, C).

This assay has the advantage of determining titer values of NMO antibody positive patients by serial dilutions of serum samples until loss of signal. However, the relevance of these titer levels remains controversial. As the AQP4 transmembrane protein is either expressed as full length M1 or as 23 amino acid shorter M23 AQP4 (Figure 5) (Neely et al., 1999; Furman et al., 2003), many studies lack the information regarding the usage of the AQP4 isoform. Recently, our group demonstrated that anti-AQP4 antibodies primarily target the shorter M23 AQP4 isoform, whereas antibodies to full length AQP4 were developed with increasing disease duration and number of relapses (Mader et al., 2010). For this purpose we used a live cell staining IF assay with transiently transfected HEK cells, resulting in 97% sensitivity for NMO and 65% for high risk NMO, with a specificity of 100% compared to controls (Mader et al., 2010). Our assay showed different staining patterns for M1 and M23 AQP4 transfected cells (Mader et al., 2010). In contrast to M1 AQP4, M23 AQP4 forms orthogonal arrays of particles (Figure 5 B), which are currently believed to be potential targets of antibody binding (Nicchia et al., 2009). Consequently the NMO IF assay yields highest sensitivity when using cell-based assay with M23 AQP4 transfected cells.

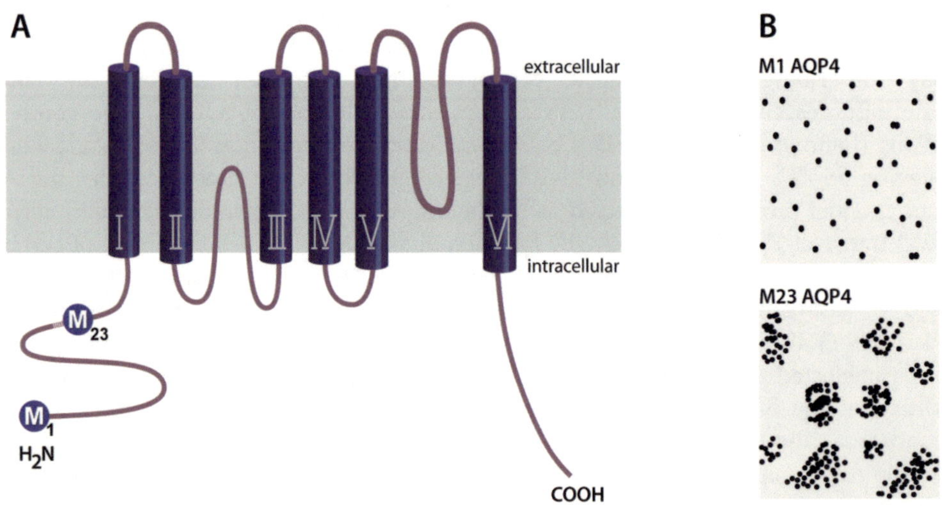


Fig. 5. Structure (A) and expression pattern (B) of the M1 and M23 AQP4 isoforms.

### 3.3 "Anti-AQP4 seronegative NMO"

The terminus "anti-AQP4 seronegative NMO" should be handled with care, as several factors contribute to the antibody serostatus. A broad range of antibody assays is available resulting in diverse sensitivity and specificity. Consequently, the percentage of seronegative NMO patients is fluctuating depending on the methodology approach. Cell-based assays using the M1 or M23 AQP4 isoform have an impact on the number of seronegative NMO patients. A negative antibody status might be credited to an administered therapy prior to testing. A depletion of antibodies below a detectable threshold could explain a negative serostatus. Although, anti-AQP4 antibodies have been detected up to ten years before disease onset (Nishiyama et al., 2009), we have analyzed a small number of patients who were initially negative for NMO IgG and turned out to be low titer positive in longitudinal samples (unpublished results). For this reasons, one has to be careful when dealing with the term "seronegative NMO". Moreover, seronegative NMO might resemble another disease course with overlapping clinical features. Particularly, pediatric NMO can present itself with diverse clinical features, and therefore stratification from MS can be difficult especially at disease onset (Lotze et al., 2008). The diagnosis might further be supported by analyzing CSF of patients. Recently, glial fibrillar acidic protein (GFAP), a marker of astrocytic damage, was shown to be significantly elevated in the CSF of NMO patients compared to classical MS (Misu et al., 2009), however this increase was primarily detectable during relapse (Misu et al., 2009). In conclusion, the anti-AQP4 antibody serostatus should be repeatedly analyzed in NMOSD using highly sensitive and specific cell based assays. The absence of anti-AQP4 antibodies over a long time interval indicates a different disease pathomechanism compared to patients with "AQP4 autoimmune channelopathy". Consequently ongoing research should focus on the discovery of new biomarkers for anti-AQP4 seronegative patients with NMO.

### 3.4 NMO-spectrum disorders

Apart from clinical definite NMO, anti-AQP4 IgG antibodies are frequently detected in limited forms of NMO (Wingerchuk et al., 2007). These patients do not fulfill the complete diagnostic criteria of NMO, but harbor a high risk of developing clinically definite NMO (Pittock et al., 2008; Mader et al., 2010). Therefore, NMO and high risk NMO patients represent the group of NMOSD, suffering either from monophasic bilateral or recurrent ON or LETM (idiopathic, isolated or recurrent) (Wingerchuk et al., 2007). Currently NMO IgG positive patients with recurrent ON were shown to have a poor visual outcome and were more likely to develop NMO in a longitudinal study (Matiello et al., 2008). Anti-AQP4 IgG seropositivity predicted a relapse in patients with a first episode of LETM event extending over three or more vertebral segments (Weinshenker et al., 2006). In 50% of these anti-AQP4 IgG seropositive LETM patients either ON occurred or LETM relapsed within half a year (Weinshenker et al., 2006). Furthermore, anti-AQP4 antibodies have been frequently detected in systemic autoimmune disorders presenting themselves with ON or LETM, such as neuropsychiatric systemic lupus erythematosus (SLE), Sjogren's syndrome, myasthenia gravis or thyroiditis (Wingerchuk et al., 2007). However, anti-AQP4 antibodies were detected exclusively in systemic autoimmune disorders in combination with NMO or High Risk NMO symptoms. The presence of anti-AQP4 antibodies could indicate a coexistence of systemic autoimmune disorders with NMO (Pittock et al., 2008; Wandinger et al., 2010), rather than an epiphenomenon (Pittock et al., 2008; Wandinger et al., 2010), yet their relationship remains unidentified.

### 3.5 Serum titer levels of anti-AQP4 IgG antibodies

The role of serum anti-AQP4 antibody titers remains controversially described. Takahashi and his group showed an involvement of AQP4-IgG antibody titers in disease pathogenesis, detecting a correlation with spinal cord lesion length (Takahashi et al., 2006). This study analyzed 148 serum samples of Japanese patients including 35 patients with NMO-spectrum disorders and demonstrated elevated AQP4-IgG titer levels in patients with permanent complete blindness, LETM and extensive or large cerebral lesions (Takahashi et al., 2006). In addition, a longitudinal study of eight NMO-IgG positive patients reported a correlation of serum anti-AQP4 Ig with clinical disease activity (Jarius et al., 2008a), demonstrating a threefold intra-individual increase of AQP4 IgG titers during relapse, which was not accompanied by other serum antibodies (Takahashi et al., 2006). Some papers suggest an effect of treatment on antibody titers, showing a reduction of NMO antibody titer levels after immunosuppressive treatment (Takahashi et al., 2006; Jarius et al., 2008a). Recently, an increase of anti-AQP4 antibody titers was described in one NMO patient following immunomodulatory treatment with IFN-ß (Palace et al., 2010). Applying conventional immunosuppressive therapy, the antibody titers decreased again in this patient (Palace et al., 2010), high lightening the importance of an early stratification of MS and NMO.

### 3.6 AQP4-IgM antibodies

Although, IgM antibodies binding to AQP4 were described at NMO lesion sites (Lucchinetti et al., 2002; Roemer et al., 2007), their role in the disease course remains unresolved. Most studies investigating autoantibodies against AQP4 refer to IgG antibodies. We addressed this issue in a recent study analyzing IgG and IgM antibodies directed to M23 AQP4 in serum of patients with NMO-spectrum disorders and in other disease groups using a live cell staining IF assay (Mader et al., 2010). In contrast to NMO IgG, which was exclusively detected in 97% of NMO patients and 65% of suspected NMO, M23 IgM antibodies were elevated in NMO (27%) and high risk NMO (12%). However, IgM antibodies to M23 AQP4 were additionally present in NMO IgG seronegative patients with isolated myelitis, MS (4%) and OND (4%). Furthermore, titer levels were much lower for IgM than for IgG AQP4. Antibodies of subtype IgM that bind to full length AQP4 were present in 10% of NMO and 8% of High Risk NMO, but not in any controls (Mader et al., 2010). This is in accordance with a study of Jarius et al. detecting IgM antibodies in almost 10% of NMO patients (4 /42) but not in any controls (Jarius et al., 2010a). Larger studies are warranted to further analyze anti-AQP4 IgG and IgM double positive patients. As anti-AQP4 IgM antibodies are more potent to activate the complement cascade, it would be tempting to further investigate the clinical parameters of anti-AQP4 IgM positive patients with NMOSD.

### 3.7 Cerebrospinal fluid anti-AQP4 antibodies

Several studies are available concerning anti-AQP4 antibodies in serum samples of patients with NMO-spectrum disorders. In contrast, few studies focused on the presence and relevance of NMO antibodies in the CSF (Takahashi et al., 2007; Klawiter et al., 2009; Jarius et al., 2010b; Dujmovic et al., 2011). Klawiter and colleges reported the presence of CSF anti-AQP4 antibodies in three seronegative NMO patients (Klawiter et al., 2009), which could not be reproduced in other publications. Recently, Jarius et al., detected CSF anti-AQP4 antibodies in NMO-IgG seropositive patients exceeding anti-AQP4 antibody serum titers ≥ 1:250, but not in anti-AQP4 antibody negative patients (Jarius et al., 2010b). In cooperation with Dujmovic we analyzed the temporal dynamics of CSF anti-AQP4 antibodies in 12 patients with NMOSD (Dujmovic et al., 2011). Thereby, we could show that longitudinal CSF anti-AQP4 IgG correlated with clinical parameters. CSF AQP4-IgG were present in patients with high serum titers and correlated with spinal MRI lesion length and CSF parameters. Moreover, clinical improvement was associated with a decrease in CSF, but not serum, anti-AQP4 IgG titers. Summarizing, CSF AQP4-IgG were associated with clinical activity and neuroinflammation (Dujmovic et al., 2011).

### 3.8 Pathogenic role of anti-AQP4 antibodies and T cells in NMO

In order to address the pathogenic relevance of anti-AQP4 antibodies, several *in vitro* and *in vivo* studies have been performed so far. Tissue sections showed the distribution of anti-AQP4 antibodies and products of complement activation surrounding hyalinized blood vessels in a rosette-like pattern (Lucchinetti et al., 2002). This deposition of NMO antibodies and complement on astrocytes at the glia limitans was accompanied by a loss of the AQP4 water channel protein (Lennon et al., 2004; Roemer et al., 2007). The cytotoxic effect of anti-AQP4 antibodies has been demonstrated in several studies so far (Jarius et al., 2008b; Hinson et al., 2009; Sabater et al., 2009; Kinoshita et al., 2010). The binding of the anti-AQP4 antibody led to an activation of the classical complement cascade, resulting in lysis of NMO antibody opsonized and AQP4-transfected cells and astrocytes (Jarius et al., 2008b). The pathogenic role of anti-AQP4 antibodies has been further supported by several *in vivo* studies using rat and mouse models (Bennett et al., 2009; Bradl et al., 2009; Kinoshita et al., 2009; Saadoun et al., 2010). Therefore, NMO-IgG antibodies were purified from the plasma exchange material of AQP4-IgG positive and negative NMO patients, MS patients and control subjects and then injected into animal models (Bradl et al., 2009). Three studies demonstrated the formation of NMO-like lesions in Lewis rats following injection of isolated human NMO-IgG in the presence of acute T cell mediated CNS inflammation (Bennett et al., 2009; Bradl et al., 2009; Kinoshita et al., 2009). In contrast, Saadoun proved the formation of NMO like lesions after injection of NMO-IgG into mouse brain only in the presence of complement, thus by-passing the damage of the blood brain barrier (Saadoun et al., 2010). In order to confirm that the NMO like pathology in the animals was due to the anti-AQP4 IgG and not based on other antibodies in the plasma exchange material, pre-absorption experiments using cells expressing AQP4 were performed (Bradl et al., 2009). This pre-absorption experiment resulted in a massive decrease of lesion size and was associated with less astrocytic damage, confirming the pathogenicity of anti-AQP4 autoantibodies (Bradl et al., 2009). As anti-AQP4 antibodies are not sufficient to induce NMO like lesions without support of T cells (Bradl et al., 2009) and/or complement (Saadoun et al., 2010), the role of T cell mediated immune responses against AQP4 is currently an issue of interest (Nelson et al., 2010; Kalluri et al., 2011; Pohl et al., 2011). Supporting evidence for a possible pathogenic role of T cells comes from observations showing no formation of NMO like lesions in immature rats after injection of anti-AQP4 autoantibodies, although these animals posses a leaky blood brain barrier (Bradl et al., 2009). Latest findings by Pohl et al. showed that AQP4 specific T cells are capable of inducing brain inflammation mainly in astrocytic glia limitans and therefore enable an entry of anti-AQP4 autoantibodies (Pohl et al., 2011). As anti-AQP4 antibodies are detectable more than ten years before disease onset (Nishiyama et al., 2009), the time point when these antibodies lead to NMO symptoms remains unresolved. It is tempting to speculate that anti-AQP4 antibodies are not harmful if they circulate peripherally and as long as they are excluded from the blood brain barrier. Whether a large amount of anti-AQP4 autoantibodies is necessary for the patients to develop symptoms remains to be investigated. Having access to the blood brain barrier, anti-AQP4 autoantibodies bind to their target antigen and result in complement activation. This leads to vascular hyalinization, necrosis, demyelination and axonal injury (Wingerchuk et al., 2007). The titer levels seem to have an impact on the disease pathogenesis as antibodies in the CSF are only detectable in high titer seropositive patients (Jarius et al., 2010b; Dujmovic et al., 2011). Latest findings indicated an influx of systemically produced anti-AQP4 antibodies through the area postrema (Popescu et al., 2011). This was supported by findings of patients suffering from intractable vomiting and nausea as initial symptoms of NMO (Popescu et al., 2011).

## 4. NMDA-receptor encephalomyelitis

### 4.1 Anti-NMDA-receptor encephalitis

The role of autoantibodies to the ionotropic NMDA (N-methyl-D-aspartate) glutamate receptor (NMDA-R; Figure 6) is well established in limbic encephalitis (Graus et al., 2010; Vincent et al., 2010; Dalmau et al., 2011).

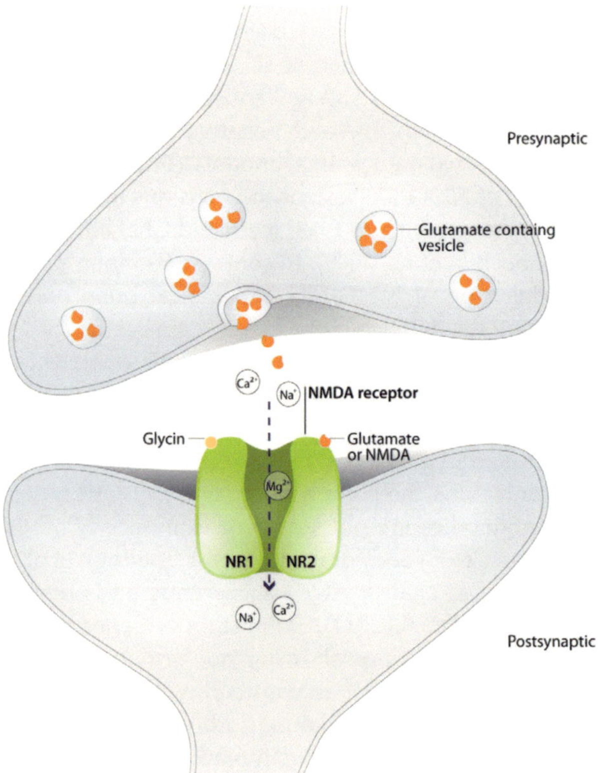


Fig. 6. NMDA-receptor expression on the postsynaptic terminal of neurons.

These novel autoantibodies were first described by Dalmau et al. in serum samples of young women presenting with a subacute-onset encephalopathy often associated with movement disorders and an underlying ovarian teratoma (Dalmau et al., 2007; Dalmau et al., 2008). The presence of neuronal tissue expressing NMDA-R within the tumour was thought to trigger the production of paraneoplastic autoantibodies. However, the origin of the autoantibodies remains unresolved, as recent publications reported numerous of non-teratoma associated cases. Among some adults, most of these non-paraneoplastic NMDA-R encephalitis cases occurred in children (Dale et al., 2009; Florance et al., 2009; Irani et al., 2010). Anti-NMDA-R encephalitis is associated with a strong female predominance (female:male ratio is 8:1) occurring primarily at a median age of 23 years (Dalmau et al., 2008).

The characteristic symptoms of anti-NMDA-R positive patients are of prominent psychiatric and behavioral nature, including rapid memory loss, seizures, abnormal movements (dyskinesias), hypoventilation and autonomic instability. This disease usually progresses from initial neuropsychiatric symptoms into a state of unresponsiveness with catatonic features, commonly associated with abnormal movements, and autonomic- and breathing instability. Additionally, most patients show prodomal symptoms such as headache, fever, nausea, vomiting, diarrhea or upper respiratory-tract symptoms. Brain MRI data show no or only minor changes which usually occur transiently despite severity of symptoms. Concerning CSF parameters, 60% of patients show OCB and mild lymphocyte pleocytosis (Dalmau et al., 2011). Interestingly, intrathecal NMDA-R antibody synthesis was observed in a majority of patients and CSF titer levels were more likely to correlate with clinical severity, compared to serum titers (Dalmau et al., 2008; Dale et al., 2009; Florance et al., 2009; Irani et al., 2010).

Although the disease can be lethal in some rare cases and despite the severity of the symptoms, more than 70% of patients recover after treatment and less than 30% of patients show incomplete recovery with memory, cognitive and motor deficits. Treatment options include immunotherapy (corticosteroids, intravenous immunoglobulin or plasma exchange) and/or tumor removal with the aim to reduce anti-NMDA-R autoantibody levels. Recent studies showed that antibodies to the NMDA-R were predominantly of the IgG1 subclass and are able to activate complement on NMDA-R expressing human embryonic kidney cells (Irani et al., 2010). However, the role of complement activation remains controversial as other findings indicated a complement-independent mode of action. Several studies have addressed the issue regarding the binding site of the autoantibodies and possible functional consequences on the targeted NMDA-R. Dalmau et al. described the NR1 isoform or NR1/NR2 heterodimers of the NMDA-R as recognition site of anti-NMDA-R antibodies (Dalmau et al., 2011). Providing further insight into the mode of action, *in vitro* and *in vivo* studies nicely demonstrated that antibodies from patients with anti-NMDA-R encephalitis caused a rapid and reversible loss of surface NMDA-R by antibody-mediated capping and internalization, resulting in abrogation of NMDA-R-mediated synaptic function (Dalmau et al., 2008; Hughes et al., 2010).

Thus, similar to the role of anti-AQP4 IgG antibodies in NMO, anti-NMDA-R antibodies helped to define a new clinical syndrome, anti-NMDA receptor encephalitis (Dalmau et al., 2011).

### 4.2 Anti-NMDA receptor antibodies in neuropsychiatric SLE

Several reports confirmed the presence of autoantibodies to NMDA-R, particularly the NR2 isoform, in the majority of patients with neuropsychiatric SLE (DeGiorgio et al., 2001; Emmer et al., 2006; Hanly et al., 2006; Kowal et al., 2006; Lapteva et al., 2006; Arinuma et al., 2008; Fragoso-Loyo et al., 2008). These autoantibodies were not only detected in serum, but also in the CSF and brain parenchyma of some SLE patients. Furthermore, CSF titers correlate with neuropsychiatric symptoms. In SLE, anti-NMDA-R antibodies were demonstrated to bind to a small peptide (DWEYS) present in the extracellular, amino-terminal domain of NR2A and NR2B subunits (DeGiorgio et al., 2001; Gielen et al., 2009). Injection of murine or human monoclonal antibodies against this peptide into the hippocampus and cerebral cortex of mice resulted in local loss of neurons and induced activation of caspase-3 in cultured human and murine neurons (DeGiorgio et al., 2001; Kowal et al., 2006; Gielen et al., 2009). Furthermore, several experimental studies in mice demonstrated a causal relationship between anti-NMDA-R autoantibodies with impairment in cognition and behavior (Diamond et al., 2009). A recent study provided evidence of a positive modulating effect on receptor function by low concentrations of anti-NMDA-R antibodies, resulting in an increase of NMDA-R mediated excitatory postsynaptic potentials. However, at high concentrations, these antibodies promote excitotoxicity through enhanced mitochondrial permeability transition. These findings might be an explanation for the either transient or permanent neuropsychiatric clinical course observed in SLE patients. In conclusion, antibodies to the NR2 isoform of NMDA-R could play an important role in the pathogenesis of neuropsychiatric lupus.

Many studies focusing on the detection of antibodies to the NMDA-R NR2A and NR2B subunits in SLE have used the ELISA technique. It is now essential that studies regarding antibody specificity in patient serum/CSF are confirmed using live cell-based assays expressing native NMDA-R or single subunits.

### 4.3 Anti-NMDA receptor antibodies in inflammatory demyelinating diseases

Interestingly, antibodies against NMDA-type glutamate receptors were also detected in both serum and CSF of patients with NMOSD (Ishikawa et al., 2007; Kruer et al., 2010). As previously described, the discovery of anti-AQP4 IgG antibodies in the serum of patients with NMOSD enables an early diagnosis and specific treatment of the disease. Despite the high percentage of AQP4-IgG seropositive NMO patients, several studies report on AQP4-IgG seronegative NMO patients who, however, show no differences in their clinical presentation. It might well be that AQP4-IgG seronegative patients represent a distinct subgroup of NMO patients, in whom the disease is triggered by other autoantibodies, such as antibodies to NMDA-R or yet unknown targets. So far, in literature there is a lack of information regarding the presence of anti-NMDA-R antibodies in other CNS demyelinating diseases, such as MS. Up to now, one case report speculates on a possible association of the rarely occurring epileptic seizures in MS (Catenoix et al., 2010) with anti-NMDA-R antibody seropositivity (Johnston et al., 2010).

## 5. Conclusion

The discovery of autoantibodies in different CNS diseases can support an early diagnosis and treatment monitoring. Moreover, antibodies can contribute to a better understanding of the disease pathogenesis. However, an antibody seronegative result should be handled with care, as this can be linked to the assay methodology, study population or to therapeutic intervention. In contrast to the high sensitivity and specificity of anti-AQP4 autoantibodies in NMO patients, antibodies to MOG are discovered "only" in a subgroup of ADEM patients. Hence, there is a lack of a specific biomarker for more than half of patients diagnosed with ADEM. Future studies focusing on these seronegative patients might facilitate a reclassification of CNS diseases through the identification of novel biomarkers. Finally, antibodies to NMDA-R are highly specific for NMDA-receptor encephalitis, whereas their role in other neurological diseases has to be confirmed by specific assays.

## 6. Acknowledgment

The authors wish to thank the ARGE NMO Austria for excellent co-operation and Kathrin Schanda and Viktoria Gredler for their help and encouragement. This work was financially supported by Innsbruck Medical University and the Austrian MS society.

## 7. References


Adelmann, M., Wood, J., Benzel, I., Fiori, P., Lassmann, H., Matthieu, J.M., Gardinier, M.V., Dornmair, K., and Linington, C. (1995). The N-terminal domain of the myelin oligodendrocyte glycoprotein (MOG) induces acute demyelinating experimental autoimmune encephalomyelitis in the Lewis rat. *J Neuroimmunol*, 63, 1, Dec, 17-27.

Amor, S., Groome, N., Linington, C., Morris, M.M., Dornmair, K., Gardinier, M.V., Matthieu, J.M., and Baker, D. (1994). Identification of epitopes of myelin oligodendrocyte glycoprotein for the induction of experimental allergic encephalomyelitis in SJL and Biozzi AB/H mice. *J Immunol*, 153, 10, Nov 15, 4349-4356.

Arinuma, Y., Yanagida, T., and Hirohata, S. (2008). Association of cerebrospinal fluid anti-NR2 glutamate receptor antibodies with diffuse neuropsychiatric systemic lupus erythematosus. *Arthritis and rheumatism*, 58, 4, Apr, 1130-1135.

Bar-Or, A., and Antel, J. (2008). Cross-reactivity between epidemiology and immunology in multiple sclerosis. *Neurology*, 71, 15, Oct 7, 1132-1133.

Bennett, J.L., Lam, C., Kalluri, S.R., Saikali, P., Bautista, K., Dupree, C., Glogowska, M., Case, D., Antel, J.P., Owens, G.P., Gilden, D., Nessler, S., Stadelmann, C., and Hemmer, B. (2009). Intrathecal pathogenic anti-aquaporin-4 antibodies in early neuromyelitis optica. *Ann Neurol*, 66, 5, Nov, 617-629.

Berger, T., Rubner, P., Schautzer, F., Egg, R., Ulmer, H., Mayringer, I., Dilitz, E., Deisenhammer, F., and Reindl, M. (2003). Antimyelin antibodies as a predictor of clinically definite multiple sclerosis after a first demyelinating event. *N Engl J Med*, 349, 2, Jul 10, 139-145.

Bonnan, M., Valentino, R., Olindo, S., Mehdaoui, H., Smadja, D., and Cabre, P. (2009). Plasma exchange in severe spinal attacks associated with neuromyelitis optica spectrum disorder. *Mult Scler*, 15, 4, Apr, 487-492.

Bradl, M., Misu, T., Takahashi, T., Watanabe, M., Mader, S., Reindl, M., Adzemovic, M., Bauer, J., Berger, T., Fujihara, K., Itoyama, Y., and Lassmann, H. (2009). Neuromyelitis optica: pathogenicity of patient immunoglobulin in vivo. *Ann Neurol*, 66, 5, Nov, 630-643.

Braley, T., and Mikol, D.D. (2007). Neuromyelitis optica in a mother and daughter. *Arch Neurol*, 64, 8, Aug, 1189-1192.

Brilot, F., Dale, R.C., Selter, R.C., Grummel, V., Kalluri, S.R., Aslam, M., Busch, V., Zhou, D., Cepok, S., and Hemmer, B. (2009). Antibodies to native myelin oligodendrocyte glycoprotein in children with inflammatory demyelinating central nervous system disease. *Ann Neurol*, 66, 6, Dec, 833-842.

Brunner, C., Lassmann, H., Waehneldt, T.V., Matthieu, J.M., and Linington, C. (1989). Differential ultrastructural localization of myelin basic protein, myelin/oligodendroglial glycoprotein, and 2',3'-cyclic nucleotide 3'-phosphodiesterase in the CNS of adult rats. *J Neurochem*, 52, 1, Jan, 296-304.

Cabre, P. (2009). Environmental changes and epidemiology of multiple sclerosis in the French West Indies. *J Neurol Sci*, 286, 1-2, Nov 15, 58-61.

Cabrera-Gomez, J.A., Kurtzke, J.F., Gonzalez-Quevedo, A., and Lara-Rodriguez, R. (2009). An epidemiological study of neuromyelitis optica in Cuba. *J Neurol*, 256, 1, Jan, 35-44.

Callen, D.J., Shroff, M.M., Branson, H.M., Li, D.K., Lotze, T., Stephens, D., and Banwell, B.L. (2009). Role of MRI in the differentiation of ADEM from MS in children. *Neurology*, 72, 11, Mar 17, 968-973.

Catenoix, H., Marignier, R., Ritleng, C., Dufour, M., Mauguiere, F., Confavreux, C., and Vukusic, S. (2010). Multiple sclerosis and epileptic seizures. *Multiple sclerosis (Houndmills, Basingstoke, England)*, Sep 22.

Collongues, N., Marignier, R., Zephir, H., Papeix, C., Blanc, F., Ritleng, C., Tchikviladze, M., Outteryck, O., Vukusic, S., Fleury, M., Fontaine, B., Brassat, D., Clanet, M., Milh, M., Pelletier, J., Audoin, B., Ruet, A., Lebrun-Frenay, C., Thouvenot, E., Camu, W., Debouverie, M., Creange, A., Moreau, T., Labauge, P., Castelnovo, G., Edan, G., Le Page, E., Defer, G., Barroso, B., Heinzlef, O., Gout, O., Rodriguez, D., Wiertlewski, S., Laplaud, D., Borgel, F., Tourniaire, P., Grimaud, J., Brochet, B., Vermersch, P., Confavreux, C., and de Seze, J. (2010). Neuromyelitis optica in France: a multicenter study of 125 patients. *Neurology*, 74, 9, Mar 2, 736-742.

Colombo, M., Dono, M., Gazzola, P., Roncella, S., Valetto, A., Chiorazzi, N., Mancardi, G.L., and Ferrarini, M. (2000). Accumulation of clonally related B lymphocytes in the cerebrospinal fluid of multiple sclerosis patients. *J Immunol*, 164, 5, Mar 1, 2782-2789.

Cree, B. (2008). Neuromyelitis optica: diagnosis, pathogenesis, and treatment. *Curr Neurol Neurosci Rep*, 8, 5, Sep, 427-433.

Cree, B.A., Lamb, S., Morgan, K., Chen, A., Waubant, E., and Genain, C. (2005). An open label study of the effects of rituximab in neuromyelitis optica. *Neurology*, 64, 7, Apr 12, 1270-1272.

Dale, R.C., de Sousa, C., Chong, W.K., Cox, T.C., Harding, B., and Neville, B.G. (2000). Acute disseminated encephalomyelitis, multiphasic disseminated encephalomyelitis and multiple sclerosis in children. *Brain*, 123 Pt 12, Dec, 2407-2422.

Dale, R.C., Irani, S.R., Brilot, F., Pillai, S., Webster, R., Gill, D., Lang, B., and Vincent, A. (2009). N-methyl-D-aspartate receptor antibodies in pediatric dyskinetic encephalitis lethargica. *Annals of neurology*, 66, 5, Nov, 704-709.

Dalmau, J., Gleichman, A.J., Hughes, E.G., Rossi, J.E., Peng, X., Lai, M., Dessain, S.K., Rosenfeld, M.R., Balice-Gordon, R., and Lynch, D.R. (2008). Anti-NMDA-receptor encephalitis: case series and analysis of the effects of antibodies. *Lancet neurology*, 7, 12, Dec, 1091-1098.

Dalmau, J., Lancaster, E., Martinez-Hernandez, E., Rosenfeld, M.R., and Balice-Gordon, R. (2011). Clinical experience and laboratory investigations in patients with anti-NMDAR encephalitis. *Lancet neurology*, 10, 1, Jan, 63-74.

Dalmau, J., Tuzun, E., Wu, H.Y., Masjuan, J., Rossi, J.E., Voloschin, A., Baehring, J.M., Shimazaki, H., Koide, R., King, D., Mason, W., Sansing, L.H., Dichter, M.A., Rosenfeld, M.R., and Lynch, D.R. (2007). Paraneoplastic anti-N-methyl-D-aspartate receptor encephalitis associated with ovarian teratoma. *Annals of neurology*, 61, 1, Jan, 25-36.

DeGiorgio, L.A., Konstantinov, K.N., Lee, S.C., Hardin, J.A., Volpe, B.T., and Diamond, B. (2001). A subset of lupus anti-DNA antibodies cross-reacts with the NR2 glutamate receptor in systemic lupus erythematosus. *Nature medicine*, 7, 11, Nov, 1189-1193.

Di Pauli, F., Mader, S., Rostasy, K., Schanda, K., Bajer-Kornek, B., Ehling, R., Deisenhammer, F., Reindl, M., and Berger, T. (2011). Temporal dynamics of anti-MOG antibodies in CNS demyelinating diseases. *Clin Immunol*, 138, 3, Mar, 247-254.

Diamond, B., Huerta, P.T., Mina-Osorio, P., Kowal, C., and Volpe, B.T. (2009). Losing your nerves? Maybe it's the antibodies. *Nat Rev Immunol*, 9, 6, Jun, 449-456.

Dujmovic, I., Mader, S., Schanda, K., Deisenhammer, F., Stojsavljevic, N., Kostic, J., Berger, T., Drulovic, J., and Reindl, M. (2011). Temporal dynamics of cerebrospinal fluid anti-aquaporin-4 antibodies in patients with neuromyelitis optica spectrum disorders. *J Neuroimmunol*, Feb 10.

Emmer, B.J., van der Grond, J., Steup-Beekman, G.M., Huizinga, T.W., and van Buchem, M.A. (2006). Selective involvement of the amygdala in systemic lupus erythematosus. *PLoS Med*, 3, 12, Dec, e499.

Florance, N.R., Davis, R.L., Lam, C., Szperka, C., Zhou, L., Ahmad, S., Campen, C.J., Moss, H., Peter, N., Gleichman, A.J., Glaser, C.A., Lynch, D.R., Rosenfeld, M.R., and Dalmau, J. (2009). Anti-N-methyl-D-aspartate receptor (NMDAR) encephalitis in children and adolescents. *Annals of neurology*, 66, 1, Jul, 11-18.

Fragoso-Loyo, H., Cabiedes, J., Orozco-Narvaez, A., Davila-Maldonado, L., Atisha-Fregoso, Y., Diamond, B., Llorente, L., and Sanchez-Guerrero, J. (2008). Serum and cerebrospinal fluid autoantibodies in patients with neuropsychiatric lupus erythematosus. Implications for diagnosis and pathogenesis. *PloS one*, 3, 10, e3347.

Franciotta, D., Columba-Cabezas, S., Andreoni, L., Ravaglia, S., Jarius, S., Romagnolo, S., Tavazzi, E., Bergamaschi, R., Zardini, E., Aloisi, F., and Marchioni, E. (2008). Oligoclonal IgG band patterns in inflammatory demyelinating human and mouse diseases. *J Neuroimmunol*, 200, 1-2, Aug 30, 125-128.

Freedman, M.S., Thompson, E.J., Deisenhammer, F., Giovannoni, G., Grimsley, G., Keir, G., Ohman, S., Racke, M.K., Sharief, M., Sindic, C.J., Sellebjerg, F., and Tourtellotte, W.W. (2005). Recommended standard of cerebrospinal fluid analysis in the diagnosis of multiple sclerosis: a consensus statement. *Arch Neurol*, 62, 6, Jun, 865-870.

Furman, C.S., Gorelick-Feldman, D.A., Davidson, K.G., Yasumura, T., Neely, J.D., Agre, P., and Rash, J.E. (2003). Aquaporin-4 square array assembly: opposing actions of M1 and M23 isoforms. *Proc Natl Acad Sci U S A*, 100, 23, Nov 11, 13609-13614.

Gaertner, S., de Graaf, K.L., Greve, B., and Weissert, R. (2004). Antibodies against glycosylated native MOG are elevated in patients with multiple sclerosis. *Neurology*, 63, 12, Dec 28, 2381-2383.

Genain, C.P., Cannella, B., Hauser, S.L., and Raine, C.S. (1999). Identification of autoantibodies associated with myelin damage in multiple sclerosis. *Nature medicine*, 5, 2, Feb, 170-175.

Genain, C.P., Nguyen, M.H., Letvin, N.L., Pearl, R., Davis, R.L., Adelman, M., Lees, M.B., Linington, C., and Hauser, S.L. (1995). Antibody facilitation of multiple sclerosis-like lesions in a nonhuman primate. *The Journal of clinical investigation*, 96, 6, Dec, 2966-2974.

Gielen, M., Siegler Retchless, B., Mony, L., Johnson, J.W., and Paoletti, P. (2009). Mechanism of differential control of NMDA receptor activity by NR2 subunits. *Nature*, 459, 7247, Jun 4, 703-707.

Goverman, J. (2009). Autoimmune T cell responses in the central nervous system. *Nat Rev Immunol*, 9, 6, Jun, 393-407.

Graus, F., Saiz, A., and Dalmau, J. (2010). Antibodies and neuronal autoimmune disorders of the CNS. *J Neurol*, 257, 4, Apr, 509-517.

Greeve, I., Sellner, J., Lauterburg, T., Walker, U., Rosler, K.M., and Mattle, H.P. (2007). Anti-myelin antibodies in clinically isolated syndrome indicate the risk of multiple sclerosis in a Swiss cohort. *Acta Neurol Scand*, 116, 4, Oct, 207-210.

Hanly, J.G., Robichaud, J., and Fisk, J.D. (2006). Anti-NR2 glutamate receptor antibodies and cognitive function in systemic lupus erythematosus. *J Rheumatol*, 33, 8, Aug, 1553-1558.

Hauser, S.L., Waubant, E., Arnold, D.L., Vollmer, T., Antel, J., Fox, R.J., Bar-Or, A., Panzara, M., Sarkar, N., Agarwal, S., Langer-Gould, A., and Smith, C.H. (2008). B-cell depletion with rituximab in relapsing-remitting multiple sclerosis. *N Engl J Med*, 358, 7, Feb 14, 676-688.

Hinson, S.R., McKeon, A., Fryer, J.P., Apiwattanakul, M., Lennon, V.A., and Pittock, S.J. (2009). Prediction of neuromyelitis optica attack severity by quantitation of complement-mediated injury to aquaporin-4-expressing cells. *Arch Neurol*, 66, 9, Sep, 1164-1167.

Hughes, E.G., Peng, X., Gleichman, A.J., Lai, M., Zhou, L., Tsou, R., Parsons, T.D., Lynch, D.R., Dalmau, J., and Balice-Gordon, R.J. (2010). Cellular and synaptic mechanisms of anti-NMDA receptor encephalitis. *J Neurosci*, 30, 17, Apr 28, 5866-5875.

Hynson, J.L., Kornberg, A.J., Coleman, L.T., Shield, L., Harvey, A.S., and Kean, M.J. (2001). Clinical and neuroradiologic features of acute disseminated encephalomyelitis in children. *Neurology*, 56, 10, May 22, 1308-1312.

Irani, S.R., Bera, K., Waters, P., Zuliani, L., Maxwell, S., Zandi, M.S., Friese, M.A., Galea, I., Kullmann, D.M., Beeson, D., Lang, B., Bien, C.G., and Vincent, A. (2010). N-methyl-D-aspartate antibody encephalitis: temporal progression of clinical and paraclinical observations in a predominantly non-paraneoplastic disorder of both sexes. *Brain : a journal of neurology*, 133, Pt 6, Jun, 1655-1667.

Ishikawa, N., Tajima, G., Hyodo, S., Takahashi, Y., and Kobayashi, M. (2007). Detection of autoantibodies against NMDA-type glutamate receptor in a patient with recurrent optic neuritis and transient cerebral lesions. *Neuropediatrics*, 38, 5, Oct, 257-260.

Jacob, A., Weinshenker, B.G., Violich, I., McLinskey, N., Krupp, L., Fox, R.J., Wingerchuk, D.M., Boggild, M., Constantinescu, C.S., Miller, A., De Angelis, T., Matiello, M., and Cree, B.A. (2008). Treatment of neuromyelitis optica with rituximab: retrospective analysis of 25 patients. *Arch Neurol*, 65, 11, Nov, 1443-1448.

Jarius, S., Aboul-Enein, F., Waters, P., Kuenz, B., Hauser, A., Berger, T., Lang, W., Reindl, M., Vincent, A., and Kristoferitsch, W. (2008a). Antibody to aquaporin-4 in the long-term course of neuromyelitis optica. *Brain*, 131, Pt 11, Nov, 3072-3080.

Jarius, S., Franciotta, D., Bergamaschi, R., Wildemann, B., and Wandinger, K.P. (2010a). Immunoglobulin M antibodies to aquaporin-4 in neuromyelitis optica and related disorders. *Clin Chem Lab Med*, 48, 5, May, 659-663.

Jarius, S., Franciotta, D., Paul, F., Ruprecht, K., Bergamaschi, R., Rommer, P.S., Reuss, R., Probst, C., Kristoferitsch, W., Wandinger, K.P., and Wildemann, B. (2010b). Cerebrospinal fluid antibodies to aquaporin-4 in neuromyelitis optica and related disorders: frequency, origin, and diagnostic relevance. *J Neuroinflammation*, 7, 52.

Jarius, S., Paul, F., Franciotta, D., Aktas, O., Hohlfeld, R., Zipp, F., and Vincent, A. (2007). Revised diagnostic criteria for neuromyelitis optica--incorporation of NMO-IgG status. *Nat Clin Pract Neurol*, 3, 5, May, E1.

Jarius, S., Paul, F., Franciotta, D., Waters, P., Zipp, F., Hohlfeld, R., Vincent, A., and Wildemann, B. (2008b). Mechanisms of disease: aquaporin-4 antibodies in neuromyelitis optica. *Nature clinical practice*, 4, 4, Apr, 202-214.

Johnston, J., Ali, K., Pearson, O.R., Rickards, C., and Vincent, A. (2010). POI14 Multiple sclerosis: a potential association with anti-N-methyl-d-aspartate receptor encephalitis. *J Neurol Neurosurg Psychiatry*, 81, 11, Nov, e56.

Kabat, E.A., Glusman, M., and Knaub, V. (1948). Quantitative estimation of the albumin and gamma globulin in normal and pathologic cerebrospinal fluid by immunochemical methods. *Am J Med*, 4, 5, May, 653-662.

Kalluri, S.R., Rothhammer, V., Staszewski, O., Srivastava, R., Petermann, F., Prinz, M., Hemmer, B., and Korn, T. (2011). Functional characterization of aquaporin-4 specific T cells: towards a model for neuromyelitis optica. *PLoS One*, 6, 1, e16083.

Kerlero de Rosbo, N., Honegger, P., Lassmann, H., and Matthieu, J.M. (1990). Demyelination induced in aggregating brain cell cultures by a monoclonal antibody against myelin/oligodendrocyte glycoprotein. *J Neurochem*, 55, 2, Aug, 583-587.

Kesselring, J., Miller, D.H., Robb, S.A., Kendall, B.E., Moseley, I.F., Kingsley, D., du Boulay, E.P., and McDonald, W.I. (1990). Acute disseminated encephalomyelitis. MRI findings and the distinction from multiple sclerosis. *Brain*, 113 ( Pt 2), Apr, 291-302.

Kinoshita, M., Nakatsuji, Y., Kimura, T., Moriya, M., Takata, K., Okuno, T., Kumanogoh, A., Kajiyama, K., Yoshikawa, H., and Sakoda, S. (2009). Neuromyelitis optica: Passive transfer to rats by human immunoglobulin. *Biochemical and biophysical research communications*, 386, 4, Sep 4, 623-627.

Kinoshita, M., Nakatsuji, Y., Kimura, T., Moriya, M., Takata, K., Okuno, T., Kumanogoh, A., Kajiyama, K., Yoshikawa, H., and Sakoda, S. (2010). Anti-aquaporin-4 antibody induces astrocytic cytotoxicity in the absence of CNS antigen-specific T cells. *Biochem Biophys Res Commun*, 394, 1, Mar 26, 205-210.

Kira, J. (2006). [Epidemiology of multiple sclerosis in Japanese: with special reference to opticopsinal multiple sclerosis]. *Rinsho Shinkeigaku*, 46, 11, Nov, 859-862.

Kira, J., Kanai, T., Nishimura, Y., Yamasaki, K., Matsushita, S., Kawano, Y., Hasuo, K., Tobimatsu, S., and Kobayashi, T. (1996). Western versus Asian types of multiple sclerosis: immunogenetically and clinically distinct disorders. *Ann Neurol*, 40, 4, Oct, 569-574.

Klawiter, E.C., Alvarez, E., 3rd, Xu, J., Paciorkowski, A.R., Zhu, L., Parks, B.J., Cross, A.H., and Naismith, R.T. (2009). NMO-IgG detected in CSF in seronegative neuromyelitis optica. *Neurology*, 72, 12, Mar 24, 1101-1103.

Kowal, C., Degiorgio, L.A., Lee, J.Y., Edgar, M.A., Huerta, P.T., Volpe, B.T., and Diamond, B. (2006). Human lupus autoantibodies against NMDA receptors mediate cognitive impairment. *Proceedings of the National Academy of Sciences of the United States of America*, 103, 52, Dec 26, 19854-19859.

Kruer, M.C., Koch, T.K., Bourdette, D.N., Chabas, D., Waubant, E., Mueller, S., Moscarello, M.A., Dalmau, J., Woltjer, R.L., and Adamus, G. (2010). NMDA receptor encephalitis mimicking seronegative neuromyelitis optica. *Neurology*, 74, 18, May 4, 1473-1475.

Krupp, L.B., Banwell, B., and Tenembaum, S. (2007). Consensus definitions proposed for pediatric multiple sclerosis and related disorders. *Neurology*, 68, 16 Suppl 2, Apr 17, S7-12.

Kuhle, J., Lindberg, R.L., Regeniter, A., Mehling, M., Hoffmann, F., Reindl, M., Berger, T., Radue, E.W., Leppert, D., and Kappos, L. (2007a). Antimyelin antibodies in clinically isolated syndromes correlate with inflammation in MRI and CSF. *J Neurol*, 254, 2, Feb, 160-168.

Kuhle, J., Pohl, C., Mehling, M., Edan, G., Freedman, M.S., Hartung, H.P., Polman, C.H., Miller, D.H., Montalban, X., Barkhof, F., Bauer, L., Dahms, S., Lindberg, R., Kappos, L., and Sandbrink, R. (2007b). Lack of association between antimyelin antibodies and progression to multiple sclerosis. *N Engl J Med*, 356, 4, Jan 25, 371-378.

Lalive, P., Hausler, M., Maurey, H., Mikaeloff, Y., Tardieu, M., Wiendl, H., Schroeter, M., Hartung, H., Kieseier, B., and Menge, T. (2011). Highly reactive anti-myelin oligodendrocyte glycoprotein antibodies differentiate demyelinating diseases from viral encephalitis in children. *Mult Scler*, 17, 3, Mar, 297-302.

Lalive, P.H., Menge, T., Delarasse, C., Della Gaspera, B., Pham-Dinh, D., Villoslada, P., von Budingen, H.C., and Genain, C.P. (2006). Antibodies to native myelin oligodendrocyte glycoprotein are serologic markers of early inflammation in multiple sclerosis. *Proceedings of the National Academy of Sciences of the United States of America*, 103, 7, Feb 14, 2280-2285.

Lapteva, L., Nowak, M., Yarboro, C.H., Takada, K., Roebuck-Spencer, T., Weickert, T., Bleiberg, J., Rosenstein, D., Pao, M., Patronas, N., Steele, S., Manzano, M., van der Veen, J.W., Lipsky, P.E., Marenco, S., Wesley, R., Volpe, B., Diamond, B., and Illei, G.G. (2006). Anti-N-methyl-D-aspartate receptor antibodies, cognitive dysfunction, and depression in systemic lupus erythematosus. *Arthritis and rheumatism*, 54, 8, Aug, 2505-2514.

Leake, J.A., Albani, S., Kao, A.S., Senac, M.O., Billman, G.F., Nespeca, M.P., Paulino, A.D., Quintela, E.R., Sawyer, M.H., and Bradley, J.S. (2004). Acute disseminated encephalomyelitis in childhood: epidemiologic, clinical and laboratory features. *Pediatr Infect Dis J*, 23, 8, Aug, 756-764.

Lennon, V.A., Kryzer, T.J., Pittock, S.J., Verkman, A.S., and Hinson, S.R. (2005). IgG marker of optic-spinal multiple sclerosis binds to the aquaporin-4 water channel. *The Journal of experimental medicine*, 202, 4, Aug 15, 473-477.

Lennon, V.A., Wingerchuk, D.M., Kryzer, T.J., Pittock, S.J., Lucchinetti, C.F., Fujihara, K., Nakashima, I., and Weinshenker, B.G. (2004). A serum autoantibody marker of neuromyelitis optica: distinction from multiple sclerosis. *Lancet*, 364, 9451, Dec 11-17, 2106-2112.

Linington, C., Berger, T., Perry, L., Weerth, S., Hinze-Selch, D., Zhang, Y., Lu, H.C., Lassmann, H., and Wekerle, H. (1993). T cells specific for the myelin oligodendrocyte glycoprotein mediate an unusual autoimmune inflammatory response in the central nervous system. *Eur J Immunol*, 23, 6, Jun, 1364-1372.

Lotze, T.E., Northrop, J.L., Hutton, G.J., Ross, B., Schiffman, J.S., and Hunter, J.V. (2008). Spectrum of pediatric neuromyelitis optica. *Pediatrics*, 122, 5, Nov, e1039-1047.

Lucchinetti, C., Bruck, W., Parisi, J., Scheithauer, B., Rodriguez, M., and Lassmann, H. (2000). Heterogeneity of multiple sclerosis lesions: implications for the pathogenesis of demyelination. *Ann Neurol*, 47, 6, Jun, 707-717.

Lucchinetti, C.F., Bruck, W., Rodriguez, M., and Lassmann, H. (1996). Distinct patterns of multiple sclerosis pathology indicates heterogeneity on pathogenesis. *Brain Pathol*, 6, 3, Jul, 259-274.

Lucchinetti, C.F., Mandler, R.N., McGavern, D., Bruck, W., Gleich, G., Ransohoff, R.M., Trebst, C., Weinshenker, B., Wingerchuk, D., Parisi, J.E., and Lassmann, H. (2002). A role for humoral mechanisms in the pathogenesis of Devic's neuromyelitis optica. *Brain*, 125, Pt 7, Jul, 1450-1461.

Mader, S., Lutterotti, A., Di Pauli, F., Kuenz, B., Schanda, K., Aboul-Enein, F., Khalil, M., Storch, M.K., Jarius, S., Kristoferitsch, W., Berger, T., and Reindl, M. (2010). Patterns of antibody binding to aquaporin-4 isoforms in neuromyelitis optica. *PloS one*, 5, 5, e10455.

, R., De Seze, J., Vukusic, S., Durand-Dubief, F., Zephir, H., Vermersch, P., Cabre, P., Cavillon, G., Honnorat, J., and Confavreux, C. (2008). NMO-IgG and Devic's neuromyelitis optica: a French experience. *Mult Scler*, 14, 4, May, 440-445.

Matiello, M., Kim, H.J., Kim, W., Brum, D.G., Barreira, A.A., Kingsbury, D.J., Plant, G.T., Adoni, T., and Weinshenker, B.G. (2010). Familial neuromyelitis optica. *Neurology*, 75, 4, Jul 27, 310-315.

Matiello, M., Lennon, V.A., Jacob, A., Pittock, S.J., Lucchinetti, C.F., Wingerchuk, D.M., and Weinshenker, B.G. (2008). NMO-IgG predicts the outcome of recurrent optic neuritis. *Neurology*, 70, 23, Jun 3, 2197-2200.

Mikaeloff, Y., Adamsbaum, C., Husson, B., Vallee, L., Ponsot, G., Confavreux, C., Tardieu, M., and Suissa, S. (2004). MRI prognostic factors for relapse after acute CNS inflammatory demyelination in childhood. *Brain*, 127, Pt 9, Sep, 1942-1947.

Mikaeloff, Y., Caridade, G., Husson, B., Suissa, S., and Tardieu, M. (2007). Acute disseminated encephalomyelitis cohort study: prognostic factors for relapse. *Eur J Paediatr Neurol*, 11, 2, Mar, 90-95.

Minagar, A., Alexander, J.S., Fowler, M.R., Long, A.C., and Kelley, R.E. (2002). Devic disease: clinical course, pathophysiology, and management. *Pathophysiology*, 9, 1, Oct, 33.

Mirsattari, S.M., Johnston, J.B., McKenna, R., Del Bigio, M.R., Orr, P., Ross, R.T., and Power, C. (2001). Aboriginals with multiple sclerosis: HLA types and predominance of neuromyelitis optica. *Neurology*, 56, 3, Feb 13, 317-323.

Misu, T., Takano, R., Fujihara, K., Takahashi, T., Sato, S., and Itoyama, Y. (2009). Marked increase in cerebrospinal fluid glial fibrillar acidic protein in neuromyelitis optica: an astrocytic damage marker. *J Neurol Neurosurg Psychiatry*, 80, 5, May, 575-577.

Neely, J.D., Christensen, B.M., Nielsen, S., and Agre, P. (1999). Heterotetrameric composition of aquaporin-4 water channels. *Biochemistry*, 38, 34, Aug 24, 11156-11163.

Nelson, P.A., Khodadoust, M., Prodhomme, T., Spencer, C., Patarroyo, J.C., Varrin-Doyer, M., Ho, J.D., Stroud, R.M., and Zamvil, S.S. (2010). Immunodominant T cell determinants of aquaporin-4, the autoantigen associated with neuromyelitis optica. *PLoS One*, 5, 11, e15050.

Nicchia, G.P., Mastrototaro, M., Rossi, A., Pisani, F., Tortorella, C., Ruggieri, M., Lia, A., Trojano, M., Frigeri, A., and Svelto, M. (2009). Aquaporin-4 orthogonal arrays of particles are the target for neuromyelitis optica autoantibodies. *Glia*, 57, 13, Oct, 1363-1373.

Nicchia, G.P., Nico, B., Camassa, L.M., Mola, M.G., Loh, N., Dermietzel, R., Spray, D.C., Svelto, M., and Frigeri, A. (2004). The role of aquaporin-4 in the blood-brain barrier development and integrity: studies in animal and cell culture models. *Neuroscience*, 129, 4, 935-945.

Nielsen, S., Nagelhus, E.A., Amiry-Moghaddam, M., Bourque, C., Agre, P., and Ottersen, O.P. (1997). Specialized membrane domains for water transport in glial cells: high-resolution immunogold cytochemistry of aquaporin-4 in rat brain. *J Neurosci*, 17, 1, Jan 1, 171-180.

Nishiyama, S., Ito, T., Misu, T., Takahashi, T., Kikuchi, A., Suzuki, N., Jin, K., Aoki, M., Fujihara, K., and Itoyama, Y. (2009). A case of NMO seropositive for aquaporin-4 antibody more than 10 years before onset. *Neurology*, 72, 22, Jun 2, 1960-1961.

Noseworthy, J.H., Lucchinetti, C., Rodriguez, M., and Weinshenker, B.G. (2000). Multiple sclerosis. *N Engl J Med*, 343, 13, Sep 28, 938-952.

O'Connor, K.C., McLaughlin, K.A., De Jager, P.L., Chitnis, T., Bettelli, E., Xu, C., Robinson, W.H., Cherry, S.V., Bar-Or, A., Banwell, B., Fukaura, H., Fukazawa, T., Tenembaum, S., Wong, S.J., Tavakoli, N.P., Idrissova, Z., Viglietta, V., Rostasy, K., Pohl, D., Dale, R.C., Freedman, M., Steinman, L., Buckle, G.J., Kuchroo, V.K., Hafler, D.A., and Wucherpfennig, K.W. (2007). Self-antigen tetramers discriminate between myelin autoantibodies to native or denatured protein. *Nature medicine*, 13, 2, Feb, 211-217.

Osuntokun, B.O. (1971). The pattern of neurological illness in tropical Africa. Experience at Ibadan, Nigeria. *J Neurol Sci*, 12, 4, Apr, 417-442.

Owens, G.P., Ritchie, A.M., Burgoon, M.P., Williamson, R.A., Corboy, J.R., and Gilden, D.H. (2003). Single-cell repertoire analysis demonstrates that clonal expansion is a prominent feature of the B cell response in multiple sclerosis cerebrospinal fluid. *J Immunol*, 171, 5, Sep 1, 2725-2733.

Palace, J., Leite, M.I., Nairne, A., and Vincent, A. (2010). Interferon Beta treatment in neuromyelitis optica: increase in relapses and aquaporin 4 antibody titers. *Arch Neurol*, 67, 8, Aug, 1016-1017.

Papais-Alvarenga, R.M., Miranda-Santos, C.M., Puccioni-Sohler, M., de Almeida, A.M., Oliveira, S., Basilio De Oliveira, C.A., Alvarenga, H., and Poser, C.M. (2002). Optic neuromyelitis syndrome in Brazilian patients. *J Neurol Neurosurg Psychiatry*, 73, 4, Oct, 429-435.

Papeix, C., Vidal, J.S., de Seze, J., Pierrot-Deseilligny, C., Tourbah, A., Stankoff, B., Lebrun, C., Moreau, T., Vermersch, P., Fontaine, B., Lyon-Caen, O., and Gout, O. (2007). Immunosuppressive therapy is more effective than interferon in neuromyelitis optica. *Mult Scler*, 13, 2, Mar, 256-259.

Paul, F., Jarius, S., Aktas, O., Bluthner, M., Bauer, O., Appelhans, H., Franciotta, D., Bergamaschi, R., Littleton, E., Palace, J., Seelig, H.P., Hohlfeld, R., Vincent, A., and Zipp, F. (2007). Antibody to Aquaporin 4 in the Diagnosis of Neuromyelitis Optica. *PLoS Med*, 4, 4, Apr 17, e133.

Pavone, P., Pettoello-Mantovano, M., Le Pira, A., Giardino, I., Pulvirenti, A., Giugno, R., Parano, E., Polizzi, A., Distefano, A., Ferro, A., Pavone, L., and Ruggieri, M. (2010). Acute disseminated encephalomyelitis: a long-term prospective study and meta-analysis. *Neuropediatrics*, 41, 6, Dec, 246-255.

Pellkofer, H.L., Suessmair, C., Schulze, A., Hohlfeld, R., and Kuempfel, T. (2009). Course of neuromyelitis optica during inadvertent pregnancy in a patient treated with rituximab. *Mult Scler*, 15, 8, Aug, 1006-1008.

Pittock, S.J., Lennon, V.A., de Seze, J., Vermersch, P., Homburger, H.A., Wingerchuk, D.M., Lucchinetti, C.F., Zephir, H., Moder, K., and Weinshenker, B.G. (2008). Neuromyelitis optica and non organ-specific autoimmunity. *Arch Neurol*, 65, 1, Jan, 78-83.

Pittock, S.J., Weinshenker, B.G., Lucchinetti, C.F., Wingerchuk, D.M., Corboy, J.R., and Lennon, V.A. (2006). Neuromyelitis optica brain lesions localized at sites of high aquaporin 4 expression. *Arch Neurol*, 63, 7, Jul, 964-968.

Pohl, M., Fischer, M.T., Mader, S., Schanda, K., Kitic, M., Sharma, R., Wimmer, I., Misu, T., Fujihara, K., Reindl, M., Lassmann, H., and Bradl, M. (2011). Pathogenic T cell responses against aquaporin 4. *Acta Neuropathol*, Apr 6.

Popescu, B.F., Lennon, V.A., Parisi, J.E., Howe, C.L., Weigand, S.D., Cabrera-Gomez, J.A., Newell, K., Mandler, R.N., Pittock, S.J., Weinshenker, B.G., and Lucchinetti, C.F. (2011). Neuromyelitis optica unique area postrema lesions: Nausea, vomiting, and pathogenic implications. *Neurology*, Mar 2.

Qin, Y., Duquette, P., Zhang, Y., Talbot, P., Poole, R., and Antel, J. (1998). Clonal expansion and somatic hypermutation of V(H) genes of B cells from cerebrospinal fluid in multiple sclerosis. *The Journal of clinical investigation*, 102, 5, Sep 1, 1045-1050.

Rash, J.E., Yasumura, T., Hudson, C.S., Agre, P., and Nielsen, S. (1998). Direct immunogold labeling of aquaporin-4 in square arrays of astrocyte and ependymocyte plasma membranes in rat brain and spinal cord. *Proc Natl Acad Sci U S A*, 95, 20, Sep 29, 11981-11986.

Rauer, S., Euler, B., Reindl, M., and Berger, T. (2006). Antimyelin antibodies and the risk of relapse in patients with a primary demyelinating event. *J Neurol Neurosurg Psychiatry*, 77, 6, Jun, 739-742.

Reindl, M., Khalil, M., and Berger, T. (2006). Antibodies as biological markers for pathophysiological processes in MS. *J Neuroimmunol*, 180, 1-2, Nov, 50-62.

Rivera, V.M., and Cabrera, J.A. (2001). Aboriginals with multiple sclerosis: HLA types and predominance of neuromyelitis optica. *Neurology*, 57, 5, Sep 11, 937-938.

Roemer, S.F., Parisi, J.E., Lennon, V.A., Benarroch, E.E., Lassmann, H., Bruck, W., Mandler, R.N., Weinshenker, B.G., Pittock, S.J., Wingerchuk, D.M., and Lucchinetti, C.F. (2007). Pattern-specific loss of aquaporin-4 immunoreactivity distinguishes neuromyelitis optica from multiple sclerosis. *Brain*, 130, Pt 5, May, 1194-1205.

Rust, R.S. (2000). Multiple sclerosis, acute disseminated encephalomyelitis, and related conditions. *Semin Pediatr Neurol*, 7, 2, Jun, 66-90.

Saadoun, S., Waters, P., Bell, B.A., Vincent, A., Verkman, A.S., and Papadopoulos, M.C. (2010). Intra-cerebral injection of neuromyelitis optica immunoglobulin G and human complement produces neuromyelitis optica lesions in mice. *Brain*, 133, Pt 2, Feb, 349-361.

Sabater, L., Giralt, A., Boronat, A., Hankiewicz, K., Blanco, Y., Llufriu, S., Alberch, J., Graus, F., and Saiz, A. (2009). Cytotoxic effect of neuromyelitis optica antibody (NMO-IgG) to astrocytes: an in vitro study. *J Neuroimmunol*, 215, 1-2, Oct 30, 31-35.

Schwarz, S., Mohr, A., Knauth, M., Wildemann, B., and Storch-Hagenlocher, B. (2001). Acute disseminated encephalomyelitis: a follow-up study of 40 adult patients. *Neurology*, 56, 10, May 22, 1313-1318.

Sellner, J., Boggild, M., Clanet, M., Hintzen, R.Q., Illes, Z., Montalban, X., Du Pasquier, R.A., Polman, C.H., Sorensen, P.S., and Hemmer, B. (2010). EFNS guidelines on diagnosis and management of neuromyelitis optica. *Eur J Neurol*, 17, 8, Aug, 1019-1032.

Sospedra, M., and Martin, R. (2005). Immunology of multiple sclerosis. *Annual review of immunology*, 23, 683-747.

Storch, M.K., Piddlesden, S., Haltia, M., Iivanainen, M., Morgan, P., and Lassmann, H. (1998). Multiple sclerosis: in situ evidence for antibody- and complement-mediated demyelination. *Ann Neurol*, 43, 4, Apr, 465-471.

Stuve, O., Nessler, S., Hartung, H.P., Hemmer, B., Wiendl, H., and Kieseier, B.C. (2005). [Acute disseminated encephalomyelitis. Pathogenesis, diagnosis, treatment, and prognosis]. *Nervenarzt*, 76, 6, Jun, 701-707.

Takahashi, T., Fujihara, K., Nakashima, I., Misu, T., Miyazawa, I., Nakamura, M., Watanabe, S., Ishii, N., and Itoyama, Y. (2006). Establishment of a new sensitive assay for anti-human aquaporin-4 antibody in neuromyelitis optica. *Tohoku J Exp Med*, 210, 4, Dec, 307-313.

Takahashi, T., Fujihara, K., Nakashima, I., Misu, T., Miyazawa, I., Nakamura, M., Watanabe, S., Shiga, Y., Kanaoka, C., Fujimori, J., Sato, S., and Itoyama, Y. (2007). Anti-aquaporin-4 antibody is involved in the pathogenesis of NMO: a study on antibody titre. *Brain*, 130, Pt 5, May, 1235-1243.

Tenembaum, S., Chamoles, N., and Fejerman, N. (2002). Acute disseminated encephalomyelitis: a long-term follow-up study of 84 pediatric patients. *Neurology*, 59, 8, Oct 22, 1224-1231.

Tomassini, V., De Giglio, L., Reindl, M., Russo, P., Pestalozza, I., Pantano, P., Berger, T., and Pozzilli, C. (2007). Anti-myelin antibodies predict the clinical outcome after a first episode suggestive of MS. *Mult Scler*, 13, 9, Nov, 1086-1094.

Vincent, A., Irani, S.R., and Lang, B. (2010). The growing recognition of immunotherapy-responsive seizure disorders with autoantibodies to specific neuronal proteins. *Curr Opin Neurol*, 23, 2, Apr, 144-150.

Wandinger, K.P., Stangel, M., Witte, T., Venables, P., Charles, P., Jarius, S., Wildemann, B., Probst, C., Iking-Konert, C., and Schneider, M. (2010). Autoantibodies against aquaporin-4 in patients with neuropsychiatric systemic lupus erythematosus and primary Sjogren's syndrome. *Arthritis Rheum*, 62, 4, Apr, 1198-1200.

Warabi, Y., Matsumoto, Y., and Hayashi, H. (2007). Interferon beta-1b exacerbates multiple sclerosis with severe optic nerve and spinal cord demyelination. *J Neurol Sci*, 252, 1, Jan 15, 57-61.

Watanabe, S., Nakashima, I., Misu, T., Miyazawa, I., Shiga, Y., Fujihara, K., and Itoyama, Y. (2007). Therapeutic efficacy of plasma exchange in NMO-IgG-positive patients with neuromyelitis optica. *Mult Scler*, 13, 1, Jan, 128-132.

Waters, P., and Vincent, A. (2008). Detection of anti-aquaporin-4 antibodies in neuromyelitis optica: current status of the assays. *Int MS J*, 15, 3, Sep, 99-105.

Weinshenker, B.G., Wingerchuk, D.M., Vukusic, S., Linbo, L., Pittock, S.J., Lucchinetti, C.F., and Lennon, V.A. (2006). Neuromyelitis optica IgG predicts relapse after longitudinally extensive transverse myelitis. *Ann Neurol*, 59, 3, Mar, 566-569.

Weissert, R., Wallstrom, E., Storch, M.K., Stefferl, A., Lorentzen, J., Lassmann, H., Linington, C., and Olsson, T. (1998). MHC haplotype-dependent regulation of MOG-induced EAE in rats. *The Journal of clinical investigation*, 102, 6, Sep 15, 1265-1273.

Wingerchuk, D.M. (2009). Neuromyelitis optica: effect of gender. *J Neurol Sci*, 286, 1-2, Nov 15, 18-23.

Wingerchuk, D.M., Hogancamp, W.F., O'Brien, P.C., and Weinshenker, B.G. (1999). The clinical course of neuromyelitis optica (Devic's syndrome). *Neurology*, 53, 5, Sep 22, 1107-1114.

Wingerchuk, D.M., Lennon, V.A., Lucchinetti, C.F., Pittock, S.J., and Weinshenker, B.G. (2007). The spectrum of neuromyelitis optica. *Lancet Neurol*, 6, 9, Sep, 805-815.

Wingerchuk, D.M., and Weinshenker, B.G. (2003). Neuromyelitis optica: clinical predictors of a relapsing course and survival. *Neurology*, 60, 5, Mar 11, 848-853.

Zaffaroni, M. (2004). Cerebrospinal fluid findings in Devic's neuromyelitis optica. *Neurol Sci*, 25 Suppl 4, Nov, S368-370.

Zhou, D., Srivastava, R., Nessler, S., Grummel, V., Sommer, N., Bruck, W., Hartung, H.P., Stadelmann, C., and Hemmer, B. (2006). Identification of a pathogenic antibody response to native myelin oligodendrocyte glycoprotein in multiple sclerosis. *Proceedings of the National Academy of Sciences of the United States of America*, 103, 50, Dec 12, 19057-19062.

# 10

# Preclinical and Predictive Algorithms in Monitoring Patients with Autoimmune Diseases and Their Relatives-at-Risks

Sergey Suchkov[1,2], Dmitry Kostyushev[1], Dmitry Gnatenko[1], Sevindzh Gadzhieva[1] and Mikhail Paltsev[3]
[1]*I.M. Sechenov First Moscow State Medical University*
[2]*Moscow State Medical Dentistry University, National*
[3]*Research Center "Kurchatov Institute"*
*Russia*

## 1. Introduction

Millions of people all round the world suffer from various autoimmune disorders. T1D, MS, SLE, autoimmune diseases of the heart, liver, intestine and other internal organs, etc., all represent severe manifestations, which deteriorate the quality of life and cause physical disability and even death in patients with chronic illnesses. Every year, the largest world economies incur megabuck losses associated with medical services, insurance and drug procurement, not to mention the ever decreasing size of the able-bodied population. The development of preclinical diagnostic algorithms for autoimmune diseases, their implementation and introduction into routine clinical practice will help detect tissue or organ pathologies at the stages where their reversal is still possible. Early implementation of causal therapy allows the physician to compensate for the lack of one or another organ and ensures complete recovery or significant improvement of the patient's health status. However, in developing updated preventive protocols, the investigator is faced with a necessity to solve fundamental problems in order to understand:

- Who should be selected for examination?
- What exactly needs to be checked?
- When should the examination be performed?
- And, last but not least, what are the analytical procedures for mass-scale monitoring?

While constructing preclinical monitoring algorithms, one should also take into consideration the diseases suffered by patients' relatives. One of the cornerstones in preventive and predictive medicine is screening for genetic abnormalities or hereditary predisposition. All-encompassing analysis of gene units and construction of individual genetic maps not only facilitate the assessment of individual risks for each concrete patient, but also allows prediction of disease development in first-degree-relatives. Therefore, today's objective demands include not only large-scale monitoring of definite cohorts of the general population, but, rather, identification of high risk cohorts coupled with genetic abnormalities and/or shifts and social factors (residence, place of employment, occupation, living conditions, etc.). However, even a comprehensive analysis is inadequate without a set of criteria providing high accuracy and reliability of state-of-health data. By illustration, it has long been believed that the same gene loci are specific for definite diseases including integer disease-related clusters. T1D, celiac disease, rheumatoid arthritis, multiple sclerosis, etc., they exist in close linkage with one another and often form polyglandular syndromes. Being a positively provisional discipline, genetics provides a fairly accurate prognosis for an individual; however, genetic tributes cannot always be adequately understood by reason of their ability to provoke extremely severe diseases. It should be taken into consideration that deleterious environmental (exogenous or endogenous) factors may strongly destabilize the physiological status of the organism by triggering pathological processes even in the presence of protective genes, and *vice versa*.

Therefore, screening of patients for the presence and evolution of biomarkers should be included into all preventive medicine protocols alongside with the patient's individual genetic map.

Even an unambiguous allocation of patients into risk groups, selection of basic state-of-art (additional, individual, etc.) screening criteria and personalized approaches to every new patient will hardly be successful without selection of optimal conditions and methods for obtaining reliable and reproducible clinical data on a mass scale.

The practical realization of these principles will enable the physician to diagnose abnormalities and/or disorders at the very earliest stages and to predict their outcome. However, suspension or blockade of pathological processes presents a formidable challenge to the medical community. In designing therapeutic strategies for autoimmune diseases, two important issues, namely, targets for autoimmune attacks and depth of morphofunctional deficiency of an organ or a tissue, should be taken into consideration. The first issue is more or less clear, since immunosuppressors with specific or nonspecific activities have long been used in the clinical practice, while the second one is not so apparent. Restoration of the structure and function of affected tissues can successfully be achieved through practical realization of the following strategies:

- allogeneic or xenogeneic transplantation. The main challenges include high risk of so-called "graft-versus-host" responses and rejection of transplanted tissues (graft rejection);
- medical products with regenerative resources. This technology seems to hold especially great promise in modern medicine. Some medicinal drugs (e.g., IgM for MS) are widely employed in the clinical practice, while others (e.g., peptide-based drugs for MS, rheumatoid arthritis, T1D) are under intensive development. The main obstacles on the way to large-scale application of such drugs are low efficiency, particularly due to organism's addiction to their active substances (reduced number of receptors, downregulation, etc.), and hyperactivation of the excretory system (augmented synthesis of liver microsomal enzymes, hyperexcretion with urine, faeces or sweat, etc.);
- stem cell technology. This trend is especially actively debated by the medical community because of its high relevance to ethic problems and legal prohibitions, on the one hand, and inability to maintain "stemness" for sufficiently long periods of time and differentiation of stem cells into "undesirable" pools, on the other. Similar problems arise at virtually every stage, viz.: search for and isolation of stem cells from the organism; enhanced accumulation of biological material, which may be critical under conditions of fulminant progression of the disease and pronounced deficit of time; necessity to maintain the pluripotent state of cells for sufficiently long periods of time without malignization *in vitro;* delivery of SC; provisional differentiation and

acquisition of high-quality material *in vitro* and control over differentiation into desired cellular pools *in vivo*.

Taking into consideration the foregoing and being guided by the Major Preventive and Preventive Medicine Principle, we developed an original protocol for screening and postscreening management of patients, which includes:

Comprehensive genetic analysis for estimating potential risks for patient's (or his/her relatives') individuality and design of protocols for diagnostic assessment and preventive treatment;

Proteomic analysis and detection of metabolic shifts including identification of biomarkers (e.g., autoAbs in case of autoimmune disorders); monitoring of evolutional and spectral characteristics of biomarkers; control over emergence of new biomarkers for updating prophylactic and preventive treatment protocols and maintenance of high curability standards;

Persistent control over predisposing factors including identification of factors potentiating specific pathologies (analysis of bacterial and virus-borne infections, monitoring compliance with regimen and other preventive measures, etc.);

Psychologic doctor-patient cooperation, strict compliance with doctor's recommendations and requirements through elucidation of disease severity (including the preclinical stage).

The use of advanced screening strategies and early implementation of specific therapy ensure substantial reduction of morbidity and mortality from autoimmune disorders and, as a consequence, significant improvement of life quality and minimization of economic losses. The same principles are embodied in the guidelines of preventive and predictive medicine. Their practical realization may culminate in the establishment of an international research network, development of novel criteria for preclinical diagnosis and treatment and validation of uniform specifications and standards for laboratory diagnostics.

## 2. The preclinical diagnosis algorithm and a new conceptual model of T1D etiology

T1D is an autoimmune disease induced by a vast variety of triggering factors. In individuals with genetic predisposition to T1D, these factors initiate autoimmune processes culminating in the appearance of autoAbs and infiltration of the pancreas with self-reactive T cells. In its turn, progressive deterioration of pancreatic functional activity leads to systemic metabolic and immune failures. These processes show a tendency for self-acceleration, aggravation by associated diseases or numerous adverse factors and formation of new linkages between immunoregulatory and immunoeffector compartments within the immune system. T1D is also distinguished for alterations at the cellular level including pathological changes in cell to-cell interactions, incompatibility of packages of secreted humoral factors, and so on. Intracellular events provoked by specific uncongenial conditions in the cell environment also play a role. Therefore, humoral factors secreted at any (cellular, tissue or organic) level and pathological changes in any link of the metabolic cascade can be regarded as highly specific *biopredictors* and valuable tools for *preclinical diagnosis* of T1D.

In the course of the autoimmune process, T1D goes through a number of sequential stages, which differ from one another by the degree of severity of the underlying pathology, functional peculiarities of affected organs and clinical manifestations of the disease. A *personalized* therapeutic approach must be based on a detailed analysis of the immune status with special reference to the patient's genetic map and is prerequisite to the construction of any early diagnosis protocol designed to indicate the pathology, to identify the stage of the autoimmune process and the functional status of the target organ and to develop, on their basis, a strictly individual treatment schedule. In addition, this approach entails early implementation of pharmacocorrective therapy and prediction of scenarios for disease progression. (Suchkov et al., 2010)

In order to follow the dynamics of T1D on the time scale and to estimate efficiency and sensitivity of innovative approaches to *preclinical diagnosis,* we developed a fundamentally new strategy of pathogenesis. Its major goal is crucial features of the disease with special emphasis on its diagnosis allowing the physician to implement adequate *preventive therapy,* to prolong the *preclinical* stage and to delay clinical manifestations of the disease.

**Stage I** is often defined as the "*genetic predisposition*" step. Its most salient feature is a repertoire of predisposition genes (predominantly, MHC class II) responsible for susceptibility to autoimmune diseases and direct initiation, gradation and exacerbation of immune pathologies.

**Stage II** is often referred to as the "intervention" step. At this stage, provoking exogenous or endogenous factors interfere with the normal functioning of immune mechanisms and deplete the functional reserves of the affected organs providing the formation of the autoimmune status (e.g., postinfective autoimmune syndrome).

**Stage III** represents an "ignoring" step where progressive disturbances in immune homeostasis are unaccompanied by direct attacks at target organs. Clinical manifestations of T1D and visible lesions in the pancreas architectonics are absent in this step, while the functional activity of the pancreatic gland is unimpaired. AutoAbs are either not produced or their titers are negligibly small.

**Stage IV** is characterized by termination of the ignoring step and initiation of autoimmune processes. The main participants at this stage are molecular factors (e.g., addressins) triggering autoimmune reactions specifically directed against islet cells. At this particular level, clonal ignoring collapses and organ infiltration occur.

**Stage V** is closely associated with the development of immunological disorders. Its central event is generation of autoAbs to insulin, GAD, β-cells, heat shock protein 60 (hsp60), zinc transporter and fogrin. AutoAbs can be specific against a single antigen (Ag) or several Ags.

**Stage VI** is defined as a "transition from uncontrolled violence to chaos". Here, minor systemic failures related to immunological disregulation progress to the extent of profound disorders. Clinical symptoms are still missing at this stage, but latent tolerance to glucose develops.

**Stage VII.** This "complete overall imbalance" step occurs when β-cell destruction reaches a certain critical level (80%). This stage is characterized by hyperglucosemia and insufficient production of insulin. Metabolic processes fluctuate slightly within normal limits due to residual secretion of the C-peptide.

**Stage VIII,** often referred to not as a T1D stage, but, rather, as emerging complications, is defined as "total or genuine diabetes", since beta cell destruction is fully complete in this step. It is distinguished for steadily decreasing titers or complete disappearance of autoAbs, functional failure of the pancreas, high glucosemia and glycosylation of proteins (including hemoglobin) against the background of systemic hypoxia and metabolic collapse. Other manifestations include disturbances in water-salt metabolism, osmotic diuresis, dehydration, activation and acceleration of gluconeogenesis and ketogenesis, enhanced breakdown of proteins and lipids, impaired lipid metabolism (low HDL levels and high LDL levels) and elevation of osmotic blood pressure resulting in microvascular and nerve tissue injuries. These disturbances are usually concomitant with acute manifestations (coma) or form the basis for more distant pathologies (micro- and macroangiopathies, neuropathies, ophthalmopathies, nephropathies, etc.).

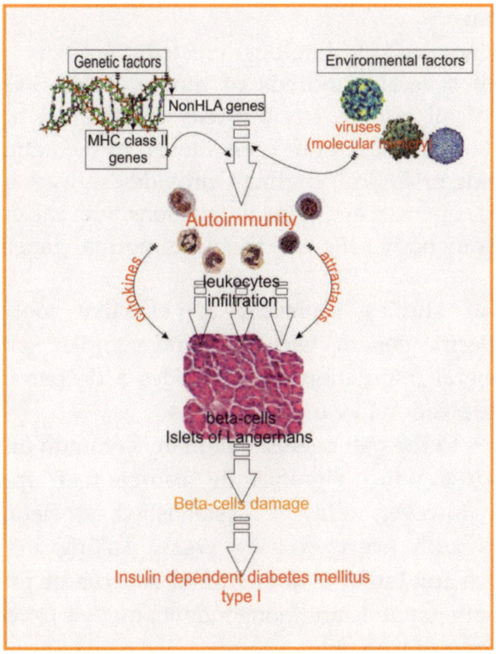


Fig. 1. The pathogenesis of T1D. Genetic and environmental factors are key elements in the susceptibility to **T1D**. Susceptible individuals develop autoimmune insulitis, which is mediated by CTL against autoAgs of *beta* cells and is characterized by enhanced production of a vast array of antiinflammatory cytokins and free radicals triggering the death (apoptosis) of *beta* cells as main targets in inflammation.

The first five stages are defined as preclinical pathology stages, while Stage VI is thought to represent a transient step. It is diagnosing T1D at stages I – V and the use of preventive treatment protocols that enable the physician to delay the progression of the underlying disease and to procure complete recovery. (Antonio Gonzalez at. al., 1996s; Matthias von Herrath at al., 2007)

## 3. The origin of genetic predisposition or "genomics: A base of preclinical medicine"

Our knowledge of pathological processes occurring in the human organism has progressed considerably in the past decades, but the mechanisms of many human diseases are still poorly understood. Recent developments in genomics made it possible to discover a wide variety of novel genes and genetic variations including clinically important ones. i.e., those triggering pathological processes in various body tissues and cells. Every year, the clinical diagnostic instrumentarium is supplemented with efficient analytical techniques for detecting single-nucleotide polymorphisms (SNP's) which determine the susceptibility of the organism to diseases, drugs and/or environmental factors. A deeper insight into gene structure and regulatory mechanisms can significantly facilitate diagnosis and treatment of individuals at risk and, in a more distant future, provide the physician with potent tools for diagnosing diseases, preventing their progression and implementing effective therapy as early as the preclinical stage.

Rapid progress in science and technology created necessary prerequisites for high-throughput screening of several hundreds of thousands of SNP variants and enabled adequate involvement of all human DNA blocks in selection of the disease associated variant provided the latter is present in the genome. From theoretical standpoint, linking of genotyping data to epidemiological findings provides a way to identification and/or characterization of gene sequences and gene interactions with the environment determining the susceptibility of various body cells and tissues to normal genetic variations and/or the underlying disease.

Genomewide association studies represent an effective tool for detecting genetic associations between specific genetic variations and complex pathological conditions in large cohorts of the general population and provides a deeper insight into mechanisms underlying genetic predisposition to various diseases.

The contribution of SNP's to the pathogenesis of many common diseases is relatively small and does not exceed 5-10%, which significantly restricts their application as markers for predicting disease risks. However, today well-established associations number in hundreds and their panel grows with every passing week. Taking into account considerable investments in the search for hitherto unidentified sources of inherited risks, it may be expected that existing (both genomic and nongenomic) models for estimating potential risks will soon be improved and rationalized.

The current need for highly multiplexed tests increases with every passing day. Innovative gene chip- and sequencing-based technologies displace rapidly traditional methods for establishing variations and mutations in the human genome. In future, the advent of improved nanotechnological sequencing protocols may further increase the accuracy and reduce the cost of genetic analysis. The idea of complete sequencing of the human genome at the cost of $1000 is becoming more and more realistic. The project, which got the name "$1000 genome", is expected to improve existing protocols through direct sequencing of individual DNA molecules. This approach is potentially oriented at elimination of the amplification step, further reduction of chemical reagents expenditure and construction of a high-precision database of genetic sequences in the foreseeable future.

The feasibility of reliable and low-cost estimation of human genetic variations put forward the idea of personalized medicine as an indispensable element of modern-day public health care. The key principle of personalized medicine is in that the health status of any human individual is most effectively controlled through implementation of individual preventive and curative treatment schedules. Although unsolvable controversies between principles of personalized medicine and populational (probative) medicine really exist, they are not inconsistent. Novel decisions are being taken in the private and public sectors, and those would enable progressive studies to provide the linkage between personalized and probative medicine.

All-round cognition of gene structure and genetic regulatory mechanisms is extremely important not only from theoretical, but also from practical point of view, particularly, for the development of state-of-art diagnostic, prognostic, preventive and therapeutic strategies for treatment of rarely occurring and common diseases.

### 3.1 IDDM1 as an example of crucial role of genomics in clinical researches

The use of high-throughput technologies in human genome studies was a step forward towards getting a deeper insight into pathogenetic mechanisms of many human diseases including insulin-dependent type 1 diabetes mellitus (T1D). Recent developments in the field of genetic factors and their pathogenetic roles suggest their high utility in the design of novel predictive strategies, stratification of patients according to disease risk and a search for new therapeutic targets. Among the immense variety of T1D strategies, two approaches are used methods of choice, viz.: (I) linkage studies of pairs of affected relatives (typically, siblings) aimed at a search for rarely occurring risk factors having large effective sizes; (II) association studies into more common risk factors having small effective sizes.

### 3.2 MHC: Genes of instability

As can be seen, identical genes can simultaneously trigger a variety of body-related autoimmune disorders. The latter form a disease-based cluster, which further develops into a polyglandular autoimmune syndrome. (Fernando MM et al., 2008)

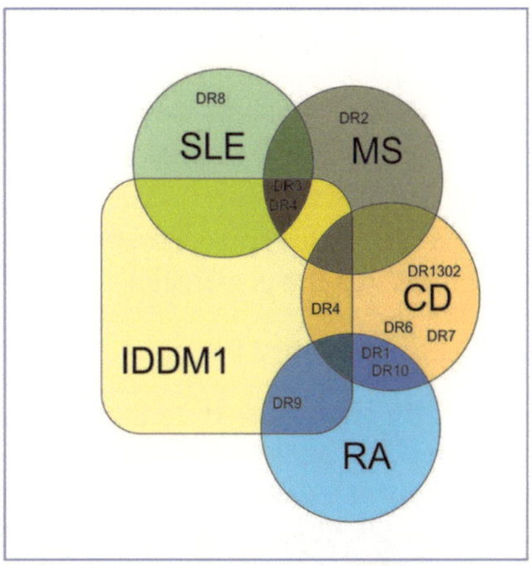


Fig. 2. The role of MHC genes in the development of diseases the key pathogenetic role in which is played by genetic predisposition. Some genes (DR7, DR8) determine the risk for only one disease (DR7, DR8), while others are responsible for two (DR1, DR10), three or even more (DR4) diseases. However, their presence is not prerequisite to the development of pathological processes, but, rather, significantly increases the likelihood of their early occurrence during the patient's lifetime.

MHC represents a large family of genes encoding molecules of three major HLA classes, viz., HLA class I, HLA class II and HLA class III. MHC plays an essential role in the functional activity of the immune system being directly involved in presentation of peptide antigens to APCs and formation of the so-called MHC restriction phenomenon. To-date, MHC is the most thoroughly investigated gene family in the human genome by virtue of its extremely close linkage to autoimmune diseases, hypersensitivity to infections and hyperbolic immune responsiveness. These genes are usually present in patients with severe autoimmune disorders and/or imbalances, e.g., rheumatoid arthritis (RA), multiple sclerosis

(MS), Crohn's disease, aneurisms of large vessels (ALV), ulcerative colitis (UC), systemic lupus erythematosus (SLE) and type 1 diabetes (T1D).

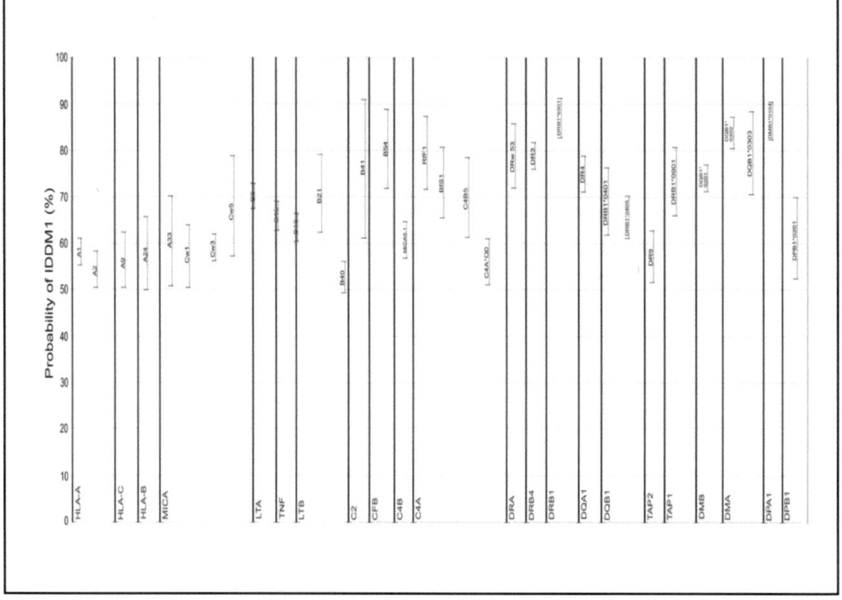


Fig. 3. The role of various MHC classes I, II and III alleles in the development of T1D. The x axis designates the continuous arrangement of some MHC 123 regions. The vertical graph segment indicates the association of an allele with a specific MHC region and the typical scatter of diabetogenicity probabilities for the given allele.

### 3.3 HLA class I: Role in T1D

Molecules of HLA class 1, jointly with HLA class II molecules and in closest association with one another afford effective protection against T1D and risks thereof. The HLA class I compartment contains both diabetoprotective genotypes (A*1101, A*3201, A*6601, B*0702, B*4403, B*3502, C*1601, C*0401) and highly associative genes (B*5701, B*3906). The diabetogenic alleles of MHC class I genes display age-related features. For example, HLA-E*0101 is predominant in patients in whom T1D developed during the first 10 years of life, while HLA-E*0103 is found in children under 10. (Hodgkinson AD et al. 2000) Apart from borderline (diabetogenic or diabetoprotective) genes, there exist several intermediate types (A*2402, A*0201, B*1801, C*0501). All of them increase the risk of diabetes, but their role in triggering autoimmune responses is insignificant. (Noble JA et al., 2010)

The increasing number of publications devoted to genes associated with T1D (Howson JM et al., 2009; Viken MK et al., 2009) and identification of reactions stimulating or potentiating beta cell destruction testify to the fact that HLA class I initiate and potentiate autoimmune destruction of beta cells and manifest close linkage to HLA class II. (Lipponen K et al., 2010) Systemic autotolerance of homogeneic CD8(+) T cells is one of the patterns subject to regulatory control of HLA class I. It is well known that T1D is concomitant with disturbances in coordinated interactions between HLA-E CD8(+) T cells and HSP60sp that are specific to them. This phenomenon is responsible for disturbances in so-called "friend or foe" identification during a switchover of normal immune processes to self-destruction. (Jiang H et al. 2010)

Some methods for early diagnosis of T1D e.g., *ex vivo* detection of GAD65 autoreactive T cell CD8(+) by HLA class I tetramers, are based on the use of HLA class 1 I antigens. (Giuliani L et al. 2009)

### 3.4 HLA class II: A wheelhorse or a time bomb?

HLA class II constitute a family of genes localized on the short arm of the 6th chromosome. These genes encode glycoproteins with an Ig-like structure and are predominantly localized on the APCs surface. Their functional role consists in presentation of Ags peptides to CD4(+) T helper cells type I. There exist several autoimmune diseases (including T1D) supported by promoting effects of HLA class II Ags.

Presumably, MHC glycoproteins modify positive and negative selection in the thymus allowing some immature autoAg-reactive T cells to escape from immune surveillance and thus avoid negative selection. However, presentation of morbid peptides to cytotoxic T lymphocytes (CTLs) or T helper cells by mature MHC seems to be more likely. Polymorphic variants (cytokin-related genes) residing in the vicinity of MHC classes I, II and III and non-MHC significantly increase the predisposition to autoimmune diseases and impart high (in comparison with healthy individuals) genomic instability. When the cells switch over their modality from Ag expression to MHC class II production, the molecules localized on the cell surface begin to form potentially autoreactive complexes and thus provoke self-reactive immune responses. Such nondiscriminating Ags were identified on the surface of beta cells of patients with T1D, on thyroid cells of patients with Grave's disease and on bile duct cells of patients with primary biliary cirrhosis. (Béatrice Faideau et al. 2005)

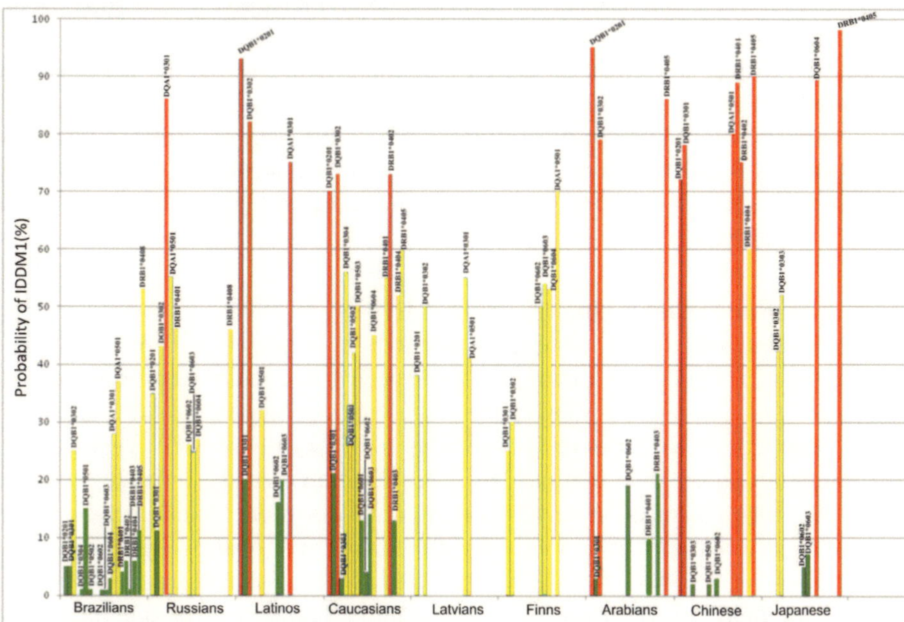


Fig. 4. The distribution of diabetogenic and protective potentials of HLA class II in different racial populations. Green columns: low risk (diabetoprotective); yellow columns: medium risk (moderately diabetogenic); red columns: highly diabetogenic. The diabetogenicity of the same alleles in different populations is either similar or radically different. It is not excluded that this parameter is controlled by environment factors.

This bar chart displays the most important T1D-predetermining haplotypes and their distribution in different populations. As can be seen, the presence of the same haplotype in two different populations contributes differentially to T1D-associated risks. For example, in Russians DQA1*0301 elicits a nearly 85% risk of T1D, whereas in Latinos the risk is less than 75%. Moreover, haplotypes spreading risks of diabetes in one population can be nonspecific for other populations. As regards DQA1*0301 its effect on acquisition of sensitivity to T1D is negligibly small in Brazilians, while in Chinese, Japanese, Arabians, Finns and Caucasians this haplotype is not associated with diabetes. These findings suggest that genetic features, haplotype frequency and contribution of specific haplotypes to susceptibility to T1D vary widely in different populations indicating different diabetogenic or protective orientation and high risk of T1D development.

Analysis of specific domains of the human genome made it possible to establish their roles in pathological processes and to get a deeper insight into molecular mechanisms responsible for instability of the human biome. The clue to the practical solution of problems in this area is to discover novel genetic markers, to secure low cost of the analysis and to ensure high accuracy of the methods employed. The totality of these factors may culminate in the construction of unique tools for subclinical diagnosis and preventive medicine.

### 3.5 HLA class III: Role in genetic predisposition

Far fewer (compared to HLA classes I and II) messages deal with contribution of HLA class III to background predisposition to T1D. In constructing a basic screening algorithm with special reference to early diagnosis potentials, one should take into consideration the crucial role of this region's genes in predisposition to T1D.

There exist about a dozen HLA class III genes manifesting a diagnostically significant association with T1D. These include NOTCH4 (rs2395106) responsible for susceptibility to rheumatoid arthritis and MSH5 (rs707915) associated with a high risk of T1D. As an overall trend, HLA classes II and III provoke diabetes at the highest levels of the odds ratio, while the effect of HLA class I on T1D is much less expressed (see Figure 3). (Valdes AM et al. 2006; Yamaji K et al.2006)

### 3.6 Non-MHC genes and their contribution to T1D

Any systemic approach to T1D diagnosis demands a large set of complementary and mutually specifying biomarkers. In addition to screening of circulating autoAbs and MHC Ags, systemic analysis of non-MHC genes is extremely important for validating the diagnosis. Though the odds ratios of the overwhelming majority of MHC genes are by one order of magnitude lower than that of MHC, identification of these gene clusters allows a qualitative description of risks for various autoimmune disorders including generation and progression of insulitis and, in a more distant perspective, objective prognosis of T1D outcomes.

In all probability (and not too surprisingly), each individual gene does not act specifically upon every component of the immune system or cell metabolism, but, rather, exerts a complex action by forming a kind of a pathological system. An immense variety of genes responsible for susceptibility to T1D are known, but their functional capabilities are either obscure or poorly investigated. Some SNPs whose role in etiology and pathogenesis of T1D leaves no doubt are described below. (Barret et. al., 2009)

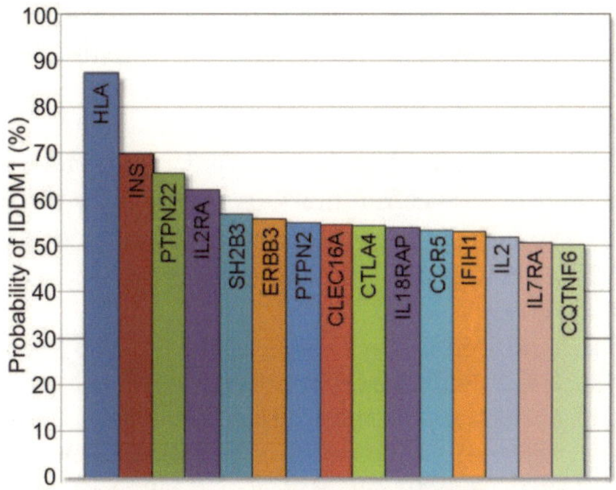


Fig. 5. A comparison of some diabetogenic non-HLA genes having mean values for HLA. The height of the column reflects the average probability of the clinical stage of type 1 diabetes (IDDM1) for the given allele. at the same time, MHC genes manifest a high degree of variation and, in some special cases, diabetoprotective activity.

**TNFAIP3 (A20),** tumor necrosis factor, alpha-induced protein 3. In the pancreas, this gene performs miscellaneous functions to include inactivation of NF-kappa B signals, prevention of inflammatory lesions of pancreatic cells, deceleration or delayed recruitment of immunocompetent cells into target organs, retardation of intercellular matrix restructuring, and so on. Studies by Liuwantara D et al. established that expression of the A20 gene is an effective mechanism of beta cell protection from TNF-induced apoptosis. Mutations in this gene and formation of SNPs initiate functional disturbances in NF-kappa B and represent the most common mechanism of disregulation and disorganization of immune reactions resulting in autoimmunity. Yet another salient feature of A20 is its ability to stimulate angiogenesis. Knockout of A20 shortens the tubule area and length in mice *in vitro.* (Grey ST et al., 2003)

A crucial role in specification of APCs and pathogenesis of T1D is played by the **ERBB3** gene known under the official name "v-erb-b2 erythroblastic leukemia viral oncogen homolog 3 (avian)". This gene encodes the family of specific receptors to the epidermal growth factor (EGFR).

Mutations in ERBB3 lead to immunoregulatory collapses coupled with continuous emergence of autoreactive cells. By virtue of its ability to provide linkage between genetic predisposition, infectious diseases and adaptive immune reactions, ERBB3 has every right to be regarded as a central molecular constituent element of the T1D-inducing complex. (Hongjie Wang et al., 2010)

**PTPN22 (LYP),** known under the official name "protein tyrosine phosphatase, non-receptor type 22 (lymphoid)", encodes lymphoid-specific intracellular phosphatase able to bind to the molecular adaptor protein CBL and thus controls its activity in the signaling pathway of the T cell receptor (TCR).

PTPN22 contains several SNPs disturbing normal operation of immune mechanisms. SNP rs2476601 is a valuable biomarker of susceptibility to autoimmune diseases, but its role in NK cell biology is not yet finally elucidated. The fact that SNP rs2476601 upsets the balance between T and NK cells *in vitro* points to the involvement of PTPN22 in immune regulation of NK function. (Douroudis et al., 2010) The PTPN22 allele 1858T worsens the function of beta cells. 1858T is associated with IAA, an autoAb participating in pancreas destruction. The 1858TT and 1858CT genotypes exhibit a steadily increasing risk for the appearance of additional autoAbs and clinical manifestations of the disease.

The primary mechanism of PTPN22 SNPs is launched upon triggering of insulin-specific autoimmune responses. SNPs produce multifarious effects: they disturb functional activity and suppress metabolic responses of beta cells to changing blood glucose levels, stimulate the transition from prediabetes to type 1 diabetes, and so on. (Fichna et al., 2010; Taniyama et al., 2010; Hermann et al., 2006)

The **IFIH1** gene (interferon induced by helicase C domain 1, also known as MDA5) encodes the DNA receptor associated with viral infections with a concomitant formation of autoreactive T cells and induction of autoimmune diabetes. Moreover, IFIH1 fulfils a protective function in hypomorphic expression of IFIH1. (Downes K et al., 2010) IFIH1 is directly involved in the destruction of Langerhans islets due to pooling and mobilization of autoreactive cells in response to viral invasion. This circumstance aggravates immune dissonance and promotes self-restructuring of targeted organs by provoking persistent deficiency of the pancreas and accelerating insulin failure. IFIH1 disturbs cell-mediated and humoral immunity by initiating selective deficiency of IgA. (Ferreira et al., 2010)

**IL2RA** (interleukin 2 receptor, alpha, also known as CD25, T1D0, TGGFR) represents, along with IL2RB and the γ-chain IL2RG, a fragment of the high-affinity receptor IL-2 (homodimerization of α-chains yields low-affinity receptors, while homodimerization of β-chains gives receptors with medium affinity). By virtue of its structural and functional peculiarities, IL2RA makes the greatest contribution to the progression of T1D. It regulates immune and inflammatory responses, exerts negative control over cell proliferation and favors differentiation of T cells. In addition, IL2RA controls apoptosis via a positive feedback mechanism. Mutations in the IL2RA gene point to IL2RA insufficiency. Genetic variations in IL2-IL21 and IL2RA/CD25 regions predetermine the susceptibility to T1D by interfering with the transcription and/or splicing of mRNA. In this way, IL2 and IL2RA exert genetic control over protein expression in different cell subpopulations. (Dendrou et al., 2008)

The **INS** (ILPR, IRDN, IDDM2, MODY) gene is a key participant in the synthesis of insulin molecules. In patients with T1D, the mutation frequency of this gene does not exceed 0.1%. (Rajasalu et al., 2007)

**CD226** (rs763361) SNPs regulate the activity of certain cells involved in immune mechanisms mediating beta cell destruction. The susceptibility to T1D is associated with SNPs rs763361 (genotype TT, OR = 2.29) and allele T (OR = 1.48). (Douroudis et al., 2009; Hafler et al., 2009)

In conclusion, we can state with assurance that nearly the overall repertoire of genes whose mutations are known to increase the risk of T1D development has been identified and characterized in terms of functional activity, which includes:

- Protection of beta cells from apoptosis (TNFAIP3);
- Secretion and metabolism of insulin (INS);
- General immunity (ERBB3, IL2RA, PTPN22, PTPN2, SH2B3, CTLA4, SUMO, ICOS;, etc.);
- Undefined function (CTSH, CLEC16A, IL7RA, CIQTNF6);
- Generation of autoAbs to beta cells (mostly, in adults) (HLA-DR3);
- Generation of autoAbs to insulin and formation of the insulin resistance syndrome (mostly, in adolescents)(HLA-DR4);

- Supporting high risks of autoimmune processes (HLA-DQ-related T1D) (NB: HLA-DR3-DQ2 and HLA-DR4-DQ8 genes are among the most popular T1D inducers in young children);
- Diabetoprotective function (HLA-DR2, DR6, DR7) (**NB**: HLA-DR1, DR5, DR8 and DR9 genes are usually identified in individuals for whom T1D is uncommon).

From the foregoing it follows that the first step of preclinical diagnosis must include identification of classical genetic biomarkers for each concrete pathology and acquisition of information from three basic resources: (i) genealogic tree, (ii) anamnesis morbid and (iii) anamnesis vita.

This approach would enable identification of individuals predisposed to a concrete disease and their distribution into risk groups with further transition to the second stage where patients are subject to investigation, using target panels of genotypic and phenotypic biomarkers and continuous monitoring of potentially affected cohorts and those predisposed to the preclinical pathology stage. The primary testing approach demands validated procedures for detecting molecular and cellular shifts in one or another cell and/or tissue function in the paradigm of the most pathogenetically significant targets. The methods employed thereupon include high-performance genomic and metagenomic scanning as well as proteomic and metabolic analyses in the paradigm of microbial colony-forming populations. Moreover, biomonitoring is based on the use of a vast array of nanotools as well as visualization and biosensoric facilities allowing comprehensive examination of "suspected" individuals and elaboration of wide-range activity-oriented treatment schedules in a real-time mode.

## 4. Proteomics: A powerful tool for predictive medicine

The role of proteomic technologies in the study of autoimmune diseases can hardly be overestimated. Virtually all currently known autoimmune diseases including diabetes mellitus, multiple sclerosis, systemic lupus erythematosus and other severe autoimmune disorders have proteomic markers of their own. At the same time, the advent of efficient high-precision diagnostic technologies opened up new opportunities in the search for novel preclinical diagnostic markers. Identification of autoAbs to immunoglobulins GADA, IAA, ICA, IA-2A and ZnT8 has become a routine procedure in T1D diagnosis. In this chapter, the main emphasis will be laid on some characteristics of specific proteins for progressive T1D.

Clusterin (apolipoprotein J) holds considerable promise as a candidate biomarker; its main function is traditionally recognized as a tool to control apoptosis. It should be noted, however, that clusterin exhibits the behaviour of an antiapoptotic chaperone when used at low concentrations; at higher concentrations (~ 12% of control), it causes disruption of mitochondria and initiates cell apoptosis by a mitochondrial mechanism. Recent reports highlighted a high regenerative potential of Clusterin, particularly, with respect to beta cells. The functional activity of this protein demands further verification and analysis, but its elevation always points to apoptosis of pancreatic beta cells. (Lee et al., 2011)

Transcortin (Corticosteroid-binding globulin, CBG) and Lumican are capable to induce pronounced (1.5–2-fold against control) upregulation. Transcortin fulfils the function of a glucocorticoid transporter and is strongly inhibited by insulin; hence, insulin deficiency is always associated with hyperproduction of Transcortin. (Fernández-Real et al., 1999) However, this protein is hardly effective as a selective biomarker for T1D, since it emerges exclusively at the latest stages of autoimmune aggression and its role in T1D etiogenesis is still unclear. Lumican, the key mediator in fibrosis-related processes, manifests an even higher degree of upregulation than Transcortin and is widely distributed in all body tissues. Its significant elevation may represent an acute response of renal tissues to high plasma levels of glucose and is also characteristic of nephropathies. However, being a convenient tool for predicting diabetic nephropathies, Lumican cannot predict associated diseases.

It may be concluded from the above-said that Clusterin is the only candidate for a selective protein biomarker for T1D, because it emerges at early stages of the disease and is more related to cause than effect.

## 5. Effects of autoAbs on the launch of autoimmune processes and pancreas deficiency: Dynamics of spectra and prognostic value in preclinical diagnosis of T1D

Today, autoantibodies (autoAbs) are the main biomarkers of diabetes mellitus. The presence of small concentrations of autoAbs in peripheral blood does not always indicate initiation of an autoimmune process, because the organism possesses a vast number of autoregulatory mechanisms. However, their collapse and significant elevation of Ab titers indicate a nearly 100% risk for diabetes in the foreseeable future. Many autoAb classes are currently known including GADA (65 and 67), IA-2Ab, INSab, HSPab, ZnT8ab, IAA, etc.

Each of these autoAbs has a prognostic value of its own and is associated with a definite type of diabetes (T1D, latent diabetes, fulminant diabetes, etc.). The factors initiating the appearance of autoAbs are also different. Among the immense diversity of causative factors, diabetogenic genes (classes I, II and III MHC) responding by activation to virus-induced inflammation (molecular mimicry) are of paramount importance. The results of in-depth studies on associativity between MHC II alleles and auto-Abs unequivocally suggest that in the present state of the problem generation of certain classes of auto-Abs and further progression of T1D can be predicted on the basis of genetic data even at the earliest stages of the disease.

### 5.1 GADA

Glutamate decarboxylase catalyzes the conversion of glutamic acid into γ-aminobutyric acid and $CO_2$ and plays a prominent role in the functional activity of the central nervous system (CNS). Its substrate (glutamic acid) is responsible for excitation, while its major metabolic product (γ-aminobutyric acid) is a key mediator of inhibition in brain neurons. The physiological role of this enzyme is confined to various aspects of insulin-dependent diabetes.

Two isoforms of GAD (GAD65 and GAD67) are encoded by two non-allelic genes localized on different chromosomes, more specifically, on the 2$^{nd}$ (GAD65) and 10$^{th}$ (GAD67) chromosomes. Both isoforms are actively expressed in CNS neurons. In human islet cells, GAD65 is a predominant isoform, while GAD67 is either present in negligibly small amounts or is not expressed at all. In contrast, in rat islet cells both GAD isoforms are expressed with a nearly equal efficiency, but the GAD67 isoform is predominant.

The prognostic significance of GADA is rather high. These autoAbs appear in circulating blood before other auto-Abs (~ 10 – 15 years before the appearance of first clinical manifestations of T1D) and are detected in 70 – 90% of cases.

Risks for T1D and Ab titers

| Autoantibody titer | 10-year risk (% ± SE) | HR (95% CI) | P |
|---|---|---|---|
| I quartile | 35 ± 9 | 1* | |
| II quartile | 22 ± 9 | 0.8 (0.3–1.9) | 0.55 |
| III quartile | 52 ± 9 | 1.7 (0.8–3.6) | 0.18 |
| IV quartile | 43 ± 10 | 1.6 (0.7–3.6) | 0.26 |

Likelihood of developing diabetes depending on the combination of epitope-specific GADA antibodies

| GADA | | | | | |
|---|---|---|---|---|---|
| Epitope combination | | | | n (T1D cases) | 10-year risk |
| MID | COOH | NH2 | 67 | | |
| + | + | + | + | 24 (8) | 39% |
| + | + | + | – | 12 (6) | 26% |
| + | + | – | + | 15 (5) | 56% |
| + | + | – | – | 62 (21) | 45% |
| + | – | + | – | 1 (0) | |
| + | – | – | – | 13 (3) | 27% |
| – | + | + | + | 1 (0) | |
| – | + | – | – | 5 (2) | 48% |
| – | – | + | – | 6 (1) | 20% |
| – | – | – | – | 10 (3) | 33% |

For GAD antibodies, MID refers to epitopes within GAD65 amino acids 235–442, COOH refers to epitopes within GAD65 amino acids 436–585, NH2 refers to epitopes within GAD65 amino acids 1–100, while GAD67 refers to epitopes present in GAD6 (combinations with no relatives are not shown). (Buzzetti et al., 2007; Mayr et al., 2007)

### 5.2 IA-2

IA-2 belongs to type 1 membrane-bound proteins containing extracellular $NH_2$-terminal glycosylated, membrane-bound and COOH-terminal cytoplasmic regions. The immune epitope of IA-2 is localized exclusively in the cytoplasmic region of IA-2 where its PTP (protein-tyrosine-phosphate)-like domain is the main recognition site for auto-Abs. The fact that the dominant T cell epitope of IA-2, also localized in the PTP-like region, is structurally similar to the VP7 region (VP7 is a major immunogenic protein of rotaviruses) provides additional evidence for the crucial role of the molecular mimicry mechanism in the pathogenesis of T1D.

IA-2β (also known as fogrin, PTP-NP, ICAAR and IAR) is structurally similar to IA-2. Its intracellular and extracellular domains are structurally identical (by 74 and 26%, respectively) to IA-2. IA-2β is predominantly localized in secretory vesicles of beta and some other neuroendocrine cells. Anti-IA-2β Abs are present in nearly 50% of patients with newly diagnosed T1D; their emergence is usually recorded several years before the appearance of the first clinical manifestations of the disease.

AutoAbs against the insulin antigen are detected in 70–90% of individuals as early as 10 - 12 years before the clinical stage of T1D.

| Auto-Ab titer | 10-year risk (% ± SE) | HR (95% CI) | P |
|---|---|---|---|
| I quartile | 20 ± 14 | 1* | |
| II quartile | 74 ± 15 | 6.0 (1.6–22.4) | 0.008 |
| III quartile | 84 ± 10 | 5.9 (1.7–21.1) | 0.006 |
| IV quartile | 71 ± 15 | 4.8 (1.3–17.9) | 0.02 |

Likelihood of developing diabetes depending on combination of epitope-specific IA-2 antibodies

| IA-2ab | | | | |
|---|---|---|---|---|
| Epitope combination | | | n (T1D cases) | 10-year risk |
| IA-2β | PTP | JM | | |
| + | + | + | 13 (8) | 81% |
| + | + | – | 12 (10) | 100% |
| + | – | + | 1 (1) | |
| + | – | – | 4 (3) | |
| – | + | + | 8 (3) | 34% |
| – | + | – | 10 (4) | 44% |
| – | – | + | 9 (2) | 41% |
| – | – | – | 4 (1) | |

For IA-2 antibodies, IA-2β refers to epitopes found in the PTP region of IA-2β and IA-2, PTP refers to epitopes found in the PTP region of IA-2 (but not IA-2β), while JM refers to epitopes within the IA-2 juxtamembrane region in amino acids 601–682 (combinations with no relatives are not shown). (Kordonouri et al., 2010; Kawasaki E et al., 2003; Hanifi-Moghaddam et al., 2003)

### 5.3 ICA

The target antigen for pancreatic islet cell antibodies has not yet been finally identified. In all probability, it represents a heterogeneous cluster of antigens expressed in beta cells. In contrast to IA-2ab, ICA is a polyclonal antibody able to interact with all populations of islet cells (α, β, γ, δ, PP) and other auto-antigens (sialoglucoconjugate, GAD, IA-2A, etc.).

Antibodies to islet cells are found in 85-90% of patients with onset T1D (cf. 0.5% in unaffected individuals) during the very first week after clinical diagnosis. Four weeks thereafter, their incidence does not exceed 50%. In patients with one-year history of T1D, antibodies to beta cells are present in only 10-20% of cases.

Similar to other cell-related Abs, ICA does not play any crucial role in beta cell degradation, but is one of key markers of cell-mediated autoimmunity. Its detection in blood serum suggests latent autoimmune diabetes (LADA) and slow degradation of beta cells.The prognostic capacity of ICA is neither high, nor low and is usually manifested 12 years prior to T1D development. Its incidence at the clinical diagnosis stage varies from 60 to 80%. Correlation between antibody titers and risks for T1D over a period of 7 years. (Achenbach et al., 2004; Williams et al., 2002)

### 5.4 IAA - AutoAbs to insulin

Insulin is a peptide hormone produced by beta cells of pancreatic Langerhans islets. The main physiological role of insulin consists in reducing glucose levels in the blood; its absolute deficiency is the main cause of T1D.Anti-insulin Abs are indispensable constituent elements of blood sera of healthy individuals where their concentrations vary from 1 to 5 µg/ml. In patients with T1D, serum concentrations of anti-insulin autoAb IgG class can reach very high levels.

Insulin antibodies are associated with many autoimmune pathologies including Graves' disease (40%), Hashimoto's disease (autoimmune thyroiditis) (20%), Addison's disease (40%), chronic hepatitis (36%), systemic lupus erythematosus (29%), etc.

Insulin-binding Ab are always present in the blood sera of insulin-treated patients. In patients with T1D, the therapeutic effect of insulin diminishes gradually with emergence of anti-insulin antibodies, especially after prolonged insulin therapy or administration of high daily doses of the hormone. Other factors, e.g., dosage form or purity of the hormonal preparation, also play a role.

Seroconversion of insulin ABS is usually recorded as early as eight years before the onset and clinical diagnosis of T1D. However, after this period high antibody titers begin to decrease gradually up to the moment of their complete elimination and are detected in only 30–60% of patients.

| Auto-Ab titers | 10-year risk (% ± SE) | HR (95% CI) | P |
|---|---|---|---|
| I quartile | 45 ± 16 | 1* | |
| II quartile | 30 ± 13 | 0.7 (0.2–2.4) | 0.55 |
| III quartile | 38 ± 17 | 0.8 (0.2–2.7) | 0.68 |
| IV quartile | 77 ± 12 | 3.0 (1.1–8.1) | 0.03 |

(Catherine Pihoker et al., 2005; Heli et al., 2009)

## 6. Metabolome as applicable to T1D management at subclinical stages to prevent or minimize the imbalance

In a recent study, a comparison of blood sera from children with type 1 diabetes (T1D), non diabetic children and children without autoimmune antibodies revealed metabolic disturbances (significant reduction of serum levels of succinate, phosphatidylcholine, phospholipin and ketoleucine, drastic elevation of glutamate, etc.) in the T1D group. , (Bougnères et al., 2008) The true reason for these disturbances is difficult to establish, since all these changes can be associated, with an equal degree of probability, with asymptomatic damage of liver and body musculature, T1D, metabolic imbalance caused by environmental factors, etc.

High lysophosphatidylcholine levels are detected in patients' blood as early as several years before the first clinical manifestations of T1D. It should be noted, however, that the aforecited studies were performed on children, but not on adults with T1D; therefore, their clinical significance is ambiguous.

Notable elevation of blood sera levels of glutamate potentiates the activity of GAD65, the major autoimmune antigen for autoAbs. The figure below shows the dynamics of the "glutamine–GABA–GADA" sequence. As can be seen, neither GADA and IAA, nor unlimited elevation of glutamine and moderate elevation of GABA take place in the initial steps. However, in the course of time the concentration of glutamic acid begins to decrease, while that of GABA increases; however, autoAbs are not generated even under these conditions. Subsequent decreases of glutamic acid and GABA are noted only against the background of increasing titers of anti-GAD65 and anti-insulin autoAbs (seroconversion). After T1D passes to the clinical diagnosis stage, auto-Abs titers begin to decrease gradually to a nearly undetectable level (this widely occurring phenomenon usually lasts 10 to 20 years).

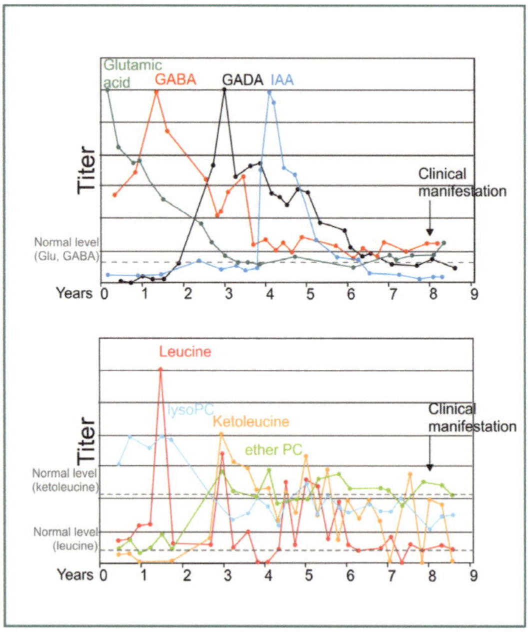


Fig. 6. The dynamics of changes in the concentrations of Glu / GABA / GADA and insulin Abs in the period between the commencement of the effect of the irreversible diabetes-inducing factor and first clinical manifestations of T1D. There is a clear seroconversion sequence Glu / GABA / GADA with a period of about 1 year. By the moment of appearance of first clinical manifestations, some antibodies detected several years theretofore, may be missing. (Noteworthy, each individual case may be different from the average).

There is evidence that in addition to the aforesaid metabolites T1D is characterized by fluctuations in the levels of succinic acid, phosphatidylcholine (even in newborns), triglycerides and phospholipids.

## 7. Environmental factors triggering T1D

Estimation of the role of environmental factors in triggering one or another pathology and development of adequate approaches to diagnosis within maximally short intervals of time is one of currently central problems in preclinical medicine. Here, it is necessary to draw a demarcation line between autoimmune disorders and background events in order to select optimal diagnostic procedures and reliable criteria, since clinical tests do not always provide unfailing results that are crucial for diagnosis. Therefore, development of strict elaborate protocols is of vital importance for identification and analysis of environmental factors.

Continuous exposure to hazardous effects of environmental factors and large-scale application of chemical substances in food industry, pharmaceutics and other sectors of national economy are harmful for human immune system, since all of them trigger pathological reactions resulting in diabetes. Furthermore, uncontrolled intake of drugs and frequent viral and bacterial infections form predisposition to allergic reactions and provoke autoagression and development of various immune disorders.

## 8. Phase 2 characteristics

### 8.1 Viral infections as triggering factors in type 1 diabetes

The large body of evidence (serological, epidemiological, biological, etc.) obtained thus far testifies to the ability of certain viruses to provoke type 1 diabetes mellitus (T1D) in human beings. Among the immense diversity of other disease-provoking factors, enteroviruses, retroviruses, reoviruses, parotiditis viruses, cytomegalovirus, Epstein-Barr virus and a clinical variant of the diabetogenic encephalomyocarditis virus are the most likely candidates for T1D-triggering factors.

Viral infections provoke diabetes by operating at different regulatory levels, e.g., by disregulating immune mechanisms, by stimulating the activity of pathological systems or by interfering with the normal course of regulatory processes occurring in the organism.

The risks of viral infection and T1D development correlate with the functional stability of the organism and its genetic and immune backgrounds. It is well known that morbidity from seasonal (especially, in the winter period) virus-borne infections correlates with very high incidence of autoimmune diseases including T1D. The reason is in shorter (in comparison with summertime) duration of the daylight period and, as a consequence, low level of vitamin D synthesis and increased morbidity from viral infections and autoimmune disorders. Additional support in favor of this hypothesis can be derived from much greater incidence of T1D in North European countries in comparison with Southern Europe.

### 8.2 Bacterial infections as triggering factors of T1D

Recent advances in immunologic research and numerous animal and human model studies shed new light on the role of enteric bacteria in triggering autoimmune reactions. It was shown, in particular, that certain bacteria (e.g., *Bacteroides ovatus*) induce diabetes in young children predisposed to T1D. The mechanisms whereby bacterial agents interfere with immune homeostasis and provoke diabetes are still poorly understood; it is known, however, that intestinal bacteria trigger autoimmune responses that initiate destructive insulitis. The strongest argument in favor of this viewpoint is an ever increasing (by 20% in comparison with control) number of affected individuals infected with sporadic variants of these bacteria. The extent of bacterial infection is especially apparent in young children whose autoimmune microbiome is the least stable and diversified. Continuous sophistication and diversification of the microbiome with ageing point to the decreasing role of bacteria in initiating diabetes in adult individuals. (Giongo et al., 2010)

### 8.3 Nutritional factors

For quite a long period of time, viruses were considered to be the only etiogenic external factors in T1D. Today, there is evidence that nutritional factors also play a role in T1D development. Although the pathogenetic mechanisms of the disease are not yet completely

understood, the role of T1D as one of the most essential links in the human immune system leaves no doubt, particularly with regard to its tolerance to food antigens.
As a rule, tolerance to food antigens largely depends on peculiarities of local immune reactions whose functional role consists in suppression of immune responses formed under the influence of several factors, viz., (i) oral tolerance, (ii) controlled chronic inflammation (so-called "physiological inflammation") and (iii) local secretion of IgA.
Disturbances in the coordinated functioning of these mechanisms stimulate the appearance of characteristic manifestations of food allergy. Measurements of blood plasma levels of Abs against various food antigens in patients with clinically confirmed T1D revealed high titers of IgA and IgG against cow's milk Ags (bovine serum albumin, BSA), beta lactoglobulin, BLG) and some other food Ags, e.g., ovalbumin, OVA. It should be noted, however, that in this particular case we deal with the so-called abuse tolerance, which can hardly be compared to food allergies associated with high levels of circulating IgE. (Kohno et al., 2002; Luopajärvi et al., 2008)

### 8.3.1 Nitrosamines

There is a statistic association between nitrosamines and diabetes as can be judged from some biochemical data on destructive effects of nitrosamines on pancreatic Langerhans islet beta cells. In a statistical study, nitrosamine levels were determined in foods consumed by children under 14 at risk of diabetes. It was found that in children with low dietary nitrosamine levels the Odds Ratio (OR) was equal to 1.0 (cf. 1.7 OR and 2.6 OR in children with medium and high levels of dietary nitrosamine). (Dahlquist et al., 1990)
Statistic analysis established a correlation between the quality and quantity of consumed food, on the one hand, and susceptibility for diabetes, on the other hand. However, this correlation is purely statistical, since biological, biochemical and immunological mechanisms responsible for this phenomenon demand further investigation and analysis. (Essien & Akpan, 2006)

## 8.4 Age

The growing tendency in the past decades is towards higher incidence of T1D in young people and children. In the first place, this is due to negative influences of environmental factors. The first peak of T1D is normally observed between the 4$^{th}$ and 6$^{th}$ years of life; the second peak is associated with hormonal transformations in the pubertal period (10–12 years).
On the other hand, there exists a special form of diabetes termed as latent autoimmune diabetes in adults (above 30) (LADA). Its most characteristic features are moderate clinical manifestations and slow progression of the autoimmune process. The finding that 6% of patients with LADA carry protective haplotypes responsible for more slow progression and less severe (in comparison with IDDM1) manifestations of the disease indicates that LADA appears to be a more widespread form of diabetes than its classical form, viz., T1D. This and the aforementioned data emphasize the need for elaborating novel effective criteria and approaches to treatment of patients with diagnosed LADA. (Bermúdez et al., 2010)

## 8.5 Gender

Analysis of sex steroids revealed that clinical manifestations of many autoimmune diseases vary widely depending on the hormonal status of the organism, e.g., menstrual cycle, administration of oral contraceptives, etc. Pregnancy should also be included in this list. The alternative hypothesis states that higher X-linked genetic predisposition of females to autoimmune diseases is a result of unbalanced X chromosome inactivation. The X-inactivation skew theory was recently corroborated for dermatosclerosis and autoimmune thyroiditis. Yet another possible mechanism is small-scale exchange of cells between mother and fetus pregnancy.

At the same time, the current views on the role of environmental factors in T1D are often diametrally opposite and many practitioners in medicine are inclined to think that the stably increasing incidence of this severe autoimmune disease is unrelated to external factors. For example, a mass-scale retrospective investigation was carried out in Saudi Arabia in the period between 1980–2009. In this study, 119 patients with T1D were divided into six groups depending on early clinical manifestations of the disease. There was no correlation between the impact of environmental factors and the incidence of T1D over a period of three decades.

## 9. Medicaments as potential T1D inducers

For many decades, it was believed that certain chemical substances including patented medicaments are harmful for the pancreas and provoke T1D. The mechanisms whereby chemical drugs exert their hazardous effects vary widely and are not clearly understood. Active drug components accumulated in body cells slow down the functional processes in different body tissues and organs and trigger pathological reactions, e.g., by providing tropism of certain pathogens or restructuring the systemic architectonics of body organs including the pancreas. The presence, in such active components, of sequestered or cryptic epitopes provokes negative phenomena, such as molecular mimicry. Not infrequently, medicinal drugs trigger a series of immunoregulatory and immunoeffector shifts, which culminate in immune disorders including autoimmune destruction of the pancreas.

## 10. T1D and vaccination: Is there a correlation between them? The role of passive immunization in T1D development

There exist quite a few hypotheses concerning the role of vaccination in triggering autoimmune diseases including T1D. This fact notwithstanding, only few instances proved to display a clearcut correlation between vaccination and development of autoimmune syndromes. (Ethan Rubinstein, 2004) In the meantime, heated discussions about association between autoimmune disorders and vaccination do not abate. Advocates of the "autoimmunization" hypothesis refer to recent flagrant global-scale spreading of autoimmune diseases with a particular on responsibility of children's vaccines manufacturers. (Classen JB & Classen DC, 1999)

There is evidence that T1D indeed develop in response to immunization. At the same time, in newborn infants vaccinated at the age of several months the incidence of T1D did not exceed the morbidity level in children immunized with a single vaccinating dose at the age of 2 years. (Karvonen et al., 1999) Mass-scale serial investigations carried out in the USA did not establish any associativity between these two events. Similarly, studies into the role of vaccination and vaccination timing as risk factors in childhood diabetes failed to establish a correlation between vaccination and the risk for autoimmune diseases. (DeStefano et al., 2001; Blom et al., 2001)

## 11. Associativity between T1D and autoimmune diseases. Polyglandular autoimmune syndromes

T1D is often concomitant with local or systemic autoimmune disturbances, which further progress to complex autoimmune diseases or polyglandular syndromes via the cross-reactivity mechanism. By illustration, in many patients T1D is associated with autoimmune thyroiditis (24.5%/autoAbs vs 47.5%), celiac disease (1.4%/autoAbs to gliadin and IgA to tissue transglutaminase vs 18.7%), MS (0.5-2%/autoAbs vs 7%), Addison's disease (1.4%/adrenal cortex autoAbs vs 0.7%), autoimmune gastritis (6.9-7.2%/parietal cell autoAbs vs 20.9%), etc. (Somers et al., 2009; Villano et al., 2009; De Block et al., 2006)
Secondary autoimmune disorders associated with later steps of T1D have a number of specific features. Thus, autoimmune thyroiditis (AIT) (autoimmune polyglandular syndrome 3A version (APS3Av)) is diagnosed in 12-15% of T1D patients; its clinical manifestations correlate positively with age, gender (AIT is more frequent in females (8.6%) than in males (3.4%)), duration of T1D (mean age of AIT patients varies between 5 and 15 years), serum levels of the thyroid-stimulating hormone (TSH), etc. Both diseases have a common familial hereditary background, but can also be present in a single individual suggesting a crucial role of genetic predisposition in the development of polyglandular syndromes. Furthermore, high incidence of AIT among first-degree relatives of T1D patients points to a significant contribution of genetic factors to immune system failures (see above). (Severinski et al., 2003; Hunger-Battefeld et al., 2009)
Noteworthy, the predominant form of AIT in patients of both sexes is hypothyroidism (8.1%), but in males with anti-thyroid Abs AIT is prevalent (85.7% vs 37.5% in females). the total incidence of hypothyroidism in T1D patients with anti-thyroid Abs is 52.2%. The interval between the onset of T1D and the appearance of first clinical manifestations of AIT varies from one year to 5–6 years, while the first thyroid autoAbs appear in the period between 6 months and 5–3 years before the onset of the disease. Blood sera of patients with APS3Av (AIT and T1D) (Hunger-Battefeld et al., 2009) contain circulating anti-thyroid peroxidase and anti-thyroglobulin Abs emerging soon after emergence of GADA (10% and 8% of cases, respectively); more than 6% of such patients contain both types of autoAbs. As mentioned earlier in this chapter, MS is also associated with T1D. In this case, morbidity from MS among male patients exceeds that in females nearly fourfold (2% vs. 0.5%). According to statistic reports, non-diabetic sisters run five times higher risks for MS than other cohorts of the general population. Consequently, adult females with T1D can be assigned to the highest risk group for associated autoimmune disorders (e.g., MS). (Bussone et al., 2009; Otto-Buczkowska et al., 2009)
The association between T1D and RA is not so apparent as in the case of T1D and MS. In depth studies established that about 13% of patients whose first-degree relatives suffer from T1D have clinical signs of RA. According to other authors, no such linkage does not exist. (Hakala et al., 1992)
Based on these findings, we can state with assurance that T1D increases the risk for autoimmune disorders through triggering the formation of autoimmune clusters and polyglandular autoimmune syndromes. As a rule, circulating autoAbs begin to appear in the blood serum as early as several years before the development of severe secondary disorders and absolute clinical manifestations of the disease. The genetic data provide the physician with a broad spectrum of autoimmune diseases that are likely to develop in patients with T1D. Time-lapse monitoring of patients' blood sera not only affords reliable

dynamic control over disease progression, but also enables the physician to estimate the efficiency of ongoing therapy, to search for early-stage biomarkers for diagnosing secondary autoimmune disorders and, last but not least, to implement adequate preventive and curative treatment.

## 12. Multiple Sclerosis (MS)

### 12.1 State-of-art models of multiple sclerosis

Multiple sclerosis (MS), a remitting and relapsing autoimmune disease of the central nervous system (CNS), represents a generalized degenerative inflammatory process. Its main causative factors are demyelination, degradation of oligodendrocytes and degeneration of axons.

The clinical course of MS includes three stages, viz., the preclinical stage, the autoimmune inflammation stage and the neurodegeneration stage. Some basically important targets (including gene-oriented ones) emerging in the course of MS evolution can be used in the design of novel preclinical diagnostic tools. Expression of gene products including functionally important transcripts is currently employed in the design of proteomes. The use of these constructs (commonly referred to as diagnostic microchips) as early as at the preclinical pathology stage allows multifarious manipulations with specific targets in the course of immune attacks. Impaired structure of the myelin sheath (demyelination) and degradation of axons take place at the very earliest stages of preclinical MS, i.e., long before the clinical onset of the disease. This generates a need for innovative preclinical diagnosis protocols and, in a more distant perspective, preventive treatment of MS. In this context, genetic tests acquire special importance as valuable analytical tools for predicting and estimating risks in MS. In terms of present-day classifications, the genes supporting predisposition to MS are divided into three main groups, viz., immune system genes (DRB1, OPN, CD44, CD24, CCR5-Δ32), myelin metabolism genes (MBP, CTLA4, ICAM1) and cytokins (TGFβ1, TNF). AutoAbs to the basic protein of myelin are amont the key autoaggression markers for demyelination-related pathologies. Some of these Abs have functional resources of their own, e.g., proteolytic activity towards the Ag substrate. The dynamics of Abs spectra in patients with MS reflect etiogenic peculiarities of MS evolution. It is now well established that pre-early stages of MS are accompanied by the appearance of specific Abs against two categories of determinants, viz., mimicking and myelin epitopes. After termination of the preclinical phase, serum titers of mimicking Abs show a tendency to decrease, while those of antimyelin and antineural autoAbs increase in contrast. This upward trend points to escalation of antitissue autoaggression and formation of a typical clinical picture of the disease including a complete set of clinical and serological criterial features of PIFAS. Early emergence and long persistence of antimyelin autoAbs in MS patients points to a correlation between serum positivity and duration of the disease. (Sepiashvili et al., 2010; Martynov et al., 2010)

## 13. Aortic aneurisms

Aortic aneurisms (AA) are related to the category of socially important diseases involving a high risk for lethality. Its main causal factors are degradation of elastin (e.g., by proteases), pronounced structural changes in medial smooth muscle cells (SMC), aortic vasculature atrophies and formation of the *preclinical* pathological syndrome. The main clinically important causes of AA established thus far can be presented as follows: (i) genetic predisposition and hereditary diseases affecting the molecular architectonics of connective tissue (e. g. Marfan's syndrome); (ii) atherosclerosis and arterial hypertension. Very often, AA is associated with atherosclerosis, especially, in patients of senior age groups. Male gender, smoking, carriage of specific infectious pathogens (herpes simplex virus, cytomegalovirus, *Chl. pneumonia,* syphilis and tuberculosis pathogens) also play a role in the pathogenesis of AA.

Long duration of the *preclinical* stage (aortal dilation to the critical level) in patients with AA provides the physician with a unique opportunity to break the pathogenetic linkage and thus to arrest the further progression of the disease on going from the preclinical to the clinical stage.

It is more expedient to perform preclinical screening in three steps in full conformity with prenosological diagnostic protocols. *(i)* identification of blood serum levels of biomarkers in the form of so-called serodiagnostic packages (matrix metalloproteinases (MMP), cystatin C, osteoprotegerin (OPG), soluble fractions of elastin (SFE) and heavy chains of myosin (HCM), antibodies against *Ch. pneumonia,* CMV and HSV). These biomarkers are used as diagnostic package components and allow maximally accurate diagnosis and, which is no less important, estimation of lesion size even at the *preclinical* stage; *(ii)* MRT or contrasting CT scanning angiography for identifying exact location of dilated vessels, viz., *topological sites* in the vascular network responsible for hypersecretion of specific biomarkers; *(iii)* biopsy of the dilated portion of the aorta containing a suspected aneurism followed by morphological, immunogenetic and molecular-biological testing of bioptats. This procedure is highly invasive and its implementation is not recommended in the absence of positive results in the first two steps. If the dilated portion of the aorta cannot be visualized directly and the first-step tests give positive results, screening for biomarkers must be repeated after a period of several months. If positive results are obtained from serological doublet tests, MRT or CT angiography must be conducted to the required extent.

Early (*preclinical*) diagnosis holds especially great promise being the most efficient step in prophylactic and preventive treatment of AA. The uniqueness and high therapeutic potentials of *preclinical* diagnosis combined with low invasiveness of the nonsurgical approach and design, on its basis, of more advanced diagnostic protocols opens up fresh opportunities for the development of rationalized and practicable innovative technologies as a breakthrough in cardio- and angiosurgery. Prospective analysis of clinical utility of *targeted* therapy as a tool for *preventive* (preoperative) treatment and/or postsurgical angiorehabilitation will also make the subject of future investigations.

## 14. Rheumatic diseases

In considering the role of pathogenetic factors in rheumatoid arthritis (RA), systemic lupus erythematosus (SLE) and ankylosing spondylitis (AS), special emphasis should be laid on risk genes and the extent to which they overlap.

According to GWA data, the contribution of MHC to RA risk can approximately be estimated as 30%, HLA-DRB1 alleles (e.g., DRB1*0401 with OR of 3) being critical for RA. Additional loci essential for estimating RA risks were identified by high-density genotyping as HLA-DP in patients with anticyclic citrullinated peptide antibodies, *(HLA-DR2(DRB1*1501))* and *DR3 (DRB1*0301)* alleles in the MHC class II region with Ors of 2, risk variants in the MHC class III cluster encoding the TNF gene and the C2 complement components C4A and C4B.

Other loci in the MHC class III region associated with SLE include: the SKIV2L gene encoding the superkiller viralicidic activity of a 2-like protein, the PTPN22 gene, TNFAIP3 and TRAF1-C5 loci (TNF-associated signalling pathway genes), Integrin-α-M (ITGAM), STAT4, IL23R and a number of other genes.

## 15. Conclusion

In-depth studies into pathogenesis and etiogenesis of autoimmune diseases and discovery of reliable biomarkers for diagnosing various pathological conditions provide a way for predicting, with a sufficiently high degree of probability, the risk of relapses and exacerbations and possible clinical manifestations of the disease. In its turn, considerable recent progress in medical science (in medical genetics, bionanomedicine and bioinformatics, in particular) provides a clue to the design of advanced protocols for preclinical screening of patients. The construction of individual genetic maps with special reference to familial predispositions and time-lapse monitoring of risk groups for pathomorphological markers have one common goal, viz., to collect information for early implementation of preventive and therapeutic intervention strategies. Moreover, dynamic control over functional activities of different body organs and tissues on the basis of well established and validated proteomic and metabolomic data enables early prediction of exacerbations and complications and implementation of preventive therapy. The latter is based on the use of state-of-art pharmacological protocols and, if surgical correction is required, of the most recent advances in transplantation and regenerative medicine.

Considerable improvement and wide-scale application of preclinical diagnosis algorithms and preventive treatment protocols for routine clinical application are among the most topical problems in today's medical practice. More urgent strategies are aimed at compensating structural and functional deficiencies of damaged organs and fragments thereof. In genetic studies combined with early detection of minor lesion foci and analysis of immune, proteomic and metabolomic disturbances open up new vistas for social welfare with the ultimate goal to improve current standards of public health care at large.

## 16. References

Achenbach, P.; Warncke, K.; Reiter, J.; Naserke, H.E.; Williams, A.J.; Bingley, P.J.; Bonifacio, E. & Ziegler, A.G. (2004) Stratification of type 1 diabetes risk on the basis of islet autoantibody characteristics. Diabetes, Vol.53, No.2 (February 2004) ISSN 384-92

Ahn, J.M.; Kim, B.G.; Yu, M.H.; Lee, I.K. & Cho, J.Y. (2010) Identification of diabetic nephropathy-selective proteins in human plasma by multi-lectin affinity chromatography and LC-MS/MS. Proteomics. Clinical applications, Vol.4, Nos.6-7 (July 2010) ISSN 644-53

Andre, I.; Gonzalez, A.; Wang, B.; Katz, J.; Benoist, C. & Mathis, D. (1996). Checkpoints in the progression of autoimmune disease: Lessons from diabetes models. Proceedings of the National Academy of Sciences of the United States of America.; Vol. 93, (March 1996), pp. 2260–2263, ISSN 2260-3

Andre, I.; Gonzalez, A.; Wang, B.; Katz, J.; Benoist, C. & Mathis, D. (1996). Checkpoints in the progression of autoimmune disease: Lessons from diabetes models. Proceedings of the National Academy of Sciences of the United States of America.; Vol. 93, (March 1996), pp. 2260–2263, ISSN 2260-3

Barrett JC, Clayton DG, Concannon P, Akolkar B, Cooper JD, Erlich HA, Julier C, Morahan G, Nerup J, Nierras C, Plagnol V, Pociot F, Schuilenburg H, Smyth DJ, Stevens H, Todd JA, Walker NM, Rich SS; Type 1 Diabetes Genetics Consortium (2009). Genome-wide association study and meta-analysis find that over 40 loci affect risk of type 1 diabetes. Nat Genet. 2009 Jun;41(6):703-7. (Epub 2009) May 10.

Blom, L.; Nystron, L. & Dahlquist, G. (1991) The Swedish childhood diabetes study: vaccinations and infections as risk determinants for diabetes in childhood. Diabetologica, Vol.34, No.3 (March 1991) ISSN 176-81

Bougnères, P. & Valleron, A.J. (2008) Causes of early-onset type 1 diabetes: toward data-driven environmental approaches. The Journal of experimental medicine, Vol.205, No.13 (December 2008) ISSN 2953-7

Bussone, G. & Mouthon, L. (2009) Autoimmune manifestations in primary immune deficiencies. Autoimmunity reviews, Vol.8, No.4 (February 2009) ISSN 332-6

Buzzetti, R.; Di Pietro, S.; Giaccari, A.; Petrone, A.; Locatelli, M.; Suraci, C.; Capizzi, M.; Arpi, M.L.; Bazzigaluppi, E.; Dotta, F. & Bosi, E. (2007) Non Insulin Requiring Autoimmune Diabetes Study Group; High titers of auto-Abs to GAD identifies a specific phenotype of adult-onset autoimmune diabetes. Diabetes Care, Vol.30, No.4 (April 2007) ISSN 932-8

Cantor, J. & Haskins, K. (2007) Recruitment and activation of macrophages by pathogenic CD4 T cells in type 1 diabetes: evidence for involvement of CCR8 and CCL1. Journal of immunology, Vol.179, No. 9 (November 2007) ISSN 5760-7

Catherine Pihoker, Lisa K. Gilliam, Christiane S. Hampe and Åke Lernmark; Auto-Abs in Diabetes. Diabetes. 2005 Dec;54 Suppl 2:S52-61.

Cherian, M.P.; Al-Kanani, K.A.; Al Qahtani, S.S.; Yesurathinam, H.; Mathew, A.A.; Thomas, V.S.; Mathew, A.M. & Abduljabbar, M.A. (2010) The rising incidence of type 1 Diabetes mellitus and the role of Environmental Factors - three Decade experience in a Primary health care center in Saudi Arabia. Journal of pediatric endocrinology and metabolism, Vol.23, No.7 (July 2010) ISSN 685-95

Chistiakov, D.A.; Voronova, N.V. & Chistiakov, P.A. (2008) The crucial role of IL-2/IL-2RA-mediated immune regulation in the pathogenesis of type 1 diabetes, an evidence coming from genetic and animal model studies. Immunology letters, Vol.118, No.1 (June 2008) ISSN 1-5

Classen, J.B. & Classen, D.C. (1999) Association between type 1 diabetes and Hib vaccine: causal relations is likely. BMJ (Clinical research ed.), Vol.319, No.7217 (October 1999) ISSN 1133

Concannon, C.; Rich, S.S. & Nepom, G.T. (2009) Mechanisms of Disease Genetics of Type 1A Diabetes. The new england journal o f medicine, (April 2009)

Dahlquist, G.G.; Blom, L.G.; Persson, L.A.; Sandström, A.I. & Wall, S.G. (1990) Dietary factors and the risk of developing insulin dependent diabetes in childhood. BMJ (Clinical research ed.), Vol.300, No.6735 (May 1990) ISSN 1302-6

Darrasse-Jèze, G.; Deroubaix, S.; Mouquet, H.; Victora, G.D.; Eisenreich, T.; Yao, K.H.; Masilamani, R.F.; Dustin, M.L.; Rudensky, A.; Liu, K. & Nussenzweig, M.C. (2009) Feedback control of regulatory T cell homeostasis by dendritic cells in vivo. The Journal of experimental medicine, Vol.206, No.9 (August 2009) ISSN 1853-62

Darrasse-Jèze, G.; Deroubaix, S.; Mouquet, H.; Victora, G.D.; Eisenreich, T.; Yao, K.H.; Masilamani, R.F.; Dustin, M.L.; Rudensky, A.; Liu, K. & Nussenzweig, M.C. (2009) Feedback control of regulatory T cell homeostasis by dendritic cells in vivo. The Journal of experimental medicine, Vol.206, No.9 (August 2009) ISSN 1853-62

De Block, C.E.; De Leeuw, I.H. & Van Gaal, L.F. (1999) High prevalence of manifestations of gastric autoimmunity in parietal cell antibody-positive type 1 (insulin-dependent) diabetic patients. The Belgian Diabetes Registry. The Journal of clinical endocrinology and metabolism, Vol.84, No.11 (November 1999) ISSN 4062-7

Dendrou, C.A. & Wicker, L.S. (2008) The IL-2/CD25 pathway determines susceptibility to T1D in humans and NOD mice. Journal of clinical immunology, Vol.28, No.6 (November 2008) ISSN 685-96

Dendrou, C.A. & Wicker, L.S. (2008) The IL-2/CD25 pathway determines susceptibility to T1D in humans and NOD mice. Journal of clinical immunology, Vol.28, No.6 (November 2008) ISSN 685-96

DeStefano, F.; Mullooly, J.P. & Okoro, C.A. et al (2001) Childhood vaccinations, vaccination timing and risk of type 1 diabetes mellitus. Pediatrics, Vol.108, No.6 (December 2001) ISSN E112

Dorman, J.S.; Steenkiste, A.R.; Burke, J.P. & Songini, M. (2003) Type 1 diabetes and multiple sclerosis: together at last. Diabetes Care, Vol.26, No.11 (2003) ISSN 3192-3

Douroudis K, Shcherbakova A, Everaus H, Aints A.; PTPN22 gene regulates natural killer cell proliferation during *in vitro* expansion.; Tissue Antigens. 2010 May 30

Douroudis, K.; Nemvalts, V.; Rajasalu, T.; Kisand, K. & Uibo, R. (2009) The CD226 gene in susceptibility of type 1 diabetes. Tissue Antigens, Vol.74, No.5 (November 2009) ISSN 417-9

Douroudis, K.; Shcherbakova, A.; Everaus, H. & Aints, A. (2010) PTPN22 gene regulates natural killer cell proliferation during in vitro expansion. Tissue antigens, Vol.76, No.4 (May 2010) ISSN 315-8

Downes, K.; Pekalski, M.; Angus, K.L.; Hardy, M.; Nutland, S.; Smyth, D.J.; Walker, N.M.; Wallace, C. & Todd, J.A. (2010) Reduced expression of IFIH1 is protective for type 1 diabetes. Public Library of Science one, Vol.5, No.9 (September 2010) ISSN e12646

Essien, A.D. & Akpan, J.O. (2006) Diabetogenic property of charred meat on litters of pregnant albino rats. Nigerian journal of physiological sciences : official publication of the Physiological Society of Nigeria, Vol.21, No.1-2 (June 2006) ISSN 37-41

Ethan Rubinstein MD (2004) Vaccination and Autoimmune Diseases: the Argument Against. IMAJ Vol.6 (July 2004); 6:433-435

Faideau, B.; Larger, E.; Lepault, F.; Carel, J.C. & Boitard. C. (2005). Role of β-Cells in Type 1 Diabetes Pathogenesis. Diabetes, Vol. 54, No.2, (December 2005) ISSN S87-S96

Favorova, O.O.; Kulakova, O.G. & Boĭko, A.N. (2010) Multiple sclerosis as a polygenic disease: an update. Genetika, Vol.46, No.3 (March 2010) ISSN 302-13

Fernando, MM.; Stevens, CR.; Walsh, EC.; De Jager, PL.; Goyette, P.; Plenge, RM.; Vyse, TJ. & Rioux, JD. (2008). Defining the role of the MHC in autoimmunity: a review and pooled analysis. Public Library of Science genetics, Vol.4, No.4, (April 2008), ISSN e1000024

Fernando, MM.; Stevens, CR.; Walsh, EC.; De Jager, PL.; Goyette, P.; Plenge, RM.; Vyse, TJ. & Rioux, JD. (2008). Defining the role of the MHC in autoimmunity: a review and pooled analysis. Public Library of Science genetics, Vol.4, No.4, (April 2008), ISSN e1000024

Ferreira, R.C.; Pan-Hammarström, Q.; Graham, R.R.; Gateva, V.; Fontán, G.; Lee, A.T.; Ortmann, W.; Urcelay, E.; Fernández-Arquero, M.; Núñez, C.; Jorgensen, G.; Ludviksson, B.R.; Koskinen, S.; Haimila, K.; Clark, H.F.; Klareskog, L.; Gregersen, P.K.; Behrens, T.W. & Hammarström, L. (2010) Association of IFIH1 and other autoimmunity risk alleles with selective IgA deficiency. Nature genetics, Vol.42, No.9 (September 2010) ISSN 777-80

Fichna, M.; Zurawek, M.; Januszkiewicz-Lewandowska, D.; Fichna, P. & Nowak, J. (2010) PTPN22, PDCD1 and CYP27B1 polymorphisms and susceptibility to type 1 diabetes in Polish patients. International journal of immunogenetics, Vol.37, No.5 (October 2010) ISSN 367-72

Fourlanos, S.; Varney, M.D.; Tait, B.D.; Morahan, G.; Honeyman, M.C.; Colman, P.G. & Harrison, L.C. (2008) The rising incidence of type 1 Diabetes is accounted for by cases with Lower-Risk Human leukocyte Antigen genotypes. Diabetes Care, Vol.31, No.8 (August 2008) ISSN 1546-9

Giongo A, Gano KA, Crabb DB, Mukherjee N, Novelo LL, Casella G, Drew JC, Ilonen J, Knip M, Hyöty H, Veijola R, Simell T, Simell O, Neu J, Wasserfall CH, Schatz D, Atkinson MA, Triplett EW.; Toward defining the autoimmune microbiome for type 1 diabetes. ISME J. 2011 Jan;5(1):82-91. Epub 2010 Jul 8

Giongo, A.; Gano, K.A.; Crabb, D.B.; Mukherjee, N.; Novelo, L.L.; Casella, G.; Drew, J.C.; Ilonen, J.; Knip, M.; Hyöty, H.; Veijola, R.; Simell, T.; Simell, O.; Neu, J.; Wasserfall, C.H.; Schatz, D.; Atkinson, M.A. & Triplett, E.W. (2011) Toward defining the autoimmune microbiome for type 1 diabetes. The ISME journal, Vol.5, No.1 (January 2011) ISSN 82-91

Giuliani, L.; Mele, R.; Di Giovine, M.; Altieri, L.; Crinò, A.; Ravà, L. & Fierabracci. A. (2009) Detection of GAD65 autoreactive T-cells by HLA class I tetramers in type 1 diabetic patients. Journal of biomedicine & biotechnology, (2009) ISSN 576219

Green, E.A.; Eynon, E.E. & Flavell, R.A. (1998) Local expression of TNFalpha in neonatal NOD mice promotes diabetes by enhancing the presentation of islet antigens. Immunity, Vol.9, No.5 (November 1998) ISSN 733-43

Grey, S.T.; Longo, C.; Shukri, T.; Patel, V.I.; Csizmadia, E.; Daniel, S.; Arvelo, M.B.; Tchipashvili, V. & Ferran, C. (2003). Genetic engineering of a suboptimal islet graft with A20 preserves beta cell mass and function. The Journal of immunology, Vol.170, No.12 (June 2003) ISSN 6250-6

Hafler, J.P.; Maier, L.M.; Cooper, J.D.; Plagnol, V.; Hinks, A.; Simmonds, M.J.; Stevens, H.E.; Walker, N.M.; Healy, B.; Howson, J.M.; Maisuria, M.; Duley, S.; Coleman, G. & Gough, S.C. (2009) CD226 Gly307Ser association with multiple autoimmune diseases. Genes and immunity, Vol.10, No.1 (January 2009) ISSN 5-10

Hanifi-Moghaddam, P.; Schloot, N.C.; Kappler, S.; Seissler, J. & Kolb, H. (2003) An Association of Autoantibody Status and Serum Cytokine Levels in Type 1 Diabetes. Diabetes, Vol.52, No.5 (May 2003) ISSN 1137-42

Hayashi, T.; Hasegawa, K.; Morimoto, M. & Onodera, T. (2003) Effect of antibodies to intercellular adhesion molecule (ICAM)-1 and lymphocyte function-associated antigen (LFA)-1 on cytokine mRNA expression in reovirus type-2-triggered autoimmune insulitis in suckling DBA/1 mice. Journal of comparative pathology, Vol.128, No.4 (May 2003) ISSN 283-8

Hayashi, T.; Morimoto, M.; Iwata, H. & Onodera, T. (1998) Interferon-gamma plays a role in pancreatic islet-cell destruction of reovirus type 2-induced diabetes-like syndrome in DBA/1 suckling mice. International journal of experimental pathology, Vol.79, No.5 (October 1998) ISSN 313-20

Heli T.A. Siljander, Satu Simell, Anne Hekkala, Jyrki Lähde, Tuula Simell, Paula Vähäsalo, Riitta Veijola, Jorma Ilonen, Olli Simell and Mikael Knip; Predictive Characteristics of Diabetes-Associated Auto-Abs Among Children With HLA-Conferred Disease Susceptibility in the General Population; December 2009 2835-2842

Hermann, R.; Lipponen, K.; Kiviniemi, M.; Kakko, T.; Veijola, R.; Simell, O.; Knip, M. & Ilonen, J. (2006) Lymphoid tyrosine phosphatase (LYP/PTPN22) Arg620Trp variant regulates insulin autoimmunity and progression to type 1 diabetes. Diabetologia, Vol.49, No.6 (June 2006) ISSN 1198-208

Herrath, M.; Sanda, S. & Herold, K. (2007). Opinion Type 1 diabetes as a relapsing-remitting desease? Nature reviews. Immunology. Vol.7, No.12, (December 2007), ISSN 988-94

Hilger, C.; Grigioni, F.; De Beaufort, C.; Michel, G.; Freilinger, J. & Hentges, F. (2001) Differential binding of IgG and IgA antibodies to antigenic determinants of bovine ser&um albumin. Clinical and experimental immunology, Vol.123, No.3 (March 2001) ISSN 387-94

Hirasawa, K.; Jun, H.S.; Han ,H.S.; Zhang, M.L.; Hollenberg, M.D. & Yoon, J.W. (1999) Prevention of encephalomyocarditis virus-induced diabetes in mice by inhibition of the tyrosine kinase signalling pathway and subsequent suppression of nitric oxide production in macrophages. Journal of virology, Vol.73, No.10 (October 1999) ISSN 8541-8

Hodgkinson, A.D.; Millward, B.A. & Demaine, A.G. (2000). The HLA-E locus is associated with age at onset and susceptibility to type 1 diabetes mellitus. Human immunology, Vol.63, No.3 (March 2000), ISSN 290-5

Hoffmann, A. & Baltimore, D. (2006) Circuitry of nuclear factor kappaB signaling. Immunological reviews, Vol.210 (April 2006) ISSN 171-86

Hongjie Wang, Yulan Jin, M. V. Prasad Linga Reddy, Robert Podolsky, Siyang Liu, Ping Yang, Bruce Bode, John Chip Reed, R. Dennis Steed, Stephen W. Anderson, Leigh Steed, Diane Hopkins, Yihua Huang, Jin-Xiong She. Genetically Dependent ERBB3 Expression Modulates Antigen Presenting Cell Function and Type 1 Diabetes Risk PLoS One. 2010 Jul 26;5(7):e11789

Howson, J.M.; Walker, N.M.; Clayton, D. & Todd, J.A. (2009) Confirmation of HLA class II independent type 1 diabetes associations in the major histocompatibility complex including HLA-B and HLA-A. Diabetes, obesity & metabolism, Suppl 1, (February 2009) ISSN 31-45

Hunger-Battefeld, W.; Fath, K.; Mandecka, A.; Kiehntopf, M.; Kloos, C.; Müller, U.A. & Wolf, G. (2009) [Prevalence of polyglandular autoimmune syndrome in patients with diabetes mellitus type 1]. [Article in German] Medizinische Klinik, Vol.104, No.3 (March 2009) ISSN 183-91

Jiang, H.; Canfield, S.M.; Gallagher, M.P.; Jiang, H.H.; Jiang, Y.; Zheng, Z. & Chess. L. (2010). HLA-E-restricted regulatory CD8(+) T cells are involved in development and control of human autoimmune type 1 diabetes. The Journal of clinical investigation, Vol. 120, No.10 (October 2010) ISSN 3641-50

Jun, H.S. & Yoon, J.W. (2001) The role of viruses in type I diabetes: two distinct cellular and molecular pathogenic mechanisms of virus-induced diabetes in animals. Diabetologia, Vol.44, No.3 (March 2001) ISSN 271-85

Kakleas, K.; Paschali, E.; Kefalas, N.; Fotinou, A.; Kanariou, M.; Karayianni, C. & Karavanaki, K. (2009) Factors for thyroid autoimmunity in children and adolescents with type 1 diabetes mellitus. Upsala journal of medical sciences, Vol.114, No.4 (2009) ISSN 214-20

Karvonen, M.; Cepaitis, Z. & Toumilheto, J. (1999) Association between type 1 diabetes and Haemophilus influenza type B vaccination: birth cohort study. BMJ (Clinical research ed.), Vol.318, No.7192 (May 1999) ISSN 1169-72

Katona-Dureković, A. (2007) The role of virus infections in the pathogenesis of type 1 diabetes--a case report. Medicinski pregled, Vol.60, No.7-8 (July 2007) ISSN 397-400

Kawasaki, E.; Nakamura, K.; Kuriya, G.; Satoh, T.; Kuwahara, H.; Kobayashi, M.; Abiru, N.; Yamasaki, H. & Eguchi. K. (2010) Autoantibodies to insulin, insulinoma-associated antigen-2, and zinc transporter 8 improve the prediction of early insulin requirement in adult-onset autoimmune diabetes. The Journal of clinical endocrinology and metabolism, Vol. 95, No.2 (February 2010) ISSN 707-13

Kim, S.J.; Jeong, D.G.; Jeong, S.K.; Yoon, T.S. & Ryu, S.E. (2007) Crystal structure of the major diabetes autoantigen insulinoma-associated protein 2 reveals distinctive immune epitopes. Diabetes, Vol.56, No.1 (January 2007) ISSN 41-8

Kohno, T.; Kobashiri, Y.; Sugie, Y.; Takai, S.; Watabe, K.; Kaino, Y. & Kida, K. (2002) Antibodies to food antigens in Japanese patients with type 1 diabetes mellitus. Diabetes research and clinical practice, Vol.55, No.1 (January 2002) ISSN 1-9

Kordonouri, O.; Hartmann, R.; Charpentier, N.; Knip, M.; Danne, T. & Ilonen, J. (2010) Genetic risk markers related to diabetes-associated auto-Abs in young patients with type 1 diabetes in berlin, Germany. Experimental and clinical endocrinology and diabetes, Vol.116, No.4 (April 2010) ISSN 245-9

Lee, M.H.; Lee, W.H.; Todorov, I. & Liu, C.P. (2010) CD4+ CD25+ regulatory T cells prevent type 1 diabetes preceded by dendritic cell-dominant invasive insulitis by affecting chemotaxis and local invasiveness of dendritic cells. The Journal of immunology : official journal of the American Association of Immunologists, Vol.185, No.4 (August 2010) ISSN 2493-501

Lipponen, K.; Gombos, Z.; Kiviniemi, M.; Siljander, H.; Lempainen, J.; Hermann, R.; Veijola, R.; Simell, O.; Knip, M. & Ilonen, J. (2010). Effect of HLA class I and class II alleles on progression from autoantibody positivity to overt type 1 diabetes in children with risk-associated class II genotypes. Diabetes, Vol.59, No.12, (December 2010) ISSN 3253-6

Liu, Y.; Stanford, S.M.; Jog, S.P.; Fiorillo, E.; Orrú, V.; Comai, L. & Bottini, N. (2009) Regulation of lymphoid tyrosine phosphatase activity: inhibition of the catalytic domain by the proximal interdomain. Biochemistry, Vol.48, No.31 (August 2009) ISSN 7525-32

Liuwantara, D.; Elliot, M.; Smith, M.W.; Yam, A.O.; Walters, S.N.; Marino, E.; McShea, A. & Grey, S.T. (2006) Nuclear factor-kappaB regulates beta-cell death: a critical role for A20 in beta-cell protection. Diabetes, Vol. 55, No.9 (September 2006) ISSN 2491-501

Martinov L.A., Salafet O.V., Kimova M.V., O. Neuhaus., Y. Shoenfeld., M.A. Paltsev., S.V. Suchkov (2010) The demyelination phenomenon and control over its progression: basic preventive protocols of the future.; Efferent and physico-chemical medicine.; (February 2010) pp. 47-52

Mayr, A.; Schlosser, M.; Grober, N.; Kenk, H.; Ziegler, A.G.; Bonifacio, E. & Achenbach, P. (2007) GAD Autoantibody Affinity and Epitope Specificity Identify Distinct Immunization Profiles in Children at Risk for Type 1 Diabetes. Diabetes, Vol.56, No.6 (June 2007) ISSN 1527-33

Metz, T.O.; Qian, W.J.; Jacobs, J.M.; Gritsenko, M.A.; Moore, R.J.; Polpitiya, A.D.; Monroe, M.E.; Camp, D.G.; Mueller, P.W. & Smith, R.D. (2008) Application of proteomics in the discovery of candidate protein biomarkers in a diabetes autoantibody standardization program sample subset. Journal of proteome research, Vol.7, No.2 (February 2008) ISSN 698-707

Noble, J.A.; Valdes, A.M.; Varney, M.D.; Carlson, J.A.; Moonsamy, P.; Fear, A.L.; Lane, J.A.; Lavant, E.; Rappner, R.; Louey, A.; Concannon, P.; Mychaleckyj, J.C. & Erlich, H.A. (2010). HLA class I and genetic susceptibility to type 1 diabetes: results from the Type 1 Diabetes Genetics Consortium. Diabetes, Vol.59, No.11 (November 2010), ISSN 2972-9

Oresic, M.; Simell, S.; Sysi-Aho, M.; Näntö-Salonen, K.; Seppänen-Laakso, T.; Parikka, V.; Katajamaa, M.; Hekkala, A.; Mattila, I.; Keskinen, P.; Yetukuri, L.; Reinikainen, A.; Lähde, J.; Suortti, T.; Hakalax, J.; Simell, T.; Hyöty, H.; Veijola, R.; Ilonen, J.; Lahesmaa, R.; Knip, M. & Simell, O. (2008) Dysregulation of lipid and amino acid metabolism precedes islet autoimmunity in children who later progress to type 1 diabetes. The Journal of experimental medicine, Vol.205, No.13 (December 2008) ISSN 2975-84

Qu, H.Q. & Polychronakos, C. (2009). The effect of the MHC locus on autoantibodies in type 1 diabetes. Journal of medical genetics, Vol.46, No.7 (July 2009), ISSN 469-71

Rajasalu, T.; Haller, K.; Salur, L.; Kisand, K.; Tillmann, V.; Schlosser, M. & Uibo, R. (2007) Insulin VNTR I/III genotype is associated with autoantibodies against glutamic acid decarboxylase in newly diagnosed type 1 diabetes. Diabetes/metabolism research and reviews, Vol.23, No.7 (October 2007) ISSN 567-71

Riachy, R.; Vandewalle, B.; Kerr Conte, J.; Moerman, E.; Sacchetti, P.; Lukowiak, B.; Gmyr, V.; Bouckenooghe, T.; Dubois, M. & Pattou, F. (2002). 1,25-dihydroxyvitamin D3 protects RINm5F and human islet cells against cytokine-induced apoptosis: implication of the antiapoptotic protein A20. Endocrinology. Vol.143, No.12 (December 2002) ISSN 4809-19

Saukkonen, T.; Virtanen, S.M.; Karppinen, M.; Reijonen, H.; Ilonen, J.; Räsänen, L.; Akerblom, H.K. & Savilahti, E. (1998) Significance of cow's milk protein antibodies as risk factor for childhood IDDM: interactions with dietary cow's milk intake and HLA-DQB1 genotype . Childhood Diabetes in Finland Study Group. Diabetologia, Vol.41, No.1 (January 2998) ISSN 72-8

Sepiashvili R.I., Kimova M.V., Kalinina E.V., Martinov L.A., D.S. Kostyushev., Y.Shoenfeld, Suchkov S.V (2010) Antibodies in the pathogenesis of demyelinating autoimmune diseases. Allergology and Immunology.; Vol. 11 No.1 pp. 20-30

Severinski, S.; Banac, S.; Severinski, N.S.; Ahel, V. & Cvijović, K. (2009) Epidemiology and clinical characteristics of thyroid dysfunction in children and adolescents with type 1 diabetes. Collegium antropologicum, Vol.33, No.1 (March 2009) ISSN 273-9

Siljander, H.T.; Simell, S.; Hekkala, A.; Lähde, J.; Simell, T.; Vähäsalo, P.; Veijola, R.; Ilonen, J.; Simell, O. & Knip, M. (2009) Predictive characteristics of diabetes-associated autoantibodies among children with HLA-conferred disease susceptibility in the general population. Diabetes, Vol. 58, No.12 (December 2009) ISSN 2835-42

Solomon, M.; Balasa, B. & Sarvetnick, N. (2010) CCR2 and CCR5 chemokine receptors differentially influence the development of autoimmune diabetes in the NOD mouse. Autoimmunity, Vol.43, No.2 (March 2010) ISSN 156-63

Somers, E.C.; Thomas, S.L.; Smeeth, L. & Hall, A.J. (2009) Are individuals with an autoimmune disease at higher risk of a second autoimmune disorder? American journal of epidemiology, Vol.169, No.6 (March 2009) ISSN 749-55

Suchkov.; L.A. Martynov.; I.A. Vinokurov.; D.S. Kostyushev.; A.A. Andreeva.; S.I. Gadzhieva.; D.A. Gnatenko.; Y. Shoenfeld.; Y.M. Lopuhin.; A. Notkins.; M.A.

Paltsev (2010) On the prospects of preclinical diagnostics within the objectives of preventive and predictive medicine. Efferent and Physico-Chemical medicine.; (March 2010)

Svejgaard, A. (2008) The immunogenetics of multiple sclerosis. Immunogenetics, Vol.60, No.6 (June 2008) ISSN 275-86

Taniyama, M.; Maruyama, T.; Tozaki, T.; Nakano, Y. & Ban, Y. (2010) Association of PTPN22 haplotypes with type 1 diabetes in the Japanese population. Human immunology, Vol.71, No.8 (August 2010) ISSN 795-8

Tavares, R.M.; Turer, E.E.; Liu, C.L.; Advincula, R.; Scapini, P.; Rhee, L.; Barrera, J.; Lowell, C.A.; Utz, P.J.; Malynn, B.A & Ma, A. (2010) The ubiquitin modifying enzyme A20 restricts B cell survival and prevents autoimmunity. Immunity, Vol.33, No.2 (August 2010) ISSN 181-91

Thrower, B.W. (2007) Clinically isolated syndromes: predicting and delaying multiple sclerosis. Neurology, Vol.68, No.24 (June 2007) ISSN S12-5

Tsai, S.J.; Sen, U.; Zhao, L.; Greenleaf, W.B.; Dasgupta, J.; Fiorillo, E.; Orrú, V.; Bottini, N. & Chen, X.S. (2009) Crystal structure of the human lymphoid tyrosine phosphatase catalytic domain: insights into redox regulation. Biochemistry, Vol.48, No.22 (June 2009) ISSN 4838-45

Valdes, A.M. & Thomson, G. (2006). Several loci in the HLA class III region are associated with T1D risk after adjusting for DRB1-DQB1. Diabetes, obesity & metabolism, Vol.11, No.1, (February 2006) ISSN 46-52

Viken, M.K.; Blomhoff, A.; Olsson, M.; Akselsen, H.E.; Pociot, F.; Nerup, J.; Kockum, I.; Cambon-Thomsen, A.; Thorsby, E.; Undlien, D.E. & Lie, B.A. (2009) Reproducible association with type 1 diabetes in the extended class I region of the major histocompatibility complex. Genes and immunity, Vol.10, No.4 (June 2009) ISSN 323-33

Villano, M.J.; Huber, A.K.; Greenberg, D.A.; Golden, B.K.; Concepcion, E. & Tomer, Y. (2009) Autoimmune thyroiditis and diabetes: dissecting the joint genetic susceptibility in a large cohort of multiplex families. The Journal of clinical endocrinology and metabolism, Vol.94, No.4 (April 2009) ISSN 1458-66

Werner, S.L.; Barken, D. & Hoffmann, A. (2005) Stimulus specificity of gene expression programs determined by temporal control of IKK activity. Science, Vol.309, No.5742 (September 2005) ISSN 1857-61

Wertz, I.E.; O'Rourke, K.M.; Zhou, H.; Eby, M.; Aravind, L.; Seshagiri, S.; Wu, P.; Wiesmann, C.; Baker, R.; Boone, D.L.; Ma, A.; Koonin, E.V. & Dixit, V.M. (2004) De-ubiquitination and ubiquitin ligase domains of A20 downregulate NF-kappaB signaling. , Nature. Vol. 430, No.7000 (August 2004) ISSN 694-9

Williams, A.J.; Bingley, P.J.; Moore, W.P. & Gale, E.A. (2002) Islet auto-Abs, nationality and gender: a multinational screening study in first-degree relatives of patients with Type I diabetes. Diabetologia, Vol.45, No.2 (February 2002) ISSN 217-23

Witas, H.W.; Jedrychowska-Dańska, K. & Zawicki, P. (2010) Changes in frequency of IDDM-associated HLA DQB, CTLA4 and INS alleles. International journal of immunogenetics, Vol.37, No.3 (June 2010) ISSN 155-8

Yamaji, K.; Ikegami, H.; Fujisawa, T.; Noso, S.; Nojima, K.; Babaya, N.; Itoi-Babaya, M.; Kobayashi, M.; Hiromine, Y.; Makino, S. & Ogihara. T. (2006). Contribution of class III MHC to susceptibility to type 1 diabetes in the NOD mouse. Annals of the New York Academy of Sciences, (October 2006) ISSN 114-7

# 11

# Application of Novel Quantitative Proteomic Technologies to Identify New Serological Biomarkers in Autoimmune Diseases

Soyoung Lee, Satoshi Serada, Minoru Fujimoto and Tetsuji Naka
*National Institute of Biomedical Innovation, Laboratory of Immune Signal*
*Japan*

## 1. Introduction

Autoimmune diseases comprise a wide variety of systemic or organ-specific inflammatory diseases, characterized by aberrant activation of immune cells that target self tissues due to misrecognizing tissue-derived proteins as foreign antigens (Hueber and Robinson, 2006; Prince, 2005). The prevalence of autoimmune diseases is approximately 2,000 ~ 3,000 per 100,000, although the prevalence varies depending on the diseases, ethnic groups and regions (Prieto and Grau, 2010). The etiology and exact pathogenesis of autoimmune diseases remain poorly understood. However, both genetic factors and environmental triggers are profoundly involved in the pathogenesis of autoimmune diseases. Notably, clinical manifestations of autoimmune disease may be different among patients, even though they have the same diagnosis, depending on the affected organs of each patient. Therefore, careful evaluation of the clinical manifestations combined with the examination of laboratory tests is required for proper diagnosis of autoimmune diseases and subsequent monitoring of the disease activity during therapy. In addition, therapeutic choices for these diseases have been limited so far and conventional therapeutics include non-steroidal anti-inflammatory drugs (NSAID), glucocorticoids, cytotoxic drugs and disease modifying anti rheumatoid drugs (DMARDs). For these reasons, autoimmune diseases have been considered to be intractable and the goal of the treatment is to control disease activity rather than to achieve remission or cure.

Recently, however, the advent of biological agents has led to the marked improvement in the treatment of rheumatoid arthritis (RA) and other inflammatory autoimmune diseases. These agents greatly contribute to improve health-related quality or daily life of patients with autoimmune diseases (Han et al., 2007; Keystone et al., 2008; Laas et al., 2009; Strand and Singh, 2007). Nevertheless, biological agents are not effective for all patients with autoimmune diseases and current biomarkers are not helpful to select an effective biological agent for individual patients. In addition, conventional inflammatory biomarkers are often inadequate to evaluate the disease activity in patients treated with biological agents. Thus, there is a growing need for the development of new biomarkers that can predict individual treatment response before starting biological therapy and evaluate the disease activity and therapeutic efficacy during therapy. In this chapter, we first outline the clinical usage and current understanding of biological agents for the treatment with autoimmune diseases and then describe our attempt to identify new biomarkers in autoimmune diseases by taking advantage of a new proteomic approach.

## 2. Biological agents for the treatment of autoimmune diseases

### 2.1 Biological agents for autoimmune therapy in clinics

The immune response is a highly coordinated process and involves complex interactions of diverse molecules including cytokines and various cell types such as lymphocytes (Figure 1). Dysregulation in immune response such as overproduction of cytokines and aberrant activation of immune cells is implicated in autoimmune disorders. Therefore, these molecules and/or cells involved in immune response have been targeted to develop therapies in autoimmune disorders (Figure 1).

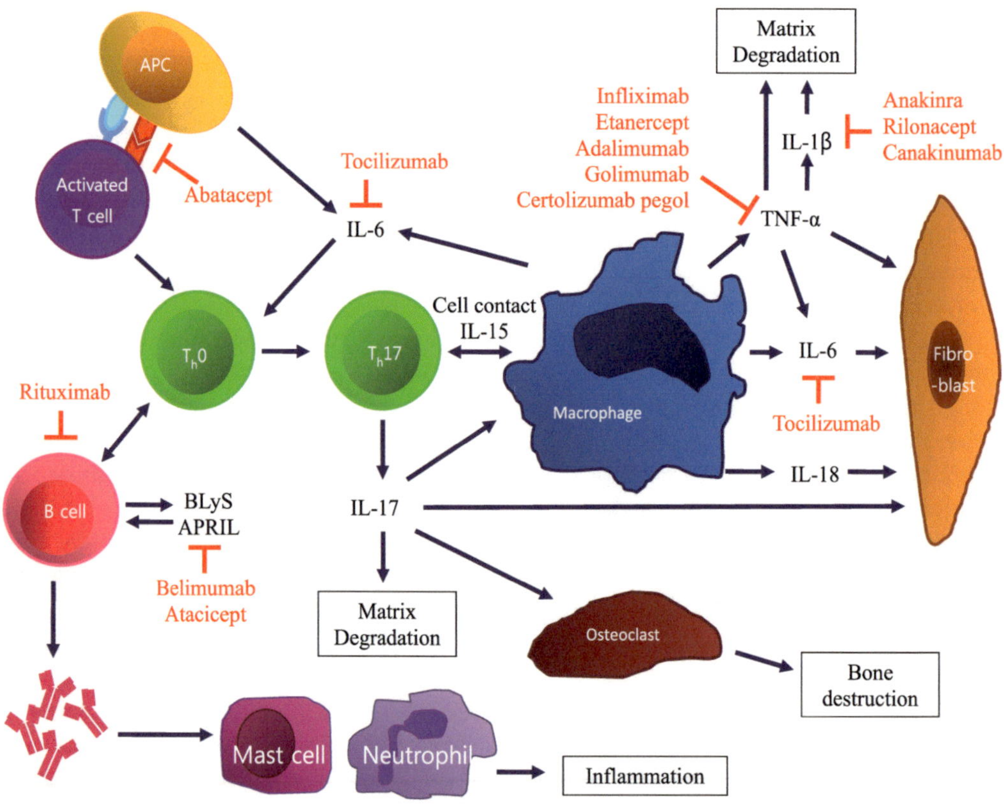


This figure summarizes the cellular interactions in the pathogenesis of RA and the interaction among antigen presenting cells (APCs), T cells, B cells, macrophages, hematopoietic cells (neutrophil, mast cell) and nonhematopoietic cells (fibroblast, connective tissue cell, and bone). These interactions are facilitated by the actions of cytokines released from the activated cells then induce the production of other pro-inflammatory and inflammatory cytokines, which contribute to the pathogenesis of RA. Also, this figure shows therapeutic biological agents proved as a RA treatment (Brennan and McInnes, 2008; McInnes and Schett, 2007).

Fig. 1. An overview of the pathogenesis of rheumatoid arthritis (RA) and the cytokine targets.

Every biological agent used in clinics today has its own specific targets and can be grouped as follows according to its aims: 1) tolerance induction, 2) inhibition of MHC, antigen, and T cell receptor interaction, 3) Inhibition of cellular function and cell-cell interaction, 4) Interference with cytokines, 5) apoptosis (Table 1). Among them, the anticytokine biological

| Strategy | Biologic Agent | Molecule | Target | Indication |
|---|---|---|---|---|
| **Tolerance induction** | Abetimus | ds-DNA | Anti-ds-DNA | SLE |
| **Inhibition of MHC, antigen, and T cell receptor interaction** | | | Under studying | |
| **Inhibition of cellular unction and cell-cell interaction** | Abatacept | CTLA4-Ig | CD80/86 | RA, JIA |
| | Rituximab | mAb to CD20 | B cells | RA, JIA |
| | Belimumab | mAb to BLyS | BLyS | SLE |
| **Interference with cytokines** | Etanercept | TNFRII/FcIgG1 | TNF-α, TNF-β | RA, PsA, Ps, AS, JIA |
| | Infliximab | mAb to TNF-α | TNF-α | RA, PsA, Ps, AS, JIA, IBD, uveitis |
| | Golimumab | mAb to TNF-α | TNF-α | RA, PsA, AS |
| | Adalimumab | mAb to TNF-α | TNF-α | RA, PsA, Ps, AS, JIA, IBD, uveitis |
| | Certolizumab pegol | Pegylated mAb to TNF-α | TNF-α | CD, RA |
| | Anakinra | IL-1 Ra | IL-1 | RA, sJIA |
| | Rilonacept | IL-1R/IL-1AcP/IgG1 | IL-1 | CAPS, sJIA |
| | Canakinumab | mAb to IL-1 | IL-1 | CAPS, sJIA |
| | Tocilizumab | mAb to IL-6R | IL-6 | JIA |
| **Apoptosis** | | mAb to Fas | Fas | |

AS: Ankylosing spondylitis, CAPS: Cryoprin-associated periodic syndrome, CD: Crohn's disease, ds-DNA: double strand-DNA, IBD: Inflammatory bowel disease, JIA: Juvenile idiopathic arthritis, mAb: Monoclonal antibody, Ps: Psoriasis, PsA: Psoriatic arthritis, RA: Rheumatoid arthritis, sJIA: Systemic-typed JIA, SLE: Systemic lupus erythematosus. (Textbook of Pediatric Rheumatology, 6th ed. 2011, Saunders)

Table 1. Summary of biological agents

agents that suppress the action of proinflammatory cytokines such as TNF, IL-1 and IL-6 are well-known and widely used in clinics. These agents were developed as therapies in RA and recommended for the treatment of patients whose disease does not respond to conventional therapies (Gomez-Reino and Carmona, 2006). RA patients treated with the anticytokine biological agents show dramatic improvement of their clinical symptoms and the levels of inflammatory biomarkers such as C-reactive protein (CRP) and erythrocyte sedimentation rate (ESR). Subsequently, these agents have been applied to the treatment of other inflammatory autoimmune diseases and have had a significant impact on patients' prognosis and survival (Andreakos et al., 2002; Efthimiou and Markenson, 2005; Maini et al., 2006; Nishimoto et al., 2009; Yokota et al., 2008).

However, it has been reported that substantial numbers of patients with autoimmune diseases still do not respond to one or more anticytokine biological agents. Among biological agents, TNF inhibitors have been extensively investigated with regard to the frequency of inadequate responders (Launois et al., 2011; Lovell et al., 2008; Maini et al., 2006; Yokota et al., 2008), because anti-TNF antibodies were the first agents approved as the therapy of RA. For example, 20~40 % of patients treated with a TNF inhibitor failed to achieve an improvement of 20 % in American College of Rheumatology criteria (Emery et al., 2008; Rubbert-Roth and Finckh, 2009). More patients lose efficacy during therapy, as shown by a report that 21 % of RA patients initially treated with etanercept no longer receive this therapy after 24 months (Feltelius et al., 2005).

Recently, patients who had an inadequate response or adverse events with one anticytokine agent are often treated with another biologic agent (Gomez-Reino and Carmona, 2006; Hyrich et al., 2007; Karlsson et al., 2008; Rubbert-Roth and Finckh, 2009). In the case of the treatment failure with the first TNF inhibitor, one survey reported that over 94 % of practicing rheumatologists in the United States of America have switched from one TNF inhibitor to another (Yazici et al., 2009). Interestingly, while some surveys reported that the efficiency of second TNF inhibitors is less than that of the first TNF inhibitor (Gomez-Reino and Carmona, 2006; Hyrich et al., 2007; Karlsson et al., 2008; Rubbert-Roth and Finckh, 2009), a large cohort study from the UK revealed that patients who switched their therapy from an initial TNF inhibitor continued to receive the second TNF inhibitor for mean length of 6 months and only 16 % of patients stopped it again due to poor response (Hyrich et al., 2007). This observation indicates that biological agents that share the common target do not always show the same effect on patients. One reason for the inefficacy of the first TNF inhibitor but not of the second one is the development of neutralizing antibody against the first agent, which may not interfere with the action of the second TNF inhibitor. Nevertheless, this observation also raises the possibility that these agents may have their own mode of action. Supporting the latter notion, there are differences in the efficacy between TNF inhibitors depending on diseases (Ackermann and Kavanaugh, 2007; Nash and Florin, 2005; Ramos-Casals et al., 2008; Sfikakis et al., 2007; Triolo et al., 2002; Veres et al., 2007). For example, while anti-TNF antibodies are effective for both RA and Crohn's disease, TNF receptor-Fc fusion protein (TNFR-Fc) is effective for RA but not for Crohn's disease.

The other treatment option after the failure with TNF inhibitors is to switch from TNF inhibitors to other biological agents with different targets. The Abatacept Trial in Treatment of Anti-TNF INadequate responders (ATTAIN) study investigated the effect of abatacept (CTLA4-Ig), an inhibitor of T cell co-stimulatory signal, on patients with active RA and an inadequate response to previous anti-TNF therapy. At 6 months, the ACR20 response rate was

50.4% in the abatacept group versus 19.5% in the placebo group and sustained improvements in ACR responses were achieved after 2 years of threatment with abatacept (Genovese et al., 2005; Rubbert-Roth and Finckh, 2009). In Randomized Evaluation of Long-Term Efficacy of Rituximab in RA (REFLEX) trial, B cell-depleting anti-CD20 antibody, rituximab, was administered to active RA patients with an inadequate response to TNF inhibitor. Among 208 patients treated with rituximab, 51 % of patients achieved an ACR20 response compared to 18 % of patients treated with placebo (Cohen et al., 2006). In addition, the patients treated with rituximab, by themselves, reported clinically meaningful and statistically improvements of pain, functional disability, and health-related quality of life (Keystone et al., 2008).
Recently, the Research on Actemra Determining efficacy after Anti-TNF failures (RADIATE) study examined the efficacy and safety of anti-IL-6 receptor (IL-6R) antibody, tocilizumab, in patients with active RA who had failed TNF inhibitor. Especially, 50.0 % of patients treated with tocilizumab at the 8 mg/kg of dose achieved ACR20 as well as rapid and sustained improvement of RA symptoms compared to 10.1 % of patients treated with placebo achieved ACR20 (Emery et al., 2008) (Figure 2). These findings are in accordance with the supposition that biological agents targeting different molecules have distinctive mechanism of action and show different effects on patients.

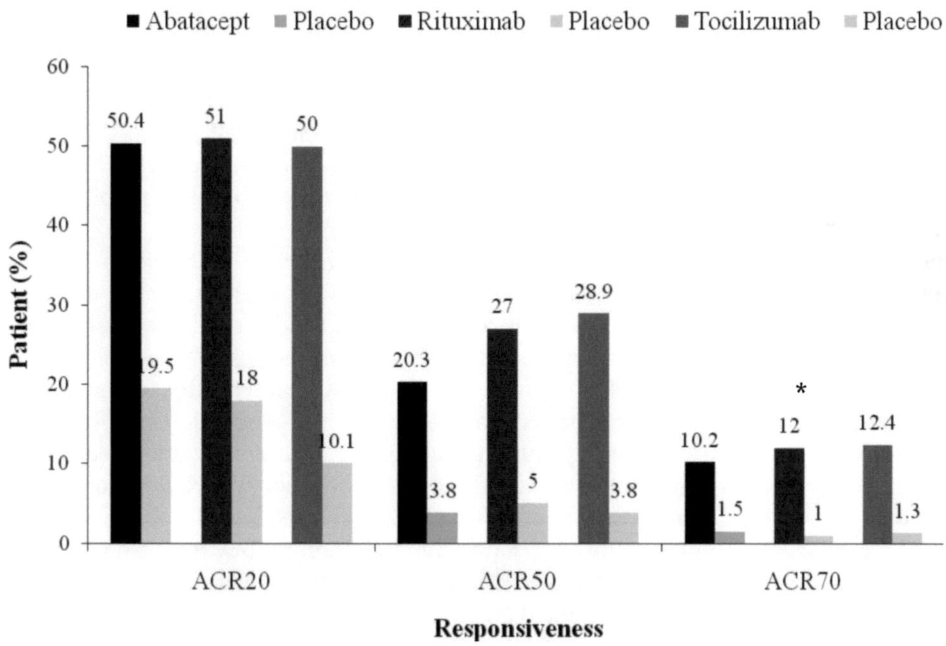


The second biological agents with other mechanisms with TNF inhibitors such as abatacept, rituximab and tocilizumab were used for patients who failed to initial TNF inhibitors. Bars show percentages of patients achieving a response according to the American College of Rheumatology 20% improvement criteria (ACR20), 50% improvement criteria (ACR50), and 70% improvement criteria (ACR70). The ACR20, ACR50, ACR70 responses in patients treated with abatacept, rituximab and tocilizumab were significantly higher than patients treated with placebo ($p<.001$, *$p=.003$).

Fig. 2. Responsiveness of treatment with the second biological agents in the patients with RA refractory to initial TNF inhibitors.

### 2.2 Biological therapeutic agents tested in animal models of autoimmune disorders

The analyses on murine disease models have contributed greatly to gain insight into pathogenesis and therapeutic strategy of autoimmune disorders. These models are also useful to clarify the detailed mechanisms of action of biological agents. We have recently investigated several disease models and reveled that anticytokine biological agents have different mechanism of action and show different effects on clinical manifestations of disease models (Fujimoto et al., 2008; Terabe et al., 2011).

We analyzed the effect of two anticytokine agents, anti-IL-6R monoclonal antibody (mAb) and TNFR-Fc, on collagen-induced arthritis (CIA), a murine model of human RA (Fujimoto et al., 2008). In accordance with the pivotal proinflammatory role of IL-6 and TNF in this arthritis model, both agents could inhibit the development of arthritis. However, while anti-IL-6R mAb potently inhibited the differentiation of Th17 cells, a highly inflammatory subset of T helper cells, TNFR-Fc exhibited no effect on Th17 cells. This observation suggests that these two agents have different action points: IL-6 blockade acts on initial phase of adoptive immune response and regulates T helper cell differentiation, whereas TNF inhibitors act much later, presumably at inflamed sites. Our study also suggests that IL-6 inhibitors may be applicable to other Th17-related autoimmune diseases. Indeed, anti-IL-6R mAb suppressed disease in a murine model of multiple sclerosis via the inhibition of Th17 cell differentiation (Serada et al., 2008). The different modes of action in anti-IL-6R mAb and TNF inhibitors may explain the difference in their efficiency in a murine model of uveoretinitis. Anti-IL-6R mAb treatment had a significant protective effect in experimental autoimmune uveoretinitis (EAU) mice, but either TNFR-Fc or anti-TNF mAb treatment did not (Hohki et al., 2010). Interestingly, in the EAU model, anti-IL-6R mAb not only suppressed Th17 cell differentiation but also suppressed autoantigen-specific Th1 cells via the generation of induced regulatory T cells, supporting the notion that IL-6 inhibitors act on initial phase of adoptive immune response (Haruta et al., 2011).

Confusingly, biological agents may act differently on different autoimmune diseases. Indeed, anti-IL-6R mAb and anti-TNF mAb, but not TNFR-Fc exerted similar effect on a murine inflammatory bowel disease (IBD) model (Terabe et al., 2011). This model is a T cell dependent colitis and is induced by the transfer of purified naïve CD4 T cells into lymphopenic mice. Both anti-IL-6R mAb and anti-TNF mAb successfully inhibited colitis, whereas TNFR-Fc did not show any protective effect on colitis. In addition, anti-IL-6R mAb and anti-TNF mAb could comparably inhibit the expansion of colitogenic T cells in this model, although like in other models, anti-IL-6R mAb additionally could modulate the profile of T helper cell differentiation (Terabe et al., 2011). Thus, anti-IL-6R mAb and anti-TNF mAb may share a similar mode of action in the inhibition of IBD. It is also notable that TNFR-Fc failed to inhibit inflammation in this colitis model (Terabe et al., 2011). Similar discrepancy in the effect of anti-TNF mAb and TNFR-Fc has been observed in human IBD. Many mechanisms have been proposed so far to explain the difference of action between these two agents. For example, anti-TNF mAb binds not only to soluble TNF-α, but also to membrane-bound TNF-α, leading to the induction of antibody-dependent and complement dependent cytotoxicity (Maini, 2004). The anti-TNF mAb may also have more capacity than TNFR-Fc to induce apoptosis via reverse signaling with cross-linking by binding firmly to transmembrane TNF(Terabe et al., 2011). Nevertheless, these hypotheses are still controversial and it remains to be explained why anti-TNF mAb and TNFR-Fc have differential effectiveness in some autoimmune diseases such as Crohn's disease. We believe that further study on this murine IBD model is useful for elucidation of this issue.

## 3. Biomarkers

### 3.1 A need for new biomarkers in the era of biological agents

Given the difference in mechanism and therapeutic effect of each biologic agent, it is desirable to select an effective biological agent on each patient before initiating therapy or after failure of the initial therapy. However, no reliable guidance is available at present for the selection of biological therapies. There is a growing need for the development of biomarkers that predict individual treatment response before therapy.

In addition, in patients treated with biological agents in whom immune response is substantially suppressed, conventional laboratory biomarkers such as CRP and ESR do not always reflect disease activity. In particular, since serum CRP is primarily dependent on liver by circulating IL-6, CRP is unable to reflect disease activity in patients treated with IL-6 inhibitors. Moreover, conventional markers may also be inadequate for the detection of inflammation unrelated to original diseases. In RA patients after joint surgery, anti-IL-6R mAb tocilizumab completely suppressed the increase in CRP and partially suppressed the rise in body temperature (Hirao et al., 2009). More importantly, biological agents may mask typical symptoms of bacterial infection and inhibit the elevation of serum biomarkers. Indeed, RA patients treated with tocilizumab did not present characteristic clinical symptoms and typical elevation of serum CRP after bacterial pneumonia and septic shock (Fujiwara et al., 2009). Even without biologic treatment, current inflammatory biomarkers are not useful to distinguish infection from flares of autoimmune diseases. This is an important issue in clinical settings, because therapeutic strategies for infection and disease flares are completely opposite. Infection must be treated primarily with antibiotics and discontinuation of biological agents should be considered. In contrast, disease flares should be treated intensively with the same or alternative biological agents. Thus, new biomarkers are needed for the detection and discrimination of inflammation by either infection or disease flares.

Even after the successful repression of disease with biologic therapies, it remains unknown yet whether biological agents can be terminated safely without disease recurrence. Therefore, a biomarker that indicates clinical remission or cure of autoimmune diseases is helpful to determine the timing to stop biological agents.

Collectively, the development of a number of novel biomarkers, such as those that can help to select biological agents before therapy, can precisely evaluate disease activity and therapeutic effect during the therapy or can instruct the timing of therapy completion after achievement of remission, are warranted for the appropriate clinical management of patients receiving biological therapies.

### 3.2 Serum proteome analysis using the new technology iTRAQ

The pathogenesis of autoimmune diseases involves alterations in the expression of genes that control pathways regulating self tolerance. However, gene transcripts may not faithfully reflect their protein levels. In addition, post-translational modifications are not amenable to the study of transcriptional profiling (Hueber and Robinson, 2006). Recently, there has been the remarkable improvement of the proteomic approaches as represented by the development of sophisticated methods of protein sample preparation and the improvement of the sensitivity, accuracy and resolution in mass spectrometer. Therefore, direct proteomic measurement may provide greater utility for the discovery of new biomarkers monitoring autoimmune diseases in the post genomic era. Current efforts to identify autoimmune disease biomarkers have focused on three groups of proteins reflective of the autoimmune disease process. These groups include 1) degradation products arising from destruction of the affected tissues, 2) enzymes that play a role in tissue degradation, and 3) cytokines and other proteins associated with immune system activation and the inflammatory response (Prince, 2005). Recent proteomics technologies have enabled us to screen these markers from proteins extracted from tissues and sera from patients (Hueber and Robinson, 2006). Accordingly, there are many proteomic studies that analyzed protein profiles and searched new biomarkers in autoimmune diseases (Dwivedi et al., 2009; Ferraccioli et al., 2010; Ling et al., 2010; Serada et al., 2010; Takeuchi et al., 2007).

The quantitative proteome analysis by mass spectrometry (MS) usually involves differential isotope labeling of proteins and peptides metabolically, enzymatically or chemically using

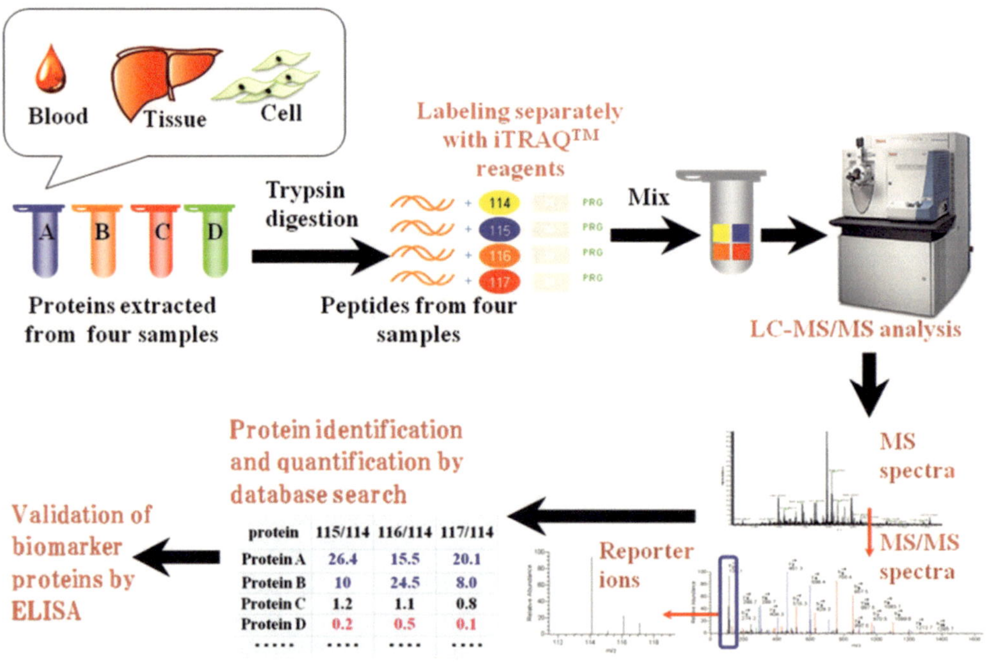


In a single experiment of iTRAQ analysis, 4 to 8 samples differentially labeled with iTRAQ reagents can be quantitatively analyzed by mass spectrometry (this figure shows a four-plex reagent experiment). First, proteins extracted from cells, tissue and/or body fluid such as blood are reduced, alkylated and digested with trypsin. Second, obtained peptides in each sample are labeled with each iTRAQTM reagent at N-terminal amino group or epsilon amino group from lysine. The iTRAQ tags are isobaric and the labeling with iTRAQ reagents results in the uniform increase in molecular weight of peptides in every sample. After labeling, samples are mixed into one tube and analyzed by liquid chromatography-tandem mass spectrometry (LC-MS/MS). Mass spectrometry is performed by full scan MS, followed by MS/MS spectra of peptides. In MS/MS spectra, iTRAQ tag-specific reporter ions (114.1, 115.1, 116.1, 117.1 in the figure) are detected in low m/z region, and these reporter ion intensities represent the abundance of the peptide from each sample. Peptide sequence information is obtained from high m/z region of MS/MS spectra and the protein is identified by database search after comparing obtained MS/MS spectra with theoretical MS/MS spectra in the database. Usually, candidate biomarker proteins obtained by iTRAQ analysis are further verified by other methods such as ELISA analysis.

Fig. 3. Flowchart of iTRAQ analysis

external reagent tags. These methods address some of the limitations faced in traditional gel-based proteomic approaches. However, these approaches still suffer from some limitations such as inability to multiplex and to quantify zero protein expression level. In contrast, a novel quantitative proteomic technology, isobaric tagging of peptides enable simultaneous identification and quantification of peptides by tandem MS and permit parallel proteome analysis of more than two samples (Aggarwal et al., 2006).

The isobaric tags for relative and absolute quantitation (iTRAQ), which is one such method commercialized, uses four amine specific isobaric reagents to label the primary amines of peptides from four to eight different biological samples. The labeled peptides from each sample are mixed, separated using two-dimensional liquid chromatography and analyzed using MS and tandem mass spectrometry (Figure 3). The isobaric tagging strategy provides multiple independent measures of the relative abundance of a protein. The capability of iTRAQ for protein quantitation has been verified by analyzing standard mixtures of proteins of known proportions (Aggarwal et al., 2006). The iTRAQ approach has now been successfully used to identify and quantify the proteins in variety of prokaryotic and eukaryotic samples (Aggarwal et al., 2006; Cong et al., 2006; DeSouza et al., 2005; Dwivedi et al., 2009; Hardt et al., 2005; Zhang et al., 2005).

### 3.3 Leucin-rich-α-2 glycoprotein as a novel biomarker

We reported for the first time that the iTRAQ technology is applicable to identify novel biomarkers in sera from patients with autoimmune diseases (Serada et al., 2010). Before we publish our results, a study was published and reported the serum proteome of RA patients treated with anti-TNF mAb therapy. They provided evidence that iTRAQ strategy can be used to obtain quantitative data that reflect changes in the serum proteome after targeted therapeutic interventions (Dwivedi et al., 2009).

We used iTRAQ technology to obtain profiles of serum proteome in RA patients before and after TNF inhibitor treatment. We then listed serum proteins that declined remarkably after treatment. Our strategy was verified by the detection of familiar biomarkers including CRP and serum amyloid A (SAA) as reduced serum proteins after treatment. Among the candidate proteins that declined after therapy, we focused on an uncharacterized protein called leucine-rich-α-2 glycoprotein (LRG) and examined further on this protein using other methods such as Western blot and ELISA. Indeed, taking advantage of ELISA analysis of many serum samples from RA patients, we found that serum levels of LRG significantly declined after therapy with TNF inhibitors and correlate well with disease activity of RA patients. In addition, LRG levels were significantly high in patients with other autoimmune diseases such as Crohn's disease and Behcet disease. As expected, the LRG correlated well with a conventional biomarker CRP in patients with these autoimmune inflammatory diseases. Interestingly, however, while CRP correlated with serum IL-6 levels, LRG did not. In accordance with this, in some Crohn's disease patients with active disease, CRP levels remained low but serum LRG concentrations were significantly elevated. Thus, LRG exhibits similarity with CRP but also has a unique property. Moreover, because serum LRG concentrations of Crohn's disease patients before starting therapy were higher in the non-responders to anti-TNF therapy than in the responders, LRG may predict therapeutic responses to TNF inhibitors in Crohn's disease patients (Serada et al., 2010).

Until now, LRG has been reported to be expressed by liver cells and neutrophils, and regulated by multiple factors and produced at local inflammatory sites. According to the previous reports, it seems that LRG is not a unique biomarker in autoimmune disease but rather is a generalized inflammatory biomarker, because serum LRG levels are reported to be increased in patients with bacterial infection and several types of cancers. Nevertheless, serum LRG satisfies the condition of an inflammatory biomarker in the point that its concentration is high at diagnosis, correlated well with disease activity and is a possible predictor of the responsiveness to biological agents. For these reasons, serum LRG is a novel inflammatory biomarker potentially surrogate for CRP. Further studies are in progress in our laboratory to determine the pathophysiological function of LRG and the clinical benefit of LRG measurement.

## 4. Conclusion

Autoimmune diseases including RA are not only rare but also difficult to treat. In the clinical field, biological agents have emerged as attractive therapeutic options for these diseases, because of their rapid and/or dramatic effectiveness to intractable diseases. However, biological agents are expensive and their usage is occasionally accompanied with severe adverse effects such as immunosuppression and fatal infection. To maximize the therapeutic potential and to minimize the adverse effects of biological agents, novel biomarkers are required for the selection of agents, monitoring of the disease activity and therapeutic efficacy or differential diagnosis of infection. In this respect, LRG we identified from iTRAQ analysis is a candidate of novel biomarkers useful for clinical practice of biological agents since it correlates with disease activity and therapeutic effectiveness of biological agents. In addition, the application of iTRAQ analysis, the novel quantitative proteomic approach, is useful for the identification of new serological biomarkers in patients with autoimmune diseases. Further studies using this approach may lead to the development of additional new biomarkers and may help to clarify the pathogenesis and identify therapeutic targets in autoimmune diseases.

## 5. References

Ackermann, C., and Kavanaugh, A. (2007). Tumor necrosis factor as a therapeutic target of rheumatologic disease. Expert Opin Ther Targets *11*, 1369-1384.

Aggarwal, K., Choe, L.H., and Lee, K.H. (2006). Shotgun proteomics using the iTRAQ isobaric tags. Brief Funct Genomic Proteomic *5*, 112-120.

Andreakos, E.T., Foxwell, B.M., Brennan, F.M., Maini, R.N., and Feldmann, M. (2002). Cytokines and anti-cytokine biologicals in autoimmunity: present and future. Cytokine Growth Factor Rev *13*, 299-313.

Brennan, F.M., and McInnes, I.B. (2008). Evidence that cytokines play a role in rheumatoid arthritis. J Clin Invest *118*, 3537-3545.

Cohen, S.B., Emery, P., Greenwald, M.W., Dougados, M., Furie, R.A., Genovese, M.C., Keystone, E.C., Loveless, J.E., Burmester, G.R., Cravets, M.W., *et al.* (2006). Rituximab for rheumatoid arthritis refractory to anti-tumor necrosis factor therapy: Results of a multicenter, randomized, double-blind, placebo-controlled, phase III trial evaluating primary efficacy and safety at twenty-four weeks. Arthritis Rheum *54*, 2793-2806.

Cong, Y.S., Fan, E., and Wang, E. (2006). Simultaneous proteomic profiling of four different growth states of human fibroblasts, using amine-reactive isobaric tagging reagents and tandem mass spectrometry. Mech Ageing Dev *127*, 332-343.

DeSouza, L., Diehl, G., Rodrigues, M.J., Guo, J., Romaschin, A.D., Colgan, T.J., and Siu, K.W. (2005). Search for cancer markers from endometrial tissues using differentially labeled tags iTRAQ and cICAT with multidimensional liquid chromatography and tandem mass spectrometry. J Proteome Res *4*, 377-386.

Dwivedi, R.C., Dhindsa, N., Krokhin, O.V., Cortens, J., Wilkins, J.A., and El-Gabalawy, H.S. (2009). The effects of infliximab therapy on the serum proteome of rheumatoid arthritis patients. Arthritis Res Ther *11*, R32.

Efthimiou, P., and Markenson, J.A. (2005). Role of biological agents in immune-mediated inflammatory diseases. South Med J *98*, 192-204.

Emery, P., Keystone, E., Tony, H.P., Cantagrel, A., van Vollenhoven, R., Sanchez, A., Alecock, E., Lee, J., and Kremer, J. (2008). IL-6 receptor inhibition with tocilizumab improves treatment outcomes in patients with rheumatoid arthritis refractory to anti-tumour necrosis factor biologicals: results from a 24-week multicentre randomised placebo-controlled trial. Ann Rheum Dis *67*, 1516-1523.

Feltelius, N., Fored, C.M., Blomqvist, P., Bertilsson, L., Geborek, P., Jacobsson, L.T., Lindblad, S., Lysholm, J., Rantapaa-Dahlqvist, S., Saxne, T., and Klareskog, L. (2005). Results from a nationwide postmarketing cohort study of patients in Sweden treated with etanercept. Ann Rheum Dis *64*, 246-252.

Ferraccioli, G., De Santis, M., Peluso, G., Inzitari, R., Fanali, C., Bosello, S.L., Iavarone, F., and Castagnola, M. (2010). Proteomic approaches to Sjogren's syndrome: a clue to interpret the pathophysiology and organ involvement of the disease. Autoimmun Rev *9*, 622-626.

Fujimoto, M., Serada, S., Mihara, M., Uchiyama, Y., Yoshida, H., Koike, N., Ohsugi, Y., Nishikawa, T., Ripley, B., Kimura, A., *et al.* (2008). Interleukin-6 blockade suppresses autoimmune arthritis in mice by the inhibition of inflammatory Th17 responses. Arthritis Rheum *58*, 3710-3719.

Fujiwara, H., Nishimoto, N., Hamano, Y., Asanuma, N., Miki, S., Kasayama, S., and Suemura, M. (2009). Masked early symptoms of pneumonia in patients with rheumatoid arthritis during tocilizumab treatment: a report of two cases. Mod Rheumatol *19*, 64-68.

Genovese, M.C., Becker, J.C., Schiff, M., Luggen, M., Sherrer, Y., Kremer, J., Birbara, C., Box, J., Natarajan, K., Nuamah, I., *et al.* (2005). Abatacept for rheumatoid arthritis refractory to tumor necrosis factor alpha inhibition. N Engl J Med *353*, 1114-1123.

Gomez-Reino, J.J., and Carmona, L. (2006). Switching TNF antagonists in patients with chronic arthritis: an observational study of 488 patients over a four-year period. Arthritis Res Ther *8*, R29.

Han, C., Smolen, J.S., Kavanaugh, A., van der Heijde, D., Braun, J., Westhovens, R., Zhao, N., Rahman, M.U., Baker, D., and Bala, M. (2007). The impact of infliximab treatment on quality of life in patients with inflammatory rheumatic diseases. Arthritis Res Ther *9*, R103.

Hardt, M., Witkowska, H.E., Webb, S., Thomas, L.R., Dixon, S.E., Hall, S.C., and Fisher, S.J. (2005). Assessing the effects of diurnal variation on the composition of human parotid saliva: quantitative analysis of native peptides using iTRAQ reagents. Anal Chem *77*, 4947-4954.

Haruta, H., Ohguro, N., Fujimoto, M., Hohki, S., Terabe, F., Serada, S., Nomura, S., Nishida, K., Kishimoto, T., and Naka, T. (2011). Blockade of interleukin-6 signaling suppresses not only th17 but also interphotoreceptor retinoid binding protein-specific Th1 by promoting regulatory T cells in experimental autoimmune uveoretinitis. Invest Ophthalmol Vis Sci 52, 3264-3271.

Hirao, M., Hashimoto, J., Tsuboi, H., Nampei, A., Nakahara, H., Yoshio, N., Mima, T., Yoshikawa, H., and Nishimoto, N. (2009). Laboratory and febrile features after joint surgery in patients with rheumatoid arthritis treated with tocilizumab. Ann Rheum Dis *68*, 654-657.

Hohki, S., Ohguro, N., Haruta, H., Nakai, K., Terabe, F., Serada, S., Fujimoto, M., Nomura, S., Kawahata, H., Kishimoto, T., and Naka, T. (2010). Blockade of interleukin-6 signaling suppresses experimental autoimmune uveoretinitis by the inhibition of inflammatory Th17 responses. Exp Eye Res *91*, 162-170.

Hueber, W., and Robinson, W.H. (2006). Proteomic biomarkers for autoimmune disease. Proteomics *6*, 4100-4105.

Hyrich, K.L., Lunt, M., Watson, K.D., Symmons, D.P., and Silman, A.J. (2007). Outcomes after switching from one anti-tumor necrosis factor alpha agent to a second anti-tumor necrosis factor alpha agent in patients with rheumatoid arthritis: results from a large UK national cohort study. Arthritis Rheum *56*, 13-20.

Karlsson, J.A., Kristensen, L.E., Kapetanovic, M.C., Gulfe, A., Saxne, T., and Geborek, P. (2008). Treatment response to a second or third TNF-inhibitor in RA: results from the South Swedish Arthritis Treatment Group Register. Rheumatology (Oxford) *47*, 507-513.

Keystone, E., Burmester, G.R., Furie, R., Loveless, J.E., Emery, P., Kremer, J., Tak, P.P., Broder, M.S., Yu, E., Cravets, M., *et al.* (2008). Improvement in patient-reported outcomes in a rituximab trial in patients with severe rheumatoid arthritis refractory to anti-tumor necrosis factor therapy. Arthritis Rheum *59*, 785-793.

Laas, K., Peltomaa, R., Puolakka, K., Kautiainen, H., and Leirisalo-Repo, M. (2009). Early improvement of health-related quality of life during treatment with etanercept and adalimumab in patients with rheumatoid arthritis in routine practice. Clin Exp Rheumatol *27*, 315-320.

Launois, R., Avouac, B., Berenbaum, F., Blin, O., Bru, I., Fautrel, B., Joubert, J.M., Sibilia, J., and Combe, B. (2011). Comparison of Certolizumab Pegol with Other Anticytokine Agents for Treatment of Rheumatoid Arthritis: A Multiple-treatment Bayesian Metaanalysis. J Rheumatol.

Ling, X.B., Park, J.L., Carroll, T., Nguyen, K.D., Lau, K., Macaubas, C., Chen, E., Lee, T., Sandborg, C., Milojevic, D., *et al.* (2010). Plasma profiles in active systemic juvenile idiopathic arthritis: Biomarkers and biological implications. Proteomics *10*, 4415-4430.

Lovell, D.J., Reiff, A., Ilowite, N.T., Wallace, C.A., Chon, Y., Lin, S.L., Baumgartner, S.W., Giannini, E.H., and Pediatric Rheumatology, C. (2008). Safety and efficacy of up to eight years of continuous etanercept therapy in patients with juvenile rheumatoid arthritis. Arthritis and Rheumatism *58*, 1496-1504.

Maini, R.N., Taylor, P.C., Szechinski, J., Pavelka, K., Broll, J., Balint, G., Emery, P., Raemen, F., Petersen, J., Smolen, J., *et al.* (2006). Double-blind randomized controlled clinical trial of the interleukin-6 receptor antagonist, tocilizumab, in European patients with rheumatoid arthritis who had an incomplete response to methotrexate. Arthritis Rheum *54*, 2817-2829.

Maini, S.R. (2004). Infliximab treatment of rheumatoid arthritis. Rheum Dis Clin North Am *30*, 329-347, vii.

McInnes, I.B., and Schett, G. (2007). Cytokines in the pathogenesis of rheumatoid arthritis. Nat Rev Immunol *7*, 429-442.

Nash, P.T., and Florin, T.H. (2005). Tumour necrosis factor inhibitors. Med J Aust *183*, 205-208.

Nishimoto, N., Miyasaka, N., Yamamoto, K., Kawai, S., Takeuchi, T., and Azuma, J. (2009). Long-term safety and efficacy of tocilizumab, an anti-IL-6 receptor monoclonal antibody, in monotherapy, in patients with rheumatoid arthritis (the STREAM study): evidence of safety and efficacy in a 5-year extension study. Ann Rheum Dis *68*, 1580-1584.

Prieto, S., and Grau, J.M. (2010). The geoepidemiology of autoimmune muscle disease. Autoimmun Rev *9*, A330-334.

Prince, H.E. (2005). Biomarkers for diagnosing and monitoring autoimmune diseases. Biomarkers *10 Suppl 1*, S44-49.

Ramos-Casals, M., Brito-Zeron, P., Soto, M.J., Cuadrado, M.J., and Khamashta, M.A. (2008). Autoimmune diseases induced by TNF-targeted therapies. Best Pract Res Clin Rheumatol *22*, 847-861.

Rubbert-Roth, A., and Finckh, A. (2009). Treatment options in patients with rheumatoid arthritis failing initial TNF inhibitor therapy: a critical review. Arthritis Res Ther *11 Suppl 1*, S1.

Serada, S., Fujimoto, M., Ogata, A., Terabe, F., Hirano, T., Iijima, H., Shinzaki, S., Nishikawa, T., Ohkawara, T., Iwahori, K., *et al.* (2010). iTRAQ-based proteomic identification of leucine-rich alpha-2 glycoprotein as a novel inflammatory biomarker in autoimmune diseases. Ann Rheum Dis *69*, 770-774.

Sfikakis, P.P., Markomichelakis, N., Alpsoy, E., Assaad-Khalil, S., Bodaghi, B., Gul, A., Ohno, S., Pipitone, N., Schirmer, M., Stanford, M., *et al.* (2007). Anti-TNF therapy in the management of Behcet's disease--review and basis for recommendations. Rheumatology (Oxford) *46*, 736-741.

Strand, V., and Singh, J.A. (2007). Improved health-related quality of life with effective disease-modifying antirheumatic drugs: evidence from randomized controlled trials. Am J Manag Care *13 Suppl 9*, S237-251.

Takeuchi, T., Nakanishi, T., Tabushi, Y., Hata, A., Shoda, T., Kotani, T., Shimizu, A., Takubo, T., Makino, S., and Hanafusa, T. (2007). Serum protein profile of rheumatoid arthritis treated with anti-TNF therapy (infliximab). J Chromatogr B Analyt Technol Biomed Life Sci *855*, 66-70.

Terabe, F., Fujimoto, M., Serada, S., Shinzaki, S., Iijima, H., Tsujii, M., Hayashi, N., Nomura, S., Kawahata, H., Jang, M.H., *et al.* (2011). Comparative analysis of the effects of anti-IL-6 receptor mAb and anti-TNF mAb treatment on CD4+ T-cell responses in murine colitis. Inflamm Bowel Dis *17*, 491-502.

Triolo, G., Vadala, M., Accardo-Palumbo, A., Ferrante, A., Ciccia, F., Giardina, E., Citarrella, P., Lodato, G., and Licata, G. (2002). Anti-tumour necrosis factor monoclonal antibody treatment for ocular Behcet's disease. Ann Rheum Dis *61*, 560-561.

Veres, G., Baldassano, R.N., and Mamula, P. (2007). Infliximab therapy for pediatric Crohn's disease. Expert Opin Biol Ther *7*, 1869-1880.

Yazici, Y., Krasnokutsky, S., Barnes, J.P., Hines, P.L., Wang, J., and Rosenblatt, L. (2009). Changing patterns of tumor necrosis factor inhibitor use in 9074 patients with rheumatoid arthritis. J Rheumatol *36*, 907-913.

Yokota, S., Imagawa, T., Mori, M., Miyamae, T., Aihara, Y., Takei, S., Iwata, N., Umebayashi, H., Murata, T., Miyoshi, M., *et al.* (2008). Efficacy and safety of tocilizumab in patients with systemic-onset juvenile idiopathic arthritis: a randomised, double-blind, placebo-controlled, withdrawal phase III trial. Lancet *371*, 998-1006.

Zhang, Y., Wolf-Yadlin, A., Ross, P.L., Pappin, D.J., Rush, J., Lauffenburger, D.A., and White, F.M. (2005). Time-resolved mass spectrometry of tyrosine phosphorylation sites in the epidermal growth factor receptor signaling network reveals dynamic modules. Mol Cell Proteomics *4*, 1240-1250.

# Part 3

## Therapeutic Interventions

# 12

# Application of Monoclonal Antibody Therapies in Autoimmune Diseases

Adrienn Angyal[1], Jozsef Prechl[2], Gyorgy Nagy[3] and Gabriella Sarmay[1]
[1]*Dept. of Immunology, Eotvos Lorand University, Budapest,*
[2]*Immunology Research Group of the Hungarian Academy of Sciences, at Eotvos Lorand University, Budapest,*
[3]*Buda Hospital of Hospitaller Brothers of St. John, Budapest*
*Hungary*

## 1. Introduction

A better understanding of the pathogenesis of autoimmunity makes it possible to select more specific therapeutic targets and design biological agents that can replace or enhance the effect of immunosuppressive drugs; these include monoclonal antibodies, soluble receptors and molecular mimetics. This chapter aims to give a brief summary on different protein-based medications: first on the biologicals targeting cytokines that induce inflammatory responses, then on drugs depleting B cells via CD20 and CD22 and finally, on agents that inhibit cell-cell contacts and block cell survival factors. Immunogenicity of these protein preparations causes a significant problem therefore the last section gives an overview of biotechnological approaches aiming to reduce this effect.

## 2. The blockade of cytokines inducing inflammatory responses

*TNFα-blocking agents (Etanercept, Adalimumab, Infliximab)*

Currently, there are 3 major TNFα-blockers available for patients who do not react well to standard therapies like methotrexate or other disease modifying anti-rheumatic drugs (DMARDs), these are: etanercept, infliximab and adalimumab. Most common side effects of anti-TNFα therapy are a higher susceptibility for infections and possible flares of TB.

Etanercept, a fusion protein consisting of two extracellular binding domains of the TNF ⟨ receptor 2 and the Fc-part of a human IgG1 molecule is acting like a soluble decoy receptor by inhibiting ligand-binding to TNF-receptors, only with an extended in vivo half-life due to the presence of the Fc-part. It is licensed by the FDA for the treatment of RA, polyarticular juvenile idiopathic arthritis (JIA), psoritic arthritis, ankylosing spondylitis and plaque psoriasis (1).

Infliximab (Remicade) is a chimeric monoclonal antibody specific for TNFα that was approved by the FDA in 1998 for the treatment of Crohn's disease (2). Its use has been extended since then to the treatment of psoriasis, ankylosing spondylitis, psoriatic arthritis, rheumatoid arthritis and ulcerative colitis.

Adalimumab (Humira), another monoclonal antibody of fully human origin was derived by a phage display library and used to treat RA patients first. Since then, clinical trials proved its effectiveness in psoriatic arthritis, ankylosing spondylitis, Crohn's disease, psoriasis and juvenile idiopathic arthritis (3).

Infliximab and adalimumab were shown to neutralize biological activity of TNFα by binding to its soluble, membrane- or receptor-bound forms, while etanercept is unable to neutralize the receptor-bound form of TNFα due to its structural features. Additionally, the anti-TNF monoclonal antibodies can induce Fc-receptor-mediated cell lysis and infliximab has been also shown to induce apoptosis of lamina propria T cells in Crohn's patients in a TNFα-dependent manner.

In a follow-up comparative study Bacquet-Deschryver et al. evaluated the effects of the 3 different anti-TNFα biologics on the re-emerginig of anti-nuclear antibodies (ANA), anti-dsDNA antibodies, RF and anti-CCP in rheumatoid arthritis and spondyloarthropathy patients (3). They found that the response to treatment is independent of the induction of ANA production and anti-dsDNA autoantibody variations regardless of the rheumatism and the anti-TNFα treatment prescribed.

Another study conducted in human TNFα transgenic mice showed that in a strictly TNFα-driven model of RA the number of $CD3^{+}CD25^{+}FoxP3^{+}$ Treg cells is initially lower than in wild-type counterparts, but gets elevated during the course of the disease. This population of regulatory T cells is attenuated in its suppressor activity, which can be restored with either passive (infliximab treatment) or active (TNF-K immunization) TNFα-blocking approaches. Moreover, the differentiation of a $CD62L^{-}$ regulatory T cell population is induced (4).

*Blockade of IL-6 (tocilizumab)*

IL-6 is a widely expressed pleiotropic cytokine, best known as main mediator of fever and acute phase reactions alongside IL-1 and TNFα. In hepatocytes it strongly induces production of acute phase proteins e.g. C-reactive protein, mannan-binding lectin, or serum amyloid protein A, and it also causes immobilization of neutrophil granulocytes from the bone marrow. Besides supporting B cell differentiation into antibody plasma cells, it has been shown to be essential in Th17 cell differentiation as well. The IL-6R consists of two chains, the 80-kDa IL-6-binding subunit and the 130-kDa membrane glycoprotein gp130 that is responsible for signal transduction (5). The expression of membrane bound IL6R is restricted to only few cell types including macrophages, neutrophils, some T-cell subpopulations and hepatocytes. On the other hand, gp130 is ubiquitously expressed. IL-6R is either shed from the cell surface by matrix metalloproteases or in human, expressed as a result of alternative splicing. Association of the IL-6/sIL-6R complex to gp130 mediates agonistic signaling events (trans-signaling) (6).

Excessive levels of the IL-6/IL-6R complex can be detected in the synovial fluid of many RA patients, which could highly contribute to osteoclast-like cell formation and therefore, joint destruction (7). Also, IL-6 production of synovial fibroblasts induces excess production of vascular endothelial growth factor (VEGF) resulting in enhanced angiogenesis and increased vascular permeability of synovial tissue. Serum IL-6 levels were found elevated in other autoimmune conditions e.g. in SLE as well (8).

Tocilizumab is a humanized IL6R-specific monoclonal antibody that blocks IL-6 mediated signal transduction via the inhibition of ligand-binding to the IL-6Rs. Phase III clinical studies showed a remarkable inhibition of radiological damage of joints. It has been approved as a therapeutic drug for the treatment of RA and in Japan for Castelman's disease and systemic juvenile idiopathic arthritis. Tocilizumab is a potential candidate drug for the therapy of several other disorders including SLE, Crohn's disease or multiple sclerosis (9).

*Inhibition of the IL-1 mediated responses with a recombinant IL-1R antagonist (anakinra)*

Like TNFα or IL-6, IL-1α and β also induce a wide spectrum of biological responses that contribute to fight infections: these include the production of acute phase proteins, raising body temperature (hence the term endogenous pyrogens) or mobilization of neutrophils, thus promoting microbe clearance by phagocytosis. The main source for IL-1α and β are macrophages and epithelial cells, whereas IL-1Ra, a naturally occurring IL-1R antagonist is released also by monocytes and hepatocytes (10). The IL-1 receptors CD121a and b are expressed on different subsets of lymphocytes, monocytes and macrophages.

Recombinant IL-1a (anakinra) is an approved therapeutic drug for RA that mimics the effects of endogenous IL-1Ra, thus blocking the IL-1 binding site on the receptor without inducing any further signaling events. The treatment with anakinra is well tolerated, with less occurring opportunistic infections than in case of TNFα blockage, and it was shown to improve joint swelling, pain and inflammation, although with less efficacy (11, 12, 13).

*Induction of alterations in IL-21 mediated cellular responses*

IL-21 is a type I cytokine expressed by activated $CD4^+$ T cells and NKT cells (14), and induces the differentiation and activation of NK cells, promotes NKT proliferation, enhances the differentiation of Th17 cells and was found to regulate mature B cell responses depending on the type of co-stimulation (within a wide range of inducing proliferation to cell death) (15). $IL21R^{-/-}$mice showed no defects in B cell development, but had severe problems with class-switch to IgG1 and IgG2b, and the down-regulation of the germinal center reaction. As a consequence they experienced a decrease in the number of plasma cells and an increase in memory B cells (16).

Although IL-21 fulfills a complex role in the immune regulation, experimental animal models indicate that its targeting could be of therapeutic benefits. In MRL/lpr mice inhibition of IL-21 improved symptoms of the disease, the mice showing a reduction in proteinuria, skin lesions, circulating dsDNA autoantibodies and lymphadenopathy (17). In collagen-induced arthritis and in adjuvant-induced arthritis, the blockade of IL-21R with an IL-21R-Fc fusion protein reversed clinical disease activity, most probably via the down-regulation of TNFα and production of IL-17 (18). In RA patients, IL-21R is expressed in the synovial macrophages and fibroblasts. In addition, a significantly higher percentage of IL-21R is to be found in the blood and synovial fluid of these individuals, where it might contribute to an increase in TNFα and IFNγ secretion upon T cell activation, thus, in up-regulating the pro-inflammatory response (19, 20).

## 3. B cell depletion therapies mediated via CD20 and CD22

While initially systemic autoimmunity was considered as a T cell-driven condition, multiple functions of B cells have been described in orchestrating autoimmune disorders, including self-reactive antibody production, auto-antigen presentation and co-stimulation of T lymphocytes, formation of ectopic lymphoid structures (neo-organogenesis) in the end-target organs and pro-inflammatory cytokine production.

*CD20-mediated B cell depletion*

Due to their central role in the immune pathogenesis of systemic autoimmunity and the observation that patients treated with non-Hodgkin's lymphoma and coexisting RA showed improvements in symptoms of RA after anti-CD20 (Rituximab) treatment, several therapies target B cells.

Physiological autoimmunity, thus the production of auto-antibodies in healthy individuals emerges upon infection and facilitates the clearing of apoptotic cells at the site of inflammation. Defects in down-regulation of this response can lead to the development of pathologic conditions. One of the several criteria by the diagnosis of autoimmunity is the presence of self-reactive antibodies in the circulation that are often present decades before the onset of clinical symptoms. During the course of B cell development, many checkpoints exist to prevent the escape of self-reactive B cells to the periphery these include receptor revision, clonal deletion and anergy (21, 22). Once an auto-reactive B cell is activated though by a self-structure first extra-follicular short-lived plasma cells are formed that produce low-affinity antibodies. Some of these auto-reactive cells also enter the germinal centers where they undergo affinity maturation and class switch, and develop into long-lived auto-reactive memory cells.

Antibodies can contribute to disease pathogenesis in two different ways: direct action by binding to its target e.g. in myasthenia gravis where anti-acetylcholine receptor antibodies bind post-synaptic receptors and compromise motor functions in neurons (23), or in Graves' disease, where the anti-thyroid stimulating hormone (TSH) receptor auto-antibodies can act as receptor agonists (24). The indirect contribution of auto-antibodies to autoimmunity consists of the formation of immune complexes inducing Fc-receptor mediated phagocytosis and/or activation of the complement system and production of pro-inflammatory cytokines, thus leading to tissue damage.

In addition to antibody production B cells also have an important role as antigen presenting cells. B cell deficiency in mice results in a disrupted lymphoid structure in the spleen, lack of follicular dendritic cell network and absence of Peyer's patches (25). B cell depletion studies in mice showed a defect in CD4+ T cell priming in the absence of B cell co-stimulation, especially when the antigen is available only at low concentrations. B cells not only provide support to T cells via direct cell-cell contact, but also shape the immune response by producing either pro-inflammatory cytokines including IL-6, IFNγ and LTα. Certain subsets are also able to produce IL-10 that has a regulatory function and contributes to the attenuation of the disease (26).

Tertiary ectopic lymphoid structures have been described at the end-organ in several autoimmune disorders: in the synovium of RA patients organized zones of B, T and follicular dendritic cells can be found in more than 50% of the cases, while kidneys of SLE patients also often contain such organized structures. B cell depletion or the blockade of B cell-T cell contacts has been proved to disrupt these ectopic lymphoid follicles and attenuate disease severity in several animal models of autoimmunity (27).

One of the most effective disease modifying anti-rheumatic drugs (DMARDs) is rituximab, a human CD20-specific chimeric monoclonal antibody. CD20 is a 35-37kDa tetra-spanning integral membrane protein first expressed on late pre-B cells in the bone marrow, present on naïve and mature B cells, down-regulated on antibody-secreting plasmablasts and extinguishing on plasma cells. It has been shown to regulate early steps of cell cycle progression, B cell proliferation and apoptosis. Upon cell activation, it gets trans-located to membrane lipid rafts, where it can act as a $Ca^{2+}$-channel (28). CD20 is also expressed on a small subset of basally activated IL1β- and TNF α–producing T cells (0.1-6.8% in healthy individuals) that showed enhanced susceptibility to apoptosis (29). Within an hour Rituximab treatment induces a ~90% reduction of the pre-treatment state in circulating $CD20^+$ B cell numbers that lasts for at least 3 months and also mediates a decrease in the number of resident $CD20^+$ B cells in the damaged tissues, although with variable efficacy: 70% of cells residing in the spleen and lymph nodes are depleted after 24 hours, while access to peritoneal B cells is limited (30, 31). Success of the depletion also varies among B cell subpopulations: splenic marginal zone B cells, germinal center B cells and peritoneal B1 cells are significantly more protected.

The reemerging of the B cell population usually occurs in the majority of the patients after 4-6 months and follows a definite pattern by immature $CD5^+$ $CD38^{high}$ transitional B cells and re-circulating plasmablasts appearing first and later circulating naïve B cells.

Monitoring of serum antibody levels in rituximab treated patients revealed that while titers of RF and anti-CCP antibodies significantly dropped, the humoral immune response towards most pathogens remained unaffected (e.g. pneumococcal capsular polysaccharide, tetanus toxoid) (32). Reduction in IgM-RF levels reflected to changes in total serum IgM levels, but the levels of IgA-RF, IgG-RF, and IgG anti-CCP antibodies decreased significantly more than those of their corresponding total serum immunoglobulin classes, which suggests that rituximab induces a selective reduction of short-lived autoantibody-secreting plasma cells. Two independent studies investigating changes in the synovial tissue composition of RA patients before and after rituximab treatment showed a significant decrease in B cell numbers in the synovium indicating that efficacy of the treatment lies in the disruption of extrafollicular lymphoid structures and the inhibition of B-T cell interactions (33).

Data about the efficacy of B cell depletion in SLE are contradictory: several studies involving only a small group of patients reported a significant clinical improvement upon rituximab treatment, while phase II/III trials showed no difference in BILAG scores. In contrast, B cell deficient lupus-prone MRL/lpr mice do not develop nephritis due to the reduced activation of the T cell compartment while transgenic mice expressing only membrane bound BCR on the cell surface (mIgM.MRL/lpr) still develop the disease (34). Another study found that mouse strains prone to develop autoimmunity are a lot more resistant to B cell depletion. These data indicate a more complex role for B cells in SLE than the production of auto-reactive antibodies. CD20-mediated B cell depletion at an early age in pristane-primed NZB/W F1 mice resulted in acceleration of the onset of disease, possibly due to the lack of IL-10 production by regulatory B cells. Treatment following the outbreak of symptoms on the other hand attenuated the intensity of the disease (35).

*CD22-mediated B cell depletion*

Another B lymphocyte restricted target is the Ig-superfamily member CD22, a 135kDa glycoprotein that is first detected in the cytoplasm of pro- and pre-B cells, becoming present on the cell surface of mature peripheral B cells. It remains expressed on germinal center B cells but is absent on plasmablasts and terminally differentiated plasma cells. Known ligands of CD22 include the tyrosine phosphatase CD45 and the lectin CD33, both binding through $\alpha$2,6-linked sialic acid motifs. While CD22 was reported to inhibit BCR-mediated cell activation *in vitro* via the recruitment of SHP-1 phosphatase to its cytoplasmic ITIM sequences upon phosphorylation by the tyrosine kinase Lyn (36), its *in vivo* role is less clarified. CD22-deficient mice develop hyper-proliferative B-lymphocytes and in consequence increased levels of auto-antibodies.

Epratuzumab, a humanized monoclonal IgG1 CD22-specific antibody recognizes a non-ligand-binding site of the CD22 molecule. It is predicted to alter BCR-signaling by inducing disruption of cell surface signaling complexes and antibody-mediated depletion of B cells (37). Epratuzumab is shown to cause phosphorylation and internalization of CD22 on peripheral B cells *in vitro*. On a small cohort of SLE-patients, when administered four times every second week it was reported to improve clinical symptoms in all of the patients based on the 6-, 10- or 18-week assessments (38).

## 4. Inhibition of cell-cell contacts and survival factors

Several other monoclonal antibodies currently under clinical trial target B cell survival factors and cytokines like B-cell activating factor (BAFF), a proliferation inducing ligand (APRIL), IL-6 or IL-10.

*Inhibition of the B cell survival factors BAFF and APRIL*

BAFF and APRIL are members of the TNF superfamily that maintain peripheral B cell- and plasma cell homeostasis by supporting cell survival. Access to BAFF modifies the stringency of negative selection of naïve B cells, as auto-reactive B cells depend more on BAFF relative to naïve mature cells. BAFF is produced by neutrophil granulocytes, monocytes, macrophages, dendritic cells and T cells as a trans-membrane protein and cleaved from the cell surface by the protease furin (39). In the serum, BAFF and APRIL are found as both homo- and hetero-trimers. The expression of receptors for soluble BAFF (BR3/BAFFR, TACI and BCMA) varies depending on the B-cell developmental stage. Highest levels of BR3/BAFFR are observed on primary and activated follicular and marginal B cells, while expression is decreased but still detectable on germinal center B cells. BR3/BAFFR is reduced or absent on antibody producing plasma cells, whereas TACI and BCMA are abundantly expressed on these cells. Memory B cells express all three BAFF-receptors. Neutralizing antibodies against BAFF cause a loss of transitional-2, marginal zone and follicular B cells *in vivo*, but transitional-1, B1 B cells, and plasma cells are not affected because latter cells receive survival signals by TACI as well (40).

| Monoclonal antibody | Type | Target molecule | Autoimmune disease |
|---|---|---|---|
| Adalimumab (Humira) | human | TNFα | RA, psoriatic arthritis, ankylosing spondylitis, Crohn's disease, psoriasis, juvenile idiopathic arthritis |
| Belimumab (Benlysta) | human | BAFF | SLE |
| Certolizumab pegol (Cimzia) | humanized | TNFα | RA, Crohn's disease |
| Epratuzumab | humanized | CD22 | SLE |
| Infliximab (Remicade) | chimeric | TNFα | Crohn's disease, psoriasis, ankylosing spondylitis, psoriatic arthritis, RA, ulcerative colitis |
| Natalizumab (Tysabri) | humanized | α4 integrin | Multiple sclerosis, Crohn's disease |
| Rituximab (Rituxan) | chimeric | CD20 | RA |
| Tocilizumab (Actemra) | humanized | IL-6R | RA, Castelman's disease |

Table 1. Examples of therapeutic antibodies for the treatment of autoimmune disorders approved by the FDA

In the serum of patients with active SLE and Sjogren's syndrome, the expression levels of soluble BAFF have been found elevated. Therefore, it is a potential target molecule in autoimmune disorders. Belimumab a humanized IgG1 monoclonal antibody blocks BAFF-binding to its receptors, thereby inhibiting the persistence of antibody producing B cells by mediating apoptotic cell death of early plasmablasts, naïve B cells and activated B cells (41) (42). Restriction of BAFF levels might facilitate the function of regulatory B cell populations. Atacicept is a fully human chimeric molecule consisting of the TACI ligand-binding extracellular domain fused to the Fc-portion of a human IgG1. It blocks both TACI- and BAFF-binding to their receptors and resulted to be successful in phase I clinical trials for the treatment of RA (43, 44, 45).

*Inhibition of B-T cell interactions*

For RA patients who give an inadequate response to anti-TNFα therapy, there is an increasing number of DMARDs that offer improvement of clinical symptoms by the inhibition of T cell-antigen presenting cell (APC) interactions.

Activation of T cells by antigens not only requires TCR-binding to the specific peptide-MHC complex on the APC, but also the ligation of co-stimulatory molecules like CD40, inducible T cell co-stimulator (ICOS) and CD28. Therefore, biologics that block these interactions may interfere with sufficient helper T cell activation and inhibit B cell differentiation into antibody producing plasma cells.

Abatacept is a soluble, fully human fusion protein of the extracellular domain of CTLA-4 and the hinge region, the CH2 and CH3 domains of a human IgG1 molecule. It recognizes B7 (CD80/86) with a high affinity and blocks its interaction with CD28, this way selectively inhibiting T cell activation. Abatacept is approved for the treatment of RA and juvenile idiopathic arthritis, and in a phase I trial it was shown to improve the clinical symptoms of psoriasis patients via the reduction of the size of the intralesional T cell population. Combination of abatacept with TNFα-blockers is not advised as it increases the occurrence of infections and provides no additional benefits (11).

Although the role of ICOS in T cell signaling has not been completely resolved yet, experimental data demonstrate that ICOS/ICOSL is an important regulator of T cell activation. It is expressed on resting T cells only at low amounts, while it gets strongly up-regulated upon activation. Highest level of expression is observed on T follicular helper cells. Blockade of ICOS/ICOSL interactions with monoclonal antibodies has been reported to improve collagen-induced arthritis and murine models of lupus (46). At the early stage of experimental autoimmune encephalomyelitis (EAE), a mouse model of sclerosis multiplex, inhibition of the ICOS/ICOSL interaction seemed to aggravate the disease, while it induced an improvement when administered at later phases (47). In glucose-6-phosphate isomerase (G6PI)-induced arthritis, early ICOSL-specific monoclonal antibody treatment resulted in significant loss of disease severity, but treatment at later stages of arthritis reduced symptoms only marginally. The number of G6PI-specific T helper cells decreased, but there was no difference in the antigen-specific antibody levels in the sera of the animals (48).

## 5. Biotechnical approaches for the reduction of immunogenicity in monoclonal antibody therapies

By the application of recombinant proteins in human medicine immunogenicity is one of the major concerns as several examples (insulin-, growth hormone-, factor VIII treatment or muronomab itself) had already shown us (49). The immune system may recognize these structures as foreign and develop an antibody response towards them, which may result in reduction of bioactivity. Factors like the sequence of the antibody, the secondary structure, the purity of the product, the dosage and frequency of administration, the diversity in MHC alleles within the population, the site of injection and the physical status of the individual all contribute to the outcome of the immunological response towards the protein-based medication (50, 51).

The clinical effects of the antibodies raised against the therapeutic protein depend on the epitope they recognize, their affinity and titer: some cause no reduction in bioactivity while others induce complications besides affecting the therapeutic benefits. These complications include increased risk of infusion reactions such as fever or rashes, pure red-cell aplasia or even cardiopulmonary and anaphylactic-like adverse events (52). In general, the emerging antibody response can inhibit the binding of the ligand to the receptor, or change the conformation and therefore the affinity and signaling properties of the soluble mediator (e.g. in case of IFNβ treatment). Immunological responses against monoclonal antibodies often enhance clearance by complex formation or block target recognition by binding to the variable region (idiotype). Rituximab, a mouse-human chimeric antibody induces the development of human anti-chimeric antibodies (HACA) in 1-5% of Non Hodgin's lymphoma and RA patients and in 65% of SLE patients, resulting in a reduction of the efficacy of B cell depletion and often in hypersensitivity reactions (53, 54).

Several different techniques exist to attenuate the break-through of tolerance against monoclonal antibodies, these include:

a. The replacement of murine constant regions with human sequences, where the specificity of the antibody remains intact (chimera design)

   The hybridoma technology enabled us to produce monoclonal murine antibodies in large quantities (55). On the other hand, generation of human hybridomas is difficult because they produce only small amounts of IgM and are very unstable. Recombinant DNA techniques make it possible to change the constant regions of murine immunoglobulins to human domains (56). The heavy and light chain genes are clustered into exons that represent the domain structures, which facilitates domain exchanges in antibody molecules. The vector selection is a critical step in the *in vitro* production of these monoclonal antibody constructs, as glycosylation patterns highly vary between species. Mammalian non-immune cells (HeLa or CHO cells) or certain myeloma cell lines are frequently used for this purpose. (57)

   The choice of the heavy chain isotype frequently defines the mechanism of action: IgG1 is binding with high affinity to FcγRs, therefore, the therapeutic antibody of such isotype is more likely to cause additional cell depletion via antibody-dependent cell-mediated cytotoxicity (ADCC). On the other hand IgG2 interacts only weakly with low affinity FcγRs, so the therapeutic effects observed are mainly attributed to the capacity of the antibody for blocking or altering cellular signaling through the targeted receptor.

b. Humanization or reshaping of the variable region, thus partial exchange of framework residues to human sequences

   The antigen specificity of the antibody is defined by only a few amino acids that are exposed to the surface of the antigen-binding pocket (paratope) and interact with the antigen. By transferring this set of residues from a nonhuman origin to a human frame (FR), the specificity of the antibody should remain (58).

The engrafting of the complementary determining regions (CDR) consists of different steps: the determination of the sequences in the nonhuman antibody that participate in the specific recognition of the antigen, the selection of the fitting human frame to engraft it in, and finally, the assembly of the nonhuman CDR and the human FR to a functional antibody via the insertion of back mutations. In order to minimize the presence of nonhuman sequences within the humanized antibody construct, several methods e.g. specificity determining residue (SDR) engrafting or superhumanization had been proposed. While the first is based on the computational analysis of the three-dimensional structure of the antigen-antibody complex, suggesting that only 20-33% of CDR residues are in contact with the antigen, the latter relies on the *in silico* selection of the best matching canonical structures of both the nonhuman and human sequences (59, 60).

For the engraftment, most frequently human germline sequences are used to minimize potential immunogenicity (61). The objective of the back mutations by establishing the functional antibody is to maintain, or if possible, even improve the affinity of the antibody. To obtain this several methods exist, such as e.g. error-prone PCR with low fidelity polymerases under nonstandard conditions or pooling random DNA fragments after digestion of the variable region with DNase I (62, 63).

Despite the fact that humanized antibodies retain less than 5% of the murine sequences, a significant anti-drug response can still be observed in 0.1-9% of the treated patients (64, 65, 66).

c. Selection of human antibody V regions using a phage library screen based on the affinity towards the antigen.

Besides attempts to avoid immunogenicity, antigen display also provides the best method to overcome limitations of the hybridoma technology concerning toxic or highly conserved antigen structures. Several display systems that apply insertion of variable region fragments to the phage genome have been developed for phage T7 (67), phage λ (68, 69, 70) and the Ff class (genus Inovirus) of the filamentous phage f1, fd, and M13 (71). The source for antibody fragments can either be a naive, a semi-synthetic or an entirely synthetic library. Naive libraries are generated by mRNA isolation and cDNA synthesis from B cells (naïve or antigen exposed cells), and the variable region genes are either expressed separately with a two or three step cloning strategy or fused as an scFv in a polymerase chain reaction (PCR). If the assembly PCR is involving randomization of the CDR3 region, namely the usage of oligonucleotide primers encoding various CDR3 and J gene segments (72), a semi-synthetic library is established. Entirely synthetic libraries use various different $V_H$ and $V_L$ germline master frameworks, combined with synthetically created CDR cassettes.

The pIII minor coat protein of the filamentous phage M13 is widely used to fuse the antibody fragment of interest with, thus resulting in the expression of the antibody fragment on the surface of the phage. High affinity binding constructs can be then selected by panning, a method that consists of incubation cycles (2-5) with surface-bound antigen, followed by a restricting washing to remove non-specific clones. Specificity of selected constructs can be evaluated then using enzyme-linked immunosorbent assay (ELISA).

As a final step for the generation of therapeutic antibodies, the selected variable region genes need to be inserted into a human frame sequence.

Clinical data show that despite the fully human sequence, many of the monoclonal antibodies produced by phage display technology e.g. the TNFα-specific adalimumab are still immunogenic (73). An explanation for this could be that *in vitro* affinity maturation lacks several control steps, as there is an additional *in vivo* selection for attributes such as stability and aggregation besides molecular recognition.

d. Human antibody production of transgenic mice expressing human immunoglobulin genes

Strategies to establish mouse strains with germ line modifications in their immunoglobulin genes usually aim for homologous recombination in mouse embryonic stem cells that disrupt endogenous Ig heavy and light chains, and introduce the human transgenes. In the past, different technologies were successfully applied to produce and deliver the human sequence transgenes: Lonberg et al. used pronuclear microinjection to introduce reconstructed minilocus transgenes (74), while Green et al. established transgenes with yeast artificial chromosome (YAC) (75). Initially, mouse heavy and κ light chain sequences were 'replaced' for several different $V_H$, $D_H$ and $J_H$ regions with $\gamma 1$, $\mu$ or $\delta$ heavy chain constant region fragments and $V_\kappa$, all five $J_\kappa$ and the $C_\kappa$ light chain genes. These transgenic animals were able to mount human antibodies in response to a targeted antigen.

There have been many initiatives undertaken since then to broaden the size of the V-region repertoire, as it has a strong influence on multiple checkpoints in B cell development and therefore the size of the mature B cell population (76). Following selection of the most efficient clones, for large-scale production usually a recombinant expression system is established to reduce costs (77).

In contrast to chimeric, humanized or *in vitro* generated therapeutic monoclonal antibodies, there are no reported cases of the generation of anti-human Ig responses towards transgenic therapeutic antibodies. Table 1 summarizes the currently available monoclonal constructs and their origin.

## 6. Conclusions

Since the development of the hybridoma technique several monoclonal antibodies have been approved for the treatment of autoimmune diseases. Immunogenicity of murine sequences caused initial complications, which could be attenuated and finally overcome by the production of chimeric and humanized antibodies and with the generation of transgenic mouse strains for human Ig-sequences. One of the crucial steps by the design of a monoclonal antibody for therapeutic applications is the selection of the right target molecule. In autoimmune disorders several options exist: the blockade of the pro-inflammatory cytokines TNFα, IL-1 or IL-6, the inhibition of T cell-B cell interactions, B cell depletion to reduce autoantibody production and the establishment of ectopic lymphoid structures or the blockade of B cell survival factors. Although we still need to face adverse events upon the application of these therapeutic antibodies, targeting specific molecules will help us to reduce the severity of occurring side effects and provide more efficient medications.

## 7. Acknowledgement

This work was supported by a grant from the Research and Technology Innovation Fund (KTIA-OTKA 80689) and the National Innovation Office (NIH)-ANR bilateral grant.

## 8. References


[1] Sethi, G., B. Sung, A. B. Kunnumakkara, and B. B. Aggarwal. 2009. Targeting TNF for Treatment of Cancer and Autoimmunity. *Adv Exp Med Biol* 647: 37-51.

[2] Colombel, J. F., E. V. J. Loftus, W. J. Tremaine, L. J. Egan, W. S. Harmsen, C. D. Schleck, A. R. Zinsmeister, and W. J. Sandborn. 2004. The safety profile of infliximab in patients with Crohn's disease: the Mayo clinic experience in 500 patients. *Gastroenterology* 126: 19-31.

[3] Bacquet-Deschryver, H., F. Jouen, M. Quillard, J. F. Menard, V. Goeb, T. Lequerre, O. Mejjad, A. Daragon, F. Tron, X. Le Loet, and O. Vittecoq. 2008. Impact of three anti-TNFalpha biologics on existing and emergent autoimmunity in rheumatoid arthritis and spondylarthropathy patients. *J Clin Immunol* 28: 445-455.

[4] Biton, J., L. Semerano, L. Delavallee, D. Lemeiter, M. Laborie, G. Grouard-Vogel, M. C. Boissier, and N. Bessis. 2011. Interplay between TNF and Regulatory T Cells in a TNF-Driven Murine Model of Arthritis. *J Immunol*

[5] Hibi, M., M. Murakami, M. Saito, T. Hirano, T. Taga, and T. Kishimoto. 1990. Molecular cloning and expression of an IL-6 signal transducer, gp130. *Cell* 63: 1149-1157.

[6] Kishimoto, T. 2005. Interleukin-6: from basic science to medicine--40 years in immunology. *Annu Rev Immunol* 23: 1-21.

[7] Nishimoto, N., K. Terao, T. Mima, H. Nakahara, N. Takagi, and T. Kakehi. 2008. Mechanisms and pathologic significances in increase in serum interleukin-6 (IL-6) and soluble IL-6 receptor after administration of an anti-IL-6 receptor antibody, tocilizumab, in patients with rheumatoid arthritis and Castleman disease. *Blood* 112: 3959-3964.

[8] Grondal, G., I. Gunnarsson, J. Ronnelid, S. Rogberg, L. Klareskog, and I. Lundberg. 2000. Cytokine production, serum levels and disease activity in systemic lupus erythematosus. *Clin Exp Rheumatol* 18: 565-570.

[9] Tanaka, T., M. Narazaki, and T. Kishimoto. 2011. Anti-interleukin-6 receptor antibody, tocilizumab, for the treatment of autoimmune diseases. *FEBS Lett*

[10] Hannum, C. H., C. J. Wilcox, W. P. Arend, F. G. Joslin, D. J. Dripps, P. L. Heimdal, L. G. Armes, A. Sommer, S. P. Eisenberg, and R. C. Thompson. 1990. Interleukin-1 receptor antagonist activity of a human interleukin-1 inhibitor. *Nature* 343: 336-340.

[11] Smolen, J. S., D. Aletaha, M. Koeller, M. H. Weisman, and P. Emery. 2007. New therapies for treatment of rheumatoid arthritis. *Lancet* 370: 1861-1874.

[12] O'Dell, J. R. 2004. Therapeutic strategies for rheumatoid arthritis. *N Engl J Med* 350: 2591-2602.

[13] Goldbach-Mansky, R. 2009. Blocking interleukin-1 in rheumatic diseases. *Ann N Y Acad Sci* 1182: 111-123.

[14] Coquet, J. M., K. Kyparissoudis, D. G. Pellicci, G. Besra, S. P. Berzins, M. J. Smyth, and D. I. Godfrey. 2007. IL-21 is produced by NKT cells and modulates NKT cell activation and cytokine production. *J Immunol* 178: 2827-2834.

[15] Leonard, W. J., and R. Spolski. 2005. Interleukin-21: a modulator of lymphoid proliferation, apoptosis and differentiation. *Nat Rev Immunol* 5: 688-698.

[16] Ozaki, K., R. Spolski, C. G. Feng, C. F. Qi, J. Cheng, A. Sher, H. C. r. Morse, C. Liu, P. L. Schwartzberg, and W. J. Leonard. 2002. A critical role for IL-21 in regulating immunoglobulin production. *Science* 298: 1630-1634.

[17] Herber, D., T. P. Brown, S. Liang, D. A. Young, M. Collins, and K. Dunussi-Joannopoulos. 2007. IL-21 has a pathogenic role in a lupus-prone mouse model and its blockade with IL-21R.Fc reduces disease progression. *J Immunol* 178: 3822-3830.

[18] Young, D. A., M. Hegen, H. L. Ma, M. J. Whitters, L. M. Albert, L. Lowe, M. Senices, P. W. Wu, B. Sibley, Y. Leathurby, T. P. Brown, C. Nickerson-Nutter, J. C. J. Keith, and M. Collins. 2007. Blockade of the interleukin-21/interleukin-21 receptor pathway ameliorates disease in animal models of rheumatoid arthritis. *Arthritis Rheum* 56: 1152-1163.

[19] Li, J., W. Shen, K. Kong, and Z. Liu. 2006. Interleukin-21 induces T-cell activation and proinflammatory cytokine secretion in rheumatoid arthritis. *Scand J Immunol* 64: 515-522.

[20] Jungel, A., J. H. Distler, M. Kurowska-Stolarska, C. A. Seemayer, R. Seibl, A. Forster, B. A. Michel, R. E. Gay, F. Emmrich, S. Gay, and O. Distler. 2004. Expression of interleukin-21 receptor, but not interleukin-21, in synovial fibroblasts and synovial macrophages of patients with rheumatoid arthritis. *Arthritis Rheum* 50: 1468-1476.

[21] Monroe, J. G., and K. Dorshkind. 2007. Fate decisions regulating bone marrow and peripheral B lymphocyte development. *Adv Immunol* 95: 1-50.

[22] von Boehmer, H., and F. Melchers. 2010. Checkpoints in lymphocyte development and autoimmune disease. *Nat Immunol* 11: 14-20.

[23] Ruff, R. L., and V. A. Lennon. 2008. How myasthenia gravis alters the safety factor for neuromuscular transmission. *J Neuroimmunol* 201-202: 13-20.

[24] Brown, R. S. 2009. Autoimmune thyroid disease: unlocking a complex puzzle. *Curr Opin Pediatr* 21: 523-528.

[25] Ngo, V. N., R. J. Cornall, and J. G. Cyster. 2001. Splenic T zone development is B cell dependent. *J Exp Med* 194: 1649-1660.

[26] Yanaba, K., J. D. Bouaziz, K. M. Haas, J. C. Poe, M. Fujimoto, and T. F. Tedder. 2008. A regulatory B cell subset with a unique CD1dhiCD5+ phenotype controls T cell-dependent inflammatory responses. *Immunity* 28: 639-650.

[27] Weyand, C. M., Y. M. Kang, P. J. Kurtin, and J. J. Goronzy. 2003. The power of the third dimension: tissue architecture and autoimmunity in rheumatoid arthritis. *Curr Opin Rheumatol* 15: 259-266.

[28] Tedder, T. F., and P. Engel. 1994. CD20: a regulator of cell-cycle progression of B lymphocytes. *Immunol Today* 15: 450-454.

[29] Wilk, E., T. Witte, N. Marquardt, T. Horvath, K. Kalippke, K. Scholz, N. Wilke, R. E. Schmidt, and R. Jacobs. 2009. Depletion of functionally active CD20+ T cells by rituximab treatment. *Arthritis Rheum* 60: 3563-3571.

[30] Hamaguchi, Y., J. Uchida, D. W. Cain, G. M. Venturi, J. C. Poe, K. M. Haas, and T. F. Tedder. 2005. The peritoneal cavity provides a protective niche for B1 and conventional B lymphocytes during anti-CD20 immunotherapy in mice. *J Immunol* 174: 4389-4399.

[31] Uchida, J., Y. Hamaguchi, J. A. Oliver, J. V. Ravetch, J. C. Poe, K. M. Haas, and T. F. Tedder. 2004. The innate mononuclear phagocyte network depletes B lymphocytes through Fc receptor-dependent mechanisms during anti-CD20 antibody immunotherapy. *J Exp Med* 199: 1659-1669.

[32] Bingham, C. O. r., R. J. Looney, A. Deodhar, N. Halsey, M. Greenwald, C. Codding, B. Trzaskoma, F. Martin, S. Agarwal, and A. Kelman. 2010. Immunization responses in rheumatoid arthritis patients treated with rituximab: results from a controlled clinical trial. *Arthritis Rheum* 62: 64-74.
[33] Lund, F. E., and T. D. Randall. 2010. Effector and regulatory B cells: modulators of CD4(+) T cell immunity. *Nat Rev Immunol* 10: 236-247.
[34] Chan, O. T., L. G. Hannum, A. M. Haberman, M. P. Madaio, and M. J. Shlomchik. 1999. A novel mouse with B cells but lacking serum antibody reveals an antibody-independent role for B cells in murine lupus. *J Exp Med* 189: 1639-1648.
[35] Haas, K. M., R. Watanabe, T. Matsushita, H. Nakashima, N. Ishiura, H. Okochi, M. Fujimoto, and T. F. Tedder. 2010. Protective and pathogenic roles for B cells during systemic autoimmunity in NZB/W F1 mice. *J Immunol* 184: 4789-4800.
[36] Carnahan, J., P. Wang, R. Kendall, C. Chen, S. Hu, T. Boone, T. Juan, J. Talvenheimo, S. Montestruque, J. Sun, G. Elliott, J. Thomas, J. Ferbas, B. Kern, R. Briddell, J. P. Leonard, and A. Cesano. 2003. Epratuzumab, a humanized monoclonal antibody targeting CD22: characterization of in vitro properties. *Clin Cancer Res* 9: 3982S-3990S.
[37] Carnahan, J., R. Stein, Z. Qu, K. Hess, A. Cesano, H. J. Hansen, and D. M. Goldenberg. 2007. Epratuzumab, a CD22-targeting recombinant humanized antibody with a different mode of action from rituximab. *Mol Immunol* 44: 1331-1341.
[38] Dorner, T., J. Kaufmann, W. A. Wegener, N. Teoh, D. M. Goldenberg, and G. R. Burmester. 2006. Initial clinical trial of epratuzumab (humanized anti-CD22 antibody) for immunotherapy of systemic lupus erythematosus. *Arthritis Res Ther* 8: R74.
[39] Bodmer, J. L., P. Schneider, and J. Tschopp. 2002. The molecular architecture of the TNF superfamily. *Trends Biochem Sci* 27: 19-26.
[40] O'Connor, B. P., V. S. Raman, L. D. Erickson, W. J. Cook, L. K. Weaver, C. Ahonen, L. L. Lin, G. T. Mantchev, R. J. Bram, and R. J. Noelle. 2004. BCMA is essential for the survival of long-lived bone marrow plasma cells. *J Exp Med* 199: 91-98.
[41] Furie, R., W. Stohl, E. M. Ginzler, M. Becker, N. Mishra, W. Chatham, J. T. Merrill, A. Weinstein, W. J. McCune, J. Zhong, W. Cai, and W. Freimuth. 2008. Biologic activity and safety of belimumab, a neutralizing anti-B-lymphocyte stimulator (BLyS) monoclonal antibody: a phase I trial in patients with systemic lupus erythematosus. *Arthritis Res Ther* 10: R109.
[42] Stohl, W., J. L. Scholz, and M. P. Cancro. 2011. Targeting BLyS in rheumatic disease: the sometimes-bumpy road from bench to bedside. *Curr Opin Rheumatol* 23: 305-310.
[43] Seyler, T. M., Y. W. Park, S. Takemura, R. J. Bram, P. J. Kurtin, J. J. Goronzy, and C. M. Weyand. 2005. BLyS and APRIL in rheumatoid arthritis. *J Clin Invest* 115: 3083-3092.
[44] Bracewell, C., J. D. Isaacs, P. Emery, and W. F. Ng. 2009. Atacicept, a novel B cell-targeting biological therapy for the treatment of rheumatoid arthritis. *Expert Opin Biol Ther* 9: 909-919.
[45] Nestorov, I., A. Munafo, O. Papasouliotis, and J. Visich. 2008. Pharmacokinetics and biological activity of atacicept in patients with rheumatoid arthritis. *J Clin Pharmacol* 48: 406-417.

[46] Nurieva, R. I., P. Treuting, J. Duong, R. A. Flavell, and C. Dong. 2003. Inducible costimulator is essential for collagen-induced arthritis. *J Clin Invest* 111: 701-706.

[47] Galicia, G., A. Kasran, C. Uyttenhove, K. De Swert, J. Van Snick, and J. L. Ceuppens. 2009. ICOS deficiency results in exacerbated IL-17 mediated experimental autoimmune encephalomyelitis. *J Clin Immunol* 29: 426-433.

[48] Matsumoto, I., H. Zhang, T. Yasukochi, K. Iwanami, Y. Tanaka, A. Inoue, D. Goto, S. Ito, A. Tsutsumi, and T. Sumida. 2008. Therapeutic effects of antibodies to tumor necrosis factor-alpha, interleukin-6 and cytotoxic T-lymphocyte antigen 4 immunoglobulin in mice with glucose-6-phosphate isomerase induced arthritis. *Arthritis Res Ther* 10: R66.

[49] Schellekens, H., and N. Casadevall. 2004. Immunogenicity of recombinant human proteins: causes and consequences. *J Neurol* 251 Suppl 2: II4-9.

[50] Hermeling, S., D. J. Crommelin, H. Schellekens, and W. Jiskoot. 2004. Structure-immunogenicity relationships of therapeutic proteins. *Pharm Res* 21: 897-903.

[51] Cohen, B. A., J. Oger, A. Gagnon, and G. Giovannoni. 2008. The implications of immunogenicity for protein-based multiple sclerosis therapies. *J Neurol Sci* 275: 7-17.

[52] Edwards, J. C., L. Szczepanski, J. Szechinski, A. Filipowicz-Sosnowska, P. Emery, D. R. Close, R. M. Stevens, and T. Shaw. 2004. Efficacy of B-cell-targeted therapy with rituximab in patients with rheumatoid arthritis. *N Engl J Med* 350: 2572-2581.

[53] Saito, K., M. Nawata, S. Iwata, M. Tokunaga, and Y. Tanaka. 2005. Extremely high titer of anti-human chimeric antibody following re-treatment with rituximab in a patient with active systemic lupus erythematosus. *Rheumatology (Oxford)* 44: 1462-1464.

[54] Sabahi, R., and J. H. Anolik. 2006. B-cell-targeted therapy for systemic lupus erythematosus. *Drugs* 66: 1933-1948.

[55] Kohler, G., and C. Milstein. 1975. Continuous cultures of fused cells secreting antibody of predefined specificity. *Nature* 256: 495-497.

[56] Jones, P. T., P. H. Dear, J. Foote, M. S. Neuberger, and G. Winter. 1986. Replacing the complementarity-determining regions in a human antibody with those from a mouse. *Nature* 321: 522-525.

[57] Whittle, N., J. Adair, C. Lloyd, L. Jenkins, J. Devine, J. Schlom, A. Raubitschek, D. Colcher, and M. Bodmer. 1987. Expression in COS cells of a mouse-human chimaeric B72.3 antibody. *Protein Eng* 1: 499-505.

[58] Studnicka, G. M., S. Soares, M. Better, R. E. Williams, R. Nadell, and A. H. Horwitz. 1994. Human-engineered monoclonal antibodies retain full specific binding activity by preserving non-CDR complementarity-modulating residues. *Protein Eng* 7: 805-814.

[59] Gonzales, N. R., E. A. Padlan, R. De Pascalis, P. Schuck, J. Schlom, and S. V. Kashmiri. 2003. Minimizing immunogenicity of the SDR-grafted humanized antibody CC49 by genetic manipulation of the framework residues. *Mol Immunol* 40: 337-349.

[60] Tan, P., D. A. Mitchell, T. N. Buss, M. A. Holmes, C. Anasetti, and J. Foote. 2002. "Superhumanized" antibodies: reduction of immunogenic potential by complementarity-determining region grafting with human germline sequences: application to an anti-CD28. *J Immunol* 169: 1119-1125.

[61] Gonzales, N. R., E. A. Padlan, R. De Pascalis, P. Schuck, J. Schlom, and S. V. Kashmiri. 2004. SDR grafting of a murine antibody using multiple human germline templates to minimize its immunogenicity. *Mol Immunol* 41: 863-872.

[62] Neylon, C. 2004. Chemical and biochemical strategies for the randomization of protein encoding DNA sequences: library construction methods for directed evolution. *Nucleic Acids Res* 32: 1448-1459.

[63] Stemmer, W. P. 1994. Rapid evolution of a protein in vitro by DNA shuffling. *Nature* 370: 389-391.

[64] Pendley, C., A. Schantz, and C. Wagner. 2003. Immunogenicity of therapeutic monoclonal antibodies. *Curr Opin Mol Ther* 5: 172-179.

[65] Hwang, W. Y., and J. Foote. 2005. Immunogenicity of engineered antibodies. *Methods* 36: 3-10.

[66] Bartelds, G. M., C. L. Krieckaert, M. T. Nurmohamed, P. A. van Schouwenburg, W. F. Lems, J. W. Twisk, B. A. Dijkmans, L. Aarden, and G. J. Wolbink. 2011. Development of antidrug antibodies against adalimumab and association with disease activity and treatment failure during long-term follow-up. *JAMA* 305: 1460-1468.

[67] Danner, S., and J. G. Belasco. 2001. T7 phage display: a novel genetic selection system for cloning RNA-binding proteins from cDNA libraries. *Proc Natl Acad Sci U S A* 98: 12954-12959.

[68] Huse, W. D., L. Sastry, S. A. Iverson, A. S. Kang, M. Alting-Mees, D. R. Burton, S. J. Benkovic, and R. A. Lerner. 1989. Generation of a large combinatorial library of the immunoglobulin repertoire in phage lambda. *Science* 246: 1275-1281.

[69] Mullinax, R. L., and J. A. Sorge. 2003. Preparing lambda libraries for expression of proteins in prokaryotes or eukaryotes. *Methods Mol Biol* 221: 271-287.

[70] Kang, A. S., T. M. Jones, and D. R. Burton. 1991. Antibody redesign by chain shuffling from random combinatorial immunoglobulin libraries. *Proc Natl Acad Sci U S A* 88: 11120-11123.

[71] McCafferty, J., A. D. Griffiths, G. Winter, and D. J. Chiswell. 1990. Phage antibodies: filamentous phage displaying antibody variable domains. *Nature* 348: 552-554.

[72] Akamatsu, Y., M. S. Cole, J. Y. Tso, and N. Tsurushita. 1993. Construction of a human Ig combinatorial library from genomic V segments and synthetic CDR3 fragments. *J Immunol* 151: 4651-4659.

[73] Aarden, L., S. R. Ruuls, and G. Wolbink. 2008. Immunogenicity of anti-tumor necrosis factor antibodies-toward improved methods of anti-antibody measurement. *Curr Opin Immunol* 20: 431-435.

[74] Lonberg, N., L. D. Taylor, F. A. Harding, M. Trounstine, K. M. Higgins, S. R. Schramm, C. C. Kuo, R. Mashayekh, K. Wymore, J. G. McCabe, and a. et. 1994. Antigen-specific human antibodies from mice comprising four distinct genetic modifications. *Nature* 368: 856-859.

[75] Green, L. L., M. C. Hardy, C. E. Maynard-Currie, H. Tsuda, D. M. Louie, M. J. Mendez, H. Abderrahim, M. Noguchi, D. H. Smith, Y. Zeng, and a. et. 1994. Antigen-specific human monoclonal antibodies from mice engineered with human Ig heavy and light chain YACs. *Nat Genet* 7: 13-21.

[76] Green, L. L., and A. Jakobovits. 1998. Regulation of B cell development by variable gene complexity in mice reconstituted with human immunoglobulin yeast artificial chromosomes. *J Exp Med* 188: 483-495.
[77] Lonberg, N. 2005. Human antibodies from transgenic animals. *Nat Biotechnol* 23: 1117-1125.

13

# The Emerging Role of Monoclonal Antibodies in the Treatmentof Systemic Lupus Erythematosus

Ewa Robak and Tadeusz Robak
*Medical University of Lodz*
*Poland*

## 1. Introduction

Systemic lupus erythematosus (SLE) is an autoimmune disease characterized by B cell hyperactivity and defective T-cell function, with production of high titer autoantibodies and clinical involvement in multiple organ systems. Patients with mild SLE can generally be maintained on a combination of non-steroidal anti-inflammatory drugs and antimalarials. Corticosteroids, azathioprine and cyclophosphamide remain important for long term management of most patients with active disease and even those in clinical remission. However, these agents have considerable side effects and are not effective in all patients with SLE. Novel immunological therapies include both B and T cell directed treatments, anticytokine and complement directed therapies. These modalities enable more specific immunosuppression, and include cyclosporin, high-dose intravenous immunoglobulin, mycophenolate mofetil, tacrolimus and new purine nucleoside analogs (Schröder and Zeunerorts 2009).

In recent years, clinical studies have been undertaken with selected monoclonal antibodies (mAbs) in the treatment of several hematological diseases, especially in malignant disorders. However, some clinical observations indicate that mAbs may be an important alternative for the conventional therapy of some autoimmune disorders (Robak 2004).

B-lymphocytes are an essential component of the acquired immune response (La Cava 2010). They randomly express cell-surface receptors which are often autoreactive and must be controlled by the process of B-cell tolerance. In SLE, the number of B-cells in the peripheral blood is often decreased, and those that are present have abnormal phenotypes indicative of activation. The important role of B cells in the pathogenesis of SLE has provided a strong rationale to target B cells in SLE. Selective therapeutic depletion of B-cells became possible with the availability of the anti-CD20 antibody rituximab.

## 2. Anti-CD20 monoclonal antibodies

The CD20 (B1) antigen is a 33–35 kDa integral membrane protein expressed on the surfaces of non-malignant and most malignant B cells (Cragg, Walshe et al. 2005). The CD20 protein consists of cytoplasmic N- and C-termini and four hydrophobic regions for anchoring the molecule in the membrane (Robak 2008). The characteristics that make CD20 a good target antigen include its relatively high level of expression and close location of the extracellular epitopes to the cell surface. The intensity of antigen expression or the number of receptor sites on the cell surface appears to correlate with the clinical response. The cytotoxic activity of mAbs directed against CD20+ cells is thought to be based on antibody-dependent cellular cytotoxicity (ADCC) via natural killer (NK) cell responses, complement-dependent cytotoxicity (CDC), or by the induction of cell signaling followed by apoptosis. At present, rituximab is the most important mAb of clinical value in patients with autoimmune disorders and B-cell lymphoid malignancies. Over the last few years, new generations of anti-CD20 mAbs have been developed for potential benefits over rituximab (Robak and Robak 2011; Lim, Beers et al. 2010). They were engineered to have augmented antitumor activity by increasing CDC or ADCC activity and increased Fc binding affinity for the low-affinity variants of the FcγRIIIa receptor (CD16) on immune effector cells. The second-generation mAbs are humanized or fully human to reduce immunogenicity, but with an unmodified Fc region. They include ofatumumab, veltuzumab, and ocrelizumab. The third-generation mAbs are also humanized but in comparison with the second-generation mAbs they also have an engineered Fc region designed to increase their effector functions by increasing binding affinity for the FcγRIIIa receptor (Ruuls, Lammerts et al. 2008). Both polymorphisms in FcγRIIIa and structure of mAb Fc can impact on the affinity between FcγRIIIa and mAb. The third-generation mAbs include AME133v, Pro13192, and GA-101.

### 2.1 Rituximab

Rituximab is an IgG-1κ immunoglobulin, containing murine light– and heavy–chain variable–region sequences and human constant region sequences. Rituximab is known as the first-generation mAb. Since approval in 1997, rituximab has become the standard of care in follicular B-cell lymphomas (FL), CLL, and aggressive lymphomas when combined with chemotherapy (Hauptrock and Hess 2008). Rituximab is administered as an intravenous infusion with a recommended dosage of 375 mg/m$^2$ given once weekly for 4 weeks. Treatment with this agent is usually well tolerated. However, infusion-related reactions occur in the majority of patients. These adverse events are typically fever, chills, rigors and rare hypotension and bronchospasm, although the incidence of these side effects decreases with subsequent rituximab infusion. Moreover, prolonged impairment of antibody production causes the increased risk of viral and bacterial infections. It should be also remembered that rituximab is a human mouse chimeric antibody and hence treated patients may be susceptible to the development of human antichimeric antibodies, which can impact on responsiveness.

A recent study has shown that treatment with rituximab affects both the cellular and humoral arm of the immune system in patients with SLE (Lu, Ng et al. 2009).

A number of prospective studies and several retrospective cohort studies of rituximab in the treatment of SLE have been reported (Cambridge, Isenbergetal. 2008). In 2005 Leonardo et al. (Leandro, Cambridge et al. 2005) described female patients with SLE who were treated with combination of rituximab, CY and prednisolone. Each patient received two infusions of rituximab (500 mg/dose), two infusions of cyclophosphamide (750 mg/dose) and 60 mg prednisolone per day for five days. Five patients were analyzed and one patient was lost to follow up after 3 months. All five patients showed an improvement in British Isles Lupus Assessment Group (BILAG) scores from a median of 14 at baseline to a median of 6 at six months. Recently, the same group reported the results of 46 patients with active SLE were treated with a 1 gm of rituximab, 750 mg of cyclophosphamide, and 100-250 mg of methylprednisolone, administered on 2 occasions 2 weeks apart (Lu, Ng et al. 2009). Twenty one patients (47%) reached partial remission after one cycle (mean followup 39.6 months). Treatment resulted in a decrease in median global BILAG scores from 12 to 5 ($P < 0.0001$) and median anti-double-stranded DNA antibody titers from 106 to 42 IU/ml ($P < 0.0001$). In addition an increase in the median C3 level from 0.81 to 0.95 mg/liter ($P < 0.02$) at 6 months was observed. Five serious adverse events were noted.

Willems et al. (Willems, Haddad et al. 2006) described the safety and efficacy of rituximab in 11 girls (mean age 13.9 years) with severe SLE including 8 girls with class IV or V lupus nephritis, 2 girls with severe autoimmune cytopenia and 1 girl with an antiprothrombin antibody. Patients received 2 to 12 intravenous infusions of rituximab (350-450 mg/$m^2$/infusion) with corticosteroids. Remission was achieved in 6 of 8 patients with lupus nephritis and in two patients with autoimmune cytopenia. However, severe adverse events occurred in 45% of the patients in this study.

Looney et al. reported the results of the first dose escalation study of rituximab for the treatment of SLE (Looney, Anolik et al. 2004). The drug was added to ongoing therapy in 18 patients with moderately active SLE. Six patients received a single infusion of 100 mg/$m^2$, six received one infusion of 375 mg/$m^2$ and six patients received four weekly doses of 375 mg/$m^2$. In this study, rituximab-induced B cell depletion was translated into a significant improvement in SLE disease activity even in the absence of substantial serologic responses. Most patients were able to decrease corticosteroid dose from 13 to 10 mg by the end of the study and three patients were able to discontinue concomitant immunosuppressives. The clinical response was most notable for rashes and arthritis.

Terrier et al. analyzed recently prospective data from the French AutoImmunity and Rituximab (AIR) registry, which includes data on patients with autoimmune disorders treated with rituximb (Terrier, Amoura et al. 2010). Overall response was observed in 80 of 113 patients (71%) by the SELENA-SLEDAI (SLE Disease Activity Index Score assessment). Efficacy was similar between patients receiving rituximab monotherapy and those receiving concomitant immunosuppressive agents. Articular, cutaneous, renal, and hematologic improvements were noted in 72%, 70%, 74%, and 88% of patients, respectively. In relapsed patients response was observed in 91% after retreatment with rituximab. Severe infections were observed in 12 patients (9%), corresponding to a rate of 6.6/100 patient-years. Most severe infections occurred within the first 3 months after the last rituximab infusion. Five patients died, due to severe infection ($n = 3$) or refractory autoimmune disease ($n = 2$).

Merrill et al reported the results of the Exploratory Phase II/III SLE Evaluation of Rituximab (EXPLORER) trial, a placebo-controlled, double-blind, multicenter study of rituximab in patients with moderately-to-severely active extrarenal SLE (Merrill, Neuwelt et al. 2010). Patients were randomized at a 2:1 ratio to receive intravenous rituximab (1,000-mg) or placebo on days 1, 15, 168, and 182, which was added to prednisone. Of the 257 patients, 88 were assigned to receive placebo, and 169 were randomized to the rituximab arm. At week 52, no difference was observed in major clinical responses or partial clinical responses between the placebo group. Decreases in the level of anti-dsDNA autoantibodies and increases in complement C3 and C4 levels were greater in the rituximab group than in the placebo group. The overall response rate was 28.4% and 29.6%, respectively. The proportion of patients in whom serious infection developed was 17% in the placebo group and 9.5% in the rituximab group.

Rituximab is also an active treatment agent in patients with lupus nephritis and central nervous system (CNS) involvement. Sfikakis et al. reported clinical response in 80% and sustained complete response in 40% of patients with class III and IV nephritis treated with rituximab and moderate doses of corticosteroids (Sfikakis, Boletis et al. 2005). In the study of Ng et al. 21 patients with renal involvement were treated with rituximab and cyclophosphamide (Ng, Cambridge et al. 2007). They had a decrease in median urinary protein creatinine ratio (PCR) from 446 to 190 mg/mmol 6 months. More recently, Pepper et al. treated 18 patients with class III/IV/V lupus nephritis with rituximab. All patients were on steroids prior to the development of lupus nephritis (Pepper, Griffith et al. 2009). The patients received mycophenolate mofetil maintenance therapy. Fourteen of 18 patients achieved complete or partial remission with a sustained response of 67% at 1 year. In addition, serum albumin increased from a mean of 29 g/L at presentation to 34 g/L at 1 year (P = 0.001). Importantly, following treatment with rituximab, 6 patients stopped prednisolone, 6 patients reduced their maintenance dose and 6 patients remained on the same dose (maximum 10 mg). No severe infections were observed.

The study performed by Tokunaga et al. showed marked improvement following rituximab therapy in patients with neuropsychiatric SLE (Tokunaga, Saito et al. 2007). A monoclonal antibody was administered at doses of 375 mg/m$^2$ once weekly for four weeks or 1000 mg once weekly for two weeks in 10 patients with refractory neuropsychiatric SLE. Treatment resulted in rapid improvement of CNS-related manifestations, particularly acute confusional state. Rituximab also improved cognitive dysfunction psychosis and seizure and reduced the SLEDAI on day 28 in all 10 patients. These effects lasted for more than a year in 5 patients. In another study, Smith et al. (Smith, Jones et al. 2006) evaluated prospectively the effects of rituximab treatment for refractory SLE and vasculitis. Patients received four weekly infusions of rituximab at a dose of 375 mg/m$^2$. Intravenous cyclophosphamide (500 mg) was administered along with the first infusion in an effort to achieve early disease control. Remission followeing rapid B cell depletion was achieved in all 11 patients including 6 complete responses and 5 partial responses. Moreover, a renal response occurred in all 6 patients with lupus nephritis. Clinical improvement was accompanied by a significant reduction in the daily dose of prednisone. Seven of 11 patients experienced a relapse, a median of 12 months after treatment. After relapse, six patients with SLE were re-treated with rituximab and all achieved remission and did so more quickly than after the primary treatment.

Rituximab is generally well tolerated. Even fewer adverse events have been observed in patients treated for SLE than in the lymphoma patients (Tokunaga, Saito et al. 2007). The most common adverse events during or following rituximab therapy are infusion related symptoms, typically fever, chills, rigors and hypotension. In patients who receive premedication consisting of antipyretic and antihistaminic drugs together with corticosteroids, infusion-related side effects are usually only mild or moderate and do not require discontinuation of rituximab administration. Occasionally, serious infections were also reported. However, these may have been related to the underlying disease and/or concomitant therapy with other immunosuppressive agents. In 2006, an FDA alert was reported after two SLE patients treated with rituximab had died from progressive multifocal leukoencephalopathy (PML) (Ermann and Bermas 2007). However, both patients had received additional treatment with cyclophosphamide. At present, it is difficult to estimate the risk of this complication in SLE patients treated with rituximab. In recent analysis, among the rheumatic diseases, 43 cases of PML (0.44%) were associated with SLE, 24 (0.25%)

with rheumatoid arthritis (RA), and 25 (0.26%) with other connective tissue diseases (CTDs) (Molloy and Calabrese 2009). Additional controlled studies with new designs are needed to define the place of rituximab in the therapeutic arsenal for SLE.

### 2.2 New generations of Anti-CD20 monoclonal antibodies

Over the last few years, new generations of anti-CD20 monoclonal antibodies have been developed for potential benefits over the classical, first-generation mAb rituximab. Compared with rituximab, new mAbs have enhanced antitumor activity resulting from increased CDC and ADCC, and increased Fc binding affinity for the low-affinity variants of the FcγRIIIa receptor (CD16) on immune effector cells (Czuczman & Gregory 2010).

#### 2.2.1 Ofatumumab

Ofatumumab (HuMax-CD20; Arzerra™, GlaxoSmithKline plc/Genmab A/S) is a second-generation, fully human, anti-CD20, IgG1 mAb in phase I, II and III trials for hematological malignancies and autoimmune diseases such as rheumatoid arthritis (RA) and multiple sclerosis. Ofatumumab specifically recognizes an epitope encompassing both the small and large extracellular loops of CD20 molecule, and is more effective than rituximab at CDC induction and killing target cells. In April 2010, the European Medicines Agency granted a conditional marketing authorization for ofatumumab, for the treatment of fludarabine-refractory CLL patients. It has been reported recently that ofatumumab, administered as 2 i.v. infusions at doses 300 mg, 700 mg, or 1,000 mg is clinically effective in patients with active RA (Østergaard , Baslund et al. 2010). Rapid and sustained peripheral B cell depletion was noted in all dose groups. Overall, 70% of patients receiving ofatumumab had a moderate or good response according to the European League Against Rheumatism (EULAR) criteria at week 24.

#### 2.2.2 Veltuzumab

Veltuzumab (IMMU-106, hA20; Immunomedics Inc., Morris Plains, NJ) is a second-generation, type 1, humanized, anti-CD20, IgG1 mAb with complementarity-determining regions (CDRs) similar to rituximab (Goldenberg, Rossi et al. 2009). This mAb is generated using the same human immunoglobulin as epratuzumab and has a >90% humanized framework. It is also very similar to rituximab in terms of antigen binding, specificity binding, and dissociation constant. Veltuzumab differs from rituximab by one amino acid (Asp101 instead of Asn101) in the CDR 3 of the variable heavy chain. Smaller murine regions may reduce infusion reactions, infusion times, and immunogenicity. This antibody has enhanced binding avidities and a stronger effect on CDC compared with rituximab in selected cell lines. Veltuzumab is safe and active agent in NHL. B cells were depleted after the first infusion of all tested doses, including dose levels less than those typically used with rituximab (Morschhauser, Leonard et al. 2009).

#### 2.2.3 Ocrelizumab

Ocrelizumab (Genentech Inc/Biogen Idec Inc/Chugai Pharmaceutical Co Ltd/Roche Holding Ag) is a second-generation, type 1, humanized, anti-CD20, IgG1 mAb with modifications of the Fc region that lead to enhanced ADCC and reduced CDC activities compared with rituximab (Kausar, Mustafa et al. 2009).This agent has the potential for enhanced efficacy compared with rituximab due to increased binding affinity for the low-affinity variants of the FcγRIIIa receptor on immune effector cells (Genovese, Kaine et al. 2008). Ocrelizumab binds to a different, but overlapping, epitope of the extracellular domain of CD20 as compared with rituximab. Ocrelizumab is a humanized mAb with the potential for enhanced efficacy in lymphoid malignancies compared with rituximab due to increased binding affinity for the low-affinity variants of the FcγRIIIa receptor (Faria & Isenberg 2010).

#### 2.2.4 GA-101

GA-101 (RO5072759) is a fully humanized, type II, IgG1 mAb derived from humanization of the parental B-Ly1 mouse antibody and subsequent glycoengineering using GlycoMab® technology. GA-101 was designed for enhanced ADCC and superior direct cell-killing properties, in comparison with currently available type I antibodies (Robak 2009). In contrast to rituximab GA101, mediated significant NK cell degranulation in whole blood samples. Thus, CDC and ADCC are believed to be the major effector mechanisms of GA101 in whole blood assays (Bologna, Gotti et al. 2011).

#### 2.2.5 TRU-015

TRU-015 (CytoxB20G, Trubion Pharmaceuticals Inc and Pfizer Inc) is a small modular immunopharmaceutical (SMIP) derived from key domains of an anti-CD20 antibody. TRU-015 represents a novel biological compound that retains Fc-mediated effector functions and is smaller than mAbs (Rubbert-Roth 2010). SMIPs belong to a novel proprietary biologic compound class that retain Fc-mediated effector functions and are smaller than mAbs (Robak, Robak et al. 2009). A SMIP molecule is a single-chain polypeptide consisting of one binding domain, one hinge domain, and one effector domain. The TRU-015 SMIP molecule is the homogeneous single-chain immunotherapeutic derived from key domains of an anti-CD20 antibody, for the potential intravenous infusion treatment of RA, SLE and B-cell lymphoid malignancies (Hayden-Ledbetter, Cerveny et al. 2009). This molecule is a compact dimer of 104 kDa that co-migrates with albumin in size exclusion chromatography and retains a long half-life *in vivo*. It is effective in mediating target cell killing in the mechanism of ADCC but has reduced CDC activity compared with rituximab. TRU-015 could represent a novel therapy for the treatment of SLE, although the efficacy, safety profile, and advantages of this compound compared with existing therapeutic options would need to be established in clinical trials (Burge, Bookbinder et al. 2008). TRU-015 has shown clinical efficacy and tolerability in phase IIa and IIb studies in patients with rheumatoid arthritis, and clinical development efforts for the treatment of lymphoma and inflammatory disease are ongoing. In the ongoing trial pharmacokinetics of TRU-015 after a single administration in subjects with membranous nephropathy secondary SLE is investigated (ClinicalTrials.gov Identifier: NCT00479622).

All new anti-CD20 mAbs are potentially useful in the treatment of SLE. However, the advantage of these new drugs over rituximab should be proven by well-designed clinical trials in rituximab-refractory patients or through head-to-head comparison.

## 3. Other B cell targeting monoclonal antibodies

### 3.1 Anti-CD22 antibody epratuzumab

Epratuzumab (Immunomedics, Inc.) is a humanized monoclonal IgG antibody that specifically targets the CD22 antigen on B cells (Leonard & Goldenberg 2007). This

monoclonal antibody is 90% to 95% of human origin thus greatly reducing the potential for immunogenicity. Unconjugated anti-CD22 antibodies only partially deplete B cells, but might deliver a negative signal by binding CD22 to the cell surface (Daridon, Blassfeld et al. 2010). Treatment of SLE patients with epratuzumab leads to a reduction of circulating CD27 negative B-cells, although epratuzumab is weakly cytotoxic to B-cells *in vitro*. Epratuzumab binding was higher on B-cells relative to T-cells. In addition, weak non-specific binding of epratuzumab on monocytes was noted. On B-cells, binding of epratuzumab was enhanced on CD27negative B-cells compared to CD27 positive B-cells, primarily related to a higher expression of CD22 on CD27negative B-cells. Epratuzumab also enhanced the migration of CD27negative B-cells towards the chemokine CXCL12.
Recently, Dorner et al. reported the results of an open-label, single-center study of 14 patients with moderately active SLE (Dörner, Kaufmann et al. 2006). Patients received 360 $mg/m^2$ of epratuzumab intravenously every 2 weeks for 4 doses with analgesic antihistamine premedication prior to each dose. Total BILAG scores decreased by ≥50% in all 14 patients at some point during the study with 92% having decrease in various amounts continuing to at least 18 weeks.
Epratuzumab toxicity consisted primarily of mild to moderate transient infusion-related events during the first infusion. These results support conducting multicenter controlled studies to examine the effects of epratuzumab in broader patient populations. A U.S. patent has been issued to Immunomedics, Inc. for epratuzumab as a potential new treatment for lupus.

### 3.2 Anti-BlyS monoclonal antibodies

The B-lymphocyte Stimulator (BLyS) and A Proliferatiave Inducing Ligand (APRIL) are ligands for receptors BAFF-R (B Cell Activation Factor), BCMA (B Cell Maturation Associate) and TACI (Transmembrane Activator and Calcium Reproducing Initiator). BLyS also known as BAFF, THANK, TALL-1 or zTNF4, is a member of TNF super-family, which stimulates immunoglobulin (Ig) production by binding to specific receptors (King and Hahn 2007). In patients with SLE, the serum levels of BLyS are elevated and its neutralization has suggested that higher levels of BLyS contribute to the generation of autoantibodies and is important in SLE pathogenesis (Toubi, Kessel et al. 2006). In consequence, neutralization of BLyS may play a role in the therapy of this disease.

#### 3.2.1 Belimumab

Belimumab (Human Genome Sciences, (Rockville, MD, USA)/Glaxo Smith Kline, (Uxbridge, UK)) is a fully human IgG1 mAb that specifically binds and inhibits the biological activity of BLyS (Wiglesworth, Ennis et al. 2010). The antibody exerts its biological activity by preventing the binding of BLyS to its receptors, resulting in autoreactive B cell apoptosis (Baker, Edwards et al. 2003). It also inhibits soluble BLyS activity at subnanomolar concentrations in a murine model. Belimumab inhibits also BLyS- induced proliferation of B-cells *in vitro* and prevents human BLyS-induced increases in splenic B-cell numbers and serum IgA titers in mice.
The safety, tolerability, immunogenicity, and pharmacology of belimumab were investigated in a phase I, randomized, placebo controlled, double-blind study in patients with SLE (Furie, Stohl et al. 2008). Seventy patients with mild to moderate disease were enrolled in this trial. Fifty-seven patients were treated with mAb and 13 with placebo. The drug was administered at 4 different doses (1.0, 4.0, 10 and 20 mg/kg) as single infusions, 21

days apart. The incidence of adverse events and laboratory abnormalities was similar among the belimumab and placebo groups. A significant reduction in the median percentage of CD20+ B-cells was noted with a one and two doses of belimumab versus placebo. However, SLE activity did not change after treatment with this mAb.

Wallace et al. assessed the safety, tolerability, biological activity, and efficacy of belimumab in combination with standard of care therapy in patients with active SLE (Wallace, Stohl et al. 2009). In this phase II, randomized trial 449 patients with SELENA-SLEDAI score ≥ 4 were randomly assigned to belimumab (1, 4, 10 mg/kg) or placebo in a 52-week study. In this study, belimumab treatment did not result in significant improvement compared with placebo. Percentage change in the SELENA-SLEDAI score at week 24, the primary endpoint of the study, was similar in both arms (19.5% in the belimumab group versus 17.2% in the placebo group). There was no significant difference in time to first SFI-defined flare over 52 weeks between the belimumab and placebo groups (67 versus 83 days, respectively). However, the median time to first SLE flare during weeks 24–52 was significantly longer with belimumab treatment (154 versus 108 days; P=0.0361). During the 52-week study and 8-week follow-up period, the incidence of AEs were similar in all treatment groups, including placebo. Only urticaria was statistically more frequent in belimumab-treated patients (4% versus 0%).

The efficacy and safety of belimumab in patients with active SLE was also assessed in a large, randomized, multicenter study recently reported by Navarra et al 2011 (Navarra, Guzmán et al. 2011). In this trial, 865 patients with scores of at least 6 on the Safety of Estrogens in Lupus Erythematosus National Assessment-Systemic Lupus Erythematosus Disease Activity Index (SELENA-SLEDAI) were randomly assigned to belimumab 1 mg/kg or 10 mg/kg, or placebo by intravenous infusion in 1 h on days 0, 14, and 28, and then every 28 days until 48 weeks, with standard of care. Significantly higher Systemic Lupus Erythematosus Responder Index (SRI) rates were noted with belimumab 1 mg/kg (51%, P=0.0129) and 10 mg/kg (58%, p=0.006) than with placebo (44%) at week 52. In addition, more patients had SELENA-SLEDAI score reduced by at least 4 points during 52 weeks with belimumab 1 mg/kg (53%, P=0.0189) and 10 mg/kg (58%, P=0.0024) than with placebo (46%). Moreover, more patients receiving belimumab 1 mg/kg (78%, P=0.1064) and 10 mg/kg (81%, P=0.0181) had no new BILAG A or no more than 1 new B flare than did those receiving placebo (73%). There was no difference in rates of adverse events in patients given belimumab 1 mg/kg and 10 mg/kg, and placebo. Serious infection was noted in 8%, 4%, and 6% patients, respectively. Severe or serious hypersensitivity reactions on an infusion day were reported in four patients.

### 3.2.2 LY2127399

Anti-BAFF monoclonal antibody LY2127399 (Eli Lilly & Company Limited) is a fully human IgG4 antibody with neutralizing activity against both membrane-bound and soluble BAFF. This may reduce the activity, proliferation and survival of B-cells. The ongoing study evaluates the efficacy, safety and tolerability of two different doses of LY2127399 administered in addition to standard of care therapy in patients with active SLE (ClinicalTrials.gov Identifier: NCT01205438).

## 4. Monoclonal antibodies inhibiting T cell costimulation

Cytotoxic lymphocyte-associated antigen-4 (CTLA-4) is a potent inhibitor of the costimulation pathway necessary to activate T cells. Abatacept (CTLA-4 immunoglobulin; CTLA4-Ig,

Orencia) is a recombinant fully humanized fusion protein, composed of the extracellular domain of human CTLA-4 and a modified Fc part of IgG-1that was engineered to prevent complement fixation (St Clair 2009). It targets T cell activation by interfering with one of the costimulatory mechanisms that are essential for cell activation. CTLA4-Ig binds to B7-1 and B7-2 on antigen presenting cells and downregulates T cell activation by disrupting CD28-B7 costimulatory interaction. Abatacept blocks the interaction between CD28 expressed on the surface of T cells and CD80/CD86 on the surface of antigen-presenting cells. The drug was approved for RA by the FDA US (Food and Drug Administration) in 2005. Abatacept was compared to placebo in a randomized, placebo controlled, phase II trial of patients with active SLE characterized by arthritis, serositis, or rash (Merrill, Burgos-Vargas et al. 2010). SLE patients were randomized at a ratio of 2:1 to receive abatacept (10 mg/kg of body weight) or placebo. Prednisone (30 mg/day or equivalent) was given for 1 month, and then the dosage was tapered. There was no difference in the percentage of patients who experienced the primary endpoint of SLE flare, as defined by BILAG, over the course of 52 weeks. However, the investigators discerned a difference in flare rates between the abatacept group (64%) and placebo group (83%). This difference was especially pronounced in the subgroup of patients with arthritis. The frequency of adverse events was comparable in the abatacept and placebo groups (90.9% versus 91.5%), but serious adverse events were higher in the abatacept group (19.8 versus 6.8%). Most serious adverse events were single, disease-related events occurring during the first 6 months. Improvements in certain exploratory measures suggest that abatacept has some efficacy in patients with non-life-threatening manifestations of SLE.

## 5. Anticytokine monoclonal antibodies

In the course of SLE, a wide variety of cytokines is dysregulated, many of which are likely to influence autoimmunity and lupus tissue inflammation (La Cava. 2010; Robak, Kulczycka et al. 2007). They are not only involved in the immune dysregulation of SLE, but also in the local inflammatory response which ultimately leads to tissue injury. Proinflammatory cytokines such as tumor necrosis factor α (TNFα), iterleukin-6 (IL-6), IL-1 and interferon-γ (IFN-γ) may play an important role in propagating the inflammatory process responsible for tissue damage. IL-12, IL-15 and IL-18 are probably also involved in pathogenesis of SLE. The possibility of blocking the proinflammatory cascade by selective inactivation of cytokines can be a successful therapy for patients with SLE.

### 5.1 Anti-IL-6 monoclonal antibodies

Data from several studies suggests that IL-6 plays an important role in the B-cell hyperactivity and immunopathology of SLE (Klashman, Martin et al. 1991). One of the most important effects of IL-6 is to induce the maturation of B lymphocytes into plasma cells and augment the imunoglobulin secretion. IL-6 binds to the IL-6 receptors which belong to the type 1 cytokine receptor superfamily that consists of two subunits, namely the IL-6 R and the gp 130. This cytokine may have a direct influence in mediating tissue damage. Elevated levels of IL-6 were detected in the serum, urine and renal glomerulli of patients with active SLE and in murine models of SLE (Grondal, Gunnarsson et al. 2000).

Tocilizumab (ACTEMRA, MRA, Roche Pharmaceuticals) is a humanized anti-human IL-6R mAb considered as a therapeutic option for patients with SLE. It is an antibody which inhibits the interleukin-6 receptor. It binds to both soluble IL-6R and transmembrane IL-6R

and inhibit IL-6 binding to its receptors, leading to the blockade of IL-6 signaling through both receptors (Jones and Ding 2010). Tocilizumab suppresses the biological activity of IL-6 and is now being used in clinical trials for RA and SLE (ClinicalTrials.gov Identifier: NCT00046774). An intraperitoneal administration of an anti-IL-6 mAb decreased the production of anti-ds DNA antibodiess in murine model of SLE and prevented the development of severe kidney disease. These results suggest that treatment with anti-IL-6 mAb has a beneficial effect on autoimmunity in murine SLE and that autoreactive B cells may be the primary target for anti-IL-6 antibody treatment (Liang, Gardner et al. 2006).
Tocilizumab is an effective agent in all the stages of RA (Jones, Sebba et al. 2010). Tocilizumab is the first agent that has been shown to be superior to methotrexate (MTX) as monotherapy for the signs and symptoms of this disease. It is also an active drug in SLE patients. Tocilizumab when used in mild to moderate lupus patient has demonstrated preliminary success and good tolerability in an open-label phase I dosage-escalation study (Illei, Shirota et al. 2010). In this trial 16 patients with mild-to-moderate disease activity were assigned to receive 1 of 3 doses of tocilizumab given intravenously every other week for total of 7 infusions: 2 mg/kg in 4 patients, 4 mg/kg in 6 patients, or 8 mg/kg in 6 patients. Patients were then monitored for an additional 8 weeks. The median decrease in anti-dsDNA antibody levels at week 14 was −9 IU/ml ($P = 0.03$). There was improvement in overall disease activity over the course of treatment. Mean SLAM scores decreased from 7.1 at baseline to 5.0 at week 14 ($P = 0.002$), and mean mSELENA–SLEDAI scores decreased from 9.5 to 5.5 ($P = 0.001$). In addition, there was no SLE flare during the treatment period. The infusions were well tolerated, without any clinically significant infusion reactions. However, the treatment induced dosage-related decreases in the absolute neutrophil count, with a median decrease of 38% in the 4 mg/kg dosage group and 56% in the 8 mg/kg dosage group. Infections were observed in 11 patients between the start of study treatment and the end of the follow up period. This study provides the first evidence that treatment with tocilizumab has an acceptable safety profile and suggests a possible immunologic and clinical benefit in SLE.

### 5.2 Anti-IL 10 monoclonal antibody

Interleukin-10 (IL-10) is a cytokine produced mainly by monocytes and lymphocytes. It impedes the activation of antigen presenting cells, down-regulates the expression of co-stimulatory molecules and blunts T cell activation and TNF-α secretion. IL-10 boosts B cell proliferation and immunoglobulin class switching resulting in enhanced antibody secretion with the capacity to enter extravascular compartments and promote inflammation in SLE (Yap & Lai 2010). The levels of IL-10 increase in the serum of patients with active SLE and correlates with disease activity. Alteration in IL-10 regulation may result in accelerated T-cell apoptosis and aberrant T-cell dependent B-cell function. In animal models of lupus nephritis, anti-IL 10 blockade offered some benefits in limiting renal damage (Ravirajan, Wang et al. 2004). The beneficial effect of a combined therapy using both anti-IL-10 and anti-C5 mAb to prevent or reduce the effect of the humoral immune response in lupus disease was also suggested. Preliminary data has shown that anti-IL-10 monoclonal antibody improved cutaneous lesions, joint symptoms, and SLEDAI in lupus patients (Llorente, Richaud-Patin et al. 2000). The anti-IL-10 monoclonal antibody was administered to six patients with steroid resistant SLE in an open label pilot study. Treatment consisted of an 20 mg/day intravenous administration of an anti-IL-10 murine mAb (B-N10) for 21 consecutive days, with a follow-up period of 6 months. Therapy was well tolerated and marked improvement in skin lesions and joint symptoms was observed in all patients over the next 6 months. Furthermore, three times lower doses of prednisone were used. The study indicates that the use of IL-10 antagonists may be beneficial in the management of refractory SLE.

## 6. Anti-CD40 and anti-CD40L monoclonal antibodies

CD40, a member of the tumor necrosis factor receptor super family, is highly expressed in normal B-cells and a variety of B-cell malignancies. CD40 ligand, also called CD154 or gp39, is a protein expressed on activated CD4+ T cells as well as on platelets, mast cells, macrophages, basophils, NK cells and B lymphocytes. An increased expression of CD40L has been found in the peripheral lymphocytes of patients with active SLE (Devi, Van Noordin et al. 1998). Moreover, serum levels of CD154 (CD40L) are higher in lupus patients than in normal persons (van Kooten & Banchereau 2000). The high expression of CD154 on T and B cells may increase production of potentially harmful auto-antibodies. The results of preclinical studies indicate that lupus-prone mice treated with anti-CD40L Abs had diminished inflammation, reduced anti-DNA autoantibody production and prolonged survival. Prolonged administration was particularly helpful in preventing fibrosis in severely nephritic mice (Kalled, Cutler et al. 2001). These results prompted the testing of anti-CD40L mAbs in human SLE.

### 6.1 Anti-CD40 monoclonal antibodies

Two mAbs directed against CD40 have been developed and investigated in preclinical studies and clinical trials, lucatumumab (HCD122) and dacetuzumab (SGN-40) (Kelley, Gelzleichter et al. 2006).

#### 6.1.1 Lucatumumab

Lucatumumab ((HCD122, CHIR-0.12.12; Novartis Pharmaceuticals) is a fully human anti-CD40 mAb directed against the B-cell surface antigen CD40. It blocks CD40/CD40L interactions *in vitro* and inhibits CD40L-induced proliferation of human peripheral blood lymphocytes without disturbing baseline lymphocyte proliferation. Lucatumumab triggers cell lysis via ADCC in cells overexpressing CD40 (Luqman, Klabunde et al. 2008).

#### 6.1.2 Dacetuzumab

Dacetuzumab (Seattle Genetics, Inc), is another humanized anti-CD40 IgG1 mAb, which induces ADCC and apoptosis of normal and malignant B-cells (Kelley, Gelzleichter et al. 2006). Dacetuzumab is able to initiate multiple signalling cascades upon ligation of CD40 on NHL cell lines. Dacetuzumab-mediated cytotoxicity is associated with up-regulation of cytotoxic ligands of the tumor necrosis factor (TNF) family including Fas/FasL, TNF-related apoptosis-inducing ligand, and TNFalpha.

### 6.2 Anti-CD40L monoclonal antibodies

#### 6.2.1 IDEC-131

IDEC-131/E6040 (Idec Pharmaceuticals Corp. San Diego) is a humanized mAb against human CD154, comprising human $\gamma 1$ heavy chains and human $\kappa$ light chains with complementarity-determining regions of murine mAb clone 24-31. In Phase I clinical trial, IDEC-131 was administered in a single intravenous infusion at doses of 0.05-15.0 mg/kg in patients with SLE. Patients were followed for 3 months to evaluate toxicity and pharmacokinetics (Davis, Totoritis et al. 2001). All patients experienced at least one adverse event. However, no infusion related cytokine-release syndrome was observed and all patients completed treatment. In a phase II, double blind, placebo-controlled, multiple-center, multiple-dose study, 85 patients with mild-to-moderately active SLE were randomized to receive 6 infusions of IDEC-131, ranging from 2.5 mg/kg to 10.0 mg/kg, or placebo over 16 weeks (Kalunian, Davis et al. 2002). At week 20, the mean change from baseline total SLEDAI scores indicated improvement in disease activity within each treatment group. In addition, the median global BILAG scores at week 20 indicated a reduction in SLE activity. However, results did not differ among the IDEC-131 treatment and placebo groups, and no dose-response relationship was noted at week 20. Moreover, the changes in levels of anti-dsDNA antibody and serum complement were not statistically significant in any group or between treatment groups and placebo. In addition, the changes in levels of anti-dsDNA antibody and serum complement were not different between treatment groups and placebo. The adverse events were also similar between the IDEC-131 and placebo groups.

### 6.2.2 BG9588

BG9588 (Biogen, Inc., Cambridge, MA) is a recombinant humanized anti-human CD40L monoclonal antibody that specifically binds to the CD40 ligand expressed on the surface of activated T lymphocytes. It blocks the CD40L/CD40 interaction between T and B cells that is required for the initiation for certain antibody responses. A short course of BG9588 treatment in patients with proliferative lupus nephritis reduced anti-dsDNA antibodies, increased C3 concentrations, and decreased hematuria (Boumpas, Furie et al. 2003). These results indicate that the drug has immunomodulatory action. Additional studies will be needed to evaluate its long-term effects.

## 7. Anticomplement antibody

Patients with SLE have widespread activation and deposition of the complement fragment in affected tissues. In murine models of SLE, the administration of the anti-C5 monoclonal antibody delayed the onset of proteinuria and prolonged survival. Moreover, pharmacological blockade of C5 receptor with a specific receptor antagonist reduces disease manifestation in experimental lupus nephritis (Cordeiro & Isenberg 2008). Furthermore, in mice with renal disease induced by a human anti-dsDNA antibody, RH-14 anti-C5 monoclonal antibody significantly reduced proteinuria.

Eculizumab (Soliris; Alexion Pharmaceuticals, Inc., Cheshire, CT) is a recombinant humanized monoclonal antibody that works by binding to complement protein C5, inhibiting its enzymatic cleavage, blocking formation of the terminal complement complex, and thus preventing red cell lysis (Parker , Kar et al. 2007). It has a molecular weight of 148 kD. Eculizumab is approved for the treatment of paroxysmal nocturnal hemoglobinuria (PNH) (Hillmen, Young et al. 2006). This antibody is potentially useful for treating patients with lupus nephritis. In this disease, the terminal components of the complement C5b-C9 play an important role in mediating the inflammation and the damage of podocytes and glomerular basement membrane (Robak & Robak 2009). Eculizumab has been recently developed and investigated in a phase I single dose study in SLE.

| MoAb | Target | Antibody characteristics |
|---|---|---|
| Rituximab | CD20 | Type I, 1st generation $IgG_{1-\kappa}$, mAb, containing murine light- and heavy-chain variable-region sequences and human constant region sequences |
| Ocrelizumab | CD20 | Type I, 2nd generation, humanized fusion $IgG_1$, binding to different CD20 epitope than rituximab, enhanced ADCC, reduced CDC, enhanced affinity for FcγRIIIa RIIIa |
| Veltuzumab (IMMU-106, hA20) | CD20 | Type I, 2nd generation, humanized $IgG_1$, binding to different CD20 epitope than rituximab, enhanced ADCC, reduced CDC, enhanced affinity for FcγRIIIa RIIIa |
| Ofatumumab (HuMax-CD20, (Arzerra) | CD20 | Type I, 2nd generation, Human $IgG_1$, binding to different CD20 epitope, more effective at CDC than rituximab |
| GA-101 (RO5072759) | CD20 | Type II, 3rdgeneration, humanized $IgG_1$, superior ADCC than rituximab and superior direct cell-killing ability |
| AME-133v (LY2469298) | CD20 | Type I, 3rd generation, humanized fusion $IgG_1$, enhanced affinity for FcγRIIIa, superior ADCC |
| PRO131921 | CD20 | Type I, 3rd generation, humanized fusion IgG1, improved binding to FcγRIIIa, better ADCC, superior anti-tumor efficacy |
| TRU-015 | CD20 | SMIP derived humanized fusion protein, ADCC and apoptosis induction |
| Epratuzumab (hLL2) | CD22 | Humanized $IgG_{1-\kappa}$, 90% to 95% of human origin , acting as an immunomodulatory agent, stimulating the CD22 molecule |
| Belimumab | BLyS | Fully human $IgG_1$ mAb that specifically binds and inhibits the biological activity of BLyS |
| Abatacept | B7-1 and B7-2 | Recombinant fully humanized fusion protein, composed of the Extracellular domain of human CTLA-4 and a modified Fc part of $IgG_1$ |
| Tocilizumab (ACTEMRA, MRA) | IL-6R | Recombinant, humanised monoclonal $IgG_1$ antihuman interleukin 6-receptor antibody |
| IDEC-131 | CD40L | IDEC-131/E6040, humanized mAb against human CD154, comprising human $\gamma_1$ heavy chains and human $\kappa$ light chains with complementarity-determining regions of murine mAb clone 24-31 |
| BG9588 | CD40L | Recombinant humanized anti-human CD40L mAb consists of the complementarity-determining regions of the murine monoclonal antibody 5c8 (anti-human CD40L antibody) with human variable-region framework residues and $IgG_1$ constant region |

| MoAb | Target | Antibody characteristics |
|---|---|---|
| Lucatumumab (HCD122, CHIR-0.12.12) | CD40 | Human $IgG_1$ mAb that blocks CD40/CD40L interactions and inducesADCC |
| Dacetuzumab (SGN-40) | CD40 | Humanized anti-CD40 $IgG_1$ mAb, which induces ADCC and apoptosis of B-cells |
| Eculizumab | Comple mentpro-tein C5 | Recombinant humanized mAb binding to complement protein C5, inhibiting its enzymatic cleavage, blocking formation of the terminal complement complex |

ADCC=antibody-dependent cellular cytotoxicity; BLyS=B-lymphocyte Stimulator;
CDC=complement-dependent cytotoxicity; mAb= monoclonal antibody;
SMIP=small modular immunopharmaceutical

Table 1. Monoclonal antibodies potentially useful in systemic lupus erythematosus

## 8. Conclusions

In recent years, clinical studies have been undertaken with selected mAbs in the treatment of SLE. The most frequently used mAb is rituximab, which is directed against CD20, a membrane protein expressed on B lymphocytes. Rituximab is effective in depleting B cells from peripheral blood, lymph nodes and bone marrow. Recent clinical studies confirm the high activity of rituximab in SLE patients, especially with lupus nephritis and neuropsychiatric involvement. Rituximab was generally well tolerated. However, occasionaly serious infections were reported. Over the last few years new generations of anti-CD20 mAbs have been developed for potential benefits over rituximab. They were engineered to have augmented antitumor activity by increasing CDC or ADCC activity and increased Fc binding affinity for the low-affinity variants of the FcγRIIIa receptor (CD16) on immune effector cells. This mAbs are are highly cytotoxic against B-cell lymphoid cells and are now being evaluated in clinical trials.

More recently, several newer mAbs have been developed and are being evaluated in phase I/II clinical trials. These include anti-cytokine therapies anti-CD40L mAbs, anti-CD-22 mAb, anti-BLys mAbs and anti- C5 mAbs. Belimumab is a fully human monoclonal antibody that binds to BLyS and inhibits its biological activity. Significantly positive results in both phase 3 studies have raised hopes that belimumab may be the long-awaited new effective therapy for SLE. Proinflammatory cytokines such as tumor necrosis factor (TNF) and interleukin- 6 (IL-6) play an important role in propagating the inflammatory process responsible for tissue damage. Blocking of these cytokines by mAbs can be also a successful therapy for patients with SLE. Finally, mAb eculizumab that specifically inhibits terminal complement activation has been recently developed and investigated in a phase I single dose study in SLE. These potentially useful agents should be further evaluated in well designed controlled trials.

## 9. Acknowledgements

This work was supported in part by the grants from the Medical University of Lodz (No 503-1093-1 and No No 503-1019-1). The authors have no conflicts of interest that are directly relevant to the content of this chapter.

## 10. References


Baker, K.P.; Edwards, B.M.; Main, S.H. et al. (2003) Generation and characterization of LymphoStat-B, a human monoclonal antibody that antagonizes the bioactivities of B lymphocyte stimulator. *Arthritis Rheum.*, Vol.48. No 11, pp. 3253-3265, ISSN 1044-2626

Bologna, L.; Gotti, E.; Manganini, M. et al. (2011). Mechanism of Action of Type II, Glycoengineered, Anti- CD20 Monoclonal Antibody GA101 in B-Chronic Lymphocytic Leukemia Whole Blood Assays in Comparison with Rituximab and Alemtuzumab. *J Immunol.*, Vol. 186, No. 6, pp. 3762-3769, ISSN 0022-1767

Boumpas, D.T.; Furie, R.; Manzi, S. et al. (2003). BG9588 Lupus Nephritis Trial Group. A short course of BG9588 (anti-CD40 ligand antibody) improves serologic activity and decreases hematuria in patients with proliferative lupus glomerulonephritis. *Arthritis Rheum.*, Vol. 48, No 3, pp. 719–727, ISSN 1044-2626

Burge, D.J.; Bookbinder, S.A.; Kivitz, A.J. et al. (2008). Pharmacokinetic and pharmacodynamic properties of TRU-015, a CD20-directed small modular immunopharmaceutical protein therapeutic, in patients with rheumatoid arthritis: a phase I, open-label, dose-escalation clinical study. *Clin Ther*, Vol. 30, No 10, pp. 1806-1816, ISSN 0149-2918

Cambridge, G.; Isenberg, D.A.; Edwards, J.C. et al. B cell depletion therapy in systemic lupus erythematosus: relationships among serum B lymphocyte stimulator levels, autoantibody profile and clinical response. *Ann Rheum Dis*,. Vol. 67, No. 7, pp. 1011-1016, ISSN 0003-4967

Cordeiro, A.C. & Isenberg, D.A. (2008). Novel therapies in lupus - focus on nephritis. *Acta Reumatol Port.*, Vol. 33, No. 2, pp. 157-169, ISSN 0303-464X

Czuczman, M.S. & Gregory SA. (2010). The future of CD20 monoclonal antibody therapy in B-cell malignancies. *Leuk Lymphoma.*, Vol. 51, No. 6, pp. 983-994, ISSN 1042-8194

Daridon, C.; Blassfeld, D. Reiter, K. et al. (2010). Epratuzumab targeting of CD22 affects adhesion molecule expression and migration of B-cells in systemic lupus erythematosus. *Arthritis Res Ther.*, Vol. 12, No. 6, pp. R204, ISSN 1478-6362

Davis, J.C. Jr.; Totoritis, MC.; Rosenberg, J. et al. (2001). Phase I clinical trial of a monoclonal antibody against CD40-ligand (IDEC-131) in patients with systemic lupus erythematosus.*J Rheumatol*, Vol. 28, No. 1, pp. 95-101, ISSN 0315-162X

Devi, B.S.; Van Noordin, S.; Krausz, T. & Davies, K.A. (1998). Peripheral blood lymphocytes in SLE—hyperexpression of CD154 on T and B lymphocytes and increased number of double negative T cells. *J Autoimmun.*, Vol. 11, No 5, pp. 471–475, ISSN 0896-8411

Dörner, T.; Kaufmann, J.; Wegener, W.A. et al. (2006). Initial clinical trial of epratuzumab (humanized anti-CD22 antibody) for immunotherapy of systemic lupus erythematosus. *Arthritis Res Ther.*, Vol. 8, No. 3, pp. R74, ISSN 1478-6362

Ermann, J.; Bermas, B.L. (2007). The biology behind the new therapies for SLE. *Int. J. Clin. Pract.*, Vol. 61, No. 12, pp. 2113-2119, ISSN 1368-5031

Faria, R.M. & Isenberg, DA. (2010). Three different B-cell depletion (anti-CD20 monoclonal antibodies) treatments for severe resistant systemic lupus erythematosus. *Lupus.*, Vol. 19, No. 10, pp. 1256-1257, ISSN 0961-2033

Furie, R.; Stohl, W.; Ginzler, E.M.; Becker, M.; Mishra, N.; Chatham, W.W, Merrill, J.T.; Weinstein, A.; McCune, W.J.; Zhong, J.; Cai, W.; Freimuth, W. (2008). Biologic activity and safety of belimumab, a neutralizing anti-B-lymphocyte stimulator (BLyS) monoclonal antibody: a phase I trial in patients with systemic lupus erythematosus. Study Group B. *Arthritis Res Ther.*, Vol 110, No 5, R109, ISSN 1478-6362

Genovese, M.C.; Kaine, J.L.; Lowenstein, M.B. et al. (2008). Ocrelizumab, a humanized anti-CD20 monoclonal antibody, in the treatment of patients with rheumatoid arthritis: a phase I/II randomized, blinded, placebo-controlled, dose-ranging study. *Arthritis Rheum*, Vol. 58, No 9, pp. 2652-2661, ISSN 1044-2626

Goldenberg, D.M.; Rossi, E.A., Stein, R. et al. (2009). Properties and structure-function relationships of veltuzumab (hA20), a humanized anti-CD20 monoclonal antibody. *Blood*, Vol. 113, No 5, pp. 1062-1070, ISSN 0006-4971

Grondal, G.; Gunnarsson, I.; Ronnelid, J. et al. (2000). Cytokine production, serum levels and disease activity in systemic lupus erythematosus. *Clin Exp Rheumatol*, Vol. 18, No 5, pp. 565–570, ISSN 0392-856X

Hayden-Ledbetter, M.S.; Cerveny, C.G.; Espling, E. et al. (2009). CD20-directed small modular immunopharmaceutical, TRU-015, depletes normal and malignant B cells. *Clin Cancer Res*, Vol. 15, No 8, pp. 2739-2746 , ISSN 1557-3265

Hauptrock, B.& Hess, G. (2009). Rituximab in the treatment of non-Hodgkin's lymphoma. *Biologics*, Vol. 2, No. 4, pp.619-633 , ISSN 1177-5491

Hillmen, P, Young NS, Schubert J, et al. (2006). The complement inhibitor eculizumab in paroxysmal nocturnal hemoglobinuria. *N Engl J Med.*, Vol. 355, No 12, pp. 1233-1243, ISSN 0028-4793

Illei, G.G; Shirota, Y.; Yarboro, C.H. et al. (2010). Tocilizumab in systemic lupus erythematosus: data on safety, preliminary efficacy, and impact on circulating plasma cells from an open-label phase I dosage-escalation study. *Arthritis Rheum.* Vol. 62, No. 2, pp. 542-552, ISSN 1044-2626

Jones, G. & Ding, C. (2010). Tocilizumab: a review of its safety and efficacy in rheumatoid arthritis. *Clin Med Insights Arthritis Musculoskelet Disord.*, Vol. 19, No. 3, pp. 81-89, ISSN 1179-5441

Jones, G.; Sebba, A.; Gu, J. et al. (2010). Comparison of TCZ monotherapy versus methotrexate monotherapy in patients with moderate to severe rheumatoid arthritis: The AMBITION study. *Ann Rheum Dis.* Vol. 69, No 1, pp. 88–96, ISSN 0003-4967

Kalled, S.L.; Cutler, A.H.; Ferrant, J.L. (2001). Long-term anti-CD154 dosing in nephritic mice is required to maintain survival and inhibit mediators of renal fibrosis. *Lupus*, Vol. 10, No 1, pp. 9–22, ISSN 0961-2033

Kalunian, K.C.; Davis, J.C. Jr.; Merrill, J.T. et al. (2002). IDEC-131 Lupus Study Group. Treatment of systemic lupus erythematosus by inhibition of T cell costimulation with anti-CD154: a randomized, double-blind, placebo-controlled trial. *Arthritis Rheum.*, Vol. 46, No 12, pp. 3251–3258, ISSN 1044-2626

Kausar, F.; Mustafa, K.; Sweis, G. et al. (2009). Ocrelizumab: a step forward in the evolution of B-cell therapy. *Expert Opin Biol Ther*, Vol. 9, No pp. 889-895, ISSN 1471-2598

Kelley, S.K.; Gelzleichter, T.; Xie, D. et al (2006). Preclinical pharmacokinetics, pharmacodynamics, and activity of a humanized anti-CD40 antibody (SGN-40) in rodents and non-human primates. *Br J Pharmacol* Vol. 148, No 8, pp. 1116-1123, ISSN 1476-5381

King, J.K. & Hahn, B.H. (2007). Systemic lupus erythematosus: modern strategies for management: a moving target. *Best Pract Res Clin Rheumatol,*. Vol. 21, No. 6, pp. 971-987, ISSN 1521-6942

Klashman, D.J.; Martin, R.A.; Martinez-Maza, O. & Stevens R.H. (1991). In vitro regulation of B cell differentiation by interleukin-6 and soluble CD23 in systemic lupus erythematosus B cell subpopulations and antigen-induced normal B cells. *Arthritis Rheum.*, Vol. 34, No. 3, pp. 276–286, ISSN 1044-2626

La Cava, A. (2010). Anticytokine therapies in systemic lupus erythematosus. *Immunotherapy,*. Vol. 2, No. 4, pp. 575-582.

La Cava, A. (2010). Targeting B cells with biologics in systemic lupus erythematosus. Expert Opinion *on Biological Therapy,* Vol. 10, No. 11, pp. 1555-1561, ISSN 1471-2598

Liang, B.; Gardner, D.B.; Griswold, D.E. et al. (2006). Anti-interleukin-6 monoclonal antibody inhibits autoimmune responses in a murine model of systemic lupus erythematosus. *Immunology,* Vol. 119, No 3, pp. 296–305, ISSN 0022-1767

Lim, S.H.; Beers, S.A.; French R.R. et al. (2010). Anti-CD20 monoclonal antibodies: historical and future perspectives. *Haematologica.,* Vol. 95, No 1, pp. 135-43, ISSN 0390-6078

Leandro, M.J.; Cambridge, G.; Edwards, J.C. et al. (2005). B-cell depletion in the treatment of patients with systemic lupus erythematosus: a longitudinal analysis of 24 patients. *Rheumatology,* Vol. 44, No. 12, pp. 1542-1545, ISSN 0315-162X

Leonard, J.P. & Goldenberg, D.M. (2007). Preclinical and clinical evaluation of epratuzumab (anti-CD22 IgG) in B-cell malignancies. *Oncogene,* Vol. 26, No. 25, pp. 3704-13, ISSN 0950-9232

Llorente, L.; Richaud-Patin, Y.; Garcia-Padilla, C. et al. (2000). Clinical and biologic effects of anti-interleukin-10 monoclonal antibody administration in systemic Lupus erythematosus. *Arthritis Rheum.* Vol. 43, No. 8, pp. 1790 - 1800, ISSN 1044-2626

Lu, T.Y.; Ng, K.P.; Cambridge, G. et al. (2009). A retrospective seven-year analysis of the use of B cell depletion therapy in systemic lupus erythematosus at University College London Hospital: the first fifty patients. *Arthritis Rheum,* Vol. 61, No.4, pp. 482-487, ISSN 1044-2626

Luqman, M.; Klabunde, S. Lin, K. et al (2008).The antileukemia activity of a human anti-CD40 antagonist antibody, HCD122, on human chronic lymphocytic leukemia cells. *Blood* , Vol. 112, No 3, pp. 711-720, ISSN 0006-4971

Merrill, J.T.; Burgos-Vargas, R., Westhovens, R. et al. (2010). The efficacy and safety of abatacept in patients with non-life-threatening manifestations of systemic lupus erythematosus: results of a twelve-month, multicenter, exploratory, phase IIb, randomized, double-blind, placebo-controlled trial. *Arthritis Rheum.* Vol.62, No.10, pp. 3077-3087, ISSN 1044-2626

Merrill, J.T.; Neuwelt, C.M.; Wallace, D.J. et al. (2010). Efficacy and safety of rituximab in moderately-to-severely active systemic lupus erythematosus: the randomized, double-blind, phase II/III systemic lupus erythematosus evaluation of rituximab trial. *Arthritis Rheum.*, Vol. 62, No. 1, pp. 222-233, ISSN 1044-2626

Molloy, E.S.& Calabrese, LH. (2008). Progressive multifocal leukoencephalopathy: a national estimate of frequency in systemic lupus erythematosus and other rheumatic diseases. *Arthritis Rheum.*, Vol. 60, No. 12, pp. 3761-5, ISSN 1044-2626

Morschhauser, F.; Leonard, J.P.; Fayad, L. et al. (2009). Humanized anti-CD20 antibody, veltuzumab, in refractory/recurrent non-Hodgkin's lymphoma: phase I/II results. *J Clin Oncol.* Vol. 27, No. 20, pp. 3346-3353, ISSN 0732-183X

Navarra, S.V.; Guzmán, R.M.; Gallacher, A.E. et al. BLISS-52 Study Group. (2011). Efficacy and safety of belimumab in patients with active systemic lupus erythematosus: a randomised, placebo-controlled, phase 3 trial. *Lancet.*, Vol. 377, No. 9767, pp. 721-731, ISSN 0140-6736

Ng, K.P.; Cambridge, G., Leandro, M.J. et al. (2007). B cell depletion therapy in systemic lupus erythematosus: long-term follow-up and predictors of response. *Ann Rheum Dis,.* Vol. 66, No. 9, pp. 1259-62, ISSN 0003-4967

Østergaard, M.; Baslund, B.; Rigby, W. et al. (2010). Ofatumumab, a human anti-CD20 monoclonal antibody, for treatment of rheumatoid arthritis with an inadequate response to one or more disease-modifying antirheumatic drugs: results of a randomized, double-blind, placebo-controlled, phase I/II study. *Arthritis Rheum.*, Vol. 62, No. 8, pp. 2227-2238, ISSN 1044-2626

Parker, C.J.; Kar, S. & Kirkpatrick, P. (2007). Eculizumab. *Nat. Rev. Drug Discov.* Vol. 6, No 7, pp. 515–625, ISSN 1474-1776

Pepper, R.; Griffith, M.; Kirwan, C. et al. (2009). Rituximab is an effective treatment for lupus nephritis and allows a reduction in maintenance steroids. *Nephrol Dial Transplant.*, Vol. 24, No. 12, pp. 3717-3723, ISSN 0931-0509

Ravirajan, C.T.; Wang, Y.; Matis, L.A. et al. (2004) Effect of neutralizing antibodies to IL-10 and C5 on the renal damage caused by a pathogenic human anti-ds DNA antibody. *Rheumatology.* Vol. 43, No 4, pp. 442–447. , ISSN 0315-162X

Robak, T. (2004). Monoclonal antibodies in the treatment of autoimmune cytopenias. *Eur J f Haematol.*, Vol. 72, No. 2, pp.79-88, ISSN 0902-4441

Robak, E.; Kulczycka, L.; Sysa-Jedrzejowska, A. et al. (2007). Circulating proangiogenic molecules PIGF, SDF-1 and sVCAM-1 in patients with systemic lupus erythematosus. *Eur Cytokine Netw.*, Vol. 18, No. 4, pp. 181-7, ISSN 1148-5493

Robak, T. (2008). Ofatumumab, a human monoclonal antibody for lymphoid malignancies and autoimmune disorders. *Curr Opin Mol Ther.*, Vol. 10, No. 3, pp. 294-309, ISSN 1355-6568

Robak, T. (2009). GA-101, a third-generation, humanized and glyco-engineered anti-CD20 mAb for the treatment of B-cell lymphoid malignancies. *Curr Opin Investig Drugs.*, Vol. 10, No. 6, pp. 588-596, ISSN 1472-4472

Robak, T.; Robak, P. & Smolewski P. (2009). TRU-016, a humanized anti-CD37 IgG fusion protein for the potential treatment of B-cell malignancies. *Curr Opin Investig Drugs,* Vol. 10, No pp. 1383-1390, ISSN 1472-4472

Robak, E. & Robak, T. (2009). Monoclonal antibodies in the treatment of systemic lupus erythematosus. *Curr Drug Targets,*, Vol. 10, No 1, pp. 26–37, ISSN 1389-4501

Robak, T & Robak, E. (2011). New anti-CD20 monoclonal antibodies for the treatment of B-cell lymphoid malignancies. *BioDrugs,* 2011 Vol. 25, No. 1, pp.13-25, ISSN 1173-8804

Rubbert-Roth, A. (2010). TRU-015, a fusion protein derived from an anti-CD20 antibody, for the treatment of rheumatoid arthritis. *Curr Opin Mol Ther.,* Vol. 12, No. 1, pp. 115-123, ISSN 1355-6568

Ruuls, S.R.; Lammerts van Bueren J.J.; van de Winkel J.G. et al. (2008). Novel human antibody therapeutics: the age of the Umabs. *Biotechnol J,* Vol. 3, No pp. 1157-1171, ISSN 0268-2575

Schröder, J.O. & Zeuner, R.A. (2009). Biologics as treatment for systemic lupus: great efforts, sobering results, new challenges. *Current Drug Discovery Technologies* , Vol.6, No. 4, pp. 252-255, ISSN 1570-1638

Sfikakis, P.P.; Boletis, J.N.; Lionaki, S. et al. (2005). Remission of proliferative lupus nephritis following B cell depletion therapy is preceded by down-regulation of the T cell costimulatory molecule CD40 ligand: an open-label trial. *Arthritis Rheum,*. Vol. 52, No. 2, pp. 501-513, ISSN 1044-2626

Smith, K.G.; Jones, R.B.; Burns, S.M. & Jayne, D.R. (2006). Long-term comparison of rituximab treatment for refractory systemic lupus erythematosus and vasculitis: Remission, relapse, and re-treatment. *Arthritis Rheum.,* Vol. 54, No. 9, pp. 2970-82, ISSN 1044-2626

St Clair, E.W. (2009). Novel targeted therapies for autoimmunity. *Curr Opin Immunol.* Vol. 21, No. 6, pp.648-657, ISSN 0952-7915

Terrier, B.; Amoura, Z.; Ravaud, P. et al. Club Rhumatismes et Inflammation. (2010). Safety and efficacy of rituximab in systemic lupus erythematosus: results from 136 patients from the French AutoImmunity and Rituximab registry. *Arthritis Rheum.,* Vol. 62, No. 8, pp. 2458-66 , ISSN 1044-2626

Tokunaga, M.; Saito, K.; Kawabata, D. et al. (2007). Efficacy of rituximab (anti-CD20) for refractory systemic lupus erythematosus involving the central nervous system. *Ann Rheum Dis.,* Vol. 66, No. 4, pp. 470-5, ISSN 0003- 4967

Toubi, E.; Kessel, A.; Rosner, I. et al. (2006). The reduction of serum B-lymphocyte activating factor levels following quinacrine add-on therapy in systemic lupus erythematosus. *Scand J Immunol.,* Vol. 63, No. 4, pp. 299-303, ISSN 0301-6323

van Kooten, C.; Banchereau, J. (2000). CD40-CD40 ligand. *J Leukoc Biol* ,Vol. 6, pp. 2-17, ISSN 0741-5400

Wallace, D.J.; Stohl, W.; Furie, R.A. et al. (2009). A phase II, randomized, double-blind, placebo-controlled, dose-ranging study of belimumab in patients with active systemic lupus erythematosus. *Arthritis Rheum.,* Vol. 61, No 9, pp. 1168–1178, ISSN 1044-2626

Wiglesworth, A.K.; Ennis, K.M. & Kockler, D.R. (2010). Belimumab: a BLyS-specific inhibitor for systemic lupus erythematosus. *Ann Pharmacother.,* Vol. 44, No.12, pp. 1955-61, ISSN 1060-0280

Willems, M.; Haddad, E.; Niaudet, P.; Koné-Paut, I. et al. French Pediatric-Onset SLE Study Group. (2006). Rituximab therapy for childhood-onset systemic lupus erythematosus. *J Pediatr.*, Vol. 148, No. 5, pp. 623-627, ISSN 0271-6798

Yap, DY.; Lai, KN. (2010). Cytokines and their roles in the pathogenesis of systemic lupus erythematosus: from basics to recent advances. *J Biomed Biotechnol,* 2010:365083. Epub 2010 May 6. ISSN 1110-7243.

# 14

# Treatment of Pediatric-Onset Lupus Nephritis: A New Option of Less Cytotoxic Immunosuppressive Therapy

Hiroshi Tanaka[1,2] and Tadaatsu Imaizumi[3]
[1]*Department of School Health Science, Faculty of Education Hirosaki University,*
[2]*Department of Pediatrics, Hirosaki University Hospital and*
[3]*Department of Vascular Biology, Hirosaki University Graduate School of Medicine*
*Japan*

## 1. Introduction

Optimal treatment for lupus nephritis in adolescents is still a great challenge. Systemic lupus erythematosus (SLE) is a chronic disease characterized by frequent disease flares for which effective and safe maintenance therapy is required (Chan et al., 2005; Lai et al., 2005). Since diffuse proliferative lupus nephritis (DPLN) is a major concern regarding treatment of young patients with SLE, the optimal immunosuppressive therapy for controlling the activity of DPLN in this population remains controversial (Niaudet, 2000; Tanaka et al., 2004, 2009). Intermittent monthly pulses of intravenous cyclophosphamide (CPA) have been reported to be effective even for patients with pediatric-onset SLE (Lehman & Onel, 2000); however, CPA is a potent immunosuppressive agent associated with myelotoxicity, gonadal toxicity, and an increased risk of secondary malignancy (Chan et al., 2000; Lai et al., 2005). Since therapy related-adverse events are a major therapeutic risk of the immunosuppressive treatment in patients with SLE, selecting a safe and effective treatment protocol poses a big dilemma for physicians treating young patients. Thus, optimal maintenance treatment for controlling the clinical activity of SLE, particularly in young patients with pediatric-onset SLE, remains to be established (Yang et al., 1994; Niaudet, 2000; Tanaka et al., 2001).
Mycofenolate mofetil (MMF) has recently been reported to be as effective as and less toxic than oral CPA or monthly intermittent pulse therapy with intravenous CPA (iv-CPA) for SLE patients (Chan et al., 2000; Lai et al., 2005; Sinclair et al., 2007). However, clinical use of MMF, in patients other than those undergoing solid organ transplantation, has not been approved by the Japanese Ministry of Health and Welfare yet. On the other hand, mizoribine (MZR), a selective inhibitor of inosine monophosphate dehydrogenase in the *de novo* pathway of purine nucleotides, which acts very similar to MMF (Burkhardt & Kalden, 1997; Yokota, 2002), has been successfully used without any serious adverse effects for the long-term treatment of young patients with lupus nephritis (Tanaka et al., 2004; Yumura et al., 2005). We hypothesized that calcineurin inhibitors, other than MZR, might be a feasible alternative treatment for patients with pediatric-onset lupus nephritis (Tanaka et al., 2007a, 2009). Tacrolimus (Tac) is a T-cell-specific calcineurin inhibitor that prevents the activation of helper T cells, thereby inhibiting the transcription of the early activation genes of interleukin (IL)-2

and suppressing the T cell-induced activation of tumor necrosis factor (TNF)-α, IL-1β and IL-6 (Kawai & Yamamoto, 2006). Therefore, Tac is an attractive therapeutic option for young patients with lupus nephritis. We believe that both MZR and Tac may be new options of less cytotoxic immunosuppressive therapy for pediatric patients with lupus nephritis. Recently, a multidrug regimen comprising prednisolone (PDN), Tac, and MMF has been reported to be safe and effective for the treatment of adult lupus (Lanta et al., 2010). We also propose that as an alternative to CPA, a multidrug therapy consisting the immunosuppressive agents, MZR and Tac, which have different modes of action, combined with PDN would be an effective and safe treatment for pediatric-onset SLE (Watanabe et al., 2011).
From our recent clinical experiences, we would like to introduce this new less cytotoxic immunosuppressive therapy for the treatment of pediatric-onset lupus nephritis. Furthermore, we would like to discuss the novel signaling pathways in mesangial cells, which may be involved in the pathogenesis of lupus nephritis.

## 2. A new option of less cytotoxic immunosuppressive therapy for pediatric-onset lupus nephritis

Recent advances in the management of lupus nephritis, together with earlier renal biopsy and selective use of aggressive immunosuppressive therapy, have contributed to a favorable outcome in children and adolescents with SLE (Yang et al., 1994; Niaudet, 2000; Tanaka et al., 2001). Nevertheless, for optimal control of the activity of lupus nephritis, we believe that more effective and less toxic treatment strategies need to be developed. Although it has been reported that iv-CPA is effective for preserving renal function in adult patients (Austin & Balow, 1999), CPA is a potent immunosuppressive agent that induces severe toxicity, including myelotoxicity, gonadal toxicity, and an increased risk of secondary malignancy (Chan et al, 2000). Thus, the optimal treatment strategy for controlling the activity of lupus nephritis, especially in children and adolescents, is still controversial (Niaudet, 2000; Tanaka et al., 2004).

### 2.1 Mizoribine, a selective inhibitor of inosine monophosphate dehydrogenase in the *de novo* pathway

The mode of action of mizoribine (MZR) is, very similar to that of MMF, owing to the selective inhibition of inosine monophosphate dehydrogenease (IMPD) in the *de novo* pathway of purine nucleotide synthesis. MZR inhibits T cell and B cell proliferation (Burkhardt & Kalden, 1997; Yokota, 2002). MZR inhibition of IMPD is competitive and different from that induced by MMF (Sonda et al., 1996). Indeed, it has been reported that the concentrations of MZR required to effectively inhibit human mixed-lymphocyte reaction, must reach peak blood levels ranging approximately from 3.0 to 6.0 μg/mL, while beyond the 6.0 μg/mL level, it may lead to myelotoxicity (Sonda et al., 1996). It has also been reported that following MZR administration, 14-3-3 proteins, that is, MZR-binding proteins in *vivo*, interact with glucocorticoid receptors to enhance the transcriptional activity of these receptors (Takahashi et al., 2000). In *vitro*, the MZR concentration required to effectively enhance steroid receptor activity has been reported to be more than 10 μM, which corresponds to a blood MZR level of approximately 2.6 μg/mL. Clinically, MZR has been successfully used without any serious adverse effects for the long-term treatment of young patients with lupus nephritis (Tanaka et al., 2004; Yumura et al., 2005). Based on previous clinical observations, the efficacy of MZR may depend on the peak serum level of the drug

(Tanaka et al., 2003; Nozu et al., 2006; Kuroda et al., 2007). In addition, it has been reported that a peak serum MZR level of at least 2.5-3.0 µg/mL may be needed to effectively suppress of serum anti-dsDNA antibody titers and attain satisfactory clinical efficacy in lupus nephritis patients (Tanaka et al., 2005). However, when using MZR with the conventional protocol of low-dose (3-4 mg/kg) daily MZR (MZR-C) in young patients with lupus nephritis, the peak blood level of the drug usually remains at around 1.0 µg/mL (Tanaka et al., 2003), which may explain the relatively mild efficacy of MZR observed in clinical practice (Kuroda et al., 2007).

In this context, we conducted a trial of relatively long-term (at least 12 months or longer) intermittent pulse therapy with oral MZR (up to 10 mg/kg as a single dose before breakfast on 2 days of the week, MZR-P), to attain increased peak blood levels of MZR, in young patients with flares of lupus nephritis (Tanaka et al., 2008a). Our results suggested that this new treatment protocol was beneficial and resulted in higher efficacy and lower toxicity, in terms of reduction of proteinuria, decrease in the serum anti-dsDNA antibody titer, recovery of hypocomplementemia, preservation serum creatinine level, and decrease in the European Consensus Lupus Activity Measurement index (ECLAM) (Masca et al., 2000) than the MZR-C (Tanaka et al., 2008a and b). The rationale for using MZR-P was as follows: 1) MZR is rapidly excreted into the urine: about 90% of the drug is completely eliminated from the circulation within about 12 hours after oral intake; thus, the accumulation of the drug is not considered to be a problem, at least under the condition of normal renal function (Yokota, 2002). Considering this point, the intermittent use of high-dose MZR may be relatively safe. 2) Higher doses of MZR increase the area under the serum concentration-time curve (AUC) in lupus patients (Yumura et al., 2005); thus, the efficacy of MZR may depend on the peak serum level of the drug, which, in turn, may be closely correlated with the AUC of the drug (Tanaka et al., 2003). 3) In an SLE mouse model, the intermittent administration (every other day) of MZR effectively reduced anti-DNA antibody production (Kamata et al., 1984). In our recent multicenter study, we confirmed that the MZR-P protocol was more effective than the MZR-C protocol, with no serious adverse events occurring during the long-term treatment of young patients with DPLN (Tanaka et al., 2008a). Also, MZR-P showed the potential usefulness of MZR-P as induction therapy in young patients even in those with DPLN (Tanaka et al., 2008a and b). Follow-up renal biopsy specimens obtained after the initiation of MZR-P revealed an apparent improvement in the 2003 classification of lupus nephritis by the International Society of Nephrology/Renal Pathology Society (ISN/RPS), with a decrease in the activity indices without a significant progression in the chronicity indices described by Austin et al. (1984). It is noteworthy that no clinical toxicity, not even amenorrhea- a serious problem in female patients, occurred in any of the study patients. This low clinical toxicity is an important advantage of MZR-P treatment, especially for long-term treatment of young patients.

Besides its immunosuppressive effects, MZR has recently been reported to suppress the progression of histologic chronicity in selected patients with lupus nephritis and IgA nephropathy (Kawasaki et al., 2004; Tanaka et al., 2007b and c; Ikezumi et al., 2008). Moreover, MZR has been reported to attenuate tubulointerstitial fibrosis in a dose-dependent manner in rat models of unilateral ureteral obstruction, non-insulin-dependent diabetes and peritoneal fibrosis via suppression of macrophage infiltration of the interstitium (Sato et al., 2001; Kikuchi et al., 2005; Takahashi et al., 2009). Interestingly, MZR has been reported to bind specifically to heat shock protein (HSP) 60, which results in interference of the chaperone activity of HSP60 *in vitro* (Itoh et al., 1999). This may, in turn, lead to suppression of the activity of α3β1-integrin, which is known to play a role in the

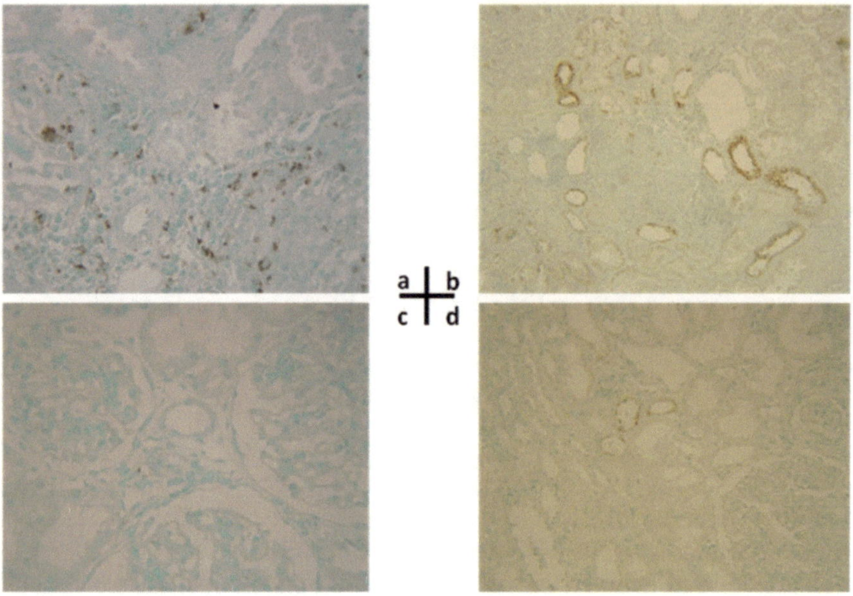


Pre-treatment renal biopsy specimen of a patient with diffuse proliferative lupus nephritis (DPLN) showing numerous CD68-positive cells (a), and the area expressing osteopontin (b) Post-MZR treatment renal biopsy specimen of a patient with DPLN who received MZR treatment showing a significant decrease in the infiltration by CD68-positive cells (c) associated with markedly decrease in the area expressing osteopontin (d)

Fig. 1. (Tanaka H, et al. Clin Rheumatol 2010)

development of interstitial fibrosis. Indeed, in a clinical setting, it has also been reported that posttreatment renal biopsy specimen from patients with severe IgA nephropathy treated with MZR, showed marked attenuation of glomerular and interstitial lesions, and significantly reduced the number of activated macropharges, associated with the expression of 14-3-3 proteins and HSP60, which are known to be MZR-binding proteins, in the inflamed glomerular cells (Ikezumi et al., 2008). Thus, it is speculated that MZR may bind directly to inflamed glomerular cells and prevent progressive damage by suppressing activated macrophages and intrinsic renal cells. Therefore, MZR itself may have a favorable effect against the progression of interstitial fibrosis in the diseased kidney. These laboratory and clinical observations suggest another beneficial mechanism of action of MZR in the treatment of renal diseases. From our recent study, we confirmed the reported beneficial histologic effects of MZR, that is, we found a significant suppression of intraglomerular macrophage infiltration accompanied with significant suppression of the chronicity indices following MZR treatment (Tanaka et al., 2010). MZR treatment also resulted in a decreasing tendency of interstitial macrophage infiltration and the expression of osteopontin, known to be a chemoattractant protein for macrophages (Fig. 1). Since the inflamed glomeruli express 14-3-3 proteins and HSP60 (Ikezumi et al., 2008), MZR may directly interact with inflamed glomerular cells, because MZR is directly excreted into the urine. Moreover, Takeuchi et al. (2010) reported that MZR directly prevented podocyte injury in experimental puromycin aminonucleoside-induced nephropathy, suggesting an anti-proteinuic effect of MZR besides its immunosuppressive effects. These beneficial mechanisms of action of MZR would warrant its use in the treatment of patients with lupus nephritis, although this theory remains speculative. We suspect that this mechanism may represent a mode of action different from that of MMF, although we could not demonstrate whether MZR was superior to MMF treatment for DPLN patients.

Further detailed studies involving a larger number of patients are needed to draw a conclusion. We believe that MZR is an attractive treatment for young patients with lupus nephritis because of attenuated histologic progression resulting from a suppressed accumulation of activated macrophages in the glomeruli. From the view point of the balance between suppression of disease activity and the adverse effects of treatment, we believe that long-term MZR treatment, including use of our MZR-P protocol, may become the new treatment of choice for young patients with lupus nephritis.

### 2.2 Tacrolimus, a calcineurin inhibitor

Some studies have recently suggested that cyclosporine A (CsA), a calcineurin inhibitor similar to Tac, might replace cytotoxic agents and reduce the dosage of concomitantly administered PDN for maintenance therapy in selected patients with lupus nephritis (Rihova et al., 2007; Moroni et al., 2008). It has been reported CsA treatment has beneficial effects in some pediatric patient with SLE resistant to conventional immunosuppressive therapy, including iv-CPA (Sakano et al., 2004; Suzuki et al., 2006). However, CsA-related nephrotoxicity, posterior reversible encephalopathy syndrome, as well as unfavorable cosmetic effects, such as hypertrichosis and gingival hypertrophy, remain major concerns for young patients with SLE, especially female adolescents.

Tacrolimus (Tac) is a T cell-specific calcineurin inhibitor that prevents activation of helper T cells, thereby inhibiting transcription of the early activation genes of IL-2 and suppressing the production of TNF-$\alpha$, IL-1$\beta$, and IL-6. Considering its effects, Tac is expected to have clinical benefits in the treatment of patients with active SLE. Indeed, to date several papers have described the efficacy and safety of Tac in patients with active SLE (Duddridge & Powell, 1997). Recently, Tac combined with PDN has been successfully administered without serious adverse effects, as induction and maintenance treatment for patients with proliferative and membranous lupus nephritis (Politt et al., 2004; Maruyama et al., 2005; Mok et al., 2005; Tse et al., 2007; Szeto et al., 2008). However, there is little information regarding the efficacy and safety of Tac in young patients with lupus nephritis (Tanaka et al., 2007a, 2009). The safety of Tac treatment is important because of its potent nephrotoxicity. Although these patients did not necessarily have permanently high blood levels of Tac (Duddridge & Powell, 1997; Tse et al., 2007), the development of an optimal Tac treatment strategy for lupus nephritis, with a dose as low as possible, is sought to minimize treatment toxicity while maintaining treatment efficacy. In this context, in Japan, Tac is usually administered once daily for patients with rheumatoid arthritis (RA) or lupus nephritis since once-daily administration of Tac is the governmental approved protocol (Kawai & Yamamoto, 2006; Tanaka et al., 2007a, 2009; Asamiya et al., 2009). Kawai and Yamamoto (2006) reported the safety of Tac administered at a dose of 1.5-3.0 mg once daily for the treatment of RA even in the elderly. Although further studies, including a histologic evaluation following Tac treatment, are needed, we consider that a once-daily regimen could shorten the exposure to Tac, would be more cost-beneficial than the conventional twice-daily protocol, and might result in better treatment compliance. Interestingly, Tac has been reported to stimulate glucocorticoid receptor (GR) transactivity through its ligands (Davies et al., 2005), which may explain the tendency to exacerbate glucose intolerance in selected patients (Mok et al., 2005). However, some patients who had experienced new flares of SLE while receiving CsA were successfully treated with Tac (Tanaka et al., 2007a, 2009). Differential control of the GR hormone-binding function by immunosuppressive ligands, such as Tac, reportedly stimulates GR transactivity beyond the effect of the ligand on hormone retention although this is not the case with CsA (Davies et al., 2005). These laboratory observations may explain the superior effect of Tac to that of CsA in selected patients with lupus, although this hypothesis remains speculative.

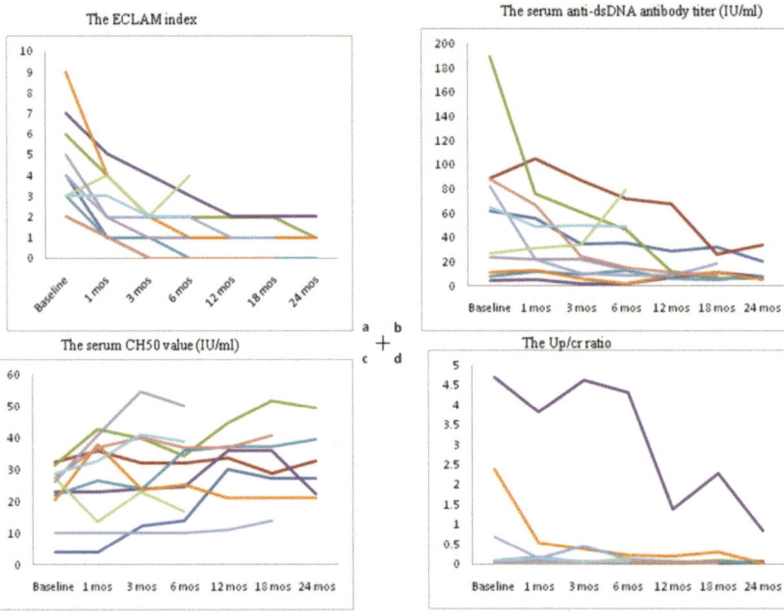


Individual changes in the ECLAM index (a), the serum anti-dsDNA antibody titer (b), the serum complement hemolytic activity (CH50) value (c) and the urinay protein/creatinone (Up/cr) ratio (d) in patients with lupus nephritis (LN) treated with tacrolimus administered once daily. A significant decrease in the ECLAM index was noted after 1 month treatment (a). A significant decrease was also noted in the serum anti-dsDNA antibody titer and the serum CH50 value after 3 months treatment (b, c). One patient with class V LN associated with massive proteinuria showed a significantly decrease in the Up/cr ratio after 12 months treatment (d).

Fig. 2. (Tanaka H, et al. Clin Nephrol 2009)

In our recent study, 11 consecutive patients with long-standing biopsy-proven lupus nephritis were recruited for at least 6 months or longer (6-24 months) as part of an open-label trial of single-daily-dose administration of Tac (3 mg/day, 0.04-0.075 mg/kg). As a result, despite the gradual tapering of the PDN dose, a marked improvement of the ECLAM index, compared with the baseline values, was observed even at 1 month after the start of treatment and in the serological parameters at 3 months. These favorable results persisted until the end of the study. Proteinuria gradually decreased and had dropped significantly by 24 months after the start of treatment (Fig. 2). After a mean of 18 months, a complete response was achieved in 8 patients (73%) and a partial response was achieved in two patients (Tanaka et al., 2009). Adverse reactions to Tac treatment were not severe and were well tolerated. Although the blood levels of Tac in the participants ranged from 1.5 ng/mL to 7.5 ng/mL, no definite relationship between the efficacy of the drug and its blood level was noted. Even though the absorption profile of Tac showed some variations among the study patients, the appropriate blood levels and doses of Tac for the treatment of young patients with lupus nephritis remains to be determined. Measuring the AUC in the pharmacokinetic profile of Tac obtained from each patient is also needed to confirm whether its efficacy depends on its blood levels. From our recent studies, although further studies involving a larger number of patients, including a histologic evaluation following Tac treatment, are needed, we believe that low-dose Tac treatment, administered once daily, may be an effective and safe method for managing selected young patients with pediatric-onset, long-standing lupus nephritis (Tanaka et al., 2007, 2009).

Tac has been reported to reduce proteinuria and mesangial alterations due to its suppressive effects on glomerular expression of IFN-γ mRNA in rat models (Ikezumi et al., 2002) In addition, it has recently been reported that Tac may overcome treatment unresponsiveness through the blockade of the drug exclusion effect of P-glycoprotein, leading to restoration of the intracellular therapeutic levels of corticosteroids and clinical improvement (Suzuki et al., 2010). These laboratory and clinical observations suggest that Tac might have other useful mechanisms of action besides its immunosuppressive effects, which would warrant its use in the treatment of patients with active and steroid-resistant SLE with lupus nephritis.

### 2.3 New multidrug therapy using tacrolimus and mizoribine

Combination therapy consisting of two immunosuppressive agents with different modes of action is useful and frequently used for immunosuppression in solid organ transplantation.The efficacy of multidrug therapy using MMF and Tac as induction therapy in patients with class V+IV lupus nephritis (DPLN with membranous lesions; Bao et al., 2008), has recently been reported. This multidrug therapy resulted in less cytotoxicity than iv-CPA therapy; the authors concluded that multidrug therapy MMF and Tac was superior to iv-CPA for inducing remission of class V+IV lupus nephritis and was well tolerated. Also, Lanta et al. (2010) reported the efficacy of adding Tac to the MMF plus PDN treatment regimen in some patients with DPLN resistant to MMF and PDN, although clinical toxicity, such as ketoacidosis, infections and muscle pain, limited the use of this combination therapy. Since the mechanisms of action of MMF and Tac are probably complementary, these clinical observations suggested the potential usefulness of multidrug therapy for the treatment of lupus nephritis. However, therapy related-adverse events remain a major therapeutic risk of the immunosuppressive treatment for patients with lupus patients.

The inhibitor of purine synthesis, MZR has reportedly exhibits relatively low clinical toxicity in patients with lupus nephritis (Tanaka et al., 2004; Yumura et al., 2005). Interestingly, aside from its immunosuppressive effect, MZR also appears to have a beneficial effect against the adverse effects of calcineurin inhibitors, such as CsA-induced intimal hyperplasia and perivascular inflammatory cell infiltration observed in rat models (Shimizu et al., 2003; Hara et al., 2009). We recently documented significant suppression of intraglomerular and interstitial macrophage infiltration accompanied by significant suppression of chronicity indices following MZR treatment in patients with lupus nephritis (Tanaka et al., 2010). Thus, we speculate that these histological observations may further support the use of MZR to treat selected patients with glomerular diseases, especially those treated with calcineurin inhibitors, such as CsA or Tac. Moreover, we hypothesized that combination therapy using low-dose Tac administered once-daily and MZR, instead of MMF, might be a beneficial alternative for the treatment of pediatric-onset refractory renal diseases including lupus nephritis (Aizawa-Yashiro et al., 2011; Watanabe et al., 2011).

We present here typical cases of pediatric-onset lupus nephritis in which the efficacy and safety of our novel multidrug therapy were observed. Patient 1 was an 11-year-old Japanese girl with a 2-year history of SLE with ISN/RPS classification class V lupus nephritis. She suddenly developed refractory epistaxis due to severe thrombocytopenia (7,000/μL) associated with serum C4 depression. The patient had been successfully managed with PDN combined with Tac. Consequently, the patient was given an emergency intravenous infusion of high-dose immunoglobulin, which transiently raised her platelet count to 36,000/μL. Because the patient was in a near-pubertal state, we avoided the use of iv-CPA. Thus, we used MZR in addition to Tac. After this combination therapy, her platelet count remained normal at 200,000/μL. The dose of concomitantly administered PDN was tapered without recurrence of thrombocytopenia. At present, 18 months after administration of this therapy, she is free of SLE signs and symptoms without therapy-related clinical toxicity (Watanabe et al., 2011). Patient 2 was a 14-year-old Japanese girl. She was treated with PDN because of hemophagocytic syndrome that she had developed 6 months earlier. When PDN was tapered, she developed malar rash, significant proteinuria/hematuria, hypocomplementemia and elevation of serum anti-dsDNA antibody titers. Percutaneous renal biopsy revealed ISN/RPS class IIIa lupus nephritis (activity index, 8; chronicity index, 2). She was administered 2 courses of methyprednisolone pulse therapy followed by multidrug therapy consisting of Tac, MZR and PDN. Because she was of pubertal age, the PDN dose was reduced to a minimum at a relative early stage. Her clinical and laboratory signs improved, and the second renal biopsy, performed 12 months after the initial biopsy, revealed marked improvement to ISN/RPS class II lupus nephritis (activity index, 4; chronicity index, 1) without any significant increase in the number of chronic lesions. At present, 36 months after the start of the administration of this therapy, she is free of SLE signs and symptoms without therapy-related clinical toxicity. In lupus nephritis patients, it is well known that flares may occur during long-term immunosuppressive treatment, even after at least a 12 month-long successful treatment with MMF or MZR (Tanaka et al., 2006; Posalski et al., 2009). Although the optimal treatment strategy for managing long-standing SLE, especially in pediatric patients, remains controversial, we believe that our treatment protocol is both effective and safe, and also easy to comply with for patients with pediatric-onset lupus. However, the long-term efficacy and safety of this regimen remains unclear. Further studies in a larger number of young patients with lupus nephritis are necessary to confirm the long-term efficacy and safety of our current protocol.

## 3. A potential new therapeutic strategy for pediatric-onset lupus nephritis: targeting the IFN regulatory factor signaling pathways

Recently, the importance of innate immunity in the pathogenesis of glomerulonephritis has been reported (Robson, 2009; Coppo et al., 2010). Toll-like receptors (TLRs), which are cell surface and intracelluar receptors for pathogen-associated molecules, play a central role in the response of both the innate and adaptive immune systems to microbial ligands (Robson, 2009). Once presumptive antigenic ligands bind to TLRs, the activation of transcriptional factors, such as interferon regulatory factors (IRF) and nuclear factor kappa B (NF-κB) is induced through intracellular signaling cascade activation. The activation results in the release of adhesion molecules, cytokines and chemokines, which play a pivotal role in the innate and adaptive immune responses (Coppo et al., 2010). Interestingly, recent studies revealed the expressions of TLRs in resident renal cells, suggesting the involvement of the TLR signaling pathway in the pathogenesis of glomerular diseases (Patole et al., 2006).

### 3.1 The retinoic acid-inducible gene-I (RIG-I) and lupus nephritis

Retinoic acid-inducible gene-I (RIG-I) encodes a DExH box protein, which is a RNA helicase. The DExH box family of proteins regulates RNA metabolism and has various biological functions. Like toll-like receptor (TLR)-3, RIG-I may detect viral RNAs and mediate immune reactions against RNA viruses (Yoneyama et al., 2004). RIG-I has also been suggested to be involved in immune and inflammatory responses in various physiological and morbid conditions (Imaizumi et al., 2009)

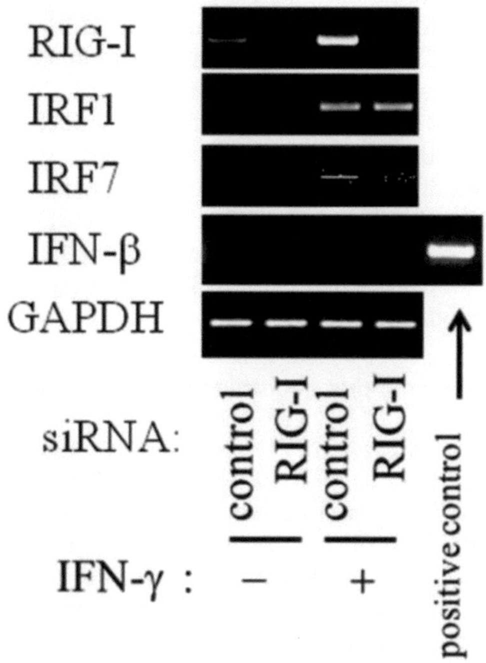


The cells were transfected with siRNA against RIG-I or a negative control non-silencing siRNA. At 24 h after the transfection, the cells were treated with 5 ng/ml IFN-γ for 24 h. RNA was extracted from the cells and RT-PCR analyses for RIG-I, IRF1, IRF7, IFN-β and GAPDH were performed.

Fig. 3. (Imaizumi et al., Lupus 2010)

In a recent study, we showed that RIG-I controlled the immune and inflammatory responses by regulating the expression of various downstream genes, including IFNs regulatory factor (IRF) genes, in mesangial cells (Imaizumi et al., 2010). We previously found RIG-I was highly expressed in the glomeruli examined in biopsy specimens from patients with lupus nephritis, and the level of expression correlated with the severity of acute inflammatory lesions (Suzuki et al., 2007). In addition, we found that the levels of RIG-I mRNA in the urinary sediment of patients with lupus nephritis were higher than those in patients with IgA nephropathy and controls (Tsugawa et al. 2008). Interestingly, repeated measurements of RIG-I mRNA in the urinary sediment of lupus patients revealed a reduction of the expression following immunosuppressive treatment (Tsugawa et al., 2008). These findings suggest that RIG-I may be involved in the acute inflammatory process in human lupus nephritis. In order to examine the involvement of RIG-I in lupus nephritis, we conducted experimental studies using human mesangial cells. Because Th1-derived cytokines are known to be key mediators in the progression of lupus-associated renal injury, and IFN-γ is one of the major Th1 type cytokines with potent proinflammatory effects that exerts its effects through the upregulation of IFN-inducible genes (Patole et al., 2006), we examined the effects of IFN-γ on the expression of RIG-I in human mesangial cells. As a result, IFN-γ treatment resulted in a concentration-dependent upregulation of the expression of RIG-I mRNA and protein in human mesangial cells. Treatment of cells with IFN-γ also induced the expression of mRNA of both IRF 1 and IRF7, which are important IFN-inducible transcriptional factors. Furthermore, knockdown of RIG-I expression by RNA interference inhibited the IFN-γ-induced expression of IRF7, but not that of IRF1. In contrast, IFN-γ did not induce the expression of IFN-β, which is known to be a target gene of IRF-7, in mesangial cells (Fig. 3) (Imaizumi et al., 2010)

Interestingly, pretreatment of cells with dexamethasone inhibited the IFN-γ-induced expression of monocyte chemoattractant protein (MCP)-1 mRNA but did not affect the induction of RIG-I or IRF7 mRNA in mesangial cells. The induction of MCP-1 mRNA by IFN-γ was not inhibited by the knockdown of NF-κB p65, indicating that the NF-κB signaling pathway was not involved. Our results suggest selective regulation of the expression of IRFs by RIG-I in human mesangial cells. The function of IRF7 has been well studied, mainly in dendritic cells and in mouse embryonic fibroblasts, and IRF7 is thought to be an important transcriptional factor that affects anti-viral responses by inducing the production of type I IFN (Honda et al., 2005).

### 3.2 Treatment of pediatric-onset lupus nephritis by direct targeting the IFN-γ/RIG-I/IRF7 pathway

Although the functional significance of IRF7 expression in mesangial cells remains to be elucidated, our recent observations suggest that the IFN-γ/RIG-I/IRF7 signaling pathways may be involved in the pathogenesis of lupus nephritis. We believe that the involvement of the newly observed IFN-γ/RIG-I/IRF7 pathway in mesangial cells may contribute to mesangial inflammation, and the intervention of this signaling pathway may lead to the development of optimal future therapeutic strategies for patients with lupus nephritis. However, further clinical and experimental issues remain to be examined in future studies.

## 4. Acknowledgements

Part of these studies was supported by a Grant from the Japan Society for the Promotion of Science (#21591259 and #22591175) and a grant from The Mother and Child Health Foundation, Osaka, Japan.

## 5. Conflict of interest statement

None declared.

## 6. References

Aizawa-Yashiro T, Tsuruga K, Watanabe S, Oki E, Ito E, Tanaka H (2011). Novel multidrug therapy for children with cyclosporine-resistant or -intolerant nephrotic syndrome. *Pediatr Nephrol* DOI: 10.1007/s00467-011-1876-z

Asamiya Y, Uchida K, Otsubo S, Takei T, Nitta K (2009). Clinical assessment of tacrolimus therapy in lupus nephritis: One-year follow-up study in a single center. *Nephron Clin Pract* 113: c330-c336.

Austin HA & Balow JE (1999) Natural history and treatment of lupus nephritis. *Semin Nephrol* 19: 2-11.

Austin HA, Muenz LR, Joyce KM, Antonnovych TT & Balow JE (1984) Diffuse proliferative lupus nephritis: Identification of specific pathologic features affecting renal outcome. *Kidney Int* 25: 689-695.

Bao H, Liu ZH, Xie HL, Hu WX, Zhang HT & Li LS (2008) Successful treatment of class V+IV lupus nephritis with multitarget therapy. *J Am Soc Nephrol* 19: 2001-2010.

Burkhardt H & Kalden JR (1997) Xenobiotic immunosuppressive agents: therapeutic effects in animal models of autoimmune diseases. *Rheumatol Int* 17: 85-90.

Chan TM, Li FK, Tang CSO, Wong RWS, Fang GX, Ji YL, Lau CS, Wong AKM, Tong MKL, Chan KW & Lai KN (2000) Efficacy of mycophenolate mofetil in patients with diffuse proliferative lupus nephritis. *N Engl J Med* 343:1156-1162

Chan TM, Tse KC, Tang CSO, Lai KN & Li FK (2005) Long-term outcome of patients with diffuse proliferative lupus nephritis treated with prednisolone and oral cyclophosphamide followed by azathioprine. *Lupus* 14: 265-272.

Coppo R, Amore A, Peruzzi L, Vergano L & Camilla R (2010). Innate immunity and IgA nephropathy. *J Nephrol* 23: 626-632.

Davies TH, Ning YM, Sanchez ER (2005) Differential control of glucocorticoid receptor hormone-binding function by tetratricopeptide repeat (TPR) proteins and immunosuppressive ligand FK506. *Biochemistry* 44: 2030-2038.

Duddridge M & Powell RJ (1997) Treatment of severe and difficult cases of systemic lupus erythematosus with tacrolimus. A report of three cases. *Ann Rheum Dis* 56: 690-692.

Hara S, Umino D, Someya T, Fujinaga S, Ohtomo Y, Murakami H & Shimizu T (2009) Protective effects of mizoribine on cyclosporine A nephropathy in rats. *Pediatr Res* 66: 524-527

Honda K, Yanai H, Negishi H, Asagiri M, Sato M, Mizutani T, Shimada N, Oba Y, Takaoka A, Yoshida N & Taniguchi T (2005). IRF-7 is the master regulator of type-I interferon-dependent immune responses. *Nature* 434: 772-777.

Ikezumi Y, Kanno K, Koike H, Tomita M, Uchiyama M, Shimizu F, Kawachi H (2002) FK506 ameliorate proteinuria and glomerular lesions induced by anti-Thy 1.1 monoclonal antibody 1-22-3. *Kidney Int* 61: 1339-1350.

Ikezumi Y, Suzuki T, Karasawa T, Kawachi H, Nikolic-Paterson DJ & Uchiyama M (2008) Use of mizoribine as a rescue drug for steroid-resistant pediatric IgA nephropathy. *Pediatr Nephrol* 23: 645-650.

Imaizumi T, Matsumiya T, Yoshida H, Naraoka T, Uesato R, Ishibashi Y, Ota K, Toh S, Fukuda S & Satoh K (2009). Tumor-necrosis factor-α induces retinoic acid-inducible gene-I in rheumatoid fibroblast-like synoviocytes. *Immunol Lett* 122: 89-93.

Imaizumi T, Tanaka H, Tajima A, Tsuruga K, Oki E, Sashinami H, Matsumiya T, Yoshida H, Inoue I & Ito E (2010) Retinoic acid-inducible gene-I (RIG-I) is induced by IFN-γ in human mesangial cells in culture: possible involvement of RIG-I in the inflammation in lupus nephritis. *Lupus* 19: 830-836.

Itoh H, Komatsuda A, Wakui H, Miura AB & Tashima Y (1999) Mammalian HSP60 is a major target for an immunosuppressant mizoribine. *J Biol Chem* 274: 35147- 35151.

Kamata K, Okubo M, Uchiyama T, Masaki Y, Kobayashi Y & Tanaka T (1984) Effect of mizoribine on lupus nephropathy of New Zealand black/white F1 hybrid mice. *Clin Immunol Immunopathol* 33: 31-38.

Kawai S & Yamamoto K (2006) Safety of tacrolimus, an immunosuppressive agent, in the treatment of rheumatoid arthritis in elderly patients. *Rheumatology* (Oxford) 45: 441-444.

Kawasaki Y, Hosoya M, Suzuki J, Onishi N, Takahashi A, Isome M, Nozawa R & Suzuki H (2004) Efficacy of multidrug therapy combined with mizoribine in children with diffuse IgA nephropathy in comparison with multidrug therapy without mizoribine and with methyprednisolone pulse therapy. *Am J Nephrol* 24: 576-581.

Kikuchi Y, Imakiire T, Yamada M, Saigusa T, Hyodo T, Hyodo N, Suzuki S & Miura S (2005) Mizoribine reduces renal injury and macropharge infiltration in non-insulin-dependent diabetic rats. *Nephrol Dial Transplant* 20: 1573-1581.

Kuroda T, Hirose S, Tanabe N, Sato H, Nakatsue T, Ajiro J, Wada Y, Murakami S, Hasegawa H, Ito S, Sakatsume M, Nakano M & Gejyo F (2007) Mizoribine therapy for patients with lupus nephritis: the association between peak mizoribine concentration and clinical efficacy. *Mod Rheumatol* 17: 206-212.

Lai KN, Tang SCW & Mok CC (2005) Treatment for lupus nephritis: a revisit. *Nephrology* (Carlton) 10: 180-188.

Lanata CM, Mahmood T, Fine DM & Petri M (2010) Combination therapy of mycophenolate mofetil and tacrolimus in lupus nephritis. *Lupus* 19: 935-940.

Lehman TJ & Onel K (2000) Intermittent intravenous cyclophosphamide arrests progression of the renal chronicity index in childhood systemic lupus erythematosus. *J Pediatr* 136: 243-247.

Maruyama M, Yamasaki Y, Sada K, Sarai A, Ujike K, Maeshima Y, Nakamura Y, Sugiyama H & Makino H (2006) Good response of membranous lupus nephritis to tacrolimus. *Clin Nephrol* 65: 276-279.

Mok CC, Tong KH, To CH, Siu YP, & Au TC (2005) Tacrolimus for induction therapy of diffuse proliferative lupus nephritis: an open-labeled pilot study. *Kidney Int* 68: 813-817.

Moroni G, Doria A & Ponticelli C. Cyclosporine (CsA) in lupus nephritis: assessing the evidence. Nephrol Dial Transplant 2009; 24: 15-20.

Mosca M, Bencivelli W, Vitali C, Carrai P, Neri R & Bombardieri S (2000) The validity of the ECLAM index for the retrospective evaluation of disease activity in systemic lupus erythematosus. *Lupus* 9: 445-450.

Niaudet P (2000) Treatment of lupus nephritis in children. *Pediatr Nephrol* 14: 158-166.

Nozu K, Iijima K, Kamioka I, Fujita T, Yoshiya K, Tanaka R, Nakanishi K, Yoshikawa N & Matsuo M (2006) High-dose mizoribine treatment for adolescents with systemic lupus erythematosus. *Pediatr Int* 48: 152-157.

Patole PS, Pawar RD, Lech M, Zecher D, Schmidt H, Segerer S, Ellwart A, Henger A, Kretzler M & Anders HJ (2006). Expression and regulation of Toll-like receptors in lupus-like immune complex glomerulomephritis of MRL-Fas (lpr) mice. *Nephrol Dial Transplant* 21: 3062-3073.

Politt D, Heintz B, Floege J & Mertens PR (2004). Tacrolimus- (FK506) based immunosuppression in severe systemic lupus erythematosus. *Clin Nephrol* 62: 49-53.

Posalski JD, Ishimori ML, Wallace DJ & Weisman MH (2009) Does mycophenolate mofetile prevent extra-renal flares in systemic lupus eruthematosus? Results from an observational study of patients in a single practice treated for up to 5 years. *Lupus* 18: 516-521.

Rihova Z, Vankova Z, Maixnerova D, Dostal C, Jancova E, Honsova E, Merta M, Rysava R & Tesar V (2007) Treatment of lupus nephritis with cyclosporine- An outcome analysis. *Kidney Blood Press Res* 30: 124-128.

Robson MG (2009). Toll-like receptors and renal disease. *Nephron Exp Nephrol* 113: e1-e7.

Sakano T, Ohta T, Kinoshita Y. Fujiwara M & Wakai M (2004) Treatment of steroid-resistant systemic lupus erythematosus with extremely low dose of cyclosporine A. *Pediatr Int* 46: 468-470.

Sato N, Shiraiwa K, Kai K, Watanabe A, Ogawa S, Kobayashi Y, Yamagishi-Imai H, Utsunomiya Y & Mitarai T (2001) Mizoribine ameliorates the tubulointerstitial fibrosis of obstructive nephropathy. *Nephron* 89: 177-185.

Shimizu H, Takahashi M, Takeda S, Tahara K, Inoue S, Nakamata Y, Kaneko T, Takeyoshi I, Morishita Y & Kobayashi E (2003) Effect of conversion from cyclosporine A to mizoribine on transplant arteriosclerosis in rat aortic allograft models. *Microsurgery* 23: 454-457

Sinclair A, Appel G, Dooley MA, Ginzler E, Isenberg D, Jayne D, Wofsy D & Solomons N (2007) Mycophenolate mofetil as induction and maintenance therapy for lupus nephritis: rationale and protocol for the randomized, controlled Aspreva Lupus Management Study (ALMS). *Lupus* 16: 972-980.

Sonda K, Takahashi K, Tanabe K, Fuchinoue S, Hayasaka Y, Kawaguchi H, Teraoka S, Toma H & Ota K (1996) Clinical pharmacokinetic study of mizoribine in renal transplantation patients. *Transplant Proc* 28: 3643-3648.

Suzuki K, Imaizumi T, Oki E, Tsugawa K, Ito E & Tanaka H (2007) Expression of retinoic acid-inducible gene-I in lupus nephritis. *Nephrol Dial Transplant* 22: 2407-2409.

Suzuki K, Saito K, Tsujimura S, Nakayamada S, Yamaoka K, Sawamukai N, Ieata S, Nawata M, Nakano K & Tanaka Y (2010) Tacrolimus, a calcineurin inhibitor, overcomes treatment unresponsiveness mediated by p-glycoprotein on lymphocytes in refractory rheumatoid arthritis. *J Rheumatol* 37: 512-520.

Suzuki K, Tanaka H, Tsugawa K & Ito E (2006) Effective treatment with cyclosporine A of a child with systemic lupus erythematosus resistant to cyclophosphamide pulse therapy. *Tohoku J Exp Med* 208: 355-359.

Szeto CC, Kwan BCH, Lai FMM, Tam LS, Li EKM, Chow KM, Gang W & Li PKT (2008) Tacrolimus for the treatment of systemic lupus erythematosus with pure class V nephritis. *Rheumatology* (Oxford) 47: 1678-1681.

Takahashi S, Taniguchi Y, Nakashima A, Arakawa T, Kawai T, Doi S, Ito T, Masaki T, Kohno N & Yorioka N (2009) Mizoribine suppresses the progression of experimental peritoneal fibrosis in a rat model. *Nephron Exp Nephrol* 112: e59-e69.

Takahashi S, Wakui H, Gustafsson JA, Zilliacus J & Itoh H (2000) Functional interaction of the immunosuppressant mizoribine with the 14-3-3 protein. *Biochem Biophys Res Commun* 274: 87-92.

Takeuchi S, Hiromura K, Tomioka M, Takahashi S, Sakairi T, Maeshima A, Kaneko Y, Kuroiwa T & Nojima Y (2010) The immunosuppressive drug mizoribine directory prevents podocyte injury in puromycin aminosucleoside nephrosis. *Nephron Exp Nephrol* 116: e3-e10

Tanaka H, Oki E, Tsuruga K, Aizawa-Yashiro T, Ito Y, Sato N, Kawasaki Y & Suzuki J (2010) Mizoribine attenuates renal injury and macrophage infiltration in patients with severe lupus nephritis. *Clin Rheumatol* 29: 1049-1054.

Tanaka H, Oki E, Tsugawa K, Nonaka K, Suzuki K & Ito E (2007a). Effective treatment of young patients with pediatric-onset, long-standing lupus nephritis with tacrolimus given as a single daily dose: An open-label pilot study. *Lupus* 16: 896-900.

Tanaka H, Oki E, Tsuruga K, Sato N, Matsukura H, Matsunaga A, Kondo Y, Suzuki J (2008a) Mizoribine treatment of young patients with severe lupus nephritis: A clinicopathologic study by the Tohoku Pediatric Study Group. *Nephron Clin Pract* 110: c73-c79.

Tanaka H, Oki Es, Tsugawa K, Suzuki K, Tsuruga K & Ito E (2007b) Long-term intermittent pulse therapy with mizoribine attenuates histologic progression in young patients with severe lupus nephritis: Report of two patients. *Nephrology* (Carlton) 12: 376-379.

Tanaka H, Oki E, Tsuruga K, Yashiro T, Hanada I & Ito E (2009) Management of young patients with lupus nephritis using tacrolimus administered as a single daily dose. *Clin Nephrol* 72: 430-436.

Tanaka H, Suzuki K, Nakahata T, Tsugawa K, Ito E & Waga S (2003) Mizoribine oral pulse therapy for patients with disease flare of lupus nephritis. *Clin Nephrol* 60: 390-394.

Tanaka H, Tateyama T & Waga S (2001) Methylprednisolone pulse therapy in Japanese children with severe lupus nephritis. *Pediatr Nephrol* 16: 817-819.

Tanaka H, Tsugawa K, Nakahata T, Kudo M, Suzuki K & Ito E (2005) Implication of peak serum level of mizoribine for control the serum anti-dsDNA antibody titer in patients with lupus nephritis. *Clin Nephrol* 63: 417-422.

Tanaka H, Tsugawa K, Oki E, Suzuki K & Ito E (2008b) Mizoribine intermittent pulse therapy for induction therapy for systemic lupus erythematosus in children: an open-label pilot study with five newly diagnosed patients. *Clin Rheumatol* 27: 85-89.

Tanaka H, Tsugawa K, Oki E, Suzuki K, Waga S & Ito E (2007c) Long-term mizoribine intermittent pulse therapy, but not azathioprine therapy, attenuated histologic progression in a patient with severe lupus nephritis. *Clin Nephrol* 68: 198-200.

Tanaka H, Tsugawa K, Suzuki K, Nakahata T & Ito E (2006) Long-term mizoribine intermittent pulse therapy for young patients with flare of lupus nephritis. *Pediatr Nephrol* 21: 962-966.

Tanaka H, Tsugawa K, Tsuruga K, Nakahata T, Suzuki K, Ito E &Waga S (2004) Mizoribine for the treatment of lupus nephritis in children and adolescents. *Clin Nephrol* 62: 412-417.

Tse KC, Lam MF, Tang SCW, Tang CSO & Chan TM (2007) A pilot study on tacrolimus treatment in membranous or quiescent lupus nephritis with proteinuria resistant to angiotensin inhibitor or blockade. *Lupus* 16: 46-51.

Tsugawa K, Oki E, Suzuki K, Imaizumi T, Ito E & Tanaka H (2008) Expression of mRNA for functional molecules in urinary sediment in glomerulonephritis. Pediatr Nephrol 23: 395-401.

Watanabe S, Tsuruga K, Aizawa-Yashiro T, Oki E, Ito E & Tanaka H (2011) Addition of mizoribine to the prednisolone plus tacrolimus treatment regimen in a patient with lupus flare. *Rheumatol Int* DOI: 10.1007/s00296-011-1858-2.

Yang LY, Chen WP & Lin CY (1994) Lupus nephritis in children. A review of 167 patients. *Pediatrics* 94:335-340

Yokota S (2002) Mizoribine: Mode of action and effects in clinical use. *Pediatr Int* 44: 196-198.

Yoneyama M, Kikuchi M, Natsukawa T, Shinobu N, Imaizumi T, Miyagishi M, Taira K, Akira S & Fujita T (2004). The RNA helicase RIG-I has an essential function in double-stranded RNA-induced innate antiviral responses. *Nat Immunol* 5: 730-737.

Yumura W, Suganuma K, Uchida K, Moriyama T, Otsubo S, Takei T, Naito M, Koike M, Nitta K & Nihei H (2005) Effects of long-term treatment with mizoribine in patients with proliferative lupus nephritis. *Clin Nephrol* 64: 28-34.

# 15

# Recent Advances in the Treatment of Neurological Autoimmune Disorders

Jagat R. Kanwar*, Bhasker Sriramoju and Rupinder K. Kanwar
*Laboratory of Immunology and Molecular Biomedical Research (LIMBR), Centre for Biotechnology and Interdisciplinary Biosciences (BioDeakin), Institute for Technology in Nanomedicine & Research Innovation, Deakin University Waurn Ponds, Geelong, Australia*

## 1. Introduction

Autoimmune diseases are a complex group of diseases arising because of the breakdown of narrow margin that exists between the immunity and tolerance. In simpler terms either T or B-cells or both are activated in the absence of a progressive infection or any other noticeable cause (Davidson & Diamond, 2001). Unable to distinguish self from non self, the renegade immune cells pose a serious threat to self molecules leading to severe destruction. The precise mechanisms that drive this event are still unclear but, most of the studies identified that genetics, environment and infections will have a role in triggering the autoimmune attack (Smith et al., 1999). An approximate of 5% of the population in western countries are currently the victims of these diseases and in this component, a major proportion of them are females displaying a higher risk of incidence (Jacobson, 1997; Kanwar, 2005). Added to this, the general ailments of the humans like atherosclerosis and gastrointestinal disturbances are found to be associated with an autoimmune component, predisposing the risk of developing an autoimmune disease (Ross, 1990, Galperin & Gershwin 1997).The influence of hormones cannot be neglected as preclinical studies have witnessed the role of oestrogen in the emergence of autoimmune diseases while testosterone was found to lower the risk in lupus prone mice (Sakic, 1998; Roubinian et al., 1978). Few epidemiological studies also revealed the preponderance of autoimmune diseases mediated by the nocturnal hormone, melatonin (Cutolo, 2003). In addition, cortisol levels and the secondary events like stress were also found to influence the autoimmune disease generation (Webster et al, 1998). Since ages, the basic principle of immunology has been the concept of clonal deletion of autoreactive immune cells and generation of a mature T & B-cell repertoire that could distinguish self from non self. The formation and survival of mature immune repertoire, always demands prolonged auto antigen exposure acknowledging the physiological importance of autoreactivity (Goldrath & Bevan, 1999; Gu et al., 1991). Though structural resemblances exist between self and non self antigens the attack is directed against self antigens under stimulatory conditions like the presence of infections, cytokines etc (Silverstein & Rose, 2000; Kanwar, 2005; Kanwar et al, 2009). Thus it is always fascinating to find answers for how the physiology of autoimmunity is turned to pathology and how the immune cells enforce their attack. This review focuses on introduction to immunity, pathology of autoimmune diseases and their treatments along with recent advancements.

## 2. Basics of immune system

The immune system comprises of a complex array of immune cells tailored to defend the body against a variety of substances that are considered as foreign including pathogenic microbes and tumors while remaining nonreactive towards the self. Immune cells are originated from the haematopoietic stem cells and are classified as lymphoid and myeloid cells comprising B & T-lymphocytes, Natural killer cells (NKs), dendritic cells and polymorphonuclear leukocytes, monocytes, mast cells, macrophages respectively (Delves, 2006). The immune cells constantly patrol the body and involve specific and non specific mechanisms in executing immune attack upon finding a foreign substance. The specificity rests particularly with T and B-cells as they display the receptors capable of recognising non self molecules from the self.

The specific attack is also complimented before by the strategic non specific immune responses generated by polymmorphonucelar cells, NKs, macrophages, co-stimulatory molecules like cytokines and serves as the initial site of attack upon finding the foreign entities. The abnormal levels of cytokines have a strong impact in the initiation and progression of autoimmune diseases. Also, therapeutic interventions with exogenous cytokines were found to be associated with the disease process, suggesting their key role in mediating the disease (Hooks et al., 1982; Trembleau et al., 1995; McKall-Faienza et al., 1998; Schattner, 1994; Kanwar et al, 1999; Kanwar et al, 2005; Kanwar et al, 2009). The complex network of immune cells is classified into subpopulations based on the expression of surface markers, functional characteristics, regions where they mature and activate. Likewise, T-cells include helper cells (Th) displaying $CD4^+$ marker and involve in modulating the immune responses. Further they comprise subsets of Th1 cells that aid other T-cells and Th2 subtype mediates the antibody generation. Cytotoxic cells (Tc) with $CD8^+$ marker are killer cells with lethal effect on intracellular pathogens, infected and tumor cells. Lastly, suppressor cells (Ts) down regulate and monitor the immune reactions. The naive T-cells undergo maturation in the thymus (hence the name T-cells) and are able to respond only to the processed antigens. Most of the nucleated cells of the mammalian system function as the antigen presenting cells (APCs) and dendrites are unique in this category expressing major histocompatibility complex proteins (MHC) and generating co stimulatory gestures for T-cell activation. APCs process the antigen and represent them in association with cell surface MHCs for T-cell recognition. These MHCs categorised as class I and Class II are crucial in the selection process of cytotoxic and helper cells respectively.

The T-cells bear an antigen recognition site on their surface called as T-cell receptor (TCR) and the initiation of T-cell mediated immunity requires the complex association of the antigen, MHC and the TCR. B-cells are specialised immune cells that act as APCs along with a prime function of antibody generation. The immature B-cells initially express a pre-B cell receptor (pre-BCR) on their surface and upon maturation they produce antibodies that act as antigen receptors towards the native antigen (Yang & Santamaria, 2006; Austyn, 2000; Roitt et al., 1998; Janeway & Travers, 1998). Both the T and B-cells express specific receptors for each antigen and this diversity is exhibited by the rearrangement of receptor gene sequences in the somatic cells rather than acquired through the inheritance (Gellert, 2002). In order to mount immune responses, the T and B-cells are activated through corresponding receptors in the presence of co-stimulatory molecules (Crow, 2004; Kanwar et al, 2000; Kanwar et al, 2003; Kanwar et al, 2005). Another essential feature of both these cells is that, upon initial exposure to an antigen both these cells generate memory cells that expand clonally. These memory cells unleash an accelerated immune attack upon antigen re-exposure (Swain, 2003; Bishop et al., 2003).

## 3. Tolerance

Because of the expression of vast diversity of antigen recognition sites on T and B-cells, molecules that are considered as self also may find chances of binding with the immune cells. Hence, a diverse range of tolerance mechanisms have been developed that train the T & B-cells to differentiate self from nonself. This process is tightly controlled in the primary lymphoid organs and is continuous to inhibit the various modes of auto reactive lymphocyte generation and activation. The basic mechanisms dealt are clonal deletion, clonal anergy and inhibition of self reactive lymphocytes (Yoshida & Gershwin, 1993; Rajewsky, 1996).

### 3.1 T and B cell tolerance

The tolerance mechanisms that develop in the primary lymphoid organs like thymus and bone marrow respectively for T and B cells constitute central tolerance. The naive T-cells originated from haematopoietic stem cells are devoid of CD4 and CD8 cell surface markers. Once migrated to the thymus, the TCR gene rearranges to develop double positive T-cells that display $CD4^+$ and $CD8^+$. Then these cells are positively selected as $CD4^+$ and $CD8^+$ cells based on their interactions with the MHC class II and Class I respectively. The cells with TCR, that fail to bind or interact MHC with little affinity undergo death and are positively selected based on weaker interactions between TCR and MHC carrying self antigens. T-cells are killed if found to interact strongly with a self antigen displayed by MHC and thus selected negatively (Palmer, 2003; Starr, 2006; Bretscher & Cohn, 1970; Kanwar et al, 2004; Kanwar, 2005). As a matter of enhanced protection from immune attack, the T-cells receiving stronger signals through TCR are deleted and this inactivation is much more sensitive compared to activation of T-cells that demand a stronger interaction between TCR and self antigen-MHC complex (Kappler, 1987; Pircher et al., 1991; Yagi & Janeway, 1990). Similar tolerance mechanisms exist for B-cell repertoire, as they are negatively selected if the BCR is found to interact strongly with the self antigens. However, active investigation is recommended to determine the existence of positive selection for B-cells. Interestingly, successful T-lymphocyte tolerance cuts down the signals for few autoreactive B-cells and thus induces B-cell tolerance (Bretscher & Cohn, 1970). During the course of their maturation, the pre B-cell receptor (BCR) cross links several avid auto-antigens. This event stimulates the rearrangement of light chain genes of the Ig's thus, driving the process of receptor editing where self antigens are replaced with non self ones (Ana et al., 2010). B-cells are deleted by apoptotic mechanism if found to interact strongly with self antigens (this happens mostly in bone marrow) and anergised if bound with little affinity (this happens mostly in periphery) (Monroe et al., 2003; Hodgkin & Basten, 1995). T-cells have a potential role in the generation and progression of chemical and spontaneously induced autoimmune diseases and the same was also demonstrated successfully in the animal studies (Singer & Theofilopoulos, 1990; Druet, 1989; Pettinelli & McFarlin, 1989; Waldor et al., 1985). Few autoreactive T-cells may escape tolerance mechanisms and spread in the periphery but, they are naive and do not hold any threat unless APCs turn active. Potential problem persists incase of molecular mimicry (where pathogenic antigens resemble self antigens) as APCs turn active and trigger T-cell attack that is indiscriminate towards self and nonself. The same also holds true for B-cells (Damian, 1964; Oldstone, 1998). On the whole, generation of autoimmune diseases is based on the narrow margin that exists between tolerance and immunity executed by deletion and survival of self reactive lymphocytes. Too much deletion compromises the immunity and too little deletion follows subsequent autoimmunity. The following figure is an ideal representation of healthy and pathologic immunity and the differentiation between tolerance and autoimmunity.

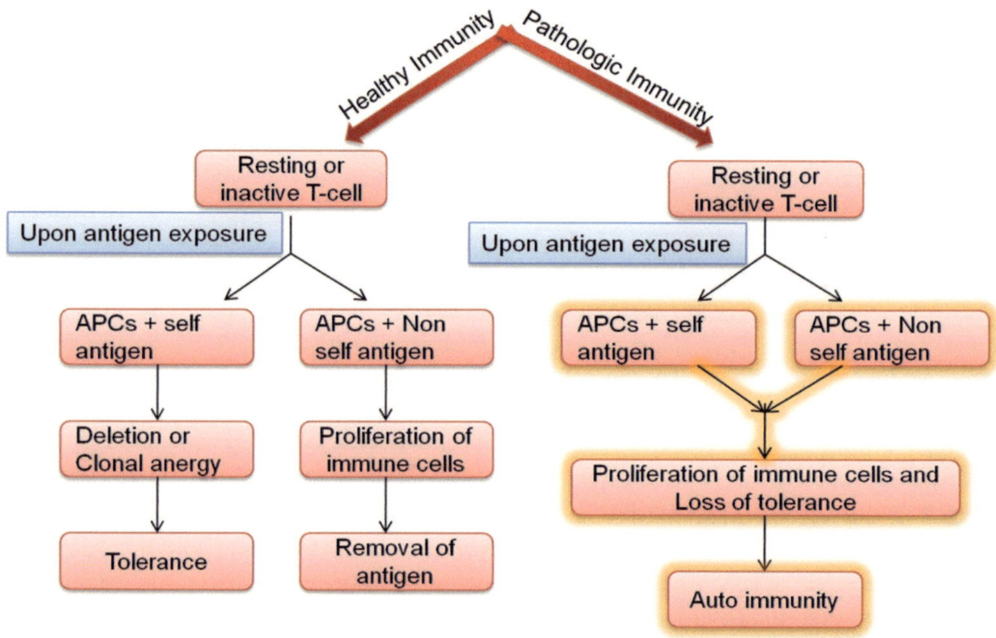


Fig. 1. Showing the comparison of healthy and pathologic immune system. A healthy T-cell upon exposure to self antigens undergo specific mechanisms of inactivation like deletion or clonal anergy constituting peripheral tolerance while an autoreactive T-cell is dysregulated with indiscriminate attack on self and non self antigens because of the lack of tolerance in autoimmunity.

## 4. Autoimmune triggers

### 4.1 Genetics

The enhanced knowledge of the mammalian immune system and the genetics lead to understanding the role of genes in autoimmune diseases. In the case of disease pathology, genetic variations are found to affect the MHC and several immunological pathways that in turn lead to the stimulation of autoimmunity. A number of studies have evidenced the potential role of genetics in the disease generation. Twin studies of multiple sclerosis (MS), rheumatoid arthritis (RA), Type- 1 diabetes and systemic lupus erythematosus (SLE) have reported a marked genetic predisposition of which the risk factor was found to be higher for monozygotic twins than the dizygotic twins. The risk of inheriting the systemic autoimmune diseases was also reported and this etiology could be due to the family history associated with the genetic vairaitons. In addition, a variety of MHC and non-MHC susceptible genes are identified in the genome wide studies of MS, SLE and RA while, few studies reported that many autoimmune diseases have a common genetic etiology operating (Glinda, 1999). Likewise, the association of intracellular tyrosine phosphatise, PTPN22 was shared in the pathologies of Type-1diabetes, RA and myasthenia gravis (Bottini, 2004; Begovich, 2004; Vandiedonck et al., 2006). In brief, genetics underscore a significant risk factor for the autoimmune etiology and presents a new area to explore.

### 4.2 Auto antigens

In the early stages of development some of the self antigens might escape recognition from the T-cell populations. This could happen because, they might not have been formed at the time of T-cell development or they might be separated from T-cell access due to remote anatomical existence (e.g. myelin basic protein) or due to the presence of membrane barriers or they might be inappropriately presented by the MHC proteins (Manoury, 1998). These cryptic antigens hinder the tolerance mechanisms and drive the autoimmune attack if they are encountered by the T-cells upon membrane barrier disruption for e.g. orchiditis upon vasectomy (Flickinger, 1994; Jarow et al., 1994) infections (Type 1 diabetes upon coxsackie B virus infection) or any other mechanism that exposes them (Yoon et al., 1979). A striking feature of auto antigens is that they are not specific to any tissue and form the integral components of all various cell types (Tan et al., 1987).

### 4.3 Role of infections

Infections have an interesting role to play in the induction of autoimmune diseases and there are several interesting mechanisms where infections mediate them. In the instances of microbial infections, immune cells cannot differentiate antigenic sequences from self proteins if structural similarities are found. This molecular mimicry unleashes the immune attack that is directed towards self and nonself leading to tissue destruction. For e.g. hepatitis B virus polymerase resembles myelin basic protein and generates auto antibodies that destroy myelin leading to multiple sclerosis (Fujinami & Oldstone, 1989; Oldstone, 1998; Fujinami & Oldstone, 1985). Infections are associated with interesting mechanisms that may enhance the severity of autoimmune diseases. Among these, epitope spreading is an instance where in an inflammatory burst, the avid APCs over process and presents the antigens to activate the large T-cell populations lowering the threshold to the disease onset. The other mechanism is termed as polyclonal activation where abundant B-cell populations are activated generating loads of antibodies along with immune complexes that pose serious threat to the tissues. The next mechanism involves the over activation and indiscriminate expansion of self reactive T-cells that are initially considered to be inefficient but can cause the disease in the presence of elevated levels of cytokines. Finally, microbes express super antigens on their surfaces that are unique in coupling T-cells with MHC complexes irrespective of their relativities (Barzilai et al., 2007a, 2007b). On the contrary when correlations were made between autoimmune diseases and infections, the incidences were found to be increased in the subjects who are at reduced risk of infections. The same holds true as autoimmune diseases have a rampant growth in western countries where the infectious incidences are lower compared to less developed nations (Bach, 2002; Patterson et al., 1996) substantiating the concept of hygiene hypothesis which states that the microbial exposure enhances the body's defence mechanisms ( Bjorksten B, 1994).

### 4.4 Role of cell adhesion molecules

The propagation of autoimmune attack desperately needs the in and out migration of the immune cells, in particular T-cells, into the susceptible environment with potent inflammatory mediation. Cell adhesion molecules provide a suitable platform for this setting and are categorised as integrins, immunoglobulins and the selectins (Ziff, 1991). An autoimmune inflammatory setting leads to the enhanced expression of vascular endothelial proteins that constitute mucosal addressin cell adhesion molecule-1 (MAdCAM-1), intercellular adhesion molecule-1 (ICAM-1) and vascular cell adhesion molecule-1 (VCAM-1). Correspondingly, the lymphocytes express the cell surface molecules P-selectin glycoprotein ligand-1 (PSGL-1), leukocyte function-associated antigen-1 (LFA-1) and very late antigen-4 (VLA-4) on their surface facilitating the adherence and entry of the immune traffic into the lesions and further enhancing the autoimmune spread (Dedrick et al., 2003; Kanwar et al., 1999).VLA-4 and LFA-1are specifically expressed by the human B cells (Alter et al, 2003) and therapeutic interventions with anti-adhesion molecule antibodies have witnessed successful termination of autoimmune disease severity in preclinical and clinical models (McMurray, 1996; Kanwar et al, 2000; Kanwar et al 2003; Kanwar, 2005; Kanwar et al 2009).

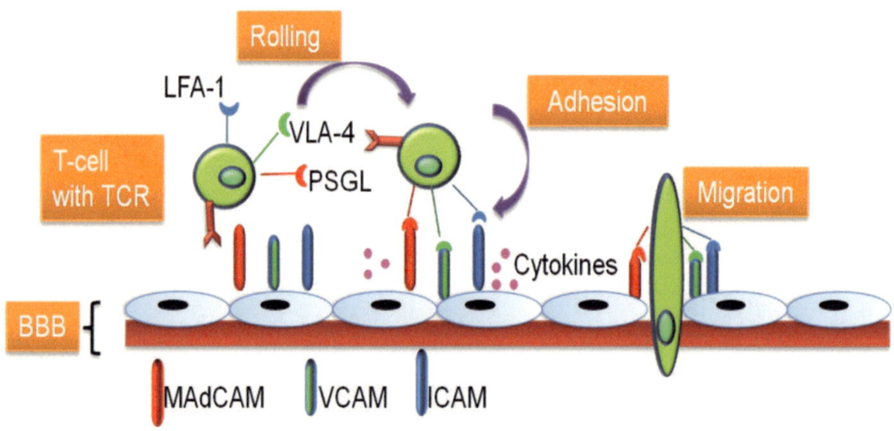


Fig. 2. Showing a typical T-cell exhibiting the phenomenon of rolling, adhesion and migration through the blood brain barrier (BBB) into the CNS. T-cell expresses PSGL-1, VLA-4 and LFA-1 on its cell surface and rolls over to adhere to the corresponding cell adhesion molecules, mucosal addressin cell adhesion molecule (MAdCAM), Vascular cell adhesion molecule (VCAM) and Intracellular cell adhesion molecule, (ICAM) respectively on the blood brain barrier capillary endothelial cells. These cell surface ligands are over expressed in an inflammatory condition facilitating the entry of T-cells into the BBB and thus initiating an autoimmune cascade.

### 4.5 Long lived plasma cells

The concept of long lived antibody secreting plasma cells were first demonstrated in a mouse model immunized with ovalbumin where in the plasma cells secreted antibodies against ovalbumin and the production was continuous independent of antigen exposure and memory cell assistance (Manz et al., 1997, 1998). The same was also observed in another mouse model infected with lymphocytic choriomeningitis virus (Slifka et al., 1998). The potential role of long lived plasma cells in the generation of autoimmune diseases was studied in NZB/W mice that served as a model for systemic lupus erythematosis (Hoyer et al, 2004). The differentiation of B-cells leading to the generation of memory cells and antibody secreting plasma cells is guided both by the antigenic and non antigenic stimuli (Tarlinton et al., 2008; Radbruch et al., 2006). However not all antibody secreting plasma cells turn long lived as it entirely depends on the antibody titre maintenance for the generation of secondary immune responses (Manz et al., 2005).

Long lived plasma cells mainly originate from the germinal centre regions and require a close reciprocation of the T and B-cells. But, once generated these cells act independently. In one of the autoimmune pathologies, it was found that self reactive B-cells are not excluded from the germinal centre region allowing the production of long lived plasma cells that were autoreactive (Cappione et al., 2005). This concept of long lived plasma cells is novel and serves as attractive targets for treating autoimmune diseases.

### 4.6 Auto antibodies

The role of auto antibodies in the pathogenesis of autoimmune diseases is often elusive but considering few autoimmune diseases like myasthenia gravis, the antibodies are specific to cell surface receptors. The basic principle for the autoantibody directed cytotoxicity is the identification of cell surface antigen followed by cell death mechanisms either through complement activated system, antibody dependent cell mediated cytotoxicity (ADCC) or by the macrophage uptake mechanism (Ohishi et al., 1995; Frisoni et al., 2005). Complement activated system is constituted by a collection of specific group of plasma proteins and are considered to be more prevailing in autoimmune diseases. The class of autoimmune haemolytic anaemia, lupus syndrome typically fall under the complement system generated autoimmune diseases (Fang et al., 2009). In the case of classical ADCC, NKs play a prime role in mediating the cell death, after the binding of antibody with the target antigen. NK's binds the Fc portions of these antibodies and induce cell death by free radical generation. Autoimmune thyroid disease is a fine example of ADCC mediated autoimmune disease (Rodien et al., 1996). Finally, macrophages execute the uptake and cell lysis processes once they find the appropriate antibody-antigen interaction (Gehrs & Friedberg, 2002). In general, the auto antibodies are directed to intracellular antigens and this understanding unveils fascinating questions of how they interact with intracellular antigens. The possible explanation could be because of the cross reaction of surface antigens with the intracellular antigens (Frisoni et al., 2005) and the exposure of intracellular components after lysis due to an impaired macrophage phagocytosis (Hansen et al., 2002). The potential significance of auto antibodies in autoimmune diseases were also demonstrated in the foetus as few of the immunoglobulin's (IgG) can cross the placenta and target the cell surface creating a havoc of tissue destruction (Clancy et al., 2004a, 2004b). Also, the apoptotic cells were found to be potent enough to generate autoantibodies if accompanied by other moieties like dendritic cells or Freunds incomplete adjuvant. These dying cells tend to activate Toll like receptors and NF-kB pathway that are associated with inflammation which in turn is linked to generation of autoantibodies (Bondanza et al., 2004), in conclusion it has to keep in mind that, auto antibodies are not always associated with the disease and few of them are valuable diagnostic aids implicated in a clinical setting.

### 4.7 Stress and autoimmune diseases

Stress of both versions physical and physiological is found to be associated with the disease generation. This was also supported from the several past studies that emotional stress was highly proportionate for predicting the disease onset. These two are related because, stress presumably shoots the neuroendochrine triggers that are predicted to alter the immune function or the cytokine levels ending up with the disease generation (Herrmann et al., 2000; Stojanovich & Marisavljevich, 2008). Also, stress induces the expression of heat shock proteins that are highly immunogenic with a potential of triggering autoimmune diseases (Kanwar et al., 2001). Therefore, therapeutic interventions for these diseases should consider management of emotions and stress.

### 4.8 Pregnancy and autoimmune diseases

In order to escape the immune attack neither the sperms nor the developing trophoblast bear the MHC proteins of either class. This peculiar feature allows the escape and survival of the sperm from the immune attack to fertilize the ovum (Johnson, 1993). Soon after fertilisation, many protective measures are adopted to protect the developing foetus and likewise it bears the human leucocyte antigen (HLA-G) marker which if otherwise would have been killed by the natural killer cells (VanVoorhis & Stovall, 1997). Also regulatory proteins from the foetus avoid the activation of complement system and its subsequent attack (Holmes & Simpson, 1992). Interesting immunological features are noticed in a pregnant woman, as changes are seen in the immune reactions that shift from Th1 to Th2 type due to the release of cytokines like TGF-beta (Raghupathy, 1997; Lim et al., 1998). This modification has a striking implication in that many of the pregnant woman experience remission of autoimmune diseases like rheumatoid arthritis (RA) and multiple sclerosis that are Th1 mediated (Allebeck et al., 1984; Cutolo & Accardo, 1991). However the risk of systemic lupus erythematosis (SLE) in pregnant woman is much higher compared to non pregnant woman and this also has drastic effects on the survival of the foetus (Khamashta et al., 1997; Cooper et al., 2002; Fraga et al., 1974).

### 4.9 T and B-cell traffic in the CNS

The migration of T-cells into the CNS adopt the same principles as they enter the peripheral tissues namely, activated T-cells migrate the tissues from the blood where as inactive ones remains in the lymph vessels (Mackay et al., 1990). To demonstrate the migration of T-cells into the CNS, Hickey et al administered labelled T-cells intravenously and observed the appearance of T-cells in the brain parenchyma soon after 3 hrs (Hickey et al., 1991). Also, T-cells in very minute levels were detected in the rat and human brains suggesting the fact that they continuously monitor the CNS (Pender, 1995). Similarly B-cells cross the BBB, perhaps more rapidly than the T-cells and differentiate into the plasma cells in response to an antigen as they do in the periphery (Knopf et al., 1998; Anthony et al., 2003; Kanwar, 2005). The following figure 3 represents the autoreactive T-cell entry and further consequences that lead to the generation of autoimmunity.

### 4.10 Co-stimulatory molecules

The phenomenon of T-cell activation and the generation of autoimmunity also depend on the involvement of several co-stimulatory molecules like B7-1, B7-2, CD28, inducible co stimulator (ICOS), OX 40 and CD40 ligand that are associated with T-cell activation. Other molecules like cytotoxic T lymphocyte antigen 4 (CTLA-4) and programmed death 1 (PD-1) regulate negative co-stimulation. Hence, effective therapeutics targeting these molecules will have a significant impact in the autoimmune disease control (Racke & Stuart, 2002; Kanwar et al 2004).

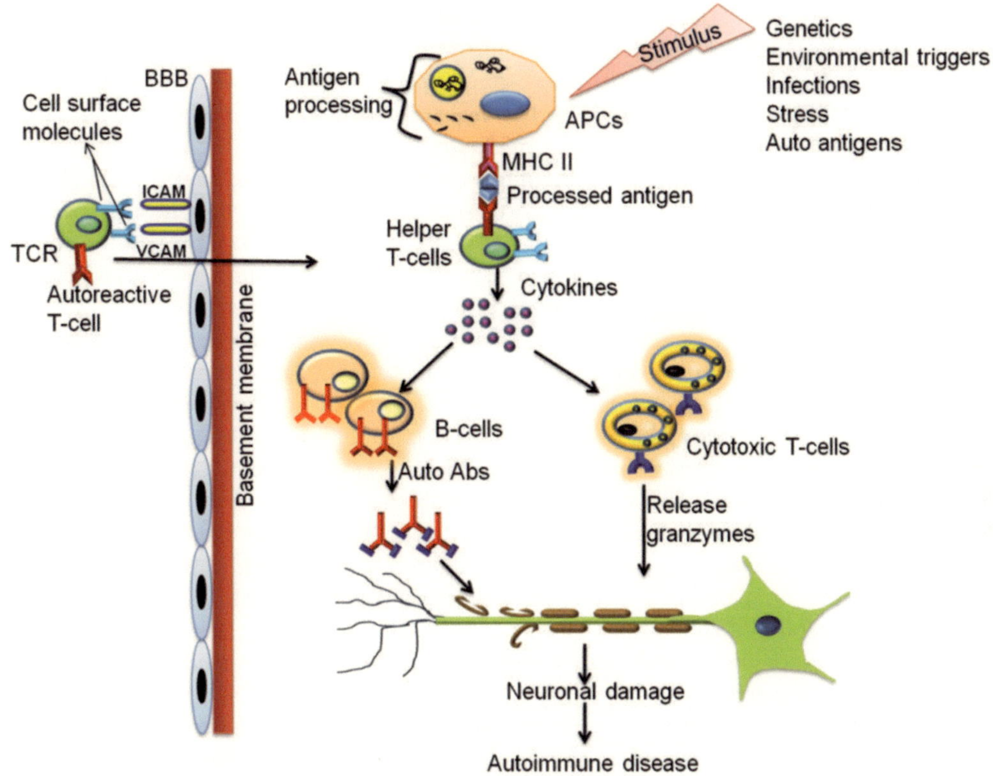


Fig. 3. Schematic representation of autoimmune attack in the CNS APCs-Antigen presenting cells; BBB-Blood brain barrier; ICAM- intercellular cell adhesion molecule; MHC-Major histocompatibility complex; TCR-T-cell receptor; VCAM- Vascular intercellular cell adhesion molecule.

The auto reactive T-cells gain entry into the CNS by the pairing of cell surface molecules leukocyte function-associated antigen-1 (LFA-1) and very late antigen-4(VLA-4) with the cell adhesion molecules, intercellular cell adhesion molecule (ICAM) and vascular cell adhesion molecule (VCAM) expressed on the brain capillary endothelium. Once after entry the helper T-cells (Th) bind with the processed peptide fragments presented along with MHC II by the antigen presenting cells (APCs).The threshold for triggering immune attack is lowered in autoimmune diseases and is stimulated by a variety of factors. The Th cells secrete a variety of cytokines that further activate the cytotoxic T-cells (Tc) and the antibody secreting B-cells. Tc cells, when activated mediate the cytotoxicity by releasing the granzymes while the B-cells differentiate into plasma cells that produce auto antibodies against a variety of targets like the myelin, nicotinic acetylcholine receptors (NAchRs), voltage gated calcium channels (VGCC), voltage gated potassium channels (VGKC), glycolipids etc mediating the corresponding neurological autoimmune disorder.

### 4.11 Autoimmunity and survivin

In an effort to address issues involved with the treatment of neurodegenerative and autoimmune diseases, the two following strategies can be employed: a neuroprotection strategy and a neuroproliferative strategy. Findings suggest that Bcl2 and IAP inducers are able to inhibit apoptosis for the purpose of neuroprotection in preclinical models (Kanwar, 2010a-d, Baratchi, 2010 a&b). Our understanding of neurodegenerative diseases has improved over the past two decades. Whereas these disorders are initiated due to a range of insults such as reactive oxygen species or misfolded proteins, all of these pathologies end with a common consequence, which is the degeneration and deterioration of neuronal cells (Kanwar et al, 2010a). Despite all of the efforts to understand and treat neurodegenerative diseases, their successful treatment has still not been achieved. A proper treatment should not only protect neural cells but should also increase their proliferation and differentiation so as to provide a promising future for an aging population and families with a history of degenerative disorders, including multiple sclerosis, Parkinson's disease and stroke. The brain's environment is the most protected part of our body and neurons are a unique cell type (Baratchi, 2011a&b). Despite playing an important role in the analysis and transfer of information to the entire body, the lack of neural self-proliferation and repair highlights the importance of their protection and proliferation. To be able to protect these cells from death and to facilitate their proliferation involves mechanisms that still need to be identified. Experimental findings achieved over the past few years have suggested that inhibitors of apoptosis (IAP), which serve a natural role in balancing cell death, might be candidate proteins with a unique potential for drug discovery (Kanwar et al, 2010). Recently we reviewed the exceptional capabilities of survivin (a unique member of IAPs) in both cell cycle and cell death pathways and its unique characteristics related to neuronal cell survival and proliferation (Baratchi, 2010a&b).

Given that this is the first report of a protective effect of SurR9-C84A following an oxidative stress injury, further work should be done to study the effects of SurR9-C84A on *in vivo* models of degenerative diseases. In summary, we reported for the first time, a recombinant, cell-permeable form of the survivin mutant protein (SurR9-C84A) efficiently enters neuronal cells, protects differentiated SK-N-SH cells from the activation of apoptosis induced by $H_2O_2$, decreases the expression of cell cycle markers, and increases antioxidant activity. Emerging nano-delivery systems could be used to bypass the blood brain barrier, facilitating drug delivery to the damaged brain. Survivin is a member of the IAP family, which has been shown to have a role in early brain development and serves a bifunctional role during mitosis and inhibition of apoptosis (Baratchi et al., 2010a; Kanwar et al., 2010). Different forms of survivin mutants (such as C84A, Δ106 and T34A) have been used for the purpose of targeting survivin overexpression in cancer cells (Cheung, 2010a&b; Kanwar et al, 2010b; (Baratchi, 2010a&b). Among the various survivin mutants, the baculovirus IAP repeat motif (C84A) was initially produced and has since been shown to have proapoptotic effects on human cancer cells. Furthermore, we previously found that SurR9-C84A has protective effects against retinoic acid induced cell toxicity (Baratchi et al., 2011b). We used the SK-N-SH cell line as a culture model of retinoic acid-induced neuronal differentiation (Baratchi, 2010a&b). We showed for the first time, the neuroprotective effect of SurR9-C84A against cytotoxic elements existing in activated T-cell supernatants such as GrB. Because GrB is a powerful pro-apoptotic member of granzymes family and is a very important mediator of damage in progressive MS and other neuro-inflammatory disorders we examined the importance of GrB released from the activated T-cells in an *in-vitro* system and compared the protective effect of SurR9-C84A with GrB inhibitor (Baratchi, 2011a&b). SurR9-C84A can be applied in neuroprotective strategies to protect differentiated neural cells from cell cycle re-entry and apoptosis. Additionally, one important advantage of this mutant over the wild type survivin is that it does not form tumour due to its pro-apoptotic effect in cancer cells. Because the over-expression of survivin has been reported in stimulated T-cells derived from patients with active MS, the neuroprotective ability of SurR9-C84A has the potential to be employed for future neurodegenerative therapies, and may also be further evaluated for targeting stimulated T-cells for the treatment of neurodegenerative diseases such as MS and other brain injuries (Baratchi, 2010a&b).

## 5. Classification of autoimmune diseases

Autoimmune diseases are characterised by the abnormal activation of the immune responses against our own tissues evidenced by the inability of the immune cells to differentiate self from non self antigens. Hence, mistakenly immune attack is directed towards our own body parts. They are categorised as systemic, involving multi target organ damage (e.g. systemic lupus erythematosis) or they can be localised involving damage to a single organ. (e.g. Type 1 diabetes) (Mackay & Rosen, 2001).
A list of autoimmune neurological diseases are included and described as follows (Dalakas, 2006).

### 5.1 Multiple sclerosis (MS)

MS is a localised neurological autoimmune disease and is marked by the characteristic inflammation and degradation of the protective nerve lining, the myelin (Lucchinetti et al., 2000; Lassmann, 2000). More than 1 million people are affected by MS with a characteristic presentation of weakness, abnormal senses, ataxia, poor balance, fatigue, vision loss and impaired cognition (Fugger et al., 2009; Kanwar et al 2004; Kanwar, 2005). Based on the histopathology multicentred inflammatory lesions were observed in the patient's brain and the spinal cord (Frohman et al, 2006). Multiple aetiological factors are involved in the preponderance of the disease and are often found to be triggered by a viral infection (Lucchinetti et al., 2000). This initiation by an infection is by the process of molecular mimicry as discussed earlier. It is rather fascinating to study the generation of inflammatory lesions and the entry mechanisms of immune cells in MS. A specific population of activated T-cells that are selective towards myelin crosses the blood brain barrier under the strong influence of chemokines while the resting T-cells are inaccessible towards the BBB due to the unfeasible environment (Charo & Ransohoff, 2006).
The cell surface molecules (integrins, selectins and cadherins) of the T-cells bind with the adhesion molecules expressed on the brain endothelial cells and finally escape into the CNS. Following their entry, the T-cells then direct the immune attack towards myelin antigen presented on their surface by the APCs (Greter et al., 2005). Along with macrophages, dendritic cells, glial cells and astrocytes present the MHC class II expression in the CSF and thus attract the T-cell traffic (Heppner et al., 2005; Greter et al., 2005). Under the influence of activated T-cells the immune attack is boosted up towards the myelin sheath and is executed by recruiting the T-cells and antibody secreting B-cells from the periphery driving the myelin assault leading to demyelination (Cepok et al., 2005; Steinman, 2002). The severity and progression of the demyelination process is influenced significantly by the B-cells as evidenced by the infiltration of macrophages and the deposition of immunoglobulins (Lucchinetti et al., 2000). The same was also supported by the observations made on clonal expansion and the presence of IgG complexes of B-cell populations in the brain and cerebrospinal fluid lesions (Qin et al., 1998; Baranzini et al., 1999; Colombo et al., 2000). The

whole process of immune attack and tissue damage is also encouraged by the active macrophages and glial cells (Brosnan & Raine,1996; Heppner et al., 2005). Interesting results were obtained from the animal model of MS, experimental autoimmune encephalomyelitis where it was found that, the pro-inflammatory T cells of Th1-type were found to be responsible for the disease exacerbations (Wekerle et al., 1986; Gold et al., 2006). There are four subtypes of MS and categorised as relapsing remitting (RR) with majority of the patients displaying recovery symptoms after disability. People who experience RR often complain a second variety of MS termed as secondary-progressive MS where the disability doesn't subside between the cycles of relapses and recoveries. The third form is the primary progressive stage where there is only progression and no remission. The last form of MS is rather rare and termed as Progressive-relapsing MS (PRMS) characterised by the severe attacks and symptoms during the remission period (Mayoclinic, 2008). More than 1 million people are affected by MS with a characteristic presentation of weakness, abnormal senses, ataxia, poor balance, fatigue, vision loss and impaired cognition. Significant contributions are being made for the disease diagnostics and management with the introduction of potential biomarkers. There are findings of glial fibrillary acidic protein (GFAP) and neurofilament light protein (NFL) (the cytoskeletal proteins of astrocytes and axons respectively) release into the CSF during the disease progression (Axelsson et al., 2010).

As per clinical data, the plasma levels of osteopontin was increased well before the induction of lesions with gadolinium (Gd) and similar profiles were observed with 7KC and 15 oxy sterol derivatives of cholesterol in MS patients. Added to this, enhanced antibody binding was reported towards these entities suggesting their potentials as biomarkers (Vogt et al., 2003; Whitaker, 1987). Also in a longitudinal cross sectional study of MS patients, it was found that levels of pentosidine, a well characterised biomarker for advanced glycation end products (AGE) were significantly elevated compared to the healthy controls. It was also observed that patients on treatment showed pentosidine down regulation compared to untreated patients. Thus, this study considers the AGE inhibitors as novel therapeutic interventions against MS. ( Sternberg et al., 2011) The recent reports on the associated tissue damage in MS patients found that it is not only limited to axons but also included significant retinal damage (Green et al., 2010).

The current therapeutic strategies for MS include the treatment for disease progression and the symptoms. Interferon's of type I (IFN-1) specifically marked as IFNb1a, IFNb1b and glatiramer acetate are considered as the first line drugs against RR form of MS but have a limited effectiveness. The mechanism of these drugs is that they down regulate the proliferation of T-cells, reduced antigen presentation, T-cell migration (interferon's in particular) and shift the immune response to Th2 type (Clerico et al., 2007; Arnon & Aharoni, 2004). Natalizumab, a humanized monoclonal antibody (mab) is found effective against MS as it inhibits the entry of T-cells into the CNS by acting against the cell surface molecule α-integrins and showed significant reduction in the relapse rate compared to the above treatment strategies (Polman et al., 2006). However, limitation exists on its indiscriminate use as it poses a serious risk of brain infection, progressive multifocal leukoencephalopathy (PML) that even causes death (Clifford et al., 2010). Corticosteroids like prednisone, prednisolone, methyl prednisolone and dexamethasone are also used against the RR and rarely against secondary progressive multiple sclerosis as they act by suppressing the immune system. They are strictly contraindicated for long term use as they are associated with a number of side effects (Merck,). Chemotherapeutics with a potential of suppressing the immune system like mitoxantrone inducing the apoptosis of lymphocytes and cyclophosphamide acting against both the T & B-cell activities, were also tried against RR and secondary progressive MS (Chan et al., 2005; Fauci et al., 1971; Multiple Sclerosis Treatments). The drugs in development for MS are Fingolimod and BG00012 that are in phase II clinical trials. Fingolimod acts by complexing the lymphocytes in the lymph nodes preventing their entry into the CNS and BG00012 is an oral formulation of Fumarate and presumed to act by neuroprotective and anti-inflammatory mechanisms inhibiting the oxidative stress (Lutterotti & Berger, 2010). Drugs in phase III clinical trials for RR form of MS are Laquinimod that acts by shifting the T-cell response to Th2 type and Teriflunomide acts by interrupting pyrimidine synthesis inhibiting the dihydro-orotate dehydrogenase and stops the expansion of T and B cells. Cladribine is efficient against both the resting and dividing T-cells and acts against the adenosine deaminase enzyme (Yang et al., 2004; Warnke et al., 2009). Monoclonal antibodies are also under evaluation and CAMPATH is tried against the CD52 expression on leukocytes. This activity depleted a majority of the lymphocytes, monocytes and dendritic cells in MS patients (Osborne, 2009; Hauser et al., 2008). A similar effect was observed with Rituximab that acts against the CD20 expression.

### 5.2 Myasthenia Gravis (MG)

In the case of myasthenia gravis the prototypic B cells produce the auto antibodies that are directed against the nicotinic acetylcholine receptor (AchR) in the neuromuscular junction (NMJ) (Drachman, 1994; Ragheb & Lisak, 1998). These antibodies from the peripherally activated B cells infiltrate the end-plate region of NMJ, and down regulate the functionally active Ach receptors either by cross linking the receptor followed by internalization or by initiating the complement-mediated immune destruction or they may make the binding site unavailable for activity (Bufler et al., 1996). Following this, the signal transmission and communication is significantly affected between the neurons and the muscles in NMJ region due to the immune attack.

Based on the symptom severity there are three subtypes of MG, Pure ocular MG characterised by weakness and fatigue of extra ocular muscles, resulting in ptosis and diplopia. Generalized MG, with extensive skeletal muscle weakness and finally myasthenia crisis, with disturbances in swallowing and respiratory failure (Hohlfeld et al., 2003). The exact role of antibodies in the pathogenesis of myasthenia gravis was confirmed from the results that, administration of myasthenic IgG antibodies generated the symptoms while the symptoms were ameliorated upon their removal (Drachman, 1994; Vincent et al., 2000). In a patient subgroup with myasthenia gravis, another variety of autoimmunity was reported with the detection of auto antibodies directed towards the muscle specific kinase. These patients were considered as seronegative to MG. (Vincent et al., 2003). The treatment modalities for MG include the acetylcholinesterase (AchE) inhibitors as the mainstay of treatment as they improve the bioavailability of Ach in the NMJ and the immune modulating agents. The AchE inhibitors of clinical significance are the pyridostigmine and neostigmine. They act by binding with AchE enzyme because of structural resemblance to Ach and slowly get hydrolysed compared to it. This improves the availability and subsequent binding of Ach to the available AchR in the NMJ. The common adverse effects associated are disturbances of GIT, respiratory system, cardiovascular system and glandular secretions (Kumar & Kaminski, 2011).

#### 5.2.1 Agents acting on immune system

Glucocorticosteroids with a potential of strong anti-inflammatory and immunosuppressive activity are tried with a successful outcome. The orally administered glucocorticoids

(prednisone in common) show a delayed onset of action and take even months to exhibit maximum therapeutic benefit (Hohlfeld et al., 2003). However, intravenous administration is recommended for the management of exacerbations (Arsura et al., 1985). Long-term treatment is not recommended due to the severe side effects featuring crushing's syndrome, obesity, precipitation of diabetes, gastrointestinal ulcers, opportunistic infections and hypertension etc. In the class of immune suppressive drugs, Azathioprine is the prominent and well tolerated drug tried against MG patients. This is a purine analogue and displays significant decrement in the levels of both T & B-cells thus monitoring the immune attack. Added to its mechanism it also exhibits anti-inflammatory actions by inhibiting promonocyte cell proliferation. It is generally given in combination to lower the dose of glucocorticoids but can also be prescribed alone for long term therapy (Mertens et al., 1981; Gold et al., 2003). Cyclosporine-A acts by binding to an intracellular protein, cyclophilin and forms a cyclosporine-cyclophilin complex. This complex exhibits immunosuppressive activity by inhibiting the phosphatase, calcineurin and prevents the cytokine formation. The clinical significance of this drug was that, it was the first drug tried in a double-blind and placebo-controlled trial MG patient population (Tindall et al., 1987). Patients with refractory MG show better responses towards cyclophosphamide, methotrexate and mycophenolate mofetil (Schneider-Gold et al., 2006). The recent advancements included are the administration of intravenous IgG that has a potential blocking activity against auto antibodies. This treatment is recommended when all the treatment modalities have failed. (Zinman et al., 2007) Advancements are made in the therapeutics of MG with the introduction of SHG2210, a novel entity with a potential to fuse with the α-subunit of the auto antibodies that are directed against AchR. This SHG2210 -autoantibody fusion complex is later cleared by the transferrin receptor mediated cellular uptake (Keefe et al., 2010).
On the whole due to the advancements made in the diagnosis and treatment, MG stands as a rear but treatable autoimmune disease.

### 5.3 Guillainbarre syndrome (GBS)

GBS is classified as an acute auto immune disease of demyelinating type mostly affecting the peripheral nervous system. Depending upon the target affected by the immune attack it is categorised to 4 subtypes. The first of its kind is the acute inflammatory demyelinating polyneuropathy (AIDP) where the immune attack is directed towards the myelin or schwann cell surface membrane. The next subtype is the acute motor axonal neuropathy (AMAN) targeting the axonal membrane in motor fibres where as both the motor and sensory nerve fibres are targeted in acute motor sensory axonal neuropathy (AMSAN). In the last subtype, distal nerve terminals and nodal regions of the ocular motor nerve are affected and termed as Miller Fisher syndrome (MFS) (Willison et al., 2002; Kuwabara, 2004). GBS is often triggered by an infection of bacterial or viral origin with auto antibodies directed against gangliosides particularly in AMAN where infections with *campylobacter jejuni* produced auto antibodies against GM1, GM1b, GD1 or GalNAc-GD1a gangliosides (Ogawara et al., 2000). There were also detectable levels of IgG and complement deposition in the nerves (Hafer-Macko et al., 1996). The distinct involvement of T and B-cells are identified in few subtypes, with the activated complement system playing a prime role in mediating demyelination and impaired conduction but still understanding the pathology of GBS remains rather elusive (Kieseier et al., 2004). The treatment for GBS is often confined to the immunomodulatory therapy where plasmapheresis and intravenous administration of immunoglobulin's IVIg are given the priority (Dalakas, 1999; Hadden et al., 1998).

Plasmapheresis is the plasma exchange where the immunoglobulins and antibodies are removed from the serum with a subsequent separation of the blood cells. Then these blood cells are isolated and added to the fresh plasma or saline to administer back into the patient. IVIg operates through multiple mechanisms that include the inhibition of antibody production, complement binding, macrophage receptor blockade and the abnormal antibody neutralisation. Both these strategies were found to have equal efficiencies in reducing the disease progression (Heather Rachel Davids).. Future therapies for GBS are directed towards the complement inhibitors. (Walgaard et al., 2011)

### 5.4 Neuromyelitis optica (NMO)

The pathology of this neurological autoimmune disorder is clear with the detection of antibodies against the aquaporin -4 water channels of the endothelial cells in the CNS (Lennon et al., 2005). In the autopsy studies, deposition of Immunoglobulins particularly of the IgM subtype were detected in the lesions with activated complimentary system leading to vascular damage. The predominant immune attack directed in this disorder is of the humoral type with majority of the attack directed towards the optic nerve and the spinal cord (Lucchinetti et al., 2002; Wingerchuk et al., 2004; Bergamaschi, 2007). Immunosuppressive therapeutics like mycophenolate mofetil, mitoxantrone and rituximab are far beneficial rather than immunomodulating agents like interferons in NMO(Bergamaschi, 2007).Eculizumab, is a new molecule under Phase I/II clinical trials and the proposed mechanism for this entity is that it inhibits the complement activation and subsequent destruction (. clinicaltrials.gov.).

### 5.5 Stiff-Man syndrome (SMS)

Stiff man or Stiff-person syndrome is also a predominant antibody directed autoimmune disease with majority of the auto antibodies directed towards the enzyme, glutamic acid decarboxylase (GAD) that is essential for the synthesis of gamma-amino butyric acid, a principal inhibitory neurotransmitter in the brain. Also, detectable levels of Immunoglobulin belonging to the subtype IgG were found in the CSF confirming the infiltration of B-cells (Dalakas et al., 2001; Ishii, 2010). The recent epidemiological studies report the existence of anti-gephyrin, anti-amphiphysin and anti-gamma-aminobutyric acid A receptor-associated protein (GABARAP) antibodies in the disease pathology. The patients experiencing this disease complain symptoms of muscular rigidity in the legs and trunk region often associated with muscle spasms (Dalakas et al., 2000). The medication for stiff man syndrome initially should begin with the skeletal muscle relaxants benzodiazepine or baclofen. Intrathecal administration of baclofen was even considered in a selected patient group. However great care has to be taken in performing this procedure as it is involved with puncturing the meninges (Duddy & Baker, 2009). Other treatment options considered are plasmapheresis and administration of Intravenous immunoglobulins like Gamimune, Gammagard, Sandoglobulin (Dalakas, 2009; Hayashi et al., 1999).

### 5.6 Paraneoplastic neurological syndromes (PNS)

The pathology associated with this autoimmune disease is quite peculiar. Antigens that are confined to the nervous system are capable of mediating an immune attack if the same antigens are expressed in the case of pathological conditions such as the breast or ovarian cancers. The immune cells that are activated against these antigens also direct their attack indiscriminately towards the antigens of the CNS that were once considered as self. A diverse range of self-antigens are identified in this setting and within this diversity, multiple epitopes are recognized within each antigen encountered. Thus, stimulated by the cancers, immune drive is targeted against the CNS evidenced by the detection of serum antibodies. The most common serum antibody detected is the anti-Hu antibody in patients coexisting with sensory neuropathy, encephalomyelitis or cerebellar ataxia (Dalmau et al., 1992; Graus et al., 2001; Darnell & Posner, 2003; Maverakis et al., 2011). Other such auto antibodies detected are anti-Yo antibodies in cerebellar degeneration (Peterson et al., 1992) anti-Ma1 and anti-Ma2 antibodies in limbic encephalitis in patients with testicular cancer (Rosenfeld et al, 2001) and antibodies in Lambert-Eaton myasthenic syndrome in small cell lung cancer patients (Carpentier & Delattre, 2001). In the paraneoplastic autoimmune CNS disorders, immune cells penetrate the blood–brain barrier and the antibody mediated destruction serves as the dominant mode of immune attack as evidenced by the localised synthesis of antibodies by the B cells (Darnell & Posner, 2003 & Pranzatelli et al., 2004). However, defining the precise mechanisms of cellular and humoral pathways in the pathophysiology is still unclear and the immune system adapts the elusive mode to identify the intracellular antigens.

The treatment for this disorder should be aimed at treating the underlying tumor with standard anticancer therapeutic regimen while the immune mediated disorder is treated by plasmapheresis or administration of immune suppressive drugs like Cyclosporine and glucocorticoids. Cyclosporine acts against both the cell and humoral mediated immune reactions and glucocorticoids are the potent anti-inflammatory and immune suppressive agents as discussed. Immune reaction suppression is even achieved by the administration of IVIg and Antithymocyte globulin is recommended in this case. It is a polyclonal IgG antibody particularly effective against T-lymphocytes and reduces the count to 85-90% (Buchwald et al., 2005; Koski & Patterson, 2006).

### 5.7 Lambert-Eaton Myasthenic Syndrome (LEMS)

Lambert-Eaton syndrome is a muscular disorder characterised by the autoantibody generation against the voltage gated calcium channels in the presynaptic nerve terminals. The communication is drastically affected between the nerves and muscles due to the inability of the nerve cells to release Ach required for muscular contraction. Hence, the symptoms of muscular rigidity and weakness are experienced in the patient population. The difference noticed between MG and LEMS is that in the latter form of the disease, with repeated contractions the muscle gets stronger for a shorter span of time instead of turning weaker (Lambert-Eaton syndrome, 2000). The primary treatment for LEMS aims to enhance the levels of Ach either by increasing its release or by inhibiting its metabolism thus making it available at the NMJ. The agents that are considered effective in this regard are Pyridostigmine bromide, 3,4-Diaminopyridine (DAP) and guanidine HCl. Pyridostigmine is an AchE inhibitor and shows symptomatic relief, while DAP and guanidine HCL acts by enhancing the release of Ach with noticeable improvement in the muscular strength. Patients who are refractory to the above treatment are prescribed with the immunosuppressive drugs as mentioned earlier (McEvoy et al., 1989; Sanders, 1995).

### 5.8 Neuromyotonia (NM)

Neuromyotonia, is a rare autoimmune disorder with antibodies directed against the voltage gated $K^+$ channels of the Shaker-type (Kv1). Based on the symptoms observed the disease is categorised as acquired neuromyotonia (NMT) with peripheral nerve hyperexcitability, fasciculations and muscle stiffness. Morvan's syndrome is associated with the symptoms of NMT along with encephalopathy and sleep disorders. The last subtype is the limbic encephalitis characterised by the CNS involvement with encephalopathic seizures, hyponatremia and abnormal electroencephalographic abnormalities. The antibodies noticed in this immune disorder were pathogenic and were confirmed by the observations of electrophysiological changes in mice, upon administration of IgG derived from patients (Kleopas et al., 2006; Buckley & Vincent, 2005; Merchut, 2010). Recently, a novel pathology was attributed to limbic encephalitis in which auto antibodies were identified against leucine-rich glioma-inactivated 1 (LGI1) protein. Previously, these auto antibodies were assumed to be acting against $K^+$ channels and hence, this disorder is now termed as limbic encephalitis associated with LGI1 antibodies (Lai et al., 2010).

Most of the patients with these disorders fairly respond when treated with immunosuppressive drugs like glucocorticosteroids. Also other recommendations include plasmapheresis and IVIg (Merchut, 2010).

### 5.9 Polyneuropathies (PN)

Polyneuropathies are divided into 3 subtypes as chronic inflammatory demyelinating polyneuropathy (CIDP), multifocal motor neuropathy (MMN) and IgM anti-myelin-associated glycoprotein (MAG) demyelinating neuropathy (Kornberg & Pestronk, 2003; Czaplinski & Steck, 2004; Kieseier et al., 2004). Both the T and B-cell mediated immune havoc is noticed in CIDP with the majority of antibodies directed towards the glycolipids GM1 (Yan et al., 2000). Similar type of antibody production is identified against GM1 in half of the patient population in MMN but the pathogenecity of these antibodies are left unidentified (Nobile-Orazio, 2001). On the contrary, the IgM antibodies generated against the myelin associated glycoprotein in anti-MAG neuropathies are identified as pathogenic with a successful transfer of the disease to the animals. The normal cellular interactions were also found to be disturbed by these anti-MAG antibodies by the complement activation towards the myelin lamellae (Latov, 1994; Dalakas & Quarles, 1996; Quarles & Weiss, 1999). The treatment options considered are mainly immunosuppressive in nature and administration of glucocorticosteroids, plasmapheresis and IVIg are in use (Shy, 2007). Figure 4 summarises the pathologies of all the neurological autoimmune diseases.

## 6. What's in the pipeline?

The role of B-cells in the autoimmune disorders is inevitable and considering this concrete paradigm researchers have now focussed targeting them with the mainstay of B-cell depletion. The targets identified were the B-lymphocyte stimulator (BLyS) protein and the CD20 expression on B-cells. Belimumab, is the humanised anti-BLyS monoclonal antibody and showed effective inhibition of invitro B-cell proliferation. (Baker et al, 2003) Also, phase I clinical trials of belimumab in SLE was well tolerated and further results are yet to be reported (Stohl, 2004). Rituximab, a chimeric anti-CD20 monoclonal antibody has the ability to deplete B-cells by multiple mechanisms and results are encouraging when it was tried against a variety of autoimmune disorders (Wylam et al., 2003; Ruegg et al., 2004; Stuve et al., 2005).. In extension ocrelizumab, a humanized version of rituximab is currently in the developing stage for targeting several autoimmune disorders (Genovese et al., 2008). The same also holds true for Epratuzumab, a humanised mab that acts by blocking CD22 and

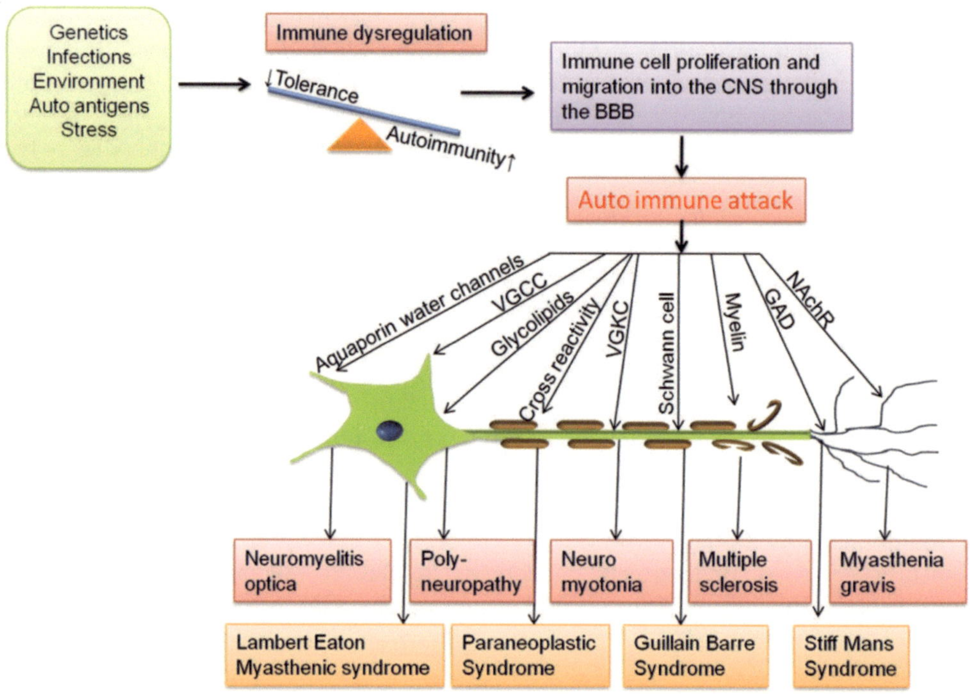


GAD-Glutamicacid decarboxylase; NAchR-Nicotinic acetylcholine receptors; VGCC- Voltage gated calcium channels; VGKC- Voltage gated potassium channels

Fig. 4. Representing the various triggers of autoimmune diseases and the different targets involved in the generation of neurological autoimmune diseases.

thereby depletes B-cell population (Dalakas, 2008). Targeting the T-cell antigens was always an area of intense interest. Researchers have made significant contributions with the development of anti-CD3 MAbs that displayed not only potent immunosuppressive activities but also the ability to restore self tolerance (Chatenoud, 2003). Progress was also presumed with the introduction of T-lymphocyte subsets, the invariant natural killer T (iNKT) cells. These unique cells stimulate a diverse range of cytokines that regulate the activities of various immune cells and thus prove to be handy for autoimmune disease therapeutics (Gabriel et al., 2010). The preclinical studies of methyl thioadenosine, a natural metabolite was found effective with its immunomodulatory activity in MS model. The results of this study showed an enhanced efficiency when it was combined with interferon's or glatiramer acetate (Moreno et al., 2010). Midkine (MK) a cytokine that binds heparin is generally involved in inflammation by promoting T-cell traffic and cytokine up regulation. The MK inhibitors are assumed to be very valuable for treating MS as an aptamer to MK was found to repress experimental autoimmune encephalitis (Muramatsu, 2011). Histone deacetylase inhibitors were also found to have a potential against MS as they are found to interfere the immune system activation empowered with neuroprotective activities (Faraco et al., 2011). Recent advancements include the application of autologous and allogenic stem cell transplantations following intense immunoablation and the former application has lower toxicities compared to the latter. Encouraging results were obtained in a group of MS patients when treated with autologous stem cells compared to the existing therapies. However, further trials are warranted for the effective use (Marmont, 2000).

| S. No | Disorder | Immune attack directed to | Current therapy | Future drugs |
|---|---|---|---|---|
| 1 | MS | Myelin | IFNb1a, IFNb1b, (Clerico et al., 2007) glatiramer acetate, (Arnon & Aharoni, 2004) natalizumab, (Polman et al., 2006) glucocorticosteroids (Merck) and chemotherapeutics (Chan et al., 2005) | Fingolimod, BG00012, (Lutterotti & Berger, 2010) Laquinimod Teriflunomide Cladribine (Yang et al., 2004; Warnke et al., 2009) Rituximab (Hauser et al., 2008) CAMPATH (Osborne, 2009) Midkine (Muramatsu, 2011) Methylthio-adenosine (Moreno et al., 2010) MAdCAM-1) antibody (Kanwar et al., 2004) Histone deacetylase inhibitors (Faraco et al., 2011) |
| 2 | MG | Nicotinic acetylcholine receptor and muscle specific kinase | AchE inhibitors, (Kumar & Kaminski, 2011) Glucocorticosteroids, (Hohlfeld et al., 2003) Azathioprine, (Mertens et al., 1981). cyclosporine, (Tindall et al., 1987) Cyclophosphamide and mycophenolate mofetil (Schneider-Gold et al., 2006) | SHG2210 (Keefe et al., 2010) |
| 3 | GBS | Myelin and axonal membrane in motor and sensory fibres | immunomodulatory therapy with plasmapheresis and IVIg (Dalakas, 1999; Hadden et al., 1998) | Complement inhibitors (Walgaard et al., 2011) |
| 4 | NMO | Aquaporin -4 water channels | interferons , mycophenolate mofetil, mitoxantrone and rituximab (Bergamaschi, 2007) | Eculizumab (clinicaltrials.gov) |

| | | | | |
|---|---|---|---|---|
| 5 | SMS | Glutamic acid decarboxylase enzyme | skeletal muscle relaxants, (Duddy & Baker, 2009) Plasmapheresis and IVIg (Dalakas, 2009; Hayashi et al., 1999) | ------- |
| 6 | PNS | Hu, Yo,Ma1 & Ma2 antibodies | Cyclosporine, glucocorticoids and Antithymocyte globulin (Buchwald et al., 2005; Koski & Patterson, 2006) | ------- |
| 7 | LEMS | Voltage gated calcium channels | Pyridostigmine bromide, 3,4-Diaminopyridine, guanidine HCl and immunosuppressive agents (McEvoy et al., 1989; Sanders, 1995) | ------- |
| 8 | NM | Voltage gated K+ channels and leucine-rich glioma-inactivated 1 protein | Glucocorticosteroids, Plasmaoheresis and IVIg (Merchut, 2010) | ------- |
| 9 | PN | Glycolipid GM1 and myelin associated glycoprotein | Glucocorticosteroids, Plasmapheresis and IVIg (Shy, 2007) | ------- |

Multiple sclerosis=MS; Myasthenia gravis=MG; Guillain-Barre syndrome=GBS; Neuromyelitis optica=NMO; Stiff-Man syndrome =SMS; Paraneoplastic neurological syndromes=PNS; Lambert-Eaton myasthenic syndrome=LEMS; Neuromyotonia=NM and Polyneuropathies=PN

Table 1. showing the disease mechanisms, current and future therapeutics for neurological autoimmune diseases.

Targeting the immune cell entry is considered to be an ideal approach and based on this concept we noticed a significant blockade of lymphocyte traffic and eventual recovery in EAE mouse model when administered with mucosal addressin cell adhesion molecule (MAdCAM-1) antibody that binds with the integrins on the lymphocyte cell surface. We also developed a combinatorial approach for this model to protect the neurons against glutamate mediated damage with the α-amino-3-hydroxy-5-methyl-4-isoxazolepropionate (AMPA)/ Kainate receptor antagonist 2,3-dihydroxy -6- nitro-7- sulfamoylbenzo (f)quinoxaline (NBQX), and the N-methyl D-aspartate (NMDA) receptor antagonist GPE(neuro protector glycine-proline-glutamic acid;N-terminal tripeptide of insulin like growth factor ). This combinatorial therapy also helps in reducing the infiltrating immune cells at the site of inflammation in the brain (Kanwar et al, 2004).. We have also patented the treatment of demyelinating diseases by administering GPE (WIPO).In addition, there are reports on the highly conserved BARF1 epitopes of Epstein Barr Virus with potent neuroprotective and mitogenic activities (Wynne et al., 2010). We, therefore anticipate conjugating antibodies with such neuroprotectors that would be definitely fruitful for treating a group of neurological autoimmune diseases. Application of nanotechnology also has a tremendous potential for their treatment, as the conjugation of nanoparticles with neuroprotectors and other therapeutics will significantly enhance the targeted delivery, bioavailability and efficacy. Finally introduction of locked nucleic acids (LNAs) has opened a new boom in the area of gene silencing. These LNAs are valuable nucleic acid analogues with striking abilities to regulate gene expression both *in vitro* and *in vivo* (Kauppinen et al., 2005). Thus, in the near future they can be suitably modified to control the genetically mediated autoimmune diseases. Table 1 shows the comparison of current and future drugs.

## 7. Conclusion

Further to conclude, the immunosuppressive and anti-inflammatory treatments considered for treating autoimmune diseases pose serious side effects upon long term administration. Hence, it is rather expected, than to hope that emerging therapies based on the advancements made in T and B-cell targeting would definitely complement or if not replace the existing therapies. It is worth mentioning to find many new novel entities that are in clinical trials for MS and other neurological autoimmune diseases. Inspite of these attractive therapeutic strategies strenuous efforts are to be made to identify the best possible candidates for effective disease control benefiting the patient population.

## 8. References

Allebeck, P., Ahlboom, A., Ljungstrom, K. & Allander, E. (1984). Do oral contraceptives reduce the incidence of rheumatoid arthritis? *Scand.J. Rheumatol*, Vol.13, pp. 140–146.

Alter, A., Duddy, M., Hebert, S., Biernacki, K., Prat, A. & Antel, J. P. (2003). Determinants of human B cell migration across brain endothelial cells. *J Immunol*, Vol.170, pp. 4497–4505.

Anthony, I.C., Crawford, D.H. & Bell, J.E. (2003). B lymphocytes in the normal brain: contrasts with HIV-associated lymphoid infiltrates and lymphomas. *Brain*, Vol.126, pp. 1058–1067.

Arnon, R. & Aharoni, R. (2004). Mechanism of action of glatiramer acetate in multiple sclerosis and its potential for the development of new applications. *Proc Natl Acad Sci USA*, Vol.101, Suppl.2, pp. 14593–14598.

*Arsura, E., Brunner, N.G., Namba, T. & Grob, D. (1985). High-dose intravenous methylprednisolone in myasthenia gravis.* Arch Neurol, *Vol.42, pp. 1149-1153.*

Austyn, J.M. (2000). Antigen-presenting Cells Experimental and Clinical Studies of Dendritic Cells. *American Journal of Respiratory and Critical Care Medicine,* Vol.162, pp.(146-150). Axelsson, M., Malmeström, C., Nilsson, S., Haghighi, S., Rosengren, L. & Lycke, J. (2010). Glial fibrillary acidic protein: a potential biomarker for progression in multiple sclerosis. *Journal of Neurology*, pp. 1-7.

Bach, J.F. (2002).The effect of infections on susceptibility to autoimmune and allergic diseases. *N Engl J Med*, Vol.347, pp. 911-920.

Baker, K.P., Edwards, B.M., Main, S.H., Choi, G.H., Wager, R.E. & Halpern, W.G. (2003). Generation and characterization of LymphoStat-B, a human monoclonal antibody that antagonizes the bioactivities of B lymphocyte stimulator. *Arthritis Rheum,* Vol.48, pp. 3253–3265.

Baranzini, S. E., Jeong, M. C., Butunoi, C., Murray, R. S., Bernard, C. C. & Oksenberg, J. R. (1999). B cell repertoire diversity and clonal expansion in multiple sclerosis brain lesions. *J Immunol,* Vol.163, pp. 5133–5144.

Baratchi, S., Kanwar, R.K., Cheung, C.H. & Kanwar, J.R. (2010a). Proliferative and protective effects of SurR9-C84A on differentiated neural cells. *J Neuroimmunol,* Vol.8, No.227, pp. 120-32.

Baratchi, S., Kanwar, R.K. & Kanwar, J.R. (2010b). Survivin: a target from brain cancer to neurodegenerative disease. *Crit Rev Biochem Mol Biol,* Vol.45, No.6, pp. 535-554.

Baratchi, S., Kanwar, R.K. & Kanwar, J.R. (2011a). Novel survivin mutant protects differentiated SK-N-SH human neuroblastoma cells from activated T-cell neurotoxicity. *J Neuroimmunol,* Vol.233, No.1-2, pp. 18-28.

Baratchi, S., Kanwar, R.K. & Kanwar, J.R. (2011b). Survivin mutant protects differentiated dopaminergic SK-N-SH cells against oxidative stress. *PLoS One,* Vol.10, No.6, pp. e15865.

Barzilai, O., Ram, M. & Shoenfeld, Y. ( 2007a). Viral infection can induce the production of autoantibodies. *Curr Opin Rheumatol,* Vol.19, pp. 636–643.

Barzilai, O., Sherer, Y., Ram, M., Izhaky, D.,Anaya, J.M. & Shoenfeld, Y. (2007b). Epstein-Barr virus and cytomegalovirus in autoimmune diseases: are they truly notorious? A preliminary report. *Ann N Y Acad Sci,* Vol.1108, pp. 567–577.

Begovich, A.B., Carlton, V.E., Honigberg, L.A., Schrodi, S.J. & Chokkalingam, A.P. (2004). Amissense singlenucleotide polymorphism in a gene encoding a protein tyrosine phos,phatase (PTPN22) is associated with rheumatoid arthritis. *Am. J. Hum. Genet,* Vol.75, pp. 330–337.

Bergamaschi, R. (2007).Immune agents for the treatment of Devic's neuromyelitis optica. *Neurol Sci* , Vol.28, pp. 238–240.

Bottini, N., Musumeci, L., Alonso, A., Rahmouni, S. & Nika, K. (2004). A functional variant of lymphoid tyrosine phosphatase is associated with type I diabetes. *Nat. Genet,* Vol.36, pp. 337–338.

Bishop, G.A., Haxhinasto, S.A., Stunz, L.L. & Hostager, B.S. (2003). Antigen-specific B-lymphocyte activation. *Crit. Rev. Immunol,* Vol.23, pp. 149–197.

Bretscher, P. & Cohn, M. A. (1970). Theory of self-nonself discrimination. *Science,* Vol.169, pp. 1042-1049.

Bjorksten, B. (1994). Risk factors in early childhood for the development of allergic disease. *Allergy,* Vol.49, pp. 400-407.

Bondanza, A., Zimmermann, V.S., Antonio, G.D., Cin, E.D., Balestrieri, G., Tincani, A., Amoura, Z., Piette, J.C., Sabbadini, M.G., Querini, P.R. & Manfred, A.A. (2004). Requirement of Dying Cells and Environmental Adjuvants for the Induction of Autoimmunity. *ARTHRITIS & RHEUMATISM,* Vol.50, No. 5, pp. 1549–1560.

Brosnan, C.F. & Raine, C.S, (1996). Mechanisms of immune injury in multiple sclerosis. *Brain Pathol,* Vol.6, pp. 243–257.

Buchwald, B., Ahangari, R., Weishaupt, A. & Toyka, K.V. (2005). Presynaptic effects of immunoglobulin G from patients with Lambert-Eaton myasthenic syndrome: their neutralization by intravenous immunoglobulins. *Muscle Nerve,* Vol.31, No.4, pp. 487-494.

Buckley, C. & Vincent, A. (2005). Autoimmune Channelopathies. *Nature Clin Pract Neurol,* Vol.1, pp. 22–32.

Bufler, J., Kahlert, S., Tzartos, S., Toyka, K.V., Maelicke, A. & Franke, C. (1996). Activation and blockade of mouse muscle nicotinic channels by antibodies directed against the binding site of the acetylcholine receptor. *J Physiol,* Vol.492, pp. 107-114.

Cappione, A., Anolik, J.H., Pugh-Bernard, A., Barnard, J., Dutcher, P., Silverman, G. & Sanz, I. (2005). Germinal center exclusion of autoreactive B cells is defective in human systemic lupus erythematosus. *J. Clin. Invest,* Vol.115, pp. 3205–3216.

Carpentier, A.F. & Delattre, J.Y. (2001). The Lambert-Eaton myasthenic syndrome, *Clin Rev Allergy Immunol,* Vol.20, pp. 155–158.

Cepok, S., Rosche., Grummel, V., Vogel, F., Zhou, D., Sayn, J., Sommer,N., Hartung, H.P. & Hemmer, B. (2005). Short-lived plasma blasts are the main B cell effector subset during the course of multiple sclerosis. *Brain,* Vol.128, pp. 1667–1676.

Chan, A., Weilbach, F.X., Toyka, K.V. & Gold, R. (2005). Mitoxantrone induces cell death in peripheral blood leucocytes of multiple sclerosis patients. *Clin Exp Immunol,* Vol.139, pp. 152-158.

Charo, I.F. & Ransohoff, R.M. (2006). The many roles of chemokines and chemokine receptors in inflammation. *N. Engl. J. Med,* Vol.354, pp. 610–621.

Chatenoud, L. (2003). CD3-specific antibody-induced active tolerance:from bench to bedside. *Nat. Rev. Immunol,* Vol.3, pp. 123–132.

Cheung, C.H., Chen, H.H., Cheng, L.T., Lyu, K.W., Kanwar, J.R. & Chang, J.Y. (2010). Targeting Hsp90 with small molecule inhibitors induces the over-expression of the anti-apoptotic molecule, survivin, in human A549, HONE-1 and HT-29 cancer cells. *Mol Cancer,* Vol.15, No.9, pp. 77.

Cheung, C.H., Sun, X., Kanwar, J.R., Bai, J.Z., Cheng, L. & Krissansen, G.W. (2010b). A cell-permeable dominant-negative survivin protein induces apoptosis and sensitizes prostate cancer cells to TNF-α therapy. *Cancer Cell Int,* Vol.1, No.10, pp. 36.

Clancy, R.M., Backer, C.B., Yin, X., Chang, M.W., Cohen, S.R. & Lee, L.A. (2004a). Genetic association of cutaneous neonatal lupus with HLA class II and tumor necrosis factor alpha: implications for pathogenesis. *Arthritis Rheum,* Vol.50, pp. 2598–2603.

Clancy, R.M., Kapur, R.P., Molad, Y., Askanase, A.D. & Buyon, J.P. (2004b). Immunohistologic evidence supports apoptosis, IgG deposition, and novel macrophage/fibroblast crosstalk in the pathologic cascade leading to congenital heart block. *Arthritis Rheum,* Vol.50, pp. 173–182.

Clerico, M., Contessa, G. & Durelli, L. (2007). Interferon-beta1a for the treatment of multiple sclerosis. *Expert Opin Biol Ther,* Vol.7, No.4, pp. 535–542.

Clifford, D.B., De Luca, A., Simpson, D.M., Arendt, G., Giovannoni, G. & Nath, A. (2010). Natalizumabassociated progressive multifocal leukoencephalopathy in patients with multiple sclerosis: lessons from 28 cases. *Lancet Neurol, Vol.9,* pp. 438–446.

Colombo, M., Dono, M., Gazzola, P., Roncella, S., Valetto, A. & Chiorazzi, N. (2000). Accumulation of clonally related B lymphocytes in the cerebrospinal fluid of multiple sclerosis patients. *J Immunol,* Vol.164, pp. 2782–2789.

Cooper, G.S., Dooley, M.A., Treadwell, E.L., St Clair, E.W. & Gilkeson, G.S. (2002). Hormonal and reproductive risk factors for development of systemic lupus erythematosus: results of a population-based, casecontrol study. *Arthritis Rheum,* Vol.46, pp. 1830–1839.

Crow, M.K. (2004). Costimulatory molecules and T-cell–B-cell interactions. *Rheum. Dis. Clin. North Am,* Vol.30, pp. 175–191.

Cutolo, M. & Accardo, S. (1991). Sex hormones and rheumatoid arthritis. *Clin. Exp. Rheumatol,* Vol.9, pp. 641–646.

Cutolo, M. (2003). Solar light effects on onset/relapses and circannual/circadian symptomatology in rheumatoid arthritis. *Clin Exp Rheumatol,*Vol.21, pp. 148–150.

Czaplinski, & Steck, A.J. (2004). Immune mediated neuropathies: an update on therapeutic strategies. *J Neurol,* Vol.251, pp. 127–137.

Dalakas, M.C. & Quarles, R.H. (1996). Autoimmune ataxic Neuropathies (sensory ganglionopathies): are glycolipids the responsible autoantigens?. *Ann Neurol,* Vol39, pp. 419–422.

Dalakas, M.C. (1999). Intravenous immunoglobulin in the treatment of autoimmune neuromuscular diseases: present status and practical therapeutic guidelines. *Muscle Nerve,* Vol.22, No.11, pp. 1479-1497.

Dalakas, M.C., Fujii, M., Li, M. & McElroy, B. (2000). The clinical spectrum of anti-GAD antibody-positive patients with stiff-person syndrome. *Neurology,* Vol.55, pp. 1531–1535.

Dalakas, M.C., Li, M., Fujii, M. & Jacobowitz, D.M. (2001). Stiff-person syndrome: quantification, specificity and intrathecal synthesis of GAD65 antibodies. *Neurology,* Vol.57, pp. 780–785.

Dalakas, M.C. (2006). B cells in the pathophysiology of autoimmune neurological disorders: A credible therapeutic target. *Pharmacology & Therapeutics,* Vol.112, No.1, pp. 57-70.

Dalakas, M.C. (2008). B cells as therapeutic targets in autoimmune neurological disorders. *Nat Clin Pract Neurol,* Vol.4, No.10, pp. 557-567.

*Dalakas, M.C. (2009). Stiff person syndrome: advances in pathogenesis and therapeutic interventions.* Curr Treat Options Neurol, Vol.11, No.2, pp. *102-110.*

Dalmau, F., Graus, M.K., Rosenblum, & Posner, J.B. (1992). Anti-Hu-associated paraneoplastic encephalomyelitis/sensory neuropathy: a clinical study of 71 patients. *Medicine (Baltimore),* Vol.71, pp. 59–72.

Damian, R.T. (1964). Molecular mimicry: antigen sharing by parasite and host and its consequences. *Am. Naturalist,* Vol.XCVIII, pp. 129–149.

Darnell, R.B. & Posner, J.B. (2003). Paraneoplastic syndromes involving the nervous system, *N Engl J Med,* Vol.349, pp. 1543–1554.

Davidson, A. & Diamond, B. (2001). Advances in Immunology. *N Engl J Med,* Vol. 345, No. 5, pp. 340-350.

Dedrick, R.L., Bodary, S. & Garovoy, M.R. (2003). Adhesion molecules as therapeutic targets for autoimmune diseases and transplant rejection. Expert Opin Biol Ther, Vol.3, No.1, pp. 85-95.

Delves, P.J. (2006). Structural and functional aspects of the innate and adaptive systems of immunity. In: Rose, NR and Mackay, IR, (eds.) *The autoimmune diseases.* pp. 9-21. Elsevier: San Diego.

Drachman, D.B. (1994). Myasthenia gravis, *N Engl J Med,* Vol.330, pp. 1797–1810.

Druet, P. (1989). Contributions of immunological reactions to nephrotoxicity. *Toxicol Lett,* Vol.46 pp. 55-64.

Duddy, M.E. & Baker, M.R. (2009). Stiff person syndrome. *Front Neurol Neurosci*, Vol.26, pp. 147-165.

Fang, C., Zhang, X., Miwa, T. & Song, W.C. (2009). Complement promotes the development of inflammatory T-helper 17 cells through synergistic interaction with Toll-like receptor signaling and interleukin-6 production. *Blood*, Vol.114, pp. 1005–1015.

Faraco, G., Cavone, L. & Chiarugi, A. (2011). The Therapeutic Potential of HDAC Inhibitors in the Treatment of Multiple Sclerosis. *Mol Med*. Feb 25. [Epub ahead of print].

Fauci, A.S., Wolff, S.M. & Johnson, J.S. (1971). Effect of cyclophosphamide upon the immune response in Wegener's granulomatosis, *N Engl J Med*, Vol.285, pp. 1493-1496.

Flickinger, C.J., Baran, M.L., Howards, S.S. & Herr, J.C. (1994). Epididymal obstruction during development results in antisperm autoantibodies at puberty in rats. *J Androl*, Vol.19, pp. 136-144.

Fraga, A., Mintz, G. & Orozco, J. (1974). Sterility and fertility rates, fetal wastage and maternal morbidity in SLE. *J. Rheumatol*, Vol.1, pp. 293–298.

Frisoni, L., McPhie, L., Colonna, L., Sriram, U., Monestier, M. & Gallucci, S. (2005). Nuclear autoantigen translocation and autoantibody opsonization lead to increased dendritic cell phagocytosis and presentation of nuclear antigens: a novel pathogenic pathway for autoimmunity? *J Immunol*, Vol.175, pp. 2692–2701.

Frohman, E.M., Racke, M.K. & Raine, C.S. (2006). Multiple sclerosis-the plaque and its pathogenesis. *N. Engl. J. Med*, Vol.354, pp. 942–955.

Fugger, L., Friese, M.A. & Bell, J.I. (2009). From genes to function: The next challenge to understanding multiple sclerosis. *Nat Rev Immunol*, Vol.9, No.6, pp. 408–417.

Fujinami, R.S. & Oldstone, M.B. (1989). Molecular mimicry as a mechanism for virus-induced autoimmunity. *Immunol Res*, Vol.8, pp. 3-15.

Fujinami, R.S.& Oldstone, M.B. (1985). Amino acid homology between the encephalitogenic site of myelin basic protein and virus: mechanism for autoimmunity. *Science*, Vol.230,No.4729, pp. 1043-1045.

Gabriel, C.L., Wu, L., Parekh, V.V. & Van Kaer, L. (2010). Invariant natural killer t cell-based therapy of autoimmune diseases. *Current Immunology Reviews*, Vol.6, No.2, pp. 88-101.

Gehrs, B.C. & Friedberg, R.C. (2002). Autoimmune hemolytic anemia. *Am J Hematol*, Vol.69, pp. 258–271.

Gellert, M. (2002). V(D)J recombination: RAG proteins, repair factors, and regulation. *Annu. Rev. Biochem*, Vol.71, pp. 101–132.

Genovese, M.C., Kaine, J.L., Lowenstein, M.B., Del Giudice, J., Baldassare, A., Schechtman, J., Fudman, E., Kohen, M., Gujrathi, S., Trapp, R.G., Sweiss, N.J., Spaniolo, G. & Dummer, W. (2008). Ocrelizumab, a humanized anti-CD20 monoclonal antibody, in the treatment of patients with rheumatoid arthritis: a phase I/II randomized, blinded, placebo-controlled, dose-ranging study. *Arthritis Rheum*, Vol.58, No.9, pp. 2652-2661.

Gold, R., Dalakas, M.C. & Toyka, K.V. (2003). Immunotherapy in autoimmune neuromuscular disorders. *Lancet Neurol*, Vol.2, pp. 22-32.

Gold, R., Linington, C. & Lassmann, H. (2006). Understanding pathogenesis and therapy of multiple sclerosis via animal models: 70 years of merits and culprits in experimental autoimmune encephalomyelitis research. *Brain*, Vol.129, pp. 1953–1971.

Goldrath, A.W. & Bevan, M.J. (1999). Selecting and maintaining a diverse T-cell repertoire. *Nature,* Vol.402, pp. 255-262.

Graus, F., Keime-Guibert, F., Rene, R., Benyahia, B., Ribalta, T. & Ascaso, C. (2001). Anti-Hu-associated paraneoplastic encephalomyelitis: analysis of 200 patients. *Brain,* Vol.24, pp. 1138–1148.

Green, A.J., McQuaid, S., Hauser, S.L., Allen I.V. & Lyness, R. (2010). Ocular pathology in multiple sclerosis: retinal atrophy and inflammation irrespective of disease duration, *Brain,* Vol.133, pp. 1591–1601.

Greter, M., Heppner, F.L., Lemos, M.P., Odermatt, B.M., Goebels, N., Laufer, T., Noelle, R.J. & Becher, B. (2005). Dendritic cells permit immune invasion of the CNS in an animal model of multiple sclerosis. *Nat. Med,* Vol.11, pp. 328–334.

Gu, H., Tarlinton, D., Muller, W., Rajewsky, K. & Forster, I. (1991). Most peripheral B cells in mice are ligand selected. *J Exp Med,* Vol.173, pp. 1357-1371.

Hadden, R.D., Cornblath, D.R., Hughes RA., Zielasek, J., Hartung, H.P., Toyka, K.V. & Swan, A.V. (1998). Electrophysiological classification of Guillain-Barre syndrome: clinical associations and outcome. Plasma Exchange/Sandoglobulin Guillain-Barre Syndrome Trial Group. *Ann Neurol,* Vol.44, No.5, pp. 780-788.

Hafer-Macko, C. E., Sheikh, K. A., Li, C. Y., Ho, T. W., Cornblath, D. R. & McKhann, G. M.. (1996). Immune attack on the Schwann cell surface in acute inflammatory demyelinating polyneuropathy. *Ann Neurol,* Vol.39, pp. 625–635.

Hauser, S.L. (2008). Multiple lessons for multiple sclerosis. *N Engl J Med,* Vol.359, No.17, pp. 1838–1841.

Hauser, S.L., Waubant, E., Arnold, D.L., Vollmer, T., Antel, J., Fox, R.J., Bar-Or, A., Panzara, M., Sarkar, N., Agarwal, S., Langer-Gould, A. & Smith, C.H. (2008) B-cell depletion with rituximab in relapsing–remitting multiple sclerosis. *N Engl J Med,* Vol.358, No.7, pp. 676–688.

Hayashi, A., Nakamagoe, K., Ohkoshi, N., Hoshino, S. & Shoji, S. (1999). Double filtration plasma exchange and immunoadsorption therapy in a case of stiff-man syndrome with negative anti-GAD antibody. *J Med,* Vol.30, No.(5-6), pp. 321-327.

Heather Rachel Davids, (Mar, 2010), Guillain-Barre Syndrome: Treatment & Medication In: *emedicine,*16.03.2011,Available from URL: emedicine.medscape.com/article/315632-treatment.

Hennies, C., Sternberg, D., Bistulfi, G.L., Kazim, L., Benedict, R.H.B., Chadha, K., Leung, C., Weinstock-Guttman, B., Munschauer, F. & Sternberg, Z. (2011). Plasma pentosidine: A potential biomarker in the management of multiple sclerosis. *Multiple Sclerosis,* Vol.17, No.2, pp. 157-163

Heppner, F.L., Greter, M., Marino, D., Falsig, J., Raivich, G., Hovelmeyer, N., Waisman, A., Rulicke, T., Prinz, M., Priller, J., Becher, B. & Aguzzi, A. (2005). Experimental autoimmune encephalomyelitis repressed by microglial paralysis. *Nat Med,* Vol.11, No.2, pp. 146–152.

Herrmann, M., Sholmerich, J. & Straub, R.H. (2000). Stress and rheumatic disease. *Rheum Dis Clin North Am,* Vol.26, No.4, pp. 737-763.

Hickey, W. F., Hsu, B. L. & Kimura, H. (1991). T-lymphocyte entry into the central nervous system. *J. Neurosci. Res,* Vol.28, pp. 254–260.

Hodgkin, P.D. & Basten, A.B. (1995). Cell activation, tolerance and antigenpresenting function. *Curr Opin Immunol,* Vol.7, pp. 121-129.

Hohlfeld, R., Melms, A., Schneider, C., Toyka, K.V. & Drachman, D.B. (2003). Therapy of myasthenia gravis and myasthenic syndromes. Brandt, T., Caplan, L.R., Dichgans, J., Diener, H.C. & Kennard, C. In: *Neurological disorders: course and treatment*, Elsevier, Stuttgart, pp. 1341-1362.

Holmes, C.H. & Simpson, K.L. (1992). Complement and pregnancy. New insights into the immunobiology of the feto maternal relationship. *Ballières Clin. Obstet. Gynecol,*Vol.6, pp.(439–460).

Hooks, J.J., Jordan, G.W., Cupps, T., Moutsopoulos, H.M., Fauci, A.S. & Notkins, A.L.. (1982). Multiple interferons in the circulation of patients with systemic lupus erythematosus and vasculitis. *Arthritis Rheum,* Vol.25, pp. 396-400.

Hoyer, B.F., Moser, K., Hauser, A.E., Peddinghaus, A., Voigt, C., Eilat, D., Radbruch, A., Manz, R.A. & Hiepe, F. (2004). Short-lived plasmablasts and long-lived plasma cells contribute to chronic humoral autoimmunity in NZB/w mice. *J. Exp.Med,* Vol.199, pp. 1577–1584.

Ishii, A. (2010). Stiff-person syndrome and other myelopathies constitute paraneoplastic neurological syndromes. *Brain Nerve,* Vol.62, No.4, pp. 377-385.

Jacobson, D.L. (1997). Epidemiology and estimated population burden of selected autoimmune disease in the United States. *Clin Immunol Immunopathol,* Vol.84, pp. 223-243.

Janeway, C. Jr. & Travers, P. (1998) Immunobiology. In: *The Immune System in Health and Disease,* pp 625-640. Garland Publishing Inc, New York Jarow, J.P., Goluboff, E.T., Chang, T.S. & Marshall, F.F. (1994). Relationship between antisperm antibodies and testicular histologic changes in humans after vasectomy. *Urology,* Vol.43, pp. 521-524.

Johnson, P.M. (1993). Reproductive and maternofetal relations, In: Gell, P.G.H. & Coombs, R.R.A, *Clinical Aspects of Immunology,* Blackwell Johnson, Oxford, pp. 755–767.

Kanwar, J.R., Harrison, J.E.B., Wang, D., Leung, E., Mueller, W., Wagner, N. & Krissansen, G.W. (1999). β7 integrins contribute to demyelinating disease of the central nervous system. *Journal of Neuroimmunology,* Vol.103, No.2000, pp. 146–152.

Kanwar, J.R., Kanwar, R.K., Wang, D. & Krissansen, G.W. (2000). Prevention of a chronic progressive form of experimental autoimmune encephalomyelitis by an antibody against mucosal addressin cell adhesion molecule-1, given early in the course of disease progression. *Immunology and Cell Biology,* Vol.78, pp. 641–645.

Kanwar, R.K., Kanwar, J.R., Wang, D., Ormrod, D.J. & Krissansen, G.W. (2001). Temporal Expression of Heat Shock Proteins 60 and 70 at Lesion-Prone Sites. *Arterioscler Thromb Vasc Biol,* Vol.21, pp. 1991-1997.

Kanwar, J.R., Berg, R.W., Yang, Y., Kanwar, R.K., Ching, L.M., Sun, X. & Krissansen, G.W. (2003). Requirements for ICAM-1 immunogene therapy of lymphoma. *Cancer Gene Ther,* Vol.10, No.6, pp. 468-476.

Kanwar, J.R., Kanwar, R.K. & Krissansen, G.W. (2004). Simultaneous neuroprotection and blockade of inflammation reverses autoimmune encephalomyelitis. *Brain,* Vol.127, No.6, pp. 131313-131331.

Kanwar. J.R. (2005). Anti-inflammatory immunotherapy for multiple sclerosis/experimental autoimmune encephalomyelitis (EAE) disease. *Curr Med Chem,* Vol.12, No.25, pp. 2947-2962.

Kanwar, J.R, Kanwar, R.K., Burrow, H. & Baratchi, S. (2009). Recent advances on the roles of NO in cancer and chronic inflammatory disorders. *Curr Med Chem*, Vol.16, No.19, pp. 2373-2394.

Kanwar, J.R., Kamalapuram, S.K. & Kanwar, R.K. (2010a). Targeting survivin in cancer: patent review. *Expert Opin Ther Pat*, Vol.20, No.12, pp. 1723-37.

Kanwar, J.R, Mahidhara, G. & Kanwar, R.K. (2010b). MicroRNA in human cancer and chronic inflammatory diseases. *Front Biosci (Schol Ed*, Vol.1, No.2, pp. 1113-1126.

Kanwar, J.R., Mohan, R.R., Kanwar, R.K., Roy, K. & Bawa, R. (2010c). Applications of aptamers in nanodelivery systems in cancer, eye and inflammatory diseases. *Nanomedicine*,Vol.5, No.9, pp. 1435-45.

Kanwar, R.K., Cheung, C.H., Chang, J.Y. & Kanwar, J.R. (2010d). Recent advances in anti-survivin treatments for cancer. *Curr Med Chem*, Vol.17, No.15, pp. 1509-1015.

Kappler, J.W., Roehm, N. & Marrack, P. (1987). T cell tolerance by clonal elimination in the thymus. *Cell*, Vol.49, pp. 273–280.

Kauppinen, S., Vester, B. & Wengel, J. (2005). Locked nucleic acid (LNA): High affinity targeting of Complementary RNA for diagnostics and therapeutics. *Drug Discovery Today: Technol*, Vol.2, pp. 287.

Keefe, D., Parng, C., Lundberg, D., Ray, S., Martineau-Bosco, J., Leng, C., Tzartos, S., Powell, J., Concino, M., Heartlein, M., Lamsa, J. & Josiah, S. (2010). In vitro characterization of an acetylcholine receptor–transferrin fusion protein for the treatment of myasthenia gravis. *Autoimmunity*, Vol.43, No.8, pp. 628–639.

Khamashta, M.A., Ruiz-Irastorza, G. & Hughes, G.R. (1997). Systemic lupus erythematosus flares during pregnancy. *Rheum. Dis. Clin. N. Am*, Vol.23, pp. 15–30.

Kieseier, B.C., Kiefer, R., Gold, R., Hemmer, B., Willison, H.J. & Hartung, H. P. (2004). Advances in understanding and treatment of immune-mediated disorders of the peripheral nervous system. *Muscle Nerve*, Vol.30, pp. 131–156.

Kleopas, A.K., Elman, L.B., Lang, B., Vincent, A. & Scherer, S.S. (2006). Neuromyotonia and limbic encephalitis sera target mature Shaker-type K+ channels: subunit specificity correlates with clinical manifestations. *Brain*, Vol.129, pp. 1570–1584.

Knopf, P. M., Harling-Berg, C. J., Cserr, H. F., Basu, D., Sirulnick, E. J. & Nolan, S. C. (1998). Antigen-dependent intrathecal antibody synthesis in the normal rat brain: tissue entry and local retention of antigen-specific B cells. *J Immunol*, Vol.161, pp. 692–701.

Kornberg, A.J. & Pestronk, A. (2003). Antibody-associated polyneuropathy syndromes: principles and treatment. *Semin Neurol*, Vol.23, pp. 181–190.

Koski, C.L. & Patterson, J.V. (2006). Intravenous immunoglobulin use for neurologic diseases. *J Infus Nurs*, Vol.29, Suppl.3, pp. S21-8.

Kumar, V. & Kaminski, H.J. (2011). Treatment of Myasthenia Gravis. *Curr Neurol Neurosci Rep*, Vol.11, pp. 89–96.

Kuwabara, S. (2004). Guillain-Barré syndrome: epidemiology, pathophysiology and management. *Drugs*, Vol.64, pp. 597–610.

Lai, M., Huijbers, M.G.M., Lancaster, E., Graus, F., Bataller, L., Balice-Gordon, R., Cowell, J.K. & Dalmau, J. (2010). Investigation of LGI1 as the antigen in limbic encephalitis previously attributed to potassium channels: A case series *The Lancet Neurology*, Vol.9, No.8, pp. 776-785.

Lambert-Eaton syndrome, In: *PubMed Health*,09.03.2011,Available from URL: www.ncbi.nlm.nih.gov/pubmedhealth/PMH0001729/.

Lennon, V.A., Kryzer, T.J., Pittock, S.J., Verkman A.S. & Hinson, S.R. (2005). IgG marker of optic-spinal multiple sclerosis binds to the aquaporin-4 water channel, *J Exp Med,* Vol.202, pp. 473–477.

Leung, E., Kanwar, R.K., Kanwar, J.R. & Krissansen, G.W. (2003). Mucosal vascular addressin cell adhesion molecule-1 is expressed outside the endothelial lineage on fibroblasts and melanoma cells. *Immunol Cell Biol,* Vol.81, No.4, pp. 320-327.

Lim, K.J.H., Odukoya, O.A. & Ajjan, R.A. (1998). Profile of cytokine mRNA expression in peri-implantation human endometrium. *Mol.Hum. Reprod,* Vol.4, pp. 77–81.

Lleo, A., Invernizzi, P., Gao, B., Podda, M. & Gershwin, M.E. (2010). Definition of human autoimmunity – autoantibodies versus autoimmune disease. *Autoimmunity Reviews,* Vol.9, pp. 259–266.

Lucchinetti, C., Bruck, W., Parisi, J., Scheithauer, B., Rodriguez, M. & Lassmann, H. (2000). Heterogeneity of multiple sclerosis lesions: implications for the pathogenesis of demyelination. *Ann Neurol,* Vol.47, pp. 707–717.

Lucchinetti, C.F., Mandler, R.N., McGavern, D., Bruck, W., Gleich, G. & Ransohoff R.M. (2002). A role for humoral mechanisms in the pathogenesis of Devic's neuromyelitis optica, *Brain,* Vol.125, pp. 1450–1461.

Lutterotti, A. & Berger, T. (2010). Advances in Multiple Sclerosis Therapy: New Oral Disease-Modifying Agents, *CML – Multiple Sclerosis,* Vol.2, No.1, pp. 1–10.

Mackay, C. R., Marston, W. L. & Dudler, L. (1990). Naive and memory T cells show distinct pathways of lymphocyte recirculation. *J. Exp. Med,* Vol. 171, No.3, pp. 801-817. Mackay, R. & Rosen, F.S. (2001). Autoimmune Diseases. *N Engl J Med,* Vol.345, pp. 340-350.

Manoury, B, Hewitt, E.W, Morrice, N, Dando, P.M, Barrett, A.J. & Watts, C. (1998). An asparaginyl endopeptidase processes a microbial antigen for class II MHC presentation. *Nature,* Vol.396, pp. 695–699.

Manz, R.A., Thiel, A. & Radbruch, A. (1997). Lifetime of plasma cells in the bone marrow.*Nature,* Vol.388, pp. 133–134.

Manz, R.A., Löhning, M., Cassese, G., Thiel, A. & Radbruch, A. (1998). Survival of long-lived plasma cells is independent of antigen. *Int. Immunol,* Vol.10, pp. 1703–1711.

Manz, R.A., Hauser, A.E., Hiepe, F. & Radbruch, A. (2005). Maintenance of serum antibody levels. *Annu. Rev. Immunol,* Vol.23, pp. 367–386.

Marmont, A.M. (2000). New horizons in the treatment of autoimmune diseases: immunoablation and stem cell transplantation. *Annu Rev Med,* Vol.51, pp. 115-134.

Maverakis, E., Goodarzi, H., Wehrli, L.N., Ono, Y. & Garcia, M.S. (2011). The Etiology of Paraneoplastic Autoimmunity. *Clin Rev Allergy Immunol,* Jan 19 [Epub ahead of print].

MayoClinic, *Multiple Sclerosis,* 25.02.2011, Available from URL: www.mayoclinic.org/multiple-sclerosis/

*McEvoy, K.M., Windebank, A.J., Daube, J.R. & Low, PA. (1989). 3,4-Diaminopyridine in the treatment of Lambert-Eaton myasthenic syndrome.* N Engl J Med, Vol.321, No.23, pp. 1567-1571.

McKall-Faienza, K.J., Kawai, K., Kundig, T.M., Odermatt, B., Bachmann, M.F., Zakarian, A., Mak, T.W. & Ohashi, P.S. (1998). Absence of TNFRp55 influences virus-induced autoimmunity despite efficient lymphocytic infiltration. *Int Immunol,* Vol.10, pp. 405-412.

McMurray, R.W. (1996). Adhesion molecules in autoimmune disease. *Semin Arthritis Rheum,* Vol.25, No.4, pp. 215-33.

Merchut, M.P. (2010). Management of voltage-gated potassium channel antibody disorders. *Neurologic Clinics,* Vol.28, No.4, pp. 941-959.

Merck, *Multiple Sclerosis (MS),* 27.02.2011, Available from URL: www.merckmanuals.com/home/sec06/ch092/ch092b.html

Mertens, H.G., Hertel, G., Reuther, P. & Ricker, K. (1981). Effect of immunosuppressive drugs (azathioprine). *Ann NY Acad Sci,* Vol.377, pp. 691-699.

Monroe, J.G., Bannish, G., Fuentes-Panana, E.M., King, L.B., Sandel, P.C., Chung, J. & Sater, R. (2003). Positive and negative selection during B lymphocyte development. *Immunol. Res,* Vol.27, pp. 427–442.

Moreno, B., Fernandez-Diez, B., Di Penta, A. & Villoslada, P. (2010). Preclinical studies of methylthioadenosine for the treatment of multiple sclerosis. *Mult Scler,* Vol.16, No.9, pp. 1102-1108.

Muramatsu, T. (2011). Midkine: a Promising Molecule for Drug Development to Treat Diseases of the Central Nervous System. *Curr Pharm Des,* Mar 4. [Epub ahead of print]. *Multiple Sclerosis Treatments,* 27.02.2011, Available from URL: www.mult-sclerosis.org/mstreatments.html Nobile-Orazio, E. (2001). Multifocal motor neuropathy. *J Neuroimmunol,* Vol.115, pp. 4–18.

Latov, N. (1994). Antibodies to glycoconjugates in neuropathy and motor neuron disease. *Prog Brain Res,* Vol.101, pp. 295–303.

Ogawara, K., Kuwabara, S., Mori, M., Hattori, T., Koga, M. & Yuki, N. (2000). Axonal Guillain-Barré syndrome: relation to anti-ganglioside antibodies and Campylobacter jejuni infection in Japan. *Ann Neurol,* Vol.48, pp. 624–631.

Ohishi, K., Kanoh, M., Shinomiya, H., Hitsumoto, Y. & Utsumi, S. (1995). Complement activation by cross-linked B cell-membrane IgM. *J Immunol,* Vol.154, pp. 3173–3179.

Oldstone, M.B.A. (1998). Molecular mimicry and immune-mediated diseases. *FASEB J,* Vol.12, pp. 1255–1265.

Osborne, R. (2009). Buzz around Campath proof-of-concept trial in MS. *Nat Biotechnol,* Vol.27, No.1, pp. 6–8.

Palmer, E. (2003). Negative selection – clearing out the bad apples from the T-cell repertoire. *Nat. Rev. Immunol,* Vol.3, pp. 383–391.

Patterson, C.C., Carson, D.J. & Hadden, D.R. (1996). Epidemiology of childhood IDDM in Northern Ireland 1989e1994: low incidence in areas with highest population density and most household crowding. *Diabetologia,* Vol.39, pp. 1063-1069.

Pender, M.P. (1995). An introduction to neuroimmunology, In: *Autoimmune neurological diseases,*Pender, M.P & McCombe, P.A, pp.16. cambridge university press.

Peterson, K., Rosenblum, M.K., Kotanides, H. & Posner, J.B. (1992). Paraneoplastic cerebellar degeneration: I. A clinical analysis of 55 anti-Yo antibody positive patients, *Neurology,* Vol.42, pp. 1931–1937.

Pettinelli, C.B. & McFarlin, D.E. (1981). Adoptive transfer of experimental allergic encephalomyelitis in SJL/J mice after in vivo activation of lymph node cells by myelin basic protein: requirement for Lyt-1+2- T lymphocytes. *J Immunol,* Vol.127, pp. 1420-1423.

Pircher, H., Rohrer, H.U., Moskophidis, D., Zinkernagel, R.M. & Hengartner, H. (1991). Lower receptor avidity required for thymic clonal deletion than for effector T cell function. *Nature,* Vol.351, pp. 482–485.

Polman, C.H., O'Connor, P.W., Havrdova, E., Hutchinson, M., Kappos, L. & Miller, D.H. (2006). A randomized, placebo-controlled trial of natalizumab for relapsing multiple sclerosis. *N Engl J Med, Vol.*354, pp. 899–910.

Pranzatelli, M.R., Travelstead, A.L., Tate, E.D., Allison, T.J., Moticka, E.J., Franz, D.N., Nigro, M.A., Parke, J.T., Stumpf, D.A. & Verhulst, S.J. (2004). B- and T-cell markers in opsoclonus-myoclonus syndrome: immunophenotyping of CSF lymphocytes, *Neurology,* Vol.62, pp. 1526–1532.

Qin, Y., Duquette, P., Zhang, Y., Talbot, P., Poole, R. & Antel, J. (1998). Clonal expansion and somatic hypermutation of VH genes of B cells from cerebrospinal fluid in multiple sclerosis. *J Clin Invest,* Vol.102, pp. 1045–1050.

Quarles, R.H. & Weiss, M.D. (1999). Autoantibodies associated with peripheral neuropathy. *Muscle Nerve,* Vol.22, pp. 800–822.

Racke, M.K & Stuart, R.W. (2002). Targeting T cell costimulation in autoimmune disease. *Expert Opin Ther Targets,* Vol.6, No.3, pp. 275-89.

Radbruch, A., Muehlinghaus, G., Luger, E.O., Inamine, A., Smith, K.G., Dörner, T. & Hiepe, F. (2006). Competence and competition: the challenge of becoming a long-lived plasma cell. *Nat. Rev. Immunol,* Vol.6, pp. 741–750.

Ragheb. & Lisak, R.P. (1998). Immune regulation and myasthenia gravis. *Ann N Y Acad Sci,* Vol.841, pp. 210–224.

Raghupathy, R. (1997). Th–1 type immunity is incompatible with successful pregnancy. *Immunol. Today,* Vol.18, pp. 478–482.

Rajewsky, K. (1996). Clonal selection and learning in the antibody system. *Nature,* Vol.381, pp.(751–758).

Rodien, P., Madec, A.M., Ruf, J., Rajas, F., Bornet, H. & Carayon, P. (1996). Antibody-dependent cell-mediated cytotoxicity in autoimmune thyroid disease: relationship to antithyroperoxidase antibodies. *J Clin Endocrinol Metab,* Vol.81, pp. 2595–2600.

Roitt, I, Brostoff, J & Male, D. (1998). Immunology, Mosby, London UK, pp. 410- 425.

Rosenfeld, M.R., Eichen, J.G., Wade, D.F., Posner, J.B. & Dalmau, J. (2001). Molecular and clinical diversity in Paraneoplastic immunity to Ma proteins. *Ann Neurol,* Vol.50, pp. 339–348.

Ross, R. (1990). Mechanisms of atherosclerosis-a review. *Adv Nephrol Necker Hosp,*Vol.19, pp.79-86.

Galperin, C & Gershwin, ME. (1997). Immunopathogenesis of gastrointestinal and hepatobiliary diseases. *JAMA,*Vol.278, pp. 1946-1955.

Roubinian, J.R., Talal, N., Greenspan, J.S., Goodman, J.R. & Siiteri, P.K. (1978).Effect of castration and sex hormone treatment on survival,anti-nucleic acid antibodies, and glomerulonephritis in NZB/NZW F1 mice. *J Exp Med,* Vol.147, pp. 1568-1583.

Ruegg, S.J., Fuhr, P. & Steck, A.J. (2004). Rituximab stabilizes multifocal motor neuropathy increasingly less responsive to IVIg. *Neurology,* Vol.63, pp. 2178–2179.

Sakic, B., Szechtman, H., Denburg, J.A., Gomy, G., Kolb, B. & Whishaw IQ. (1998).Progressive atrophy of pyramidal neuron dendrites in autoimmune MRL/lpr mice. *J Neuroimmunol,* Vol.87, pp. 162-170.

Sanders, D.B. (1995). Lambert-Eaton myasthenic syndrome: clinical diagnosis, immune-mediated mechanisms, and update on therapies. *Ann Neurol*, Vol.37, Suppl 1, pp. 63-73.

Schattner, A. (1994). Lymphokines in autoimmunity-a critical review. *Clin Immunol Immunopathol*, Vol.70, pp. 177-189.

Schneider-Gold, C., Hartung, H.P. & Gold, R. (2006). Mycophenolate mofetil and tacrolimus: New therapeutic options in neuroimmunological diseases. *Muscle & Nerve*, Vol.34, pp.284-291.

Shy, M.E. (2007). Peripheral neuropathies, Goldman L, Ausiello D. In: *Cecil Medicine*, Elsevier, Philadelphia, Pa: Saunders, pp.446.

Silverstein, A.M. & Rose, N.R. (2000).There is only one immune system! The view from immunopathology. *Semin Immunol*, Vol.12, No.173, No.8, pp. 257-344.

Singer, P.A. & Theofilopoulos, A.N. (1990).T cell receptor V) repertoire expression in murine models of SLE. *Immunol Rev*, Vol.118, pp. 103-127.

Slifka, M.K., Antia, R., whitmire, J.K. & Ahmed, R. (1998). Humoral immunity due to long-lived plasma cells. *Immunity*, Vol.8, pp. 363–372.

Smith, D.A. & Dori, R. (1999). Introduction to Immunology and Autoimmunity. *Environmental Health Perspectives*, Vol.107, Supplement. 5, pp. 661-665.

Starr, T.K., Jameson, S.C. & Hogquist, K.A. (2003). Positive and negative selection of T cells. *Annu. Rev. Immunol*, Vol.21, pp. 139–176.

Steinman, L. (2002). A few autoreactive cells in an autoimmune infiltrate control a vast population of nonspecific cells: a tale of smart bombs and the infantry. *Proc. Natl. Acad. Sci. U. S. A*, Vol.93, pp. 2253–2256.

Stohl, S.W. (2004). Targeting B lymphocyte stimulator in systemic lupus erythematosus and other autoimmune rheumatic disorders. *Expert Opin Ther Targets*, Vol.8, pp. 177–189.

Stojanovich, L. & Marisavljevich, D. (2008). Stress as a trigger of autoimmune disease *Autoimmun Rev*, Vol.7, No.3, pp. 209-213.

Stuve, O., Cepok, S., Elias, S., Saleh, A., Hartung, H.P., Hemmer, B. & Kieseier, B.C. (2005). Clinical stabilization and effective bB-lymphocyte depletion in the cerebrospinal fluid and peripheral blood of a patient with fulminant relapsing-remitting multiple sclerosis, *Arch Neurol*, Vol.62, pp. 1620–1623.

Swain, S.L. (2003). Regulation of the generation and maintenance of T-cell memory: a direct, default pathway from effectors to memory cells. *Microbes. Infect*, Vol.5, pp. 213–219

Tan, M.E., Reimer, G. & sullivan, K.(1987).Itracellularv antigens:diagnostic fingerprints but aetiological dilemmas, Evered, D & Whelan, J. In: *autoimmunity and autoimmune disease.* John Wiley & Sons Ltd, Chichester,UK, pp. 25-30.

Tarlinton, D., Radbruch, A., Hiepe, F. & Dörner, T. (2008). Plasma cell differentiation and survival. *Curr.Opin. Immunol*, Vol.20, pp. 162–169.

Tindall, R.S., Rollins, J.A., Phillips, J.T., Greenlee, R.G., Wells, L. & Belendiuk, G. (1987). Preliminary results of a double-blind, randomized, placebo-controlled trial of cyclosporine in myasthenia gravis. *N Engl J Med*, Vol.316, pp. 719-724.

Trembleau, S., Germann, T., Gately, M.K. Z. & Adorini, L. (1995).The role of IL-12 in the induction of organ-specific autoimmune diseases. *Immunol Today*, Vol.16, pp. 383-386.

Vandiedonck, C., Capdevielle, C., Giraud, M., Krumeich, S. & Jais, J.P. (2006). Association of the PTPN22*R620W polymorphism with autoimmune myasthenia gravis. *Ann. Neuro,* .Vol.59, pp. 404–407.

VanVoorhis, B.J. & Stovall, D.W. (1997). Autoantibodies and fertility: a review of the literature. *J. Reprod. Immunol.*Vol.33, pp. 239–256.

Vincent, A., Beeson, D. & Lang, B. (2000). Molecular targets for autoimmune and genetic disorders of neuromuscular transmission. *Eur J Biochem,* Vol.267, pp. 6717–6728.

Vincent, A., Bowen, J., Newsom-Davis, J. & McConville, J. (2003). Seronegative generalised myasthenia gravis: clinical features, antibodies and their targets. *Lancet Neurol,* Vol.2, pp. 99-106.

Vogt, M.H., Lopatinskaya, L., Smits, M., Polman, C.H. & Nagelkerken, L. (2003). Elevated osteopontin levels in active relapsing-remitting multiple sclerosis. *Ann Neurol,* Vol.53, No.6, pp. 819–822.

Waldor, M.K., Sriram, S., Hardy, R., Herzenberg, L.A., Herzenberg, L.A., Lanier, L., Lim, M. & Steinman, L. (1985). Reversal of experimental allergic encephalomyelitis with a monoclonal antibody to a T cell subset marker (L3T4). *Science,* Vol.15, pp. 417

Walgaard, C., Jacobs, B.C. & Van Doorn, P.A. (2011). Emerging drugs for Guillain-Barr? Syndrome. *Expert Opin Emerg Drugs,* Vol.16, No.1, pp. 105-120.

Warnke, C., Meyer, H.G., Hartung, H.P., Stuve, O. & Kieseier, B.C. (2009). Review of teriflunomide and its potential in the treatment of multiple sclerosis. *Neuropsychiatr Dis Treat,* Vol.5, pp. 333–340.

Webster, E.L., Torpy, D.J., Elenkov, I.J. & Chrousos, G.P. (1998). Corticotropinreleasing hormone and inflammation. *Ann NY Acad Sci,* Vol.840, pp. 21-32.

Wekerle, H., Linington, C., Lassmann, H. & Meyermann, R, (1986). Cellular immune reactivity within the CNS. *Trends Neurosci,* Vol.9, pp. 271–277.

Whitaker, J.N. (1987). The presence of immunoreactive myelin basic protein peptide in urine of persons with multiple sclerosis. *Ann Neurol,* Vol.22, No.5, pp. 648–655.

Willison, H. J. & Yuki, N. (2002). Peripheral neuropathies and anti-glycolipid antibodies. *Brain,* Vol.125, pp. 2591–2625.

Wingerchuk, D.M. (2004). Neuromyelitis optica: current concepts, *Front Biosci,* Vol.9, pp. 834–840.

WIPO, 28.03.2011, Available from URL: www.wipo.int/pctdb/en/fetch.jsp?LANG=ENG&DBSELECT=PCT&SERVER_TYPE=19-10&SORT=11316447-KEY&TYPE_FIELD=256&IDB=0&IDOC=1324445&C=10&ELEMENT_SET=B&RESULT=5&TOTAL=7&START=1&DISP=25&FORM=SEP-0/HITNUM,B-ENG,DP,MC,AN,PA,ABSUM-ENG&SEARCH_IA=US2001032198&QUERY=%28PA%2fJagat+AND+PA%2fKanwar%29+]

Wylam, M.E., Anderson, P.M., Kuntz, N.L. & Rodriguez, V. (2003). Successful treatment of refractory myasthenia gravis using rituximab: a pediatric case report. *J Pediatr,* Vol.143, pp. 674–677.

Wynne, A., Kanwar, R.K., Khanna, R. & Kanwar, J.R. (2010). Recent Advances on the Possible Neuroprotective Activities of Epstein- Barr Virus Oncogene BARF1 Protein in Chronic Inflammatory Disorders of Central Nervous System. *Current Neuropharmacology,* Vol.8, pp. 268-275.

Yagi, J. & Janeway, C.A. (1990). Ligand thresholds at different stages of T cell development. *Int. Immunol*, Vol.2, pp. 83–89.

Yan, W.X., Taylor, J., Andrias-Kauba, S. & Pollard, J.D. (2000). Passive transfer of demyelination by serum or IgG from chronic inflammatory demyelinating polyneuropathy patients. *Ann Neurol*, Vol.47, pp. 765–775.

Yang, J.S., Xu, L.Y., Xiao, B.G., Hedlund, G. & Link, H. (2004). Laquinimod (ABR-215062) suppresses the development of experimental autoimmune encephalomyelitis, modulates the Th1/Th2 balance and induces the Th3 cytokine TGF-beta in Lewis rats. *J Neuroimmunol*, Vol.56, pp. 3–9.

Yang, Y. & Santamaria, P. (2006). T cells and autoimmunity. In: Rose, N.R. & Mackay, I.R. *The Autoimmune Diseases*, Elsevier Academic Press, San Diego, pp. 59-82.

Yoon, J.W., Austin, M., Onodera, T. & Notkins, A.L. (1979).Virus-induced diabetes mellitus. Isolation of a virus from the pancreas of a child with diabetic ketoacidosis. *N Engl J Med*, Vol.300, pp. 1173-1179

Yoshida, S. & Gershwin M.E. (1993). Autoimmunity and selected environmental factors of disease induction. *Semin Arthritis Rheum*, Vol.22, pp. 399-419.

Ziff, M. (1991). Role of the endothelium in chronic inflammatory synovitis. *Arthritis Rheum*, Vol.34, pp. 1345-1352.

Zinman, L., Ng, E. & Bril, V. (2007). IV immunoglobulin in patients with myasthenia gravis - A randomized controlled trial. *Neurology*, Vol.68, pp. 837-841.

An Open Label Study of the Effects of Eculizumab in Neuromyelitis Optica, In: *clinical trials.gov*, 7.03.2011, Available from URL:
clinicaltrials.gov/ct2/show/NCT00904826

# 16

# Synthetic Glucocorticoids Modulate Function of Neural Cells: Implications in Autoimmune Neurological Disorders

Oscar Gonzalez-Perez, Norma A. Moy-Lopez and Jorge Guzman-Muniz
*University of Colima/ Laboratory of Neuroscience, School of Psychology*
*Mexico*

## 1. Introduction

Glucocorticoids are hormones synthesized from cholesterol in the cortex of adrenal glands. Synthetic glucocorticoids are chemical derivatives synthesized from cholic acid obtained from cattle or steroid sapogenins. The chemical structure of these drugs is very similar to that of natural glucocorticoids. Therefore, the synthetic derivatives efficiently bind to intracellular receptors of glucocorticoid and mineralocorticoid, which promote a myriad of transcriptional and non-transcriptional processes. Synthetic glucocorticoids can trigger a cascade of events including neurotransmitter modulation, protein expression, neuronal firing or neurite growth. In addition, these substances are some of the most potent antiinflammatory and immunosuppressive agents available in human medicine with a good drug safety profile in humans. Thus, they are a valuable pharmacological tool for the treatment of acute and chronic neuroinflammation, and autoimmune disorders with neurological involvement. However, increasing evidence indicates that a high-dose or a long-term delivery of synthetic glucocorticoids may promote cognitive dysfunction, memory impairment, apoptosis, systemic hypersensitivity, urticaria-angioedema, neuronal degeneration, cerebral atrophy, major depression or steroid psychosis. Yet, these major side effects are relatively infrequent, the unrestricted use of glucocorticoids has to be avoided and systematic neuropsychological assessments are recommended to detect early neurological impairment. Herein, we discuss the mechanisms by which synthetic glucocorticoids may induce neural degeneration and other pathological changes in different brain regions. In addition, we describe the role of glucocorticoids in some autoimmune neurological disorders.

## 2. Glucocorticoids

The hypothalamus-pituitary-adrenal axis exerts an important regulation on neural functions mediated by the releasing of steroid molecules named corticosteroids. These hormones are synthesized from cholesterol in the cortex of adrenal glands (Fietta et al., 2009; Nicolaides et al., 2010). Two types of corticoids have been identified: glucocorticoids and mineralocorticoids. Glucocorticoids are produced in the inner region of the adrenal cortex (fascicular zone), while mineralocorticoids are synthesized in the outer part of the adrenal cortex (glomerular zone) (Schimmer & George 1998). The name mineralocorticoid derives from early observations that associated these hormones with the homeostasis of sodium and water, whereas glucocorticoids obtained their name from initial observations that these steroids were involved in the metabolism of glucose. To date, it is well accepted that gluco- and mineralocorticoids have a number of pleiotropic and systemic effects (Figure 1) on cardiovascular system (Schimmer & George 1998; Ullian 1999), erythropoiesis (Amylon et al. 1986; King et al. 1988), calcium and bone metabolism (Thacker 2010), gastrointestinal tract (Black 1988), nitrogen excretion and glucose metabolism (Schimmer & George 1998), and exert a strong regulation in the immune system (Silverman et al. 2005). These physiological properties of glucocorticoids are useful in clinical medicine to treat and control a broad spectrum of diseases, such as: allergies, autoimmune diseases, cancer, hormonal replacement, asthma and sepsis. Nevertheless, glucocorticoids also have potentially harmful effects on several body systems, including the central nervous system. Some of these neurological impairments will be discussed below.

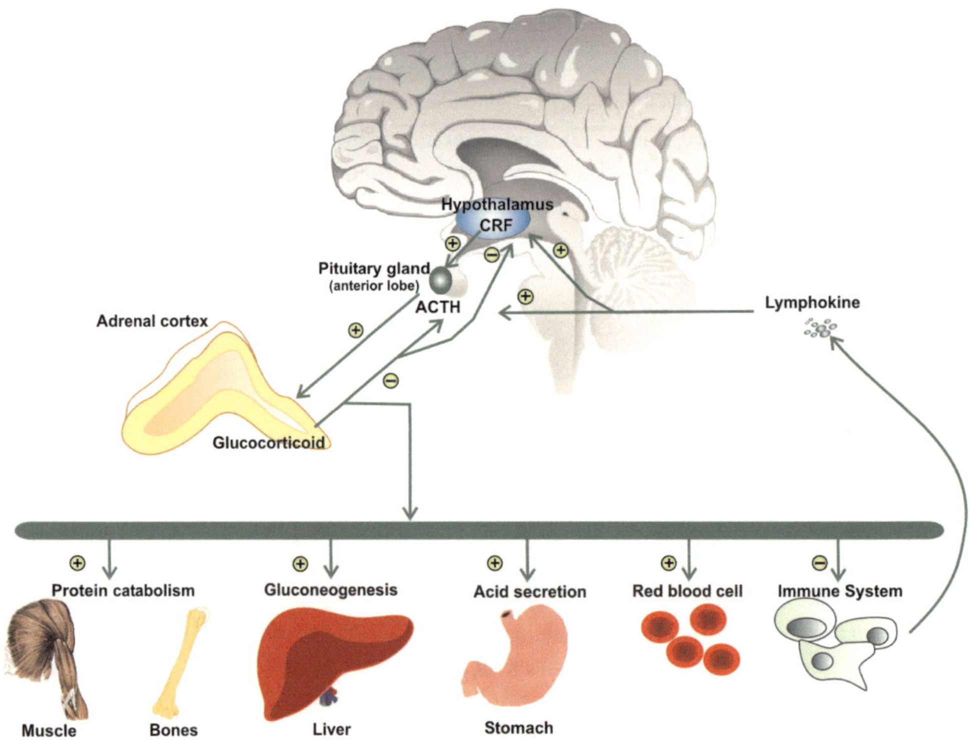


Fig. 1. Physiological effects of glucocorticoids and the hypothalamus-pituitary-adrenal axis. CRF = corticotropin-releasing factor ; ACTH = adrenocorticotrophin hormone; (+) indicates stimulation and (-) indicates inhibition.

## 3. Synthetic glucocorticoids

Synthetic glucocorticoids are usually synthesized from cholic acid obtained from cattle or steroid sapogenins found in plants. The chemical structure of these drugs is slightly different from that of natural glucocorticoids (Figure 2 A - B). For example, prednisolone differs from cortisol only by a δ-1-dihydro configuration. Instead, bexamethasone and betamethasone have additional 9-α-fluoro and 16-β- or 16-α-methyl groups, respectively (Tegethoff et al. 2009).

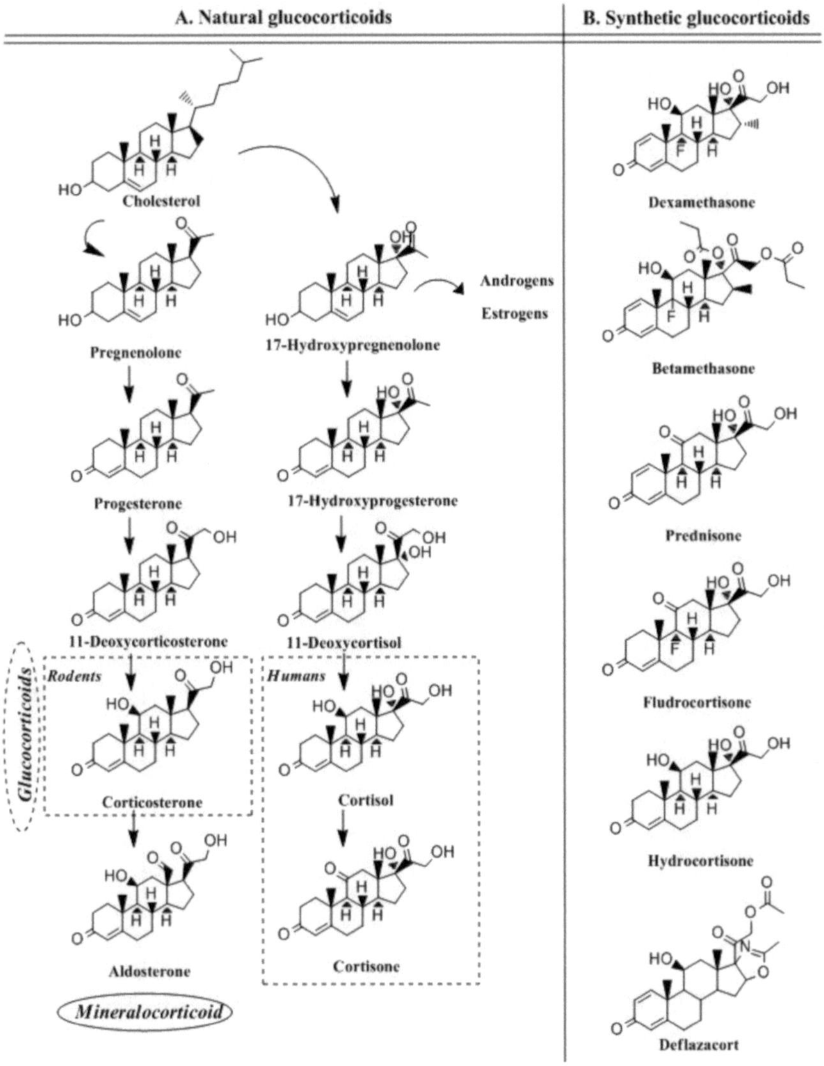


Fig. 2. Chemical structures of glucocorticoids. A. Metabolic pathways in the adrenocortical hormone biosynthesis. B. Synthetic glucocorticoids with anti-inflammatory and immunosuppressive activity.

Endogenous and synthetic glucocorticoids regulate a number of physiological and behavioural responses via intracellular receptors, which modulate the function of neural cells. In several brain regions, neural cells express two types of corticoid receptors: Type-1 receptors, also called mineralocorticoid receptors (MRs), and Type-2 receptors, also called glucocorticoid receptors (GRs) or NR3C1 (nuclear receptor subfamily 3, group C, member 1) (Fietta et al. 2009; Hoppmann et al. 2010; Marques et al. 2009; Prager et al. 2010). NR3C1 mediates the negative feedback in the HPA axis and in other limbic structures (de Kloet 2003; De Kloet et al. 1998). GRs have tenfold lesser affinity for corticosteroids than MRs (Table 1). The physiological outcome of these interactions is that GRs are mainly active during periods of abundant glucocorticoid secretion, such as circadian peak, systemic inflammation or stress. Thus, some of the functions of GRs include the regulation of energy metabolism, cellular homeostasis, stress-induced response, information storage and retrieval (de Kloet 2003; de Kloet et al. 1999; De Kloet et al. 1998). In contrast, MRs have a high affinity for corticosteroids; as a result, they are active when circulating glucocorticoid levels are relatively low. These receptors are highly expressed in hippocampus, septum, amygdala, frontal cortex, hypothalamic paraventricular nucleus and locus coeruleus (de Kloet 2003; De Kloet et al. 1998). One of the main functions of MRs is the regulation of basal HPA tone (de Kloet 2003; De Kloet et al. 1998).

| **Characteristics** | **11β-HSD1** | **11β-HSD2** |
|---|---|---|
| **Molecular mass** | 34 kDa | 40 kDa |
| **Activity (Km)** | Low affinity<br>Cortisol: 17 mM<br>Corticosterone: 20 mM<br>Cortisone: 200 mM | High affinity<br>Cortisol:12 nM<br>Corticosterone: 45 nM<br>Dexamethasone: 140 nM |
| **Inhibitors** | Glycerhetinic acid<br>Carbenoxolone | |

Table 1. Glucocorticoid affinity in type-1 (11β-HSD1) and type-2 receptors (11β-HSD2). Modified from Buckingham 2006.

| **Glucocorticoid** | **Plasma half-life** | **Potency** |
|---|---|---|
| Cortisol | **Short** | 0.8 |
| Cortisone | **$t_{1/2}$ 8-12 h** | 1 |
| Hydrocortisone | | 0.8 |
| Deflazacort | **Intermediate** | 5 |
| Prednisone | **$t_{1/2}$ 12-36 h** | 4 |
| Prednisolone | | 4 |
| Methylprednisolone | | 5 |
| Triamcinolone | | 5 |
| Dexamethasone | **Long** | 25 |
| Betamethasone | **$t_{1/2}$ 36-72 h** | 30-40 |

Table 2. Potency and plasma half-life of natural and synthetic glucocorticoids commonly used in medicine.

The pharmacological effects of natural and synthetic glucocorticoids are mediated by the same genomic and non-genomic pathways (Buckingham 2006; Lowenberg et al. 2005; Lowenberg et al. 2006). The levels of efficacy, potency and pharmacological activity of synthetic hormones are determined by their pharmacokinetic properties (Table 2) (Fietta et al. 2009; Gonzalez-Perez et al. 2007). In clinic, synthetic glucocorticoids are commonly used as anti-inflammatory drugs for the treatment of allergies, rheumatic diseases, asthma, lymphoproliferative diseases and autoimmune disorders (Liberman et al. 2010). Most, if not all, of them can bind to both MRs and GRs, but with different affinities (Gonzalez-Perez et al. 2007). Remarkably, an increasing number of pre-clinical and clinical studies indicate that synthetic glucocorticoids can modify the citoarchitecture and function of glial cells, which alter the brain homeostasis.

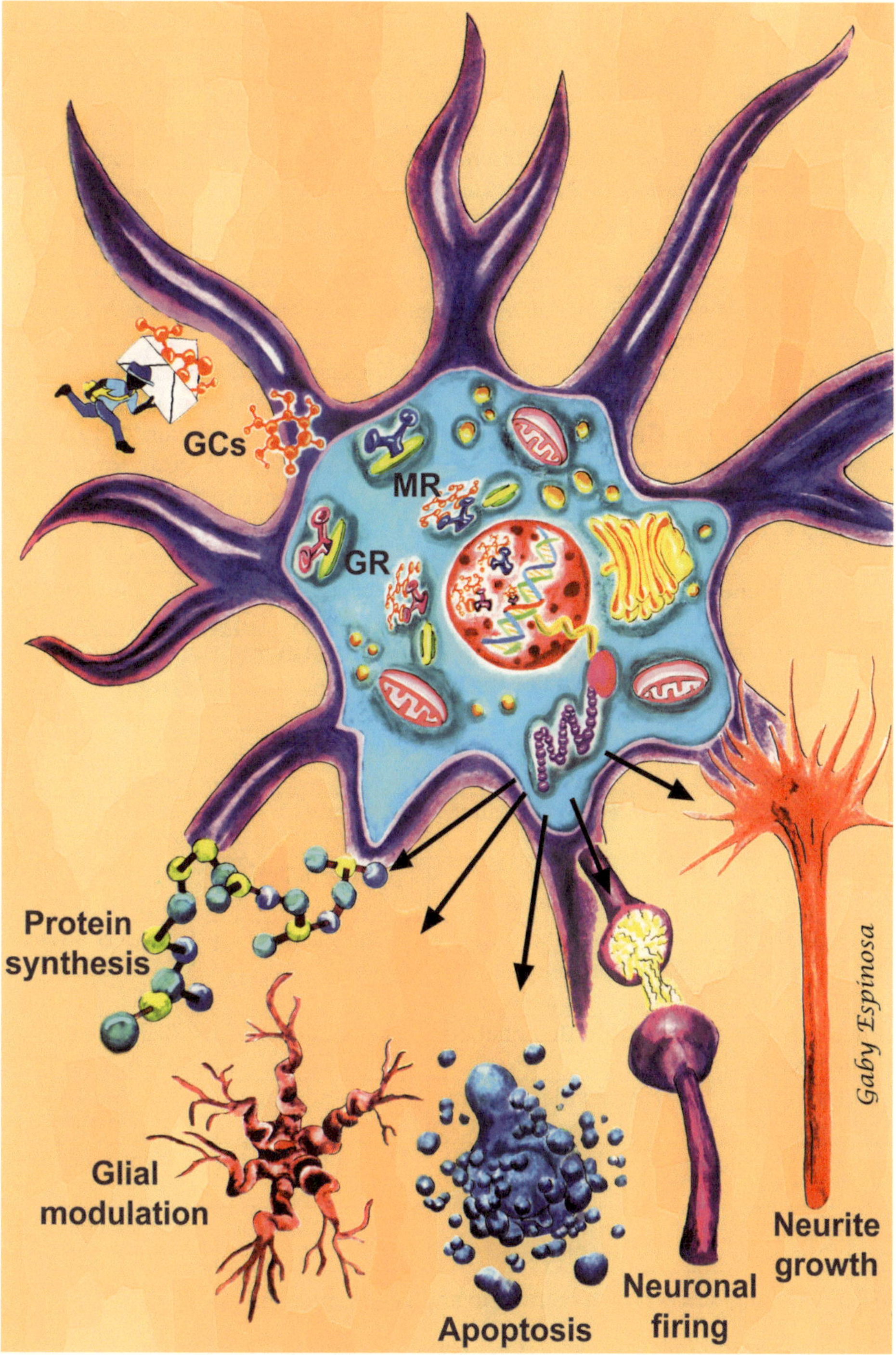


Fig. 3. Astrocytes modulate and/or promote several effects into the brain under the influence of glucocorticoids. Corticoids (GCs); glucocorticoid receptor (GR); mineralocorticoid receptor (MR).

## 4. Effects of synthetic glucocorticoids on astroglia

GRs and MRs are expressed not only by neurons, but also by glial cells or *neuroglia* (Bohn et al. 1991; Vielkind et al. 1990). Glial cells are non-neuronal cells that preserve neural homeostasis, form myelin, and provide support and protection for neurons. In fact, corticoids exert several effects into the brain by targeting glial cells that, in turn, modify the cerebral functioning (Figure 3). Astrocytes, collectively known as *astroglia,* are the most abundant glial cells and play multiple roles into the brain, such as: Neurotransmitter reuptake and release, modulation of synaptic transmission, nervous system repair, hormonal signalling, vascular tone regulation, preservation of blood–brain barrier and, in some cases, astrocytes may function as neural stem cells (Gonzalez-Perez & Alvarez-Buylla 2011; Kettenmann & Ransom 2005).
Astroglia expresses the intermediate filament glial fibrilliary acidic protein (GFAP), which is used as cellular marker of these cells (Ihrie & Alvarez-Buylla 2008). Interestingly, astrocytes contain high number of GRs and MRs; consequently, astrocyte function and their GFAP expression are highly susceptible to glucocorticoids (Lambert et al. 2000; Rozovsky et al. 1995). Some of the effects of glucocorticoids on gene and protein expression in astrocytes are summarized in the table 3.

| Protein / gene | Function | Glucocorticoid effect | Reference |
|---|---|---|---|
| Glial fibrilliary acidic protein (GFAP) | Intermediate filament protein | Upregulation | (O'Callaghan et al. 1991; Ramos-Remus et al. 2002) |
| Glial glutamate transporter (GLT-1) | Neurotransmitter recycling | Upregulation | (Reagan et al. 2004; Zschocke et al. 2005) |
| Glutamine synthetase | Neurotransmitter recycling | Upregulation | (Hansson 1989; Vardimon et al. 1999) |
| Basic fibroblast growth factor (bFGF) | Neurotrophic protein | Upregulation | (Niu et al. 1997) |
| S100β | Ca2+-binding neurotrophic protein | Upregulation | (Van den Hove et al. 2006) |
| N-myc downstream-regulated gene (Ndrg2) | Cell differentiation | Upregulation | (Nichols et al. 2005) |
| Lipocortin-1 | Anti-inflammatory protein | Upregulation | (McLeod & Bolton 1995) |
| Nerve growth factor (NGF) | Neurotrophic protein | Downregulation | (Niu et al. 1997) |
| Vimentin | Intermediate filament | Downregulation | (Avola et al. 2004) |

Table 3. Effects of glucocorticoids on protein and gene expression in astrocytes.

*In vitro* administration of dexamethasone, corticosterone or aldosterone inhibits astrocyte proliferation in a dose-dependent manner (Crossin et al. 1997). This effect seems to be mediated by neural cell adhesion molecules, which inhibit activation of mitogen-activated protein (MAP) kinase (Krushel et al. 1998). The corticoid-induced inhibition of cell proliferation and growth retardation may also be enhanced by a concomitant reduction in the production of insulin-like growth factor 1 (IGF-1) in parenchymal astrocytes (Adamo et al. 1988). On the other hand, the overexpression of GFAP and chondroitin sulfate proteoglycans in reactive astrocytes has been related to a deficient neuronal repair and less neurite outgrowth. Methylprednisolone can revert these adverse effects by downregulating astrocyte activation (Liu et al. 2008) and reducing the number of GFAP-expressing astroglia (Sabolek et al. 2006). Further studies indicate that dexamethasone can modify hippocampal neuron development and survival by decreasing the mRNA levels of nerve growth factor (NGF) (Niu et al. 1997) and GFAP in hippocampus and neocortex (Aleong et al. 2003). In contrast, other reports using corticosterone (Bridges et al. 2008), prednisone (Ramos-Remus et al. 2002) and deflazacort (Gonzalez-Castaneda et al. 2007) reported an increase in the number and cytoplasmic processes of hippocampal and cortical astrocytes. The reason for these discrepancies is not well-known, but they appear to be mediated by dose- and region-dependent phenomena (Gonzalez-Perez et al. 2001).

Glucocorticoids not only modify the function of glial cells in adult stages, but also during prenatal development. Prenatal betamethasone administration delays both astrocyte and capillary tight junction maturation (Huang et al. 2001a), as well as the myelination in the corpus callosum (Huang et al. 2001b). Remarkably, glucocorticoid effects are not limited to the modulation of cell morphology or molecular expression in neuroglia. Instead, they are key modulators of glycogen metabolism and neurotransmitter transporter homeostasis as demonstrated in several experimental models. For instance, cortical astrocytes exposed to dexamethasone show a reduction of noradrenaline-induced glycogen synthesis (Allaman et al. 2004). Prednisolone, betamethasone and dexamethasone inhibit the transporter uptake of monoamines producing effects on physiological and behavioral processes (Hill et al. 2010). The glial glutamate transporter-1 (GLT-1) is also affected by synthetic glucocorticoids. In cortical astrocytes, dexamethasone provokes a marked increase in the GLT-1 transcription and GLT-1 protein levels (Zschocke et al. 2005). GABAergic neurons are also affected by synthetic glucocorticoids that impair their rhythmic firing, which may lead to cognitive deficit (Hu et al. 2010). Taken together, this evidence indicates that synthetic glucocorticoids exert a strong modulation on neural cells by modifying protein expression, neurite growth, cell proliferation, neurotransmitter uptake, neuronal firing, vasculature function and neuronal degeneration.

### 4.1 Implications in autoimmune neurological disorders. Pathological features observed in patients upon GCs administration

One major application of synthetic glucocorticoids is the treatment of acute and chronic neuroinflammatory disorders, such as multiple sclerosis, autoimmune encephalomyelitis, immune rejection, Parkinson's disease, retinal degeneration and others. Increasing evidence indicates that the therapeutic efficacy of glucocorticoids against autoimmune disorders may rely not only on their well-known anti-inflammatory effects, but also on their properties of neuro-gliomodulation (Gonzalez-Perez et al. 2007). For instance, methylprednisolone has a synergistic effect with Nogo-66 receptor protein, which promotes functional recovery and axonal growth in a model of spinal cord contusion (Ji et al. 2005). Methylprednisolone also mediates anti-apoptotic effects on oligodendrocytes by activating STAT5 proteins, which up-regulate a splicing isoform of the bcl-x gene (Xu et al. 2009). On the other hand, prednisone contributes to attenuate experimental autoimmune encephalomyelitis by preventing the reduction of brain-derived neurotrophic factor (BDNF) and NGF mRNA expression into the brain (Chen et al. 2009). Promising results have also been obtained with dexamethasone and fluocinolone in several studies, i.e. dexamethasone reduces astroglial reactivity to implanted neuroprosthetic devices in rat cortex (Spataro et al. 2005), whereas intravitreous administration of fluocinolone attenuates retinal degeneration (Glybina et al. 2010). Further evidence suggests that dexamethasone produces immunosuppressive effects on the astrocyte response to interleukin-1-beta stimulation (Pousset et al. 1999) and counteracts blood-brain barrier failure by decreasing transendothelial permeability (Cucullo et al. 2004).

Despite synthetic glucocorticoids have demonstrated an adequate safety profile, increasing clinical experience and experimental studies indicate that corticoids are able to promote cognitive dysfunction, anxiety, cerebral atrophy, depression and steroid psychosis. One of the first studies that associated the glucocorticoid delivery with mood disorders in humans was reported in prednisone-treated asthmatic children (Bender et al. 1991). However, adults are also affected by corticoids as demonstrated in healthy volunteers that, after receiving a high-dose prednisone or dexamethasone, showed mood changes and memory impairment (Keenan et al. 1996; Schmidt et al. 1999; Wolkowitz 1994). Cerebral atrophy was reported after a long-term treatment with glucocorticoids in patients with no previous history of central nervous system affection (Bentson et al. 1978; Hara et al. 1981). Other immunologic disorders, such as systemic corticosteroid hypersensitivity (de Sousa et al. 2010; Rachid et al. 2011), toxic epidermal necrolysis (Navarro Llanos et al. 1996) or urticaria-angioedema (Gomez et al. 2002), have also been associated with the administration of glucocorticoids.

Under specific circumstances synthetic corticoids may impair or even potentiate the progress of neurological disorders as reported in experimental models of Alzheimer's disease, hypoxia or prenatal glucocorticoid delivery. This fact appears to be particularly important in neurodegenerative disorders related to oxysterol production such as Alzheimer's disease and multiple sclerosis. Oxysterols are oxidized forms of cholesterol that provokes oligodendrocyte apoptosis. Dexamethasone exacerbates the apoptotic effects of oxysterols on oligodendrocytes, resulting in secondary necrosis (Trousson et al. 2009). Cerebral vasculature is also altered by exposure to dexamethasone that may deteriorate hippocampal functions (Neigh et al. 2010). In hypoxia models, dexamethasone increases the expression of Bnip3, a pro-apoptotic Bcl-2 family, which impairs hypoxic tissue damage (Sandau & Handa 2007).

Neuronal function and survival are also affected by synthetic corticoids. Dexamethasone increases oxidative stress and expression of monoamine oxidase A and B, resulting in a higher loss of dopaminergic neurons (Arguelles et al. 2010). Oral administration of prednisone or deflazacort promotes neuronal degeneration of pyramidal neurons in CA1 and CA3 hippocampal regions (Gonzalez-Castaneda et al. 2007; Gonzalez-Perez et al. 2007; Ramos-Remus et al. 2002). Dexamethasone also decreases the number of neurons in the striatum (dorsomedial caudate-putamen) and hippocampus (dentate gyrus, CA1 and CA3 subfields), which may account for some of the cognitive deficits seen following administration of glucocorticoids to healthy volunteers (Haynes et al. 2001). Glucocorticoids also target the developing brain as reported in children exposed to synthetic glucocorticoids *in uterus,* who showed a reduction in fetal and, in some cases, newborn and infant HPA axis activity (Tegethoff et al. 2009). Other studies indicate that prenatal dexa- or betamethasone exposure also affects postnatal cognitive functions (Hauser et al. 2007; Hauser et al. 2006), reduces the survival of cholinergic neurons (Emgard et al. 2007), and produces permanent changes in the cytoarchitecture within midbrain dopamine nuclei (McArthur et al. 2005).

Taken together, this evidence indicates that synthetic glucocorticoid may have detrimental effects on glial and neuronal integrity. Therefore, some authors have proposed that uncontrolled use of glucocorticoids may predispose to the development of a range of psychiatric and neurological conditions throughout life.

## 5. Conclusion

Synthetic glucocorticoids are a valuable therapeutic strategy against neuroinflammation and autoimmune disorders with neurological involvement. In fact, anti-inflammatory strategies receive growing attention for their potential to prevent pathological deterioration in multiple sclerosis (the most prevalent chronic autoimmune disease of the central nervous system), Parkinson's disease, autoimmune encephalomyelitis and other severe neurological disorders. Nevertheless, the uncontrolled use of glucocorticoids must be avoided because of their deleterious potential on cognition, neuronal survival and apoptosis induction. Yet, in those clinical situations where glucocorticoid use is necessary, a continuous neuropsychological assessment is strongly recommended to detect a possible neurological deterioration.

## 6. Acknowledgments

This work was supported in part by grants from the Consejo Nacional de Ciencia y Tecnologia's (CB-2008-101476) and the National Institute of Neurological Disorders and Stroke (NIH R01 NS070021-01).

## 7. References

Adamo, M., Werner, H., Farnsworth, W., et al. (1988). Dexamethasone reduces steady state insulin-like growth factor I messenger ribonucleic acid levels in rat neuronal and glial cells in primary culture. *Endocrinology*, Vol.123, No.5, Nov 1988, pp. (2565-70).

Aleong, R., Aumont, N., Dea, D., et al. (2003). Non-steroidal anti-inflammatory drugs mediate increased in vitro glial expression of apolipoprotein E protein. *Eur J Neurosci*, Vol.18, No.6, Sep 2003, pp. (1428-38).

Allaman, I., Pellerin, L., & Magistretti, P.J. (2004). Glucocorticoids modulate neurotransmitter-induced glycogen metabolism in cultured cortical astrocytes. *J Neurochem*, Vol.88, No.4, Feb 2004, pp. (900-8).

Amylon, M.D., Perrine, S.P., & Glader, B.E. (1986). Prednisone stimulation of erythropoiesis in leukemic children during remission. *Am J Hematol*, Vol.23, No.2, Oct 1986, pp. (179-81).

Arguelles, S., Herrera, A.J., Carreno-Muller, E., et al. (2010). Degeneration of dopaminergic neurons induced by thrombin injection in the substantia nigra of the rat is enhanced by dexamethasone: role of monoamine oxidase enzyme. *Neurotoxicology*, Vol.31, No.1, Jan 2010, pp. (55-66).

Avola, R., Di Tullio, M.A., Fisichella, A., et al. (2004). Glial fibrillary acidic protein and vimentin expression is regulated by glucocorticoids and neurotrophic factors in primary rat astroglial cultures. *Clin Exp Hypertens*, Vol.26, No.4, May 2004, pp. (323-33).

Bender, B.G., Lerner, J.A., & Poland, J.E. (1991). Association between corticosteroids and psychologic change in hospitalized asthmatic children. *Ann Allergy*, Vol.66, No.5, May 1991, pp. (414-9).

Bentson, J., Reza, M., Winter, J., et al. (1978). Steroids and apparent cerebral atrophy on computed tomography scans. *J Comput Assist Tomogr*, Vol.2, No.1, Jan 1978, pp. (16-23).

Black, H.E. (1988). The effects of steroids upon the gastrointestinal tract. *Toxicol Pathol*, Vol.16, No.2, 1988, pp. (213-22).

Bohn, M.C., Howard, E., Vielkind, U., et al. (1991). Glial cells express both mineralocorticoid and glucocorticoid receptors. *J Steroid Biochem Mol Biol*, Vol.40, No.1-3, 1991, pp. (105-11).

Bridges, N., Slais, K., & Sykova, E. (2008). The effects of chronic corticosterone on hippocampal astrocyte numbers: a comparison of male and female Wistar rats. *Acta Neurobiol Exp (Wars)*, Vol.68, No.2, 2008, pp. (131-8).

Buckingham, J.C. (2006). Glucocorticoids: exemplars of multi-tasking. *Br J Pharmacol*, Vol.147 Suppl 1, Jan 2006, pp. (S258-68).

Crossin, K.L., Tai, M.H., Krushel, L.A., et al. (1997). Glucocorticoid receptor pathways are involved in the inhibition of astrocyte proliferation. *Proc Natl Acad Sci U S A*, Vol.94, No.6, Mar 18 1997, pp. (2687-92).

Cucullo, L., Hallene, K., Dini, G., et al. (2004). Glycerophosphoinositol and dexamethasone improve transendothelial electrical resistance in an in vitro study of the blood-brain barrier. *Brain Res*, Vol.997, No.2, Feb 6 2004, pp. (147-51).

Chen, X., Hu, X., Zou, Y., et al. (2009). Combined treatment with minocycline and prednisone attenuates experimental autoimmune encephalomyelitis in C57 BL/6 mice. *J Neuroimmunol*, Vol.210, No.1-2, May 29 2009, pp. (22-9).

de Kloet, E.R. (2003). Hormones, brain and stress. *Endocr Regul*, Vol.37, No.2, Jun 2003, pp. (51-68).

de Kloet, E.R., Oitzl, M.S., & Joels, M. (1999). Stress and cognition: are corticosteroids good or bad guys? *Trends Neurosci*, Vol.22, No.10, Oct 1999, pp. (422-6).

De Kloet, E.R., Vreugdenhil, E., Oitzl, M.S., et al. (1998). Brain corticosteroid receptor balance in health and disease. *Endocr Rev*, Vol.19, No.3, Jun 1998, pp. (269-301).

de Sousa, N.G., Santa-Marta, C., & Morais-Almeida, M. (2010). Systemic corticosteroid hypersensitivity in children. *J Investig Allergol Clin Immunol*, Vol.20, No.6, 2010, pp. (529-32).

Emgard, M., Paradisi, M., Pirondi, S., et al. (2007). Prenatal glucocorticoid exposure affects learning and vulnerability of cholinergic neurons. *Neurobiol Aging*, Vol.28, No.1, Jan 2007, pp. (112-21).

Fietta, P., Fietta, P., & Delsante, G. (2009). Central nervous system effects of natural and synthetic glucocorticoids. *Psychiatry Clin Neurosci*, Vol.63, No.5, Oct 2009, pp. (613-22).

Glybina, I.V., Kennedy, A., Ashton, P., et al. (2010). Intravitreous delivery of the corticosteroid fluocinolone acetonide attenuates retinal degeneration in S334ter-4 rats. *Invest Ophthalmol Vis Sci*, Vol.51, No.8, Aug 2010, pp. (4243-52).

Gomez, C.M., Higuero, N.C., Moral de Gregorio, A., et al. (2002). Urticaria-angioedema by deflazacort. *Allergy*, Vol.57, No.4, Apr 2002, pp. (370-1).

Gonzalez-Castaneda, R.E., Castellanos-Alvarado, E.A., Flores-Marquez, M.R., et al. (2007). Deflazacort induced stronger immunosuppression than expected. *Clin Rheumatol*, Vol.26, No.6, Jun 2007, pp. (935-40).

Gonzalez-Perez, O., & Alvarez-Buylla, A. (2011). Oligodendrogenesis in the subventricular zone and the role of epidermal growth factor. *Brain Res Rev*, Jan 12 2011, pp.

Gonzalez-Perez, O., Luquin, S., Garcia-Estrada, J., et al. (2007). Deflazacort: a glucocorticoid with few metabolic adverse effects but important immunosuppressive activity. *Adv Ther*, Vol.24, No.5, Sep-Oct 2007, pp. (1052-60).

Gonzalez-Perez, O., Ramos-Remus, C., Garcia-Estrada, J., et al. (2001). Prednisone induces anxiety and glial cerebral changes in rats. *J Rheumatol*, Vol.28, No.11, Nov 2001, pp. (2529-34).

Hansson, E. (1989). Regulation of glutamine synthetase synthesis and activity by glucocorticoids and adrenoceptor activation in astroglial cells. *Neurochem Res*, Vol.14, No.6, Jun 1989, pp. (585-7).

Hara, K., Watanabe, K., Miyazaki, S., et al. (1981). Apparent brain atrophy and subdural hematoma following ACTH therapy. *Brain Dev*, Vol.3, No.1, 1981, pp. (45-9).

Hauser, J., Dettling-Artho, A., Pilloud, S., et al. (2007). Effects of prenatal dexamethasone treatment on postnatal physical, endocrine, and social development in the common marmoset monkey. *Endocrinology*, Vol.148, No.4, Apr 2007, pp. (1813-22).

Hauser, J., Feldon, J., & Pryce, C.R. (2006). Prenatal dexamethasone exposure, postnatal development, and adulthood prepulse inhibition and latent inhibition in Wistar rats. *Behav Brain Res*, Vol.175, No.1, Nov 25 2006, pp. (51-61).

Haynes, L.E., Griffiths, M.R., Hyde, R.E., et al. (2001). Dexamethasone induces limited apoptosis and extensive sublethal damage to specific subregions of the striatum and hippocampus: implications for mood disorders. *Neuroscience*, Vol.104, No.1, 2001, pp. (57-69).

Hill, J.E., Makky, K., Shrestha, L., et al. (2010). Natural and synthetic corticosteroids inhibit uptake(2)-mediated transport in CNS neurons. *Physiol Behav*, Nov 21 2010, pp.

Hoppmann, J., Perwitz, N., Meier, B., et al. (2010). The balance between gluco- and mineralo-corticoid action critically determines inflammatory adipocyte responses. *J Endocrinol*, Vol.204, No.2, Feb 2010, pp. (153-64).

Hu, W., Zhang, M., Czeh, B., et al. (2010). Stress impairs GABAergic network function in the hippocampus by activating nongenomic glucocorticoid receptors and affecting the integrity of the parvalbumin-expressing neuronal network. *Neuropsychopharmacology*, Vol.35, No.8, Jul 2010, pp. (1693-707).

Huang, W.L., Harper, C.G., Evans, S.F., et al. (2001a). Repeated prenatal corticosteroid administration delays astrocyte and capillary tight junction maturation in fetal sheep. *Int J Dev Neurosci*, Vol.19, No.5, Aug 2001a, pp. (487-93).

Huang, W.L., Harper, C.G., Evans, S.F., et al. (2001b). Repeated prenatal corticosteroid administration delays myelination of the corpus callosum in fetal sheep. *Int J Dev Neurosci*, Vol.19, No.4, Jul 2001b, pp. (415-25).

Ihrie, R.A., & Alvarez-Buylla, A. (2008). Cells in the astroglial lineage are neural stem cells. *Cell Tissue Res*, Vol.331, No.1, Jan 2008, pp. (179-91).

Ji, B., Li, M., Budel, S., et al. (2005). Effect of combined treatment with methylprednisolone and soluble Nogo-66 receptor after rat spinal cord injury. *Eur J Neurosci*, Vol.22, No.3, Aug 2005, pp. (587-94).

Keenan, P.A., Jacobson, M.W., Soleymani, R.M., et al. (1996). The effect on memory of chronic prednisone treatment in patients with systemic disease. *Neurology*, Vol.47, No.6, Dec 1996, pp. (1396-402).

Kettenmann, H., & Ransom, B.R. (2005). Neuroglia. Oxford University Press, New York.

King, D.J., Brunton, J., & Barr, R.D. (1988). The influence of corticosteroids on human erythropoiesis. An in vivo study. *Am J Pediatr Hematol Oncol*, Vol.10, No.4, Winter 1988, pp. (313-5).

Krushel, L.A., Tai, M.H., Cunningham, B.A., et al. (1998). Neural cell adhesion molecule (N-CAM) domains and intracellular signaling pathways involved in the inhibition of astrocyte proliferation. *Proc Natl Acad Sci U S A*, Vol.95, No.5, Mar 3 1998, pp. (2592-6).

Lambert, K.G., Gerecke, K.M., Quadros, P.S., et al. (2000). Activity-stress increases density of GFAP-immunoreactive astrocytes in the rat hippocampus. *Stress*, Vol.3, No.4, Nov 2000, pp. (275-84).

Liberman, A.C., Castro, C.N., Noguerol, M.A., et al. (2010). Molecular Mechanisms of Glucocorticoids Action: From Basic Research to Clinical. *Current Immunology Reviews*, Vol.6, No.4, 2010, pp. (371-380).

Liu, W.L., Lee, Y.H., Tsai, S.Y., et al. (2008). Methylprednisolone inhibits the expression of glial fibrillary acidic protein and chondroitin sulfate proteoglycans in reactivated astrocytes. *Glia*, Vol.56, No.13, Oct 2008, pp. (1390-400).

Lowenberg, M., Tuynman, J., Bilderbeek, J., et al. (2005). Rapid immunosuppressive effects of glucocorticoids mediated through Lck and Fyn. *Blood*, Vol.106, No.5, Sep 1 2005, pp. (1703-10).

Lowenberg, M., Verhaar, A.P., Bilderbeek, J., et al. (2006). Glucocorticoids cause rapid dissociation of a T-cell-receptor-associated protein complex containing LCK and FYN. *EMBO Rep*, Vol.7, No.10, Oct 2006, pp. (1023-9).

Marques, A.H., Silverman, M.N., & Sternberg, E.M. (2009). Glucocorticoid dysregulations and their clinical correlates. From receptors to therapeutics. *Ann N Y Acad Sci*, Vol.1179, Oct 2009, pp. (1-18).

McArthur, S., McHale, E., Dalley, J.W., et al. (2005). Altered mesencephalic dopaminergic populations in adulthood as a consequence of brief perinatal glucocorticoid exposure. *J Neuroendocrinol*, Vol.17, No.8, Aug 2005, pp. (475-82).

McLeod, J.D., & Bolton, C. (1995). Dexamethasone induces an increase in intracellular and membrane-associated lipocortin-1 (annexin-1) in rat astrocyte primary cultures. *Cell Mol Neurobiol*, Vol.15, No.2, Apr 1995, pp. (193-205).

Navarro Llanos, A., Elizalde Eguinoa, J., Boto de los Bueys, B., et al. (1996). [Toxic epidermal necrolysis in a patient treated with high doses of deflazacort]. *Med Clin (Barc)*, Vol.106, No.15, Apr 20 1996, pp. (599).

Neigh, G.N., Owens, M.J., Taylor, W.R., et al. (2010). Changes in the vascular area fraction of the hippocampus and amygdala are induced by prenatal dexamethasone and/or adult stress. *J Cereb Blood Flow Metab*, Vol.30, No.6, Jun 2010, pp. (1100-4).

Nichols, N.R., Agolley, D., Zieba, M., et al. (2005). Glucocorticoid regulation of glial responses during hippocampal neurodegeneration and regeneration. *Brain Res Brain Res Rev*, Vol.48, No.2, Apr 2005, pp. (287-301).

Niu, H., Hinkle, D.A., & Wise, P.M. (1997). Dexamethasone regulates basic fibroblast growth factor, nerve growth factor and S100beta expression in cultured hippocampal astrocytes. *Brain Res Mol Brain Res*, Vol.51, No.1-2, Nov 1997, pp. (97-105).

O'Callaghan, J.P., Brinton, R.E., & McEwen, B.S. (1991). Glucocorticoids regulate the synthesis of glial fibrillary acidic protein in intact and adrenalectomized rats but do not affect its expression following brain injury. *J Neurochem*, Vol.57, No.3, Sep 1991, pp. (860-9).

Pousset, F., Cremona, S., Dantzer, R., et al. (1999). Interleukin-4 and interleukin-10 regulate IL1-beta induced mouse primary astrocyte activation: a comparative study. *Glia*, Vol.26, No.1, Mar 1999, pp. (12-21).

Prager, E.M., Brielmaier, J., Bergstrom, H.C., et al. (2010). Localization of mineralocorticoid receptors at mammalian synapses. *PLoS One*, Vol.5, No.12, 2010, pp. (e14344).

Rachid, R., Leslie, D., Schneider, L., et al. (2011). Hypersensitivity to systemic corticosteroids: an infrequent but potentially life-threatening condition. *J Allergy Clin Immunol*, Vol.127, No.2, Feb 2011, pp. (524-8).

Ramos-Remus, C., Gonzalez-Castaneda, R.E., Gonzalez-Perez, O., et al. (2002). Prednisone induces cognitive dysfunction, neuronal degeneration, and reactive gliosis in rats. *J Investig Med*, Vol.50, No.6, Nov 2002, pp. (458-64).

Reagan, L.P., Rosell, D.R., Wood, G.E., et al. (2004). Chronic restraint stress up-regulates GLT-1 mRNA and protein expression in the rat hippocampus: reversal by tianeptine. *Proc Natl Acad Sci U S A*, Vol.101, No.7, Feb 17 2004, pp. (2179-84).

Rozovsky, I., Laping, N.J., Krohn, K., et al. (1995). Transcriptional regulation of glial fibrillary acidic protein by corticosterone in rat astrocytes in vitro is influenced by the duration of time in culture and by astrocyte-neuron interactions. *Endocrinology*, Vol.136, No.5, May 1995, pp. (2066-73).

Sabolek, M., Herborg, A., Schwarz, J., et al. (2006). Dexamethasone blocks astroglial differentiation from neural precursor cells. *Neuroreport*, Vol.17, No.16, Nov 6 2006, pp. (1719-23).

Sandau, U.S., & Handa, R.J. (2007). Glucocorticoids exacerbate hypoxia-induced expression of the pro-apoptotic gene Bnip3 in the developing cortex. *Neuroscience*, Vol.144, No.2, Jan 19 2007, pp. (482-94).

Schimmer, B.P., & George, S.R. (1998). Adrenocortical steroid hormones. In *Principles of medical pharmacology*, (Kalant, H., et al., Eds.), pp. 634-646. Saunders Elsevier, Toronto.

Schmidt, L.A., Fox, N.A., Goldberg, M.C., et al. (1999). Effects of acute prednisone administration on memory, attention and emotion in healthy human adults. *Psychoneuroendocrinology*, Vol.24, No.4, May 1999, pp. (461-83).

Silverman, M.N., Pearce, B.D., Biron, C.A., et al. (2005). Immune modulation of the hypothalamic-pituitary-adrenal (HPA) axis during viral infection. *Viral Immunol*, Vol.18, No.1, 2005, pp. (41-78).

Spataro, L., Dilgen, J., Retterer, S., et al. (2005). Dexamethasone treatment reduces astroglia responses to inserted neuroprosthetic devices in rat neocortex. *Exp Neurol*, Vol.194, No.2, Aug 2005, pp. (289-300).

Tegethoff, M., Pryce, C., & Meinlschmidt, G. (2009). Effects of intrauterine exposure to synthetic glucocorticoids on fetal, newborn, and infant hypothalamic-pituitary-adrenal axis function in humans: a systematic review. *Endocr Rev*, Vol.30, No.7, Dec 2009, pp. (753-89).

Thacker, H. (2010). Glucocorticoid-induced osteoporosis. *Cleve Clin J Med*, Vol.77, No.12, Dec 2010, pp. (843; author reply 843-4).

Trousson, A., Makoukji, J., Petit, P.X., et al. (2009). Cross-talk between oxysterols and glucocorticoids: differential regulation of secreted phopholipase A2 and impact on oligodendrocyte death. *PLoS One*, Vol.4, No.11, 2009, pp. (e8080).

Ullian, M.E. (1999). The role of corticosteriods in the regulation of vascular tone. *Cardiovasc Res*, Vol.41, No.1, Jan 1999, pp. (55-64).

Van den Hove, D.L., Steinbusch, H.W., Bruschettini, M., et al. (2006). Prenatal stress reduces S100B in the neonatal rat hippocampus. *Neuroreport*, Vol.17, No.10, Jul 17 2006, pp. (1077-80).

Vardimon, L., Ben-Dror, I., Avisar, N., et al. (1999). Glucocorticoid control of glial gene expression. *J Neurobiol*, Vol.40, No.4, Sep 15 1999, pp. (513-27).

Vielkind, U., Walencewicz, A., Levine, J.M., et al. (1990). Type II glucocorticoid receptors are expressed in oligodendrocytes and astrocytes. *J Neurosci Res*, Vol.27, No.3, Nov 1990, pp. (360-73).

Wolkowitz, O.M. (1994). Prospective controlled studies of the behavioral and biological effects of exogenous corticosteroids. *Psychoneuroendocrinology*, Vol.19, No.3, 1994, pp. (233-55).

Xu, J., Chen, S., Chen, H., et al. (2009). STAT5 mediates antiapoptotic effects of methylprednisolone on oligodendrocytes. *J Neurosci*, Vol.29, No.7, Feb 18 2009, pp. (2022-6).

Zschocke, J., Bayatti, N., Clement, A.M., et al. (2005). Differential promotion of glutamate transporter expression and function by glucocorticoids in astrocytes from various brain regions. *J Biol Chem*, Vol.280, No.41, Oct 14 2005, pp. (34924-32).

17

# Intravenous Immunoglobulins in Neurological Diseases: Established and Novel Clinical Applications

Konstantina G. Yiannopoulou
*Neurological Department, Laiko General Hospital of Athens*
*Greece*

## 1. Introduction

Over the last decade, high-dose polyclonal intravenous immunoglobulin (IVIg) is used increasingly in the management of autoimmune conditions of the central and peripheral nervous system. Despite the expanded use of IVIg, the consensus on its optimal use is insufficient. Currently chronic idiopathic demyelinating polyneuropathy (CIDP), Guillain - Barre syndrome (GBS) and multifocal motor neuropathy (MMN) are the three major immune neuropathies, in which the latest evidence strongly supports the use of IVIg as a first-line therapy. In addition to these disorders, there is a rising number of other neurological indications in which IVIg has been used as a therapy, even though the available evidence-based data are relatively sparse and less convincing. Due to increasing costs of this treatment and relative shortage of products, careful selection of patients who will benefit from IVIg is extremely important (Elovaara & Hietaharju, 2010).
In this paper the current literature on the use of IVIG in treatment of neurological diseases has been reviewed and evidence-based recommendations, as well as less convincing data and future possibilities for its use in these disorders are presented.

## 2. IVIg in therapy of autoimmune neuropathies

Currently CIDP, GBS and MMN are the three major immune neuropathies, in which the latest evidence strongly supports the use of IVIg as a first-line therapy (level A recommendation). However, questions remain regarding the dose, timing and duration of IVIg treatment in these disorders. The efficacy of IVIg has been also proven in some paraneoplastic neuropathies (level B) (European Federation of Neurology Society [EFNS] task force, 2008; Elovaara & Hietaharju, 2010). There are other peripheral neuropathies in which there are reports of the efficacy of IVIg. These include diabetic amyotrophy, vasculitic peripheral neuropathy and painful sensory neuropathy associated with Sjogren's syndrome. The evidence for these conditions has been insufficient to earn a recommendation for the use of IVIg from national or international guidelines (Hughes et al, 2009).

### 2.1 Guillan-barre syndrome (GBS)

GBS is an autoimmune disorder of the peripheral nervous system. The incidence of GBS is approximately two per 100 000/year in adults. It may lead to respiratory failure requiring artificial ventilation in up to 30% of patients and about 5% die in this disease (Hughes et al, 2006).

GBS consists of four major subtypes: acute inflammatory demyelinating polyneuropathy (AIDP); acute motor axonal neuropathy (AMAN); acute motor and sensory axonal neuropathy (AMSAN); and Fisher syndrome. The subtypes can be differentiated by clinical, electrophysiological and pathological findings. Diagnosis of GBS is made in the setting of the classic clinical scenario of a monophasic illness reaching a nadir within 4 weeks with symmetric weakness and sensory loss, areflexia and elevated cerebrospinal fluid (CSF) protein without pleocytosis. Presumed antecedent inciting events, such as infections, occur in up to 80% (van Doorn P.A. et al, 2008).

Molecular mimicry probably plays an important role in the pathogenesis. Infection with a pathological agent such as *Campylobacter jejuni* leads to the formation of cross-reacting antibodies. In AIDP, such cross-reacting anti-myelin or anti-ganglioside antibodies attack Schwann cell surface epitopes of motor and sensory fibres. Subsequent complement activation and macrophage infiltration leads to multi-focal inflammatory demyelination with conduction failure and secondary axonal degeneration. AMAN and AMSAN are characterized by axonal/nodal antibody binding, complement activation, macrophage attachment at nodes, opening of the periaxonal space and macrophage infiltration in motor axons in AMAN, or in motor and sensory axons in AMSAN (van Doorn P.A. et al, 2008).

The proposed autoimmune aetiology led to the introduction of immunotherapy. Before its introduction, 10% of patients died and 20% were left seriously disabled (EFNS task force, 2008). Plasma exchange (PE) was the first treatment of GBS that was shown to offer a significant benefit in randomized controlled trials (RCT) and became. The first RCT on the use of IVIg was published in 1992, followed later by other trials.

Even though both IVIG and PE are considered as first-line therapy for GBS, IVIG is usually favored over PE due to its simplicity and better availability. Standard therapy of IVIG is 0.4 g / kg given for 5 days, but there is only limited evidence concerning the optimal dosage. There are also other unanswered questions. Additional primary treatments are needed, as up to 20% of patients with GBS die or are unable to walk after 1 year. Treatments to enhance nerve regeneration and to improve function in existing but partially repaired nerves are also required. The Inflammatory Neuropathy Consortium of the Peripheral Nerve Society defined a need for trials of IVIg treatment in mild GBS and Fisher syndrome, an IVIg dose-finding study in GBS and studies on the use of complement inhibitors and sodium channel blockers (Hughes et al, 2009).The most urgent question is whether patients who continue to deteriorate after a standard course of IVIG should receive a second course or receive some other additional treatment An international study concerning this last issue is about to be launched in the near future (Elovaara & Hietaharju, 2010).

Recommendations:

- IVIg 0.4 g/kg/day for 5 days or PE can be used as first line treatment and are considered to be equally effective (level A).
- IVIg has lesser side effects than PE and this would favour IVIg over PE treatment (level B). --IVIg treatment after PE, as standard combination, does not produce significant extra benefit and can not be recommended (level B).
- Combining high-dose intravenous methylprednisolone with IVIg may have a minor shortterm benefit (level C).
- Children, who generally have a better prognosis, should be treated with IVIg as firstline treatment (level C).

- Patients who improve after IVIg and then relapse should preferentially be retreated with a second course of IVIg (good practice point).
- In patients who seem to be unresponsive to the first course of IVIg a second course may be tried, but evidence supporting such a strategy is lacking (good practice point).
- No recommendations can be given whether mildly affected GBS patients or patients with Miller Fisher syndrome should be treated with IVIG. (EFNS task force, 2008).

### 2.2 Chronic Inflammatory Demyelinating Polyneuropathy (CIDP)

CIDP is a progressive or relapsing autoimmune disease that targets the myelin sheaths of the peripheral nerves, leading to weakness, sensory loss and impairment of gait and coordination. It has a variable clinical course causing both temporary and permanent disability. There is no definitive test for CIDP, and in most patients diagnosis is based on the clinical presentation and demonstration of demyelinating abnormalities in electrodiagnostic studies (Hughes et al, 2009).

It has been shown to respond to several therapies, including corticosteroids, PE and IVIg. The efficacy of IVIg has been assessed in five RCTs including 235 participants. In addition, there is one RCT, which has compared IVIg with PE, and one study, which has compared IVIg with prednisolone. A recently published Cochrane review summarizes the results of these studies and concludes that IVIg therapy improves disability for at least 2–6 weeks compared with placebo (Eftimov et al., 2009). During this induction period IVIg has an efficacy similar to PE and corticosteroids.

The ICE study (Hughes et al, 2008) that is included in this review is not only the largest but also the longest reported RCT ever performed in CIDP patients. Furthermore, it was the first trial aimed to assess the long-term efficacy of IVIg. The results of ICE study unequivocally demonstrated a beneficial effect on disability that is sustained up to 48 weeks.

The initial dose used in the ICE study (2 g/kg) was similar to that used in practice. This dose was shown to be more effective than 1 g/kg or 0·25 g/kg, although higher doses were not examined. The initial dose is usually given over one or several days, depending on tolerability or convenience. Patients who do not respond to an initial dose may respond to subsequent doses. In the ICE study, 44% of responders improved by 3weeks after the initial treatment, and an additional 50% of patients responded only after a second dose of 1 g/kg at week 3, as measured at week 6 of the study. However, it is not known whether even more patients would have improved if additional treatments had been given, as patients who did not show improvement, including those who were stable, were crossed-over at week 6. In clinical practice, initial responses have been seen up to 3 months into the treatment, and stabilization of previously progressive disease is considered to be a positive response (Hughes et al, 2009).

IVIg responsive patients in the ICE trial were treated with 1 g/kg every 3 weeks for up to 24 weeks, with the responsive patients re-randomized to continue treatment or placebo in phase 2 of the study for an additional 24 weeks. Continued improvement was observed in some patients at up to 32 weeks into the study. Approximately 50% of the responders in the first phase of the study suffered a relapse during phase 2 when switched to placebo. Given the goal of achieving maximal improvement, a reasonable strategy would be to continue treatment until the improvement plateaus, before stopping to see whether additional treatments are still needed. Discontinuing the treatments prior to that point would risk leaving the patient with less than optimal function.

CIDP patients with very mild symptoms may not need any treatment at all. Approximately 20% of the CIDP patients seem to improve spontaneously. Treatment should be considered for patients with moderate or severe disability. IVIg (2 g / kg in 2–5 days) or corticosteroids (1 mg / kg or 60 mg daily) are recommended as first-line treatment in sensory and motor CIDP (EFNS task force, 2008). For pure motor CIDP, IVIg treatment should be the first choice and if corticosteroids are used, patients should be monitored closely for deterioration. In patients with relapsing-remitting CIDP responding to IVIg, attempts should be made to reduce the dose in order to find out if the patient still needs IVIg and what is the adequate dose. In addition to IVIg, PE can be considered as a treatment of choice in long-term therapy of relapsing-remitting CIDP. A number of immunosuppressant and chemotherapeutic agents have been reported to be effective in open studies, but only azathioprine and interferon beta have been investigated in RCT, with negative results (Hughes et al, 2004).

CIDP is a treatable disease whose manifestations can be prevented by early diagnosis and treatment with IVIg. Additional efforts are needed, however, to develop more reliable diagnostic tests, establish optimal treatment regimens and increase awareness of this condition.

Recommendations:

- Patients with very mild symptoms which do not or only slightly interfere with activities of daily living may be monitored without treatment (good practice point).
- Treatment should be considered for patients with moderate or severe disability.
- IVIg (2 g/kg in 2–5 days) (level A) or corticosteroids (1 mg/kg or 60 mg daily) (level B) can be used as first-line treatment in sensorimotor CIDP. The presence of relative contraindications to either treatment should influence the choice (good practice point). - For pure motor CIDP IVIg treatment should be first choice and if corticosteroids are used, patients should be monitored closely for deterioration (good practice point).
- If a patient responds to IVIg, attempts should be made at intervals to reduce the dose to discover whether the patient still needs IVIg and what dose is needed (good practice point).
- It is important to avoid deterioration sometimes seen just before the next IVIg course. The treatment intervals should be such that this deterioration does not happen.
- If a patient becomes stable on intermittent IVIg the dose should be reduced before the frequency of administration is lowered (good practice point) (EFNS task force, 2008).

### 2.3 Multifocal motor neuropathy (MMN)

MMN is a rare autoimmune disorder which may cause prolonged periods of disability due to progressive weakness of one or more limbs.

There are four RCTs, which have examined the effects of IVIg vs placebo in patients with MMN. The total number of participants in these trials was only 34. A Cochrane review, however, showed that muscle strength improved in 78% of patients treated with IVIg and only in 4% of those who received placebo (van Schaik et al, 2005).

Because both prednisolone and PE have proved to be ineffective and even harmful, and cyclophosphamide, even though moderately effective, has significant side effects in long-term use, IVIg remains the only beneficial treatment for MMN.

Approximately one third of patients with MMN have a sustained remission (>12 months) with IVIg alone and approximately half of the patients need repeated IVIg infusions (Leger et al, 2008). The effect of IVIg declines during prolonged treatment, even if the dosage is increased, probably due to ongoing axonal degeneration (Terenghi et al, 2004).

There is only one RCT on the use of an immunosuppressive agent as an additional therapy (Piepers et al, 2007). This study with 28 patients showed that mycophenolate mofetil neither produced significant benefit nor reduced the need for IVIg.
Elevated anti-ganglioside GM1 antibodies and definite conduction block have been shown to be correlated with a favourable response to IVIg (class IV evidence) (EFNS task force, 2008). However, in one retrospective study, treatment with higher than normal maintenance doses of IVIg (1.6–2.0 g/kg given over 4–5 days) promoted re-innervation, decreased the number of conduction blocks and prevented axonal degeneration in 10 MMN patients for up to 12 years (Vucic et al, 2004).
Recommendations:

- As there is no other treatment of proven benefit, the recommendation is to use IVIg (2 g/kg in 2–5 days) as a first-line treatment (level A).
- If the initial IVIg treatment is effective, repeated infusions should be considered (level C).
- A considerable number of patients need prolonged treatment, but attempts should be made to decrease the dose to discover whether a patient still needs IVIg (good practice point).
- Furthermore, the frequency of maintenance therapy should be guided by the individual response, whereby typical treatment regimens are 1 g/kg every 2–4 weeks or 2 g/kg every 4–8 weeks (good practice point) (EFNS task force, 2008).

### 2.4 Paraproteinaemic demyelinating neuropathy

Paraproteinaemia, also known as monoclonal gammopathy, is characterized by the presence of abnormal immunoglobulin (M protein) produced by bone marrow cells in blood. The different types of immunoglobulin are classified according to the heavy chain class as IgG, IgA or IgM. The non-malignant paraproteinaemias are generally referred to as monoclonal gammopathy of undetermined significance (MGUS).
Paraproteins are found in up to 10% of patients with peripheral neuropathy which is not secondary to another primary illness. In about 60% of patients with MGUS-related neuropathy the paraprotein belongs to the IgM subclass. In almost 50% of patients who have IgM MGUS and a peripheral neuropathy, the M protein reacts against myelin-associated glycoprotein. The most common type of IgM MGUS related peripheral nerve involvement is a distal, symmetrical demyelinating neuropathy. Patients with IgG or IgA paraproteinaemic neuropathy usually have both proximal and distal weakness and sensory impairment that is indistinguishable from CIDP.
Two RCTs with IVIg have been performed, encompassing 33 patients with IgM paraproteinaemic demyelinating neuropathy (class II). A third randomized study was an open parallel group trial with 20 patients which compared IVIg and recombinant interferon-a (class II). The results of these three trials have been summarized in a Cochrane review, which concluded that IVIg is relatively safe and may produce some short-term benefit (Lunn & Nobile-Orazio, 2006).
No RCTs are available on the effects of IVIg in IgG or IgA paraproteinaemic neuropathy. There is one retrospective review of 20 patients with IgG MGUS neuropathy treated with IVIg; beneficial response was found in eight of them (class IV). An open prospective trial of IVIg reported clinical improvement in two of four patients with IgG MGUS (class IV). In a review which included 124 patients with IgG MGUS neuropathy, 81% of the 67 patients with a predominantly demyelinating neuropathy responded to the same immunotherapies

used for CIDP (including IVIg) as compared with 20% of those with axonal neuropathy (class IV). A Cochrane review states that observational or open trial data provides limited support for the use of immunotherapy, including IVIg, in patients with IgG and IgA paraproteinaemic neuropathy (Allen et al, 2007).

Recommendations:

- IVIg should be considered as initial treatment of demyelinating IgM MGUS-related neuropathy (level B recommendation).
- As long as long-term effects and cost-benefit aspects are not known, routine use of IVIg cannot be recommended in patients without significant disability (good practice point).
- However, in patients with significant disability or rapid worsening, IVIg may be tried, although its efficacy is not proven (good practice point).
- In patients with CIDP-like neuropathy, the detection of paraproteinaemia does not justify a different therapeutic approach from CIDP without a paraprotein. (EFNS task force, 2008).

### 2.5 Diabetic amyotrophy

Lumbosacral radiculoplexus neuropathy (LRPN) originally described in diabetic patients as diabetic amyotrophy is a distinct clinical condition characterized by debilitating pain, weakness and atrophy most commonly affecting the proximal thigh muscles asymmetrically. The syndrome is usually monophasic and preceded by significant weight loss (at least more than 10 lbs). Though a self-limited condition, recovery is gradual with some residual weakness (Bhanushai & Muley, 2008).

- There are reports and small open studies of the efficacy of IVIg in diabetic amyotrophy (Hughes et al, 2009).

Recommendations:

- The evidence for this condition has been insufficient to earn a recommendation for the use of IVIg.

### 2.6 Vasculitic peripheral neuropathy

Vasculitic neuropathy is routinely considered as a vasculitis associated with neuropathy. The consensus definition of pathologically definite vasculitic neuropathy requires that vessel wall inflammation is accompanied by vascular damage. A case definition of clinically probable vasculitic neuropathy in patients lacking biopsy proof incorporates clinical features typical of vasculitic neuropathy: sensory or sensory-motor involvement, asymmetric/multifocal pattern, lower-limb predominance, distal-predominance, pain, acute relapsing course, and non-demyelinating electrodiagnostic features (Good Practice Points from class II/III evidence). (Collins et al, 2010). There are reports of the efficacy of IVIg in vasculitic peripheral neuropathy (Hughes et al, 2009).

Recommendations:

- The evidence for this condition has been insufficient to earn a recommendation for the use of IVIg.

### 2.7 Painful sensory neuropathy of Sjogren's syndrome

Primary Sjogren's syndrome is associated with seven forms of neuropathy: sensory ataxic neuropathy, painful sensory neuropathy without sensory ataxia, multiple mononeuropathy, multiple cranial neuropathy, trigeminal neuropathy, autonomic neuropathy and radiculoneuropathy, based on the predominant neuropathic symptoms. The majority of patients are diagnosed with Sjogren's syndrome after neuropathic symptoms appearance. Painful sensory neuropathy without sensory ataxia is the second more frequent form of neuropathy associated with Sjogren's syndrome. It is characterised by chronic progression of sensory symptoms without substantial motor involvement, although the affected sensory modalities and distribution pattern vary. Autonomic symptoms, like abnormal pupils and orthostatic hypotension are often seen. Unelicited somatosensory evoked potentials and spinal cord posterior column abnormalities in MRI are observed. Sural nerve biopsy specimens reveal variable degrees of axon loss, predominantly small fibre loss (Mori et al, 2005). Patients usually suffer from severe neuropathic pain, with small-fiber neuropathy causing lancinating or burning pain which can disproportionately affect the proximal torso or extremities, and the face (ie, in a "non-length-dependent distribution") (Birnbaum, 2010).

There are reports and small open studies of the efficacy of IVIg in painful sensory neuropathy associated with Sjogren's syndrome (Hughes et al, 2009).

Recommendations:

- The evidence for this condition has been insufficient to earn a recommendation for the use of IVIg.

## 3. IVIg in therapy of myasthenia gravis (MG)

Myasthenia gravis (MG) is caused by autoantibodies against antigen in the post-synaptic neuromuscular membrane; in most patients against the acetylcholine receptor (AChR), in 5% against muscle-specific tyrosin kinase (MuSK), and in 5% against undefined antigen. A direct induction of muscle weakness by the autoantibodies has been shown.

The efficacy of IVIg in the treatment of MG has been confirmed by five controlled, prospective studies that are summarized in a Cochrane review. In acute exacerbations of MG, IVIG and PE have roughly the same efficacy, but when using IVIg the effect is slightly slower and there are less side effects (Gajdos et al, 2006).

The optimal dose of IVIG in MG has also been debated. So far no marked superiority of IVIg 2 g/kg over 2 days compared to 1 g/kg in a single day has been detected. The dose used has mostly been 2 g / kg resulting in the improvement after 3–6 days. Although IVIg is an effective treatment for acute exacerbations of MG, it is not recommended as maintenance therapy. Importantly, IVIg is often used in preparing MG patients for thymectomy or other types of surgery in case they have severe weakness, bulbar symptoms, poor pulmonary function, or a thymoma, even though there are no controlled studies justifying this practice. IVIg therapy has also been considered as rescue therapy in worsening MG, exacerbations of the disease during pregnancy and before giving birth, and neonatal MG. IVIg is considered safe in children and in elderly patients (EFNS task force, 2008).

Recommendations

- Intravenous immunoglobulin is an effective treatment for acute exacerbations of MG and for short-term treatment of severe MG (level A).
- IVIG is similar to PE regarding effect.
- This treatment is safe also for children, during pregnancy and for elderly patients with complicating disorders.
- There is not sufficient evidence to recommend IVIG for chronic maintenance therapy in MG alone or in combination with other immunoactive drugs (EFNS task force, 2008).

## 4. IVIg in therapy of inflammatory myopathies

The inflammatory myopathies are rare autoimmune diseases characterized by muscle weakness, which is usually proximal, painless and of insidious onset. The three groups of autoimmune myopathies are dermatomyositis (DM), polymyositis (PM) and inclusion body myositis (IBM). There are some controlled trials on the use of IVIg in patients with dermatomyositis (DM) and inclusion body myositis (IBM), and only one with polymyositis (PM) (EFNS task force, 2008; Hughes et al, 2008).

### 4.1 DM

DM is an inflammatory disease, affecting skin and muscle and causing varying degrees of muscle weakness, ranging from mild to severe. Prominent inflammation is observed usually at the periphery of the fascicle, leading to atrophy of the fibres around the fascicle (Hughes et al, 2008).

In a majority of DM patients a favourable response has been reported and therefore IVIg is recommended as a second line treatment in combination with prednisone for those who have not improved with corticosteroids alone. A total dose of 2 g / kg given over 2–5 days for adults and over 2 days for children is a safe initial treatment option. In severe, life-threatening DM, IVIg can be considered as the first line treatment together with other immunosuppressive therapy (Elovaara et al, 2010; EFNS task force, 2008).

Recommendations:

- IVIg is recommended as a second-line treatment in combination with prednisone for patients with DM who have not adequately responded to corticosteroids (level B).
- IVIg is recommended, in combination with immunosuppressive medication, as a measure to lower the dose of steroids in patients with DM (level C).
- IVIg is not recommended as monotherapy for DM (good practice point).
- In severe, life-threatening DM IVIg can be considered as the first-line treatment together with other immunosuppressive therapy (good practice point) (EFNS task force, 2008).

### 4.2 IBM

IBM is a progressive inflammatory skeletal muscle disease that presents with a distinctive pattern of weakness in the wrist and finger flexors and quadriceps muscles. It is characterized by inflammatory cells surrounding myofibres and rimmed vacuoles.

In IBM, the available evidence based on trials with small to moderate numbers of patients suggests an overall negative outcome even if a small number of patients reported improvement in swallowing difficulties. Therefore, IVIg cannot be recommended for the treatment of sporadic IBM (Hughes et al, 2008).

Recommendation:

- IVIg can not be recommended for the treatment of sporadic IBM (level A) (EFNS task force, 2008).

### 4.3 PM

Polymyositis is an inflammatory myopathy with no rash. It is defined by symmetric proximal muscle weakness, elevated serum muscle enzymes, myopathic changes on electromyography, characteristic muscle biopsy abnormalities and the absence of histopathologic signs of other myopathies. Muscle weakness is indeed the most common presenting feature of polymyositis. The onset is usually insidious and the distribution of weakness is typically symmetric and proximal. Myalgias occur in less than 30% of the patiens (Dalakas & Hohlfeld, 2003).

Only one non-RCT (evidence class III) and two case series (evidence class IV) on IVIg therapy for polymyositis have been published. Only the first one used IVIg exclusively in patients with polymyositis. This study reported clinical improvement in 71% of patients with significant improvement in muscle power, muscle disability scores, and creatinine kinase levels ($P < 0.01$). Steroid doses could be reduced after IVIg ($P < 0.05$) (Hughes et al, 2008).

Recommendation:

- IVIg may be considered amongst the treatment options for patients with polymyositis not responding to first line immunosuppressive treatment (level C).

## 5. IVIg in therapy of demyelinating diseases of central nervous system

### 5.1 Multiple sclerosis (MS)

Multiple sclerosis (MS) is a central nervous system chronic inflammatory disease that is characterized by an extensive and complex immune response. It is the most common demyelinating disease of the central nervous system in young adults. MS can cause a variety of symptoms, including changes in sensation, visual problems, muscle weakness, depression, difficulties with coordination and speech, severe fatigue, cognitive impairment, problems with balance, overheating, and pain. MS will cause impaired mobility and disability in more severe cases. Multiple sclerosis may take several different forms, with new symptoms occurring either in discrete attacks or slowly accruing over time. Between attacks, symptoms may resolve completely, but permanent neurologic problems often persist, especially as the disease advances. MS currently does not have a cure, though several treatments are available that may slow the appearance of new symptoms (Baumstarck-Barrau et al, 2011)

Although earlier trials on the efficacy of IVIg in Relapsing Remitting MS (RRMS) have demonstrated a reduction in relapses, a recent study investigating the prevention of relapses with IVIg (PRIVIG trial) failed to confirm these earlier observations (Fazekas et al, 2008). In this study 127 patients with RRMS participated in a double blind, placebo-controlled trial, in which 44 and 42 patients received treatment with 0.2 or 0.4 g / kg of IVIg and 42 patients received placebo every 4 weeks for 48 weeks. After 1 year, the proportion of relapse-free patients did not differ between the groups, and there was no difference in MRI activity assessed 6-weekly. The authors of the study suggested that the obtained results may be related to short disease duration and overall disease activity of the study population that was more like that observed in a population with a clinically isolated syndrome.

The efficacy of IVIg in the treatment of MS exacerbations has been addressed in small add-on type studies that could not demonstrate any additional benefits due to addition of IVIg to conventional treatment of acute exacerbations with high-dose IV methylprednisolone. However, a recent study reported that IVIg might have a beneficial effect in patients with insufficient recovery from optic neuritis, if treatment with high-dose IV methylprednisolone fails (Achiron, 2008). No clinically significant effects were seen in progressive forms of MS, and consequently IVIg is not recommended in these conditions (Elovaara et al, 2010).

Currently the main indication for the use of IVIg in MS is to reduce relapses during pregnancy or breastfeeding when other therapies may not be used safely (Haas & Homes, 2007).

Recommendations:

- IVIG could still be considered as a second or third-line therapy in RRMS if conventional immunomodulatory therapies are not tolerated because of side effects or concomitant diseases (level B), and in particular in pregnancy where other therapies may not be used (good clinical practice point).
- IVIG cannot be recommended for treatment in secondary progressive MS (level A).
- IVIg does not seem to have any valuable effect as add-on therapy to methylprednisolone for acute exacerbations (level B)
- IVIg cannot be recommended as treatment for chronic symptoms in MS (level A).
- In clinically isolated syndromes and in primary progressive MS there is not sufficient evidence to make any recommendations.

### 5.2 Neuromyelitis optica (NMO)

Neuromyelitis optica (NMO) termed also Devic's disease, is a demyelinating disease of the spinal cord and optic nerves that may manifest by recurrent attacks and tends to have a poor prognosis.
There is only one case type study suggesting that monthly IVIg was associated with cessation of relapses (class IV evidence) (Bakker & Metz, 2004).

### 5.3 Balo's concentric sclerosis

Balo's concentric sclerosis is a severe demyelinating disease with poor prognosis. There is a case report suggesting that IVIg (0.4 g/kg/daily for 5 days) and interferon-beta-1a given post-partum may result partial neurological improvement (class IV evidence) (Airas et al, 2005).

### 5.4 Acute disseminated encephalomyelitis (ADEM)

Acute-disseminated encephalomyelitis (ADEM) is a monophasic immune-mediated demyelinating disease of the central nervous system that is associated with significant morbidity and mortality. Controlled studies on therapy in ADEM are not available. Standard treatment is high-dose steroids. The use of IVIg (0.4 g/kg/day for 5 days or 1 g/kg/2 days) has been reported in case reports and small series suggesting that IVIg may have favourable effects when used as an initial therapy in both adults and children (class IV evidence). IVIg may have beneficial effects also as second line therapy (class IV evidence) [149-152] especially in patients who could not receive or failed to respond to steroids (class IV evidence) or in patients with peripheral nervous system involvement and steroid failure (class IV evidence). Alternatively combination therapy by steroids and IVIG (class IV evidence) or steroids, IVIg and PE were suggested to have favourable effects especially if given early in the course of disease (class IV evidence) (EFNS task force 2008).
Recommendations:

- IVIg may have a favourable effect in the treatment of ADEM and therefore it should be tried (0.4 g/kg/day for 4–5 consecutive days) in patients with lack of response to high-dose steroids (good practice point). The cycles may be repeated. PE could also be considered in patients with a lack of response to high-dose steroids.

## 6. IVIg in therapy of paraneoplastic syndromes

Due to the rarity of immunologically mediated paraneoplastic diseases, there are very few prospective, randomized, double-blind and placebo-controlled studies.

### 6.1 Lambert – eaton myasthenic syndrome (LEMS)

Lambert-Eaton myasthenic syndrome (LEMS) is an immune-mediated disorder of the presynaptic neuromuscular transmission, which more frequently occurs as the remote effect of a neoplasm. The clinical features described are proximal weakness, especially in the lower limbs, with diminished tendon reflexes and post-tetanic potentiation. Autonomic symptoms are often reported, including pupil abnormalities, dry eyes and mouth, and erectile dysfunction (Maddison & Newsom-Davis, 2005).

LEMS is considered to respond best to immunosupressive treatment. However, there is only one report showing the beneficial but short-term effect of IVIg on the muscle strength in LEMS (class II evidence) and there is also a recent Cochrane review that has concluded that limited data from one placebo-controlled study show improvement in muscle strength after IVIg (Maddison & Newsom-Davis, 2005).

The IVIg response regarding improvement of muscle strength does probably not differ in paraneoplastic and non-paraneoplastic LEMS.

Recommendations:

- IVIg therapy may be tried in paraneoplastic LEMS (good practice point).

### 6.2 Neuromyotonia

Acquired neuromyotonia is a condition associated with muscle hyperactivity that includes muscle stiffness, cramps, myokymia, pseudomyotonia and weakness, most common in the limbs and trunk. The typical finding on electromyography is spontaneous motor unit discharges occurring in distinctive doublets, triplets, or longer runs with high intraburst frequency (Hart et al, 2002).

Only one case report describes the beneficial effect of IVIg in patient with neuromyotonia, whilst another case report demonstrated worsening after IVIG therapy (EFNS task force, 2008).

### 6.3 Paraneoplastic opsoclonus ataxia syndrome (OMS)

Opsoclonus refers to involuntary, conjugate, multivectorial, saccadic eye movements. It can occur as an isolated neurologic anomaly but, when it occurs with involuntary multifocal jerking movements of the skeletal musculature, the phenomenon is known as opsoclonus–myoclonus syndrome (OMS). The syndrome often includes features of ataxia, or incoordination with voluntary movements. In the setting of malignancy, opsoclonus is linked most clearly to neuroblastoma, occurring in 3% of childhood cases. Anti-neuronal antibodies, usually to nuclear antigens, are considered markers of immune system activation in this disorder, detected in 81% of pediatric patients (Pittock et al, 2003).

Symptoms in paraneoplastic opsoclonus - ataxia syndrome in paediatric neuroblastoma patients are stated to improve, although data concerning the long-term benefits of the treatment is lacking (class IV evidence). In adult patients the response is less immunosuppressive, although IVIg is suggested to accelerate recovery (class IV evidence) (EFNS task force, 2008).

Recommedation:

- -IVIg therapy may be tried in opsoclonus-ataxia especially in paediatric neuroblastoma patients (good practice point).

### 6.4 Paraneoplastic cerebellar degeneration

Cerebellar dysfunction is one of the most common paraneoplastic presentations of cancer. The tumours more commonly involved are small-cell lung cancer, gynaecological and breast tumours, and Hodgkin's lymphoma. Neurological deficits are sometimes preceded by prodromal symptoms, such as a viral-like illness, dizziness, nausea, or vomiting that might be attributed to a peripheral vestibular process. These symptoms are followed by gait unsteadiness that rapidly develops into ataxia, diplopia, dysarthria, and dysphagia. Some patients have blurry vision, oscillopsia, and transient opsoclonus.Initial MRI is normal in most patients, although over time, MRI shows cerebellar atrophy and PET demonstrates hypometabolism (Dalmau & Rosenfeld, 2008).

### 6.5 Limbic encephalitis

Autoimmune limbic encephalitis (LE) can arise both by paraneoplastic and non-paraneoplastic mechanisms. Patients with LE usually have a subacute onset of memory impairment, disorientation and agitation, but can also develop seizures, hallucinations and sleep disturbance. The following investigations may aid the diagnosis: analysis of cerebrospinal fluid (CSF), electroencephalography, magnetic resonance imaging, fluorodeoxyglucose positron emission tomography and neuronal antibodies in the serum and CSF. Neuronal antibodies are sometimes, but not always, pathogenic. Autoimmune LE may respond to corticosteroids, intravenous IgG (IVIG) or plasma exchange. The cornerstone of paraneoplastic LE therapy is resection of the tumour and/or oncological treatment. Several differential diagnoses must be excluded, among them herpes simplex encephalitis (Vedeler & Storstein, 2009)

### 6.6 Paraneoplastic sensory neuronopathy (SSN)

Paraneoplastic sensory neuronopathy (SSN) is characterized by primary damage of the sensory nerve cell body of the dorsal root ganglia. A paraneoplastic origin is only one of the causes of SSN The most common low associated tumor is small cell lung carcinoma. The main clinical complains at onset are pain and paresthesias with asymmetric distribution that involves the arms rather than the legs. Later, pain is replaced by numbness, limb ataxia, and pseudoathetotic movements of the hands. The neurologic examination shows abolition of the deep tendon reflexes and involvement of all modalities of sensation with clear predominance of the joint position. Electrophysiologic studies show marked, but not restricted, involvement of the sensory fibres (Dalmau & Rosenfeld, 2008).

Evidence for the effect of IVIg in paraneoplastic cerebellar degeneration, limbic encephalitis and sensory neuropathy is scarce. In previously published reports, patients were treated with a combination of immunosupressive or immunomodulatory drugs, including IVIG, with a poor response (class IV evidence) (EFNS task force, 2008).

Recommendations:

- No clear recommendations of the effect of IVIG in paraneoplastic neuromyotonia, cerebellar degeneration, limbic encephalitis or sensory neuronopathy can be made due to lack of data (EFNS task force, 2008).

## 7. IVIg in therapy of Stiff-Person Syndrome (SPS)

Stiff-person syndrome (SPS) is characterized by muscle stiffness and episodic spasms. A significant decline of the stiffness scores was found in a randomized trial of 16 SPS patients treated with IVIg . Based on this study IVIg may be considered as a safe and effective second-line therapy for patients with SP incompletely responding to diazepam and / or baclofen and who have significant disability requiring a cane or a walker due to truncal

stiffness and frequent falls. The recommendation is to use IVIg (2 g / kg in 2-5 days) (EFNS task force, 2008).
Recommendations:

- In patients with SPS incompletely responding to diazepam and/or baclofen and with significant disability requiring a cane or a walker due to truncal stiffness and frequent falls, the recommendation is to use IVIg (2 g/kg in 2-5 days) (level A based on class I evidence).

## 8. IVIg in therapy of post-polio syndrome (PPS)

Post-polio syndrome (PPS) is characterized by new muscle weakness, muscle atrophy, fatigue and pain developing several years after acute polio. The prevalence of PPS in patients with previous polio is 20-60%.
Post-polio syndrome is caused by an increased degeneration of enlarged motor units, and some motor neurones cannot maintain all their nerve terminals. Muscle overuse may contribute. Immunological and inflammatory signs have been reported in the cerebrospinal fluid and central nervous tissue (EFNS task force, 2008).
There are two RCTs of treatment with IVIg in PPS (class I evidence) including 155 patients. In the study with highest power, a significant increase of mean muscle strength of 8.3% was reported after two IVIg treatment cycles during 3 months. Physical activity and subjective vitality also differed significantly in favour of the IVIG group (Farbu et al., 2007).
Post-polio syndrome is a chronic condition. Although a modest IVIG effect has been described short term, nothing is known about long-term effects. Responders and non-responders have not been defined.
Any relationship between the clinical response to IVIG treatment and PPS severity, cerebrospinal fluid inflammatory changes and cerebrospinal fluid changes after IVIg is unknown. Optimal dose and IVIG cycle frequency has not been examined. Cost-benefit evaluation has not been performed.
Recommendations:

- IVIG has a minor to moderate positive effect on muscle strength and some aspects of quality of life in PPS (class I evidence).
- As long as responding subgroups, long term effects, dosing schedules and cost-benefit aspects are not known, routine use of IVIG for PPS cannot be recommended (good practice point).
- However, in the very few patients with especially rapid progression of muscle weakness and atrophy, especially if there are indications of ongoing low-grade inflammation in the spinal cord, IVIg may be tried if a rigorous follow-up of muscle strength and quality of life can be undertaken (good practice point) (EFNS task force, 2008).

## 9. IVIg in therapy of drug resistant epilepsy (DRIE)

Drug-resistant infantile epilepsy (DRIE) syndromes include a number of diseases such as Landau-Kleffner syndrome (LKS), West syndrome, Lennox-Gastaut syndrome, severe myoclonic epilepsy or RE that typically manifest in childhood or adolescence and are characterized by epilepsy and progressive neurological dysfunction.

Standard treatment of RE consists of anti-epileptic drugs, high-dose steroids or PE. Surgical treatment also may be considered.
Case studies and small series have reported that some patients with RE respond in some measure to treatment with IVIG (class IV).
Approximately a hundred patients with West or Lennox-Gastaut syndromes have been treated with IVIg with widely varying results. The treatment has resulted in reduction in the number of seizures with improvement in the EEG in about half of the cases. The positive effects were noted few days to several weeks to months after treatment. Relapses have been common.
Successful use of IVIg as initial monotherapy in LKS has been reported in case studies and after initial therapy by steroids or antiepileptic drugs and steroids in only few patients. Case studies on the use of IVIg in RE have suggested that monthly IVIg therapy (0.4 g/kg for 5 days at 4-week interval followed by monthly maintenance IVIg) may ameliorate disease in patients who are refractory to antiepileptic drugs or steroids and PE (EFNS task force, 2008).
Recommendation:

- IVIg seems to have a favourable effect in RE and may be tried in selected patients that are refractory to other therapies (good practice point).
- IVIg has been administered at doses of 0.4 g/kg/day for 4–5 consecutive days, the cycles may be repeated after 2–6 weeks.

## 10. IVIg in therapy of narcolepsy with cataplexy (NC)

Narcolepsy with cataplexy (NC) is caused by substantial loss of hypocretin neurons. NC patients carry the HLA-DQB1*0602 allele suggesting that hypocretin neuron loss is due to an autoimmune attack.
There are some case studies that report that IVIg treatment initiated before 9 months disease duration has some clinical efficiency. The unaffected CSF hypocretin-1 levels and lack of autoantibodies suggest that any autoimmune process occurs very early in NC. The final IVIg effect needs to be investigated in RCTs (Knudsen et al, 2010).

## 11. IVIg in therapy of Alzheimer's disease (AD)

Alzheimer's Disease (AD) is the most common neurodegenerative disorder leading to dementia. The pathological hallmarks of AD are extracellular accumulation of Ab peptides, as senile plaques and intracellular neurofibrillary tangles composed of tau proteins.
Clinical studies of active immunization in humans with AD were complicated by the development of meningoencephalitis in 6% of the patients treated with vaccine AN1792 in a phase II clinical trial. Furthermore, only 20% of the patients immunized with AN1792 developed a twofold increase in anti-Ab antibodies.
However, progress was made with the discovery that peripheral administration of antibodies against Ab peptide could reduce amyloid burden to a similar extent as active immunization. Passive immunization had the advantage that the potentially harmful activation of host T cells could be avoided.
Based on the finding that externally administered antibodies were able to protect mice from AD, it was hypothesized that high titres of natural anti-Ab antibodies may protect humans from AD, while low levels may predispose certain individuals to the development of AD. Studies have found reduced levels of anti-Ab antibodies both in the serum and CSF of

patients with AD. Autoantibody-decorated plaques were found frequently in patients with AD and patients with low antibody-levels were shown to harbour more diffuse plaques than patients with high levels. Autoantibodies against Ab may therefore be important for maintaining plaque homeostasis.

IVIg has been shown to contain autoantibodies against many states of Ab peptide aggregation including monomers, oligomers and fibrils and may therefore have a distinct advantage over monoclonal anti-Ab until the precise pathogenic state(s) of the Ab peptide is known (Hughes et al, 2008).

Recently, commercially available IVIg have been used in small pilot trials for the treatment of patients with AD, based on the hypothesis that IVIG contains naturally occurring autoantibodies (nAbs-Abeta) that specifically recognize and block the toxic effects of Abeta. Furthermore, these nAbs-Abeta are reduced in AD patients compared with healthy controls, supporting the notion of replacement with IVIg. Beyond the occurrence of nAbs-Abeta, evidence for several other mechanisms associated with IVIg in AD has been reported in preclinical experiments and clinical studies. In 2009, a phase III clinical trial involving more than 360 AD patients was initiated and may provide conclusive evidence for the effect of IVIg as a treatment option for AD in 2011(Dodel et al, 2010).

## 12. Conclusion

IVIg is used increasingly in neurological diseases.

Its efficacy has been proved in GBS, CIDP and MMN, where it is considered as the first-line treatment. However, questions remain regarding the dose, timing and duration of IVIg treatment in these disorders.

It is also successfully used in acute exacerbations of MG and as a short-term treatment of severe MG. It is recommended in SPS, in some paraneoplastic syndromes and as a second-line treatment in combination with prednisone in dermatomyositis and a treatment option in polymyositis.

In MS, IVIg is indicated mainly in reducing disease activity during pregnancy and breastfeeding.

In addition to these major indications, IVIg is increasingly used even in such conditions where the strong evidence is currently lacking, like refractory epilepsy, narcolepsy, post polio syndrome.

According to preliminary data, IVIg might be a promising candidate for the treatment of (AD). Large-scale randomized trials are under way, and the results of these studies are awaited eagerly worldwide.

When considering treatment options, it is important to notify that uncontrolled use may lead to high costs and limited availability of IVIg. Careful selection of patients who will benefit from IVIg is extremely important.

ABBREVIATIONS:

AChR: acetylcholine receptor

AD: Alzheimer's Disease

ADEM: Acute-disseminated encephalomyelitis

AIDP: acute inflammatory demyelinating polyneuropathy

AMAN: acute motor axonal neuropathy

AMSAN: acute motor and sensory axonal neuropathy

CIDP: chronic idiopathic demyelinating polyneuropathy

CSF: cerebrospinal fluid
DM: dermatomyositis
DRIE: Drug-resistant infantile epilepsy
GBS: Guillain - Barre syndrome
IBM: inclusion body myositis
IVIg: intravenous immunoglobulin
LEMS: Lambert-Eaton myasthenic syndrome
LRPN: Lumbosacral radiculoplexus neuropathy
MGUS: monoclonal gammopathy of undetermined significance
MMN: multifocal motor neuropathy
MG: Myasthenia gravis
MS: Multiple Sclerosis
MuSK: muscle-specific tyrosin kinase
NC: Narcolepsy with cataplexy
NMO: Neuromyelitis optica
OMS : opsoclonus–myoclonus syndrome
PE: Plasma exchange
PM: polymyositis
PPS: Post-polio syndrome
RCT: randomized controlled trials
RRMS: Relapsing Remitting Multiple Sclerosis
SPS: Stiff-person syndrome
SSN: Paraneoplastic sensory neuronopathy

## 13. References


Achiron, A. (2008). Winning combination: the additive / synergistic benefits of IVIg in corticosteroid refractory optic neuritis. *Eur J Neurol*, Vol.15, pp.1145.

Airas, L., Kurki, T., Erjanti, H. & Marttila RJ. (2005). Successful pregnancy of a patient with Balo's concentric sclerosis. *Multiple Sclerosis*, Vol.11, pp. 346–348.

Allen, D., Lunn, M.P.T., Niermeijer, J. & Nobile-Orazio, E. (2007). Treatment for IgG and IgA paraproteinaemic neuropathy. *Cochrane Database of Systematic Reviews*, CD005376.

Bakker, J. & Metz, L. (2004). Devic's neuromyelitis optica treated with intravenous gamma globulin (IVIG). *Canadian Journal of Neurological Sciences*, Vol. 31, pp. 265–267.

Baumstarck-Barrau, K., Simeoni, M-C., Reuter, F., Klemina, I., Aghababian, V., Pelletier, J. & Auquier, P. (2011).Cognitive function and quality of life in multiple sclerosis patients: a cross-sectional study *BMC Neurology*,Vol.11, No.17, doi:10.1186/1471-2377

Bhanushali, M.J., Muley, S.A. (2008). Diabetic and non-diabetic lumbosacral radiculoplexus neuropathy. *Neurology India*, Vol. 56 No.4, pp.420-5.

Birnbaum, J. (2010). Peripheral nervous system manifestations of Sjφgren syndrome: clinical patterns, diagnostic paradigms, etiopathogenesis, and therapeutic strategies. *Neurologist*, Vol.16, No. 5, pp. 287-297.

Collins, M.P., Dyck, P.J., Gronseth, G.S., Guillevin, L., Hadden, R.D., Heuss, D., Lıger, J.M., Notermans, N.C., Pollard, J.D., Said, G., Sobue, G., Vrancken, A.F.& Kissel, J.T.; Peripheral Nerve Society (2010). Peripheral Nerve Society Guideline on the classification, diagnosis, investigation, and immunosuppressive therapy of non-systemic vasculitic neuropathy: executive summary. *J Peripher Nerv Syst.*, Vol.15, No.3, pp.176-84.

Dalakas, M.C., Hohlfeld, R. (2003). Polymyositis and dermatomyositis. *Lancet*, Vol.362, pp.971-982.

Dalmau, J.& Rosenfeld, M.R.(2008). Paraneoplastic syndromes of the CNS. *Lancet Neurology*, Vol. 7, No. 4, pp. 327-340.

Dodel, R., Neff, F., Noelker, C., Pul, R., Du Y, Bacher, M., Oertel, W. (2010). Intravenous immunoglobulins as a treatment for Alzheimer's disease: rationale and current evidence. *Drugs*, Vol., 26, No. 70(5), pp. 513-28.

EFNS task force on the use of intravenous immunoglobulin in treatment of neurological Diseases: Elovaara, I., Apostolski, S., van Doorn, P., Gilhus, N. E., Hietaharju, A., Honkaniemi, J. I., van Schaik, N., Scolding, N., Soelberg Sψrensen, P. & Udd, B. (2008). EFNS guidelines for the use of intravenous immunoglobulin in treatment of neurological diseases *European Journal of Neurology*, Vol.15, pp. 893–908.

Eftimov, F., Winer J.B., Vermeulen M., de Haan R., van Schaik I.N. (2009). Intravenous immunoglobulin for chronic inflammatory demyelinating polyneuropathy. *Cochrane Database Syst Rev*, Vol. 21:CD001797.

Elovaara, I. & Hietaharju, A. (2010). Can we face the challenge of expanding use of intravenous immunoglobulin in neurology? *Acta Neurologica Scandinavia*, Vol.122, pp. 309–315.

Farbu, E., Rekand, T., Vik-Mo, E., Lygren, H., Gilhus, N.E., Aarli, J.A. (2007). Post-polio syndrome patients treated with intravenous immunoglobulin: a double-blinded randomized controlled pilot study. *European Journal of Neurology*, Vol. 14, pp. 60–65.

Fazekas, F., Lublin, F.D., Li, D. Freedman, M.S., Hartung, H.P., Rieckmann, P., Sorensen P.S., Maas-Enriquez M., Sommerauer B., Hanna, K. PRIVIG Study group. UBC MR/MRI Research group. Intravenous immunoglobulin in relapsing-remitting multiple sclerosis. (2008). A dose finding trial. *Neurology*, Vol. 71, pp. 265–71.

Gajdos, P., Chevret, S., Toyka, K. (2006). Intravenous immunoglobulin for myasthenia gravis. *Cochrane Database Syst Rev*, Vol.19, No.2, CD002277.

Haas, J., Hommes, O.R. (2007). A dose comparison study of IVIG in postpartum relapsing-remitting multiple sclerosis. *Mult Scler*, Vol.13, pp. 900–908.

Hart, I.K., Maddison, P., Newsom-Davis, J., Vincent, A., Mills, K.R. (2002). Phenotypic variants of autoimmune peripheral nerve hyperexcitability. *Brain*, Vol.125, pp.1887-95.

Hughes, R.A., Swan A.V. & van Doorn P.A. (2004). Cytotoxic drugs and interferons for chronic inflammatory demyelinating polyradiculoneuropathy. *Cochrane Database Syst Rev*, Vol. 18, No.4:CD003280.

Hughes, R.A., Raphael J.C., Swan A.V. & van Doorn P.A. (2006). Intravenous immunoglobulin for Guillain-Barre' syndrome, *Cochrane Database Syst Rev*, Vol. 25, No.1,CD002063.

Hughes, R.A., Donofrio, P., Bril V., Dalakas, M.C., Deng C., Hanna K., Hartung H.P., Latov N., Merkies I.S., van Doorn P.A. ICE Study Group. (2008). Intravenous immune globulin (10% caprylate-chromatography purified) for the treatment of chronic inflammatory demyelinating polyradiculoneuropathy (ICE study): a randomised placebo-controlled trial. *Lancet Neurol*, Vol. 7, pp.136–44.

Hughes, R. A. C., Dalakas, M. C., Cornblath D. R., N. Latov, Weksler M. E. & Relkin N. (2009). Clinical applications of intravenous immunoglobulins in neurology, *Clinical and Experimental Immunology*, Vol.158, No. 1, pp. 34–42.

Knudsen, S., Mikkelsen, J.D., Bang, B., Gammeltoft, S. & Jennum P.J. (2010). Intravenous immunoglobulin treatment and screening for hypocretin neuron-specific autoantibodies in recent onset childhood narcolepsy with cataplexy. *Neuropediatrics.* Vol. 41, No. 5, pp. 217-22.

Leger, J.M., Viala, K., Cancalon, F., Maisonobe, T., Gruwez, B., Waegemans, T. & Bouche, P. (2008). Intravenous immunoglobulin as short- and long-term therapy of multifocal motor neuropathy: a retrospective study of response to IVIg and of its predictive criteria in 40 patients. *J Neurol Neurosurg Psychiatry*, Vol.79, pp.93–96.

Lunn, M.P.T. & Nobile-Orazio, E. (2006). Immunotherapy for IgM anti-myelin-associated glycoprotein paraprotein-associated peripheral neuropathies. *Cochrane Database of Systematic Reviews,* CD002827.

Maddison, P. & Newsom-Davis, J. (2005). Treatment for Lambert-Eaton myasthenic syndrome. *Cochrane Database of Systematic Reviews*, Vol. 2: CD003279.

Mori, K., Iijima, M., Koike, H., Hattori, N., Tanaka, F., Watanabe, H., Katsuno, M., Fujita, A., Aiba, I., Ogata, A., Saito, T., Asakura, K., Yoshida, M., Hirayama, M. & Sobue, G. (2005). The wide spectrum of clinical manifestations in Sjφgren's syndrome-associated neuropathy. *Brain,* Vol. 128, No. 11, pp. 2518-2534.

Piepers, S., Van den Berg-Vos, R., Van der Pol, W.L., Franssen, H., Wokke, J. & Van den Berg, L. (2007). Mycophenolate mofetil as adjunctive therapy for MMN patients: a randomized, controlled trial. Brain, Vol.130, pp.2004–10.

Pittock, S.J., Lucchinetti, C.F., Lennon, V.A. (2003). Anti-neuronal nuclear autoantibody type 2: paraneoplastic accompaniments. *Ann Neurol,* Vol. 53, pp.580–587.

Terenghi, F., Cappellari, A., Bersano, A., Carpo, M., Barbieri, S.& Nobile-Orazio, E. (2004). How long is IVIG effective in multifocal motor neuropathy? *Neurology,* Vol. 62, pp. 666–668.

van Doorn P.A., Ruts L. & Jacobs B.C. (2008). Clinical features, pathogenesis, and treatment of Guillain–Barrı syndrome, *Lancet Neurol,* Vol. 7, pp.939-950.

van Schaik, I.N., van den Berg, L.H., de Haan, R., Vermeulen, M. (2005). Intravenous immunoglobulin for multifocal motor neuropathy. *Cochrane Database Syst Rev,* Vol.18, No.2: CD004429.

Vedeler, C.A., Storstein, A.(2009). Autoimmune limbic encephalitis. *Acta neurologica Scandinavica. Supplementum.* Vol.189, pp.63-7

Vucic, S., Black, K.R., Chong, P.S.T., Cros, D. (2004). Multifocal motor neuropathy. Decrease in conduction blocks and reinnervation with long-term IVIG. *Neurology,* Vol.63, pp.1264–1269.

# 18

# Cellular Based Therapies for the Treatment of Multiple Sclerosis

James Crooks[1], Guang-Xian Zhang[2] and Bruno Gran[1]
[1]*University of Nottingham,*
[2]*Thomas Jefferson University, Philadelphia,*
[1]*United Kingdom*
[2]*USA*

## 1. Introduction

Multiple sclerosis (MS) is a chronic inflammatory autoimmune disease of the central nervous system (CNS) and the primary cause of non-traumatic neurologic disability in the western world. Infiltration of myelin-specific effector T cells into the CNS is thought to cause demyelination and loss of axons resulting in deficient signal conduction and clinical onset of the disease. Although previously thought to be initiated by T helper 1 (Th1) cells, it has become evident that Th17 cells are also involved (Cua 2003). In addition, CD8+ T cells, macrophages, and B cells are also found in inflammatory infiltrates in the CNS of affected individuals. During the initial phases of the disease, once the myelin-specific peripherally activated T cells penetrate the CNS, they are re-activated by antigen presenting cells presenting their target antigen within the CNS and act to cause damage to axonal myelin through the activation of macrophages and the release of myelin toxic substances (Aktas, Waiczies et al. 2007).

One of the main obstacles to recovery and to the treatment of MS is the relatively low efficiency of spontaneous remyelination of axons by oligodendrocytes. In the majority of cases during the early phases of the disease a large amount of oligodendrocytes and their precursors are preserved within the characteristic demyelination plaques and retain the ability to remyelinate. Despite this resident population of remyelinating cells it has been shown that over time remyelination becomes incomplete and fails, resulting in the irreversible neurological damage associated with the disease (Franklin 2002).

The direct cause of MS remains unknown but it seems most likely to be a mixture of both genetic susceptibility and environmental factors. Genetic factors had been long suspected to affect the chances of an individual developing MS. It has been known for some time that there is a familial link to the disease with a sharp increase in disease probability if a family member has the disease (Dyment, Ebers et al. 2004), with a direct correlation between how closely related the affected individual is and the probability of developing the disease. The importance of genetic factors was underscored by the fact that adopted children have no statistically significant increase in there disease susceptibility compared to the general population, even if any of their adoptive family members have the disease. Other genetic factors such as gender and race have also been shown to have an effect (Sospedra and Martin 2005).

More recently environmental factors have been highlighted by an increase in MS cases in westernised society as opposed to that of other less developed areas of the world. It is thought this may be due to the lack of exposure to infection during adolescence and childhood and has been highlighted in places such as Japan (Li, Chu et al. 2007) where a strong link may exist between the number of MS cases and the increase in sanitation. Among infectious environmental factors, Epstein Barr and other human Herpes viruses have received most attention in recent years (Levin, Munger et al. 2010). Other non-infectious environmental factors, such as latitude and sun exposure have also been linked to the disease (Sospedra and Martin 2005).

Current treatments for MS include IFN-β, glatiramer acetate and mitoxantrone which show some degree of efficacy and have potential side effects (Markowitz 2010). New more effective treatments for MS are highly desirable, in particular those able to slow disease progression in addition to reducing the frequency of clinical exacerbations. Although several pharmacological therapies are in clinical trials or have recently been approved (such as the immunosuppressive drug Fingolimoid, (Cohen and Chun 2011)), cellular treatments are attractive alternatives. They may theoretically possess the ability to modulate the immune response but also enhance spontaneous remyelination of damaged axons and thus limit or even reverse the irreversible neurological damage associated with MS. The challenge is making this theoretical potential become a reality.

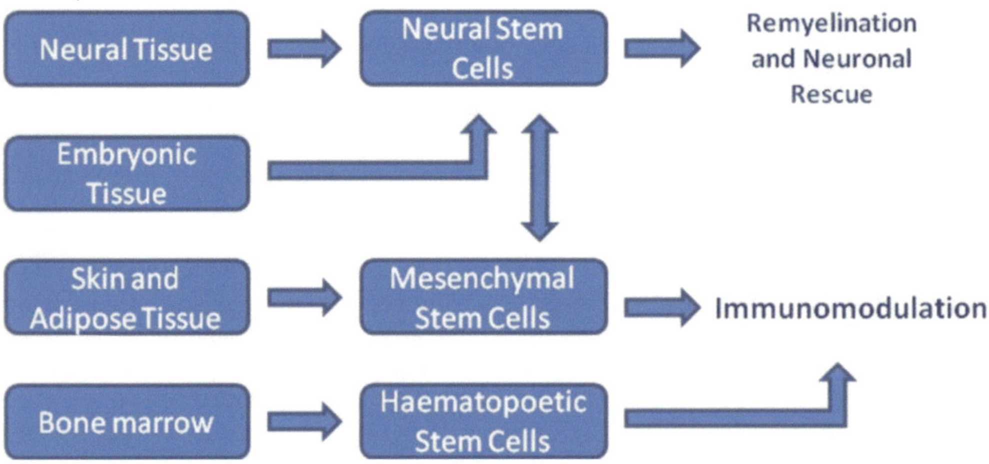


Fig. 1. Potential roles for different types of stem cells in the treatment of MS [Adapted from (Martino, Franklin et al. 2010)].

## 2. Stem cell therapies

Stem cells are the most promising treatment option in cellular therapy as they have the potential to differentiate into a multitude of cells. There are several types of stem cells which are isolated from different types of tissue which include embryonic, mesenchymal, hematopoietic and neuronal stem cells along with the relatively new discovery of fibroblast derived induced pluripotent stem cells (IPS). These different phenotypes of stem cells hold great potential in the treatment of a variety of different conditions and potentially have a range of positive effects on MS and a range of other inflammatory, traumatic and neurodegenerative CNS conditions. The fact that stem cells possess the theoretical ability, under the right conditions, to differentiate into any type of cell in the body makes them a very desirable treatment option. However significant issues arise with their use including ethics, access to the cells, and their potential side effects.

### 2.1 Embryonic stem cells

Of all the different types of stem cells, embryonic stem cells (ESC) have the largest differentiating potential and are also the best categorised but despite this their use has come up against a variety of practical and ethical hurdles due to their embryonic source. Theoretically embryonic stem cells can provide an unlimited supply of cells with vast differentiation potential. In animal models and in the right environment, they can be directed into differentiating into oligodendrocytes and successfully undertaking remyelination (Nistor, Totoiu et al. 2005). This remyelination has been shown in a number of animal models following the infusion of ESC derived glial precursors leading to a significant degree of remyelination in both the spinal column and the brain (Brustle, Jones et al. 1999). It has also been noted that the time of infusion with these cells is crucial, with some studies showing that, in the case of spinal injury, remyelination is much more effective if the embryonic stem cell derived cells are introduced soon after the damage (7 days) as opposed to later after the event (10 months) (Keirstead, Nistor et al. 2005). This suggests that in the case of neurodegenerative disease these cells may be more effective if transplanted in the earlier stages of the condition.

Not only do embryonic stem cells show the potential to remyelinate but also have an effect on EAE through the modulation of the immune system, with a number of animal models showing a down regulation of the auto-immune T-lymphocyte response against self antigen (Fandrich, Lin et al. 2002). This immunomodulatory potential has been proposed to be through both contact-dependent mechanisms and the release of soluble factors. For example $PGE_2$ was identified as one of these factors in murine models in which embryonic stem cells had been used to dampen the immune response in organ transplantation (Imberti, Casiraghi et al. 2011).

Despite the promising potential of embryonic stem cells as a therapy for multiple diseases and conditions there are several hurdles which realistically may never be fully overcome. The first of these are the ethical ramifications of work involving embryonic stem cells. The fact that embryonic stem cells would most likely have to be sourced from human embryos has raised serious concerns about the use of sources of 'potential life' as a research tool. To date, much of the work in stem cell research has been conducted using unwanted embryos originally produced for IVF treatment. However, if this became a main stream treatment embryos would have to be produced for the specific purpose of producing appropriate stem cells, which many see as unethical (de Wert and Mummery 2003). Another ethical hurdle would be the production of autologus stem cells where the nucleus from the cell of the patient would be infused into a de-nucleated oocyte in order to create a strain of stem cells specific to the patient which would help to bypass the issue of rejection (de Wert and Mummery 2003). Many believe the specific use of embryonic stem cells is not the issue; it is the precedent it would set. The ethical debate surrounding ESC is unlikely to be easily resolved.

Another issue surrounding embryonic stem cells is safety. The use of heterologus embryonic stem cells carries the risk of the formation of teratoma (tumour) within the specific organ of transplantation (Bjorklund, Sanchez-Pernaute et al. 2002; Blum and Benvenisty 2008). Altering the cells to reduce this risk may prove very difficult and may also have a detrimental effect on the cells' ability to exert the therapeutic purpose for which they are intended. This issue can be avoided with the use of autologus stem cells (mentioned above) but this leads to not only ethical but also practical issues, with every patient being treated having to be cloned to produce the stock of autologous cells for treatment.

### 2.2 Adult neuronal stem cells

Adult neural stem cells (aNSC) do not carry the same ethical burden as embryonic stem cells and have shown the ability to both remyelinate demyelinated axons and modulate the autoimmune response. These cells are generally isolated from the adult mammalian sub ventricular zone (SVZ), which makes them difficult to extract and use for clinical purposes. They can be maintained for extended periods in vitro and still retain the ability to differentiate and proliferate (Nunes, Roy et al. 2003). In EAE it has been documented that aNSC can act to aid the disease both through remyelination and through an immunomodulatory effect. In terms of remyelination, aNSC have been proposed as treatments for a multitude of different conditions such as neurodegenerative disorders including MS (Magalon, Cantarella et al. 2007), CNS traumas (Iwanami, Kaneko et al. 2005) and malignant tumours. Transplanted cells have been shown to migrate from the area of infusion to the area of inflammation (Ben-Hur, Einstein et al. 2003) especially within the white matter of the CNS, with the labelling of infused cells showing that 80% of lesions contain labelled cells within 24 hours of infusion (Politi, Bacigaluppi et al. 2007). aNSC are also seen to be durable within the body with labelled cells still detected within lesions 20 days after infusion (Politi, Bacigaluppi et al. 2007). Along with the detection of aNSC presence and migration visualised by cell labelling, remyelination and cell replacement have also been visualised in EAE with the use of electron microscopy (Pluchino, Quattrini et al. 2003). aNSC's have been shown to migrate to areas of demyelination (and not to areas of normal looking brain and CNS matter) and differentiate into oligodendrocytes capable of remyelination and thus attenuate the clinical symptoms of EAE within the tested animals.

In terms of the immunomodulatory effects of aNSC on neurodegenerative diseases such as MS there has been some debate. It has been shown that animals given an IV injection of aNSCs in the early stages of EAE show a significant immunosuppressive effect. Animals treated with aNSCs were shown to have a gathering of the infused cells at the spleen and lymph nodes and here had a profound effect on the immune response to self CNS antigen through their interaction with the T-cell populations in these areas (Einstein, Fainstein et al. 2007). T-cells isolated from the lymph nodes of mice that had been infused with aNSC's showed no activation in the presence of either CNS specific antigens or other non-specific stimulus (Einstein, Fainstein et al. 2007). It is evident that these cells, when injected intravenously at the early stages of the disease, do not penetrate the CNS or get attracted to areas of inflammation like aNSC's injected at the height of the disease but travel to areas of immune regulation such as the spleen and lymph nodes where they have an dampening effect on the peripheral immune response (Ben-Hur 2008).

The key to the use of aNSC's in therapy will be optimising the technique to allow both the immunomodulatory and the remyelinating features of the treatment to work in tandem and thus have a greater effect on the symptoms of the disease. aNSCs have several advantages over other forms of stem cells, including fewer ethical burdens, maintaining differential and proliferative ability over long periods of time, and having both immunomodulatory and remyelinating potential. Therefore, they are one of the more promising avenues of investigation into MS treatments. They also seem to pose little risk of tumour formation, which is in stark contrast to a number of other stem cell types. In all the aNSC transplant studies in both healthy and diseased animals there have been no instances of tumour formation which suggests that the potential use of this treatment in vivo would carry little if any risk in the way of tumour development.

### 2.3 Mesenchymal stem cells

Mesenchymal stem cells are stromal stem cells which can be isolated from a variety of adult tissues but predominantly from the bone marrow. The therapeutic effect of these cells on neurodegenerative diseases has previously been based mainly on immunomodulation, but recently it has been proposed that these cells may be able to induce axon remyelination. However, this is yet to be unequivocally proven. In terms of immunomodulation, bone marrow isolated mesenchymal stem cells are known to have a dampening effect of the autoimmune response to CNS self antigens in EAE. The mesenchymal cells are shown to have an inhibitory effect on the activation of encephalitogenic T cells primed against self CNS antigen, thus reducing disease severity (Kassis, Grigoriadis et al. 2008). T-cells isolated from MSC-treated animals show a reduced ability to produce inflammatory cytokines (such as IFN-$\gamma$ and TNF-$\alpha$) and do not proliferate in the presence of the EAE-inducing CNS self antigen (Gerdoni, Gallo et al. 2007). In addition to reducing T-cell function, MSCs can also modulate the proliferation and maturation of antigen presenting cells (APC) (Beyth, Borovsky et al. 2005), which in turn affect T-cell priming to self antigens.

The potential for the infusion of mesenchymal bone marrow derived stem cells to induce a degree of remyelination in animal models of MS has been reported in a few studies. Such cells removed from the bone marrow of donor mice and cultured in vitro were infused into damaged EAE spinal cords and induce both central and peripheral myelination (Akiyama, Radtke et al. 2002).

Bone marrow stem cells can also be used as a source of neural cells, bone marrow-derived neural stem cells. These cells are phenotypically identical to aNSC isolated from the SVC and express the neural stem cell marker nestin. Like aNSC's and unlike other stem cells isolated from the bone marrow, these cells show the ability to migrate into the CNS and differentiate into both oligodendrocytes and neurons at sites of CNS damage, such as inflammatory CNS lesions in MS (Kabos, Ehtesham et al. 2002). However, their differentiation into cells capable of remyelination is not the only way these cells are said to act in the repair of damaged axons. They may also promote remyelination by pre-existing cells through the release of growth factors. Bone marrow derived neuronal cells also seem to have significant immunomodulatory properties, such as in vitro suppression of T cells, B cells and natural killer (NK) cells.

### 2.4 Haematopoietic stem cells

Hematopoietic stem cells (HSC) have been extensively studied for immune replacement therapy in aggressive forms of MS. There are a number of advantages to this form of stem cell which is why research into it has been so thorough. The isolation process compared to that of other stem cells is less invasive and more ethically acceptable as the CD34+ cells can be easily isolated from peripheral blood. HSC transplantation (HCST) may be one of the most potent available forms of immunotherapy; however issues of safety have limited the advance of this approach into clinical use. Useful predictors of good therapeutic outcomes after HSCT include rigorous selection of the most suitable patients for this type of treatment and the specific treatment protocol. Patients with low to intermediate level of disability experiencing active relapses despite treatments with IFN-beta or with more potent immunosuppressive drugs, such as mitoxantrone, may show a better risk/benefit ratio than those with advanced, secondary progressive disease with higher disability (Muraro, Cassiani Ingoni et al. 2003; Burt, Cohen et al. 2005). The regime of treatment is also vital to the success of the treatment with early studies, which used myeloblative transplantation regimes, suffering high levels of toxicity and mortality (Burt, Cohen et al. 2005). The use of revised, non myeloblative HSCT conditioning protocols, seems to have had a positive effect on the mortality rates associated with the previous treatment regimes.

There are many issues when using hematopoietic stem cells as a treatment option in MS involving both ethics and safety. The risk involved in HSCT is relatively high although safety has increased over recent years. An example is the drop in mortality rate in patients suffering from autoimmune conditions treated with autologus hematopoietic stem cell transplantation, which was 7.3% between 1995 and 2000 and dropped to 1.3% in the period from 2001-2007 (Schippling, Heesen et al. 2008). The direct effect of the hematopoietic stem cells in giving rise to malignant tumours is an obvious risk but another major issue is the level of immunosupression needed during a stem cell transplantation, which leaves the patient particularly vulnerable to infections. The risk factors in this type of immunosuppressive therapy make it a last resort, with patients and treating physicians having to assess and discuss the risk/benefit ratios of such a treatment before undertaking it. Considering that many patients with MS live for many years and can, to some degree, manage and slow the progression of their illness with pharmaceutical treatments, it may be hard to justify a therapy such as AHSCT. However, as the methods and techniques involved in AHSCT improve and the favourable outcomes seen in animal models are translated into human studies (this has already been seen in the limited number of humans successfully treated with the method), this treatment could in time become a key immunomodulation technique in treating MS. As these issues are overcome large scale, long term, controlled studies will be necessary to test the true efficacy of the treatment (Mancardi and Saccardi 2008) after which HSCT treatment may be deemed safe for larger scale use.

### 2.5 Induced pluripotent stem cells

Induced pluripotent stem cells (IPS) are possibly the most exciting development in the field of stem cell therapy for the last few years. A group in Japan has shown that it is possible to generate pluripotent stem cells from fibroblast cultures with the addition of just 4 transcription factors (Oct 3/4, Sox2, Klf4 and c-Myc) under ESC culturing conditions (Takahashi, Tanabe et al. 2007). These cells represent a significant step forward as they share the morphology and many functional properties with ESCs but can be generated from fibroblasts in the laboratory. The accessibility of fibroblasts, the comparatively straight forward techniques involved in generating IPS and the removal of important ethical burdens suggests an enormous treatment potential for such a type of stem cells. These cells could become a valid treatment option in regenerative medicine not only in MS but a variety of other inflammatory, neurodegenerative, and traumatic diseases including spinal cord injury, juvenile diabetes (Thomson, Itskovitz-Eldor et al. 1998) and potentially many others.

Despite their enormous potential, IPS do raise a number of safety concerns which must be overcome before they are considered as a valid treatment in humans. Due to a large number of retroviral integration sites (retroviruses are used to insert the relevant transcription factors into target cells to induce IPS) on IPS for each of the stimulating factors they may be prone to tumourigenesis. Mouse studies showed around 20% rate of tumour formation which is thought to be due to the reactivation of the c-Myc oncogene by retrovirus (Okita, Ichisaka et al. 2007). Tumour formation caused by retroviral integration is a serious issue which must be solved before this treatment is considered in the clinic.

Other problems must be resolved as well. The yield of IPS cells from human fibroblast cultures is very low, which could represent a practical obstacle to the development of IPS as a treatment. The precise nature of IPS and their origin is still a matter of debate. Different theories suggest that the cells induced into IPS are actually undifferentiated stem cell-like cells within the fibroblast cultures. It is also possible that undetectable genetic alterations in the cells of origin may be required for IPS induction (Takahashi, Tanabe et al. 2007). For now these cells are a very useful tool within the process of understanding disease mechanisms and toxicology ex-vivo however the ultimate goal must be to develop this therapy to a point where it can be used to treat human conditions. Considering that these cells were only discovered in 2007, research into this form of pluripotent cells is still at an early stage. As time progresses it is likely some of the issues surrounding these cells will be overcome, and along with a better understanding of the mechanisms behind these cells they may become a valid treatment option in human medicine.

In summary, stem cells treatments are, and have been for some time, one of the most promising and exciting potential treatment options within human medicine. Thus far, they have failed to fulfil this immense promise having been held back by many ethical, practical and safety related hurdles. Nevertheless, stem cell research is constantly moving forward. With the discovery of new treatment protocols and new types of promising cells, such as IPS, the time when stem cells become a front line treatment for immunomodulation and neural regeneration in MS may be closer than ever.

## 3. Non-stem cell cellular therapies

It is not only stem cells which have been identified as a potential treatment option for patients suffering from MS. There are a range of possible cellular treatments which involve the infusion of cells isolated from the body with aims varying from halting the progression of the disease through immunomodulation to the active re-myelination of affected axons. Non-stem cell treatments would include the infusion of peripheral nervous system myelinating Schwann cells into the CNS as well as the use of ex vivo cultured oligodendrocytes, olfactory ensheathing cells and even cells isolated from the body's immune system such as T-cells.

### 3.1 Oligodendrocyte and oligodendrocyte precursor cells

Myelination of axons within the CNS is typically the task of oligodendrocytes and their precursors during development and in response to damage, however it has been shown that a significant proportion of these cells are lost or are deemed functionally inactive in MS, particularly in chronic phases of disease. It has been suggested that the reason for this decrease in numbers of oligodendrocytes is due to either the lack of differentiation of precursor cells into mature oligodendrocytes or the death of the oligodendrocytes once they reach a certain point within the developmental process (Wolswijk 2000).

There is a degree of debate over the stage at which oligodendrocyte precursor cells (OPC) are most effective at myelinating axons along there maturation process. It is thought that oligodendrocyte progenitor cells are responsible for generating the largest amount of myelin over the widest area and are more proficient than mature oligodendrocytes (Franklin 2002; Wolswijk 2002). There is evidence that mature oligodendrocytes when infused into a demyelinated CNS environment are less capable of migration and division at the site of demyelination than the more motile and proliferative oligodendrocyte progenitor cell. Another advantage of OPCs is their ability to react to their microenvironment. The path of maturation of these cells is affected by cytokines, chemokines and growth factors causing their maturation to a cell with remyelinating potential "in the right place at the right time", which is also aided by enhancement of the signalling matrix and removal of phagocytic debris by inflammatory cells (Zawadzka and Franklin 2007).

### 3.2 Schwann cells

Schwann cells, typically responsible for myelination within the peripheral nervous system, are seen as an alternative to oligodendrocytes and OPCs in the cellular treatment of MS and have been shown to be capable of a significant degree of axonal remyelination within the CNS of MS patients (Lavdas, Papastefanaki et al. 2008). Despite the issues surrounding the use of these cells, such as their inability to interact with astrocytes and limited survivability within the CNS, their ability to remyelinate axons and improve axonal conduction in damaged axons is not in doubt. The question is whether they can do so to such a degree that it is an effective and worthwhile treatment option for patients with MS. Schwann cells have been proposed as a treatment for CNS damage not only for MS but for other pathological conditions including the repair of spinal cord injury (Oudega 2007) where their proposed function to aid the remyelination of damaged axons remains the same. There are many positive and negative aspects to Schwann cells as a potential cellular treatment option in MS, with the main advantage being the ease of accessibility from peripheral nerve biopsies and thus the relatively simple task of culturing autologus populations of these cells. Another positive aspect is that they are less likely than oligodendrocytes to be prone to MS related autoimmune attack as this tends to be against the CNS myelinating cells due to being targeted towards mature oligodendrocyte antigens (Kohama, Lankford et al. 2001). On this note, the myelin they produce is also less likely to be susceptible to autoimmune attack due the slight differences in its make up as compared with the myelin produced by oligodendrocytes. Due to the autoimmune attack in the CNS being focused against antigens within the oligodendrocyte produced myelin, the subtle differences in the makeup of Schwann cell myelin makes it a less likely target.

As we have explained, the fact that Schwann cells are not usually resident within the CNS has its advantages in terms of not being recognised in an autoimmune attack, however the fact that these cells are out of their usual environment also has some negative ramifications. Schwann cells do not tend to migrate to areas of inflammation within the white matter of the CNS due to the inhibitory effect that astrocytes have on them. Schwann cells and astrocytes cannot coexist which poses huge problems in the treatment of MS as the majority of demyelinated plaques contain large numbers of astrocytes. Astrocytes have a number of detrimental effects on Schwann cells, effecting both their successful migration into the CNS white matter (Iwashita, Fawcett et al. 2000) and their ability to remyelinate and survive (Shields, Blakemore et al. 2000) within damaged astrocyte rich areas. It is proposed that this negative effect on Schwann cells in mediated by the release of soluble factors from the astrocytes (astrocyte conditioned medium reduced Schwann cell proliferation and remyelination (Guenard, Gwynn et al. 1994)) such as Ephrins (Afshari, Kwok et al. 2010) and also through a prolonged contact interaction between Schwann cells and the astrocytes mediated by N-Cadherin (Wilby, Muir et al. 1999). This limited ability to function within the CNS is a major drawback for the use of Schwann cells as a remyelinating treatment as any effect they do have will be short lived due to the short time span they can survive within the appropriate system. If Schwann cells are to become a widely used remyelinating treatment option in the treatment of MS work will have to be done to produce a Schwann cell-based therapy capable of migrating to sites of CNS inflammation and able to survive in the presence of astrocytes. Efforts are being made to improve the chances of Schwann cells surviving interaction with astrocytes through methods such as genetically altering the cells (Papastefanaki, Chen et al. 2007).

### 3.3 Olfactory ensheathing cell

Another type of cell that has been proposed for the remyelination of axons in multiple sclerosis is the olfactory ensheathing cell (OEC). These are a form of unique glial cell found only in the olfactory system close to the first cranial nerve. These cells are favourable over other cell based therapies for a number of properties, one of which is their ability to survive in the presence of astrocytes. Astrocytes are found around areas of MS induced CNS inflammation and as previously discussed are a major problem for Schwann cell therapy. OEC's can survive in conjunction with astrocytes and can also make the environment around the CNS inflammation more hospitable to the migration and survival of endogenous Schwann cells (Boyd, Lee et al. 2004).

Despite this ability to survive and retain function in the presence of astrocytes there are also some disadvantages to the OEC in the treatment of MS. Despite their ability to remyelinate axons and partially regenerate nerve fibres (Richter and Roskams 2008) they do not seem to have a great deal of the ability to cross the MS associated lesion and or to reconnect with neurons on the opposite side of the lesion. It is thought that due to this process of repair not being overly apparent most of the benefit for the use of OEC comes from the promotion of the growth of intact fibres. However, in the case of spinal injury it has been shown that, to at least some degree, these cells have the ability to stimulate neuroprotection, activate angiogenesis and stimulate axon re-growth as well as remyelination (Richter and Roskams 2008). Another benefit of these cells is that in some cases they have been suggested to restore a degree of functions lost due to the CNS lesions. However, there is very little immunological data to support this conclusion, which was derived mainly from behavioural tests (Barnett and Riddell 2004). It is thought that the most useful way to utilise this type of cells may be to use them in parallel with other synergistic treatments. This would produce a combination treatment with the potential to regenerate axons but also reconnect the damaged connections across the compromised areas of the CNS which OEC alone are unable to do (Barnett and Riddell 2007).

### 3.4 T-cell therapy

Another cellular treatment for MS which differs from all the previous treatments as it does not involve remyelinating cells is T-cell therapy. When thinking of ways to tackle autoimmunity one of the most obvious candidates for cellular therapy has to be regulatory T-cells due to their role in maintaining immunological self tolerance within the body. This CD4+CD25+ cell surface marker positive family of cells within the body is in part to control the immune response and therefore seem an obvious choice for cellular therapy for MS. It is known that in the peripheral blood of patients with MS there is a significant decrease in the functionality of T-regulatory cells (Viglietta, Baecher-Allan et al. 2004) when compared to healthy controls, which shows this may be a causative mechanism behind the disease and readdressing this balance may go some way to alleviating autoimmunity.

It has been shown in animal models that adoptive transfer of such T-regulatory cells has a positive effect on models of autoimmune disease (Jiang, Lechler et al. 2006), in some cases offering a significant degree of protection from the disease (Kohm, Carpentier et al. 2002) and therefore poses a degree of therapeutic potential in the treatment of MS. The therapeutic potential of these cells is based on their ability to suppress the function of auto reactive T helper cells in-vitro and to show a significant potential for in-vivo treatment as well. There is also the possibility of targeting these cells in-vivo with other drugs in an attempt to expand an antigen specific population of these cells to tackle the autoimmune response in the MS patients.

Another form of T cell therapy which has been proposed is the use of inflammatory CD4+ T cells. These cells have long been thought to have little therapeutic potential in CNS autoimmunity but it has been proposed by a group in Israel that a lack of CD4+ immune cells recruited to the CNS may affect the immunological balance in the CNS further and exacerbate inflammation within the system (Schwartz and Shechter 2010). Their theory is that these CD4+ T cells must be recruited to the CNS to modify areas of local inflammation and also to aid the protective process through the recruitment of blood-borne monocytes (Schwartz, London et al. 2009). Many current therapies for MS involve treatment with immunosuppressive drug regimes which will strongly inhibit the ability of these inflammatory T cells to perform the proposed protective function and it has thus been proposed that a boost of such a T cell response to carefully chosen CNS proteins may act to improve and not hinder the immunological response against the localised inflammation.

In summary, although cellular therapies for MS are often focused around stem cells, it is evident that non stem cell therapies have an important role to play. They do in most cases provide a safer, more ethical and more practical option of treatment compared to stem cells but may not posses as much treatment potential. However, this is not to say they are less effective than the treatments currently available. Like stem cells, the different types of these cells give non stem cell cellular therapies both remyelination and immunomodulatory potential. These cells have the potential to be used on their own or in combination with other therapies. With steps being taken to improve their efficacy (such as genetic alteration in the case of Schwann cells), they could become mainstream treatments in the fight against MS.

## 4. Conclusion

The devastating effect MS has on the lives of affected individuals and those close to them demands that this field of research be at the forefront of treatment development. The lack of current effective and curative therapies for this disease makes the advancement of cellular treatments all the more important as a new more effective line of treatment. The outstanding potential of cellular therapies to cover all bases in terms of treatment of MS including immunomodulation, neuroprotection and remyelination makes them impossible to ignore as they realistically have the most potential of any field of treatment currently available. Their potential is almost limitless with the variety of different effects the different cellular treatments can have on the disease and how these could fit the needs of individual patients and their specific disease circumstances.

The challenge to take these cellular therapies from being full of potential to being effective treatment options is one thousands of researchers around the world are working on every day. They strive to remove the issues which at the moment are holding back the clinical potential of these 'shining light' treatments in order to be able to offer patients diagnosed with MS hope that it may be possible to restore the myelin architecture within their CNS and to overcome the disease. The treatment options for MS are currently insufficient but the encouraging point is that the field is constantly moving forwards. With cellular based therapies at the forefront of this advancement it will give sufferers of the disease hope that better treatments and better prognosis may be just around the corner.

## 5. References


Afshari, F. T., J. C. Kwok, et al. (2010). "Astrocyte-produced ephrins inhibit schwann cell migration via VAV2 signaling." *J Neurosci* 30(12): 4246-4255.

Akiyama, Y., C. Radtke, et al. (2002). "Remyelination of the rat spinal cord by transplantation of identified bone marrow stromal cells." *J Neurosci* 22(15): 6623-6630.

Aktas, O., S. Waiczies, et al. (2007). "Neurodegeneration in autoimmune demyelination: recent mechanistic insights reveal novel therapeutic targets." *J Neuroimmunol* 184(1-2): 17-26.

Barnett, S. C. and J. S. Riddell (2004). "Olfactory ensheathing cells (OECs) and the treatment of CNS injury: advantages and possible caveats." *J Anat* 204(1): 57-67.

Barnett, S. C. and J. S. Riddell (2007). "Olfactory ensheathing cell transplantation as a strategy for spinal cord repair--what can it achieve?" *Nat Clin Pract Neurol* 3(3): 152-161.

Ben-Hur, T. (2008). "Immunomodulation by neural stem cells." *J Neurol Sci* 265(1-2): 102-104.

Ben-Hur, T., O. Einstein, et al. (2003). "Transplanted multipotential neural precursor cells migrate into the inflamed white matter in response to experimental autoimmune encephalomyelitis." *Glia* 41(1): 73-80.

Beyth, S., Z. Borovsky, et al. (2005). "Human mesenchymal stem cells alter antigen-presenting cell maturation and induce T-cell unresponsiveness." *Blood* 105(5): 2214-2219.

Bjorklund, L. M., R. Sanchez-Pernaute, et al. (2002). "Embryonic stem cells develop into functional dopaminergic neurons after transplantation in a Parkinson rat model." *Proc Natl Acad Sci U S A* 99(4): 2344-2349.

Blum, B. and N. Benvenisty (2008). "The tumorigenicity of human embryonic stem cells." *Adv Cancer Res* 100: 133-158.

Boyd, J. G., J. Lee, et al. (2004). "LacZ-expressing olfactory ensheathing cells do not associate with myelinated axons after implantation into the compressed spinal cord." *Proc Natl Acad Sci U S A* 101(7): 2162-2166.

Brustle, O., K. N. Jones, et al. (1999). "Embryonic stem cell-derived glial precursors: a source of myelinating transplants." *Science* 285(5428): 754-756.

Burt, R. K., B. Cohen, et al. (2005). "Hematopoietic stem cell transplantation for multiple sclerosis." *Arch Neurol* 62(6): 860-864.

Cohen, J. A. and J. Chun (2011). "Mechanisms of fingolimod's efficacy and adverse effects in multiple sclerosis." *Ann Neurol* 69(5): 759-777.

Cua, D. J. (2003). "Interleukin-23 rather than Interleukin-12 is the critical cytokine for autoimmune inflammation of the brain." *Nature* 421: 744-748.

de Wert, G. and C. Mummery (2003). "Human embryonic stem cells: research, ethics and policy." *Hum Reprod* 18(4): 672-682.

Dyment, D. A., G. C. Ebers, et al. (2004). "Genetics of multiple sclerosis." *Lancet Neurol* 3(2): 104-110.

Einstein, O., N. Fainstein, et al. (2007). "Neural precursors attenuate autoimmune encephalomyelitis by peripheral immunosuppression." *Ann Neurol* 61(3): 209-218.

Fandrich, F., X. Lin, et al. (2002). "Preimplantation-stage stem cells induce long-term allogeneic graft acceptance without supplementary host conditioning." *Nat Med* 8(2): 171-178.

Franklin, R. J. (2002). "Remyelination of the demyelinated CNS: the case for and against transplantation of central, peripheral and olfactory glia." *Brain Res Bull* 57(6): 827-832.

Franklin, R. J. (2002). "Why does remyelination fail in multiple sclerosis?" *Nat Rev Neurosci* 3(9): 705-714.

Gerdoni, E., B. Gallo, et al. (2007). "Mesenchymal stem cells effectively modulate pathogenic immune response in experimental autoimmune encephalomyelitis." *Ann Neurol* 61(3): 219-227.

Guenard, V., L. A. Gwynn, et al. (1994). "Astrocytes inhibit Schwann cell proliferation and myelination of dorsal root ganglion neurons in vitro." *J Neurosci* 14(5 Pt 2): 2980-2992.

Imberti, B., F. Casiraghi, et al. (2011). "Embryonic stem cells, derived either after in vitro fertilization or nuclear transfer, prolong survival of semiallogeneic heart transplants." *J Immunol* 186(7): 4164-4174.

Iwanami, A., S. Kaneko, et al. (2005). "Transplantation of human neural stem cells for spinal cord injury in primates." *J Neurosci Res* 80(2): 182-190.

Iwashita, Y., J. W. Fawcett, et al. (2000). "Schwann cells transplanted into normal and X-irradiated adult white matter do not migrate extensively and show poor long-term survival." *Exp Neurol* 164(2): 292-302.

Jiang, S., R. I. Lechler, et al. (2006). "CD4+CD25+ regulatory T-cell therapy." *Expert Rev Clin Immunol* 2(3): 387-392.

Kabos, P., M. Ehtesham, et al. (2002). "Generation of neural progenitor cells from whole adult bone marrow." *Exp Neurol* 178(2): 288-293.

Kassis, I., N. Grigoriadis, et al. (2008). "Neuroprotection and immunomodulation with mesenchymal stem cells in chronic experimental autoimmune encephalomyelitis." *Arch Neurol* 65(6): 753-761.

Keirstead, H. S., G. Nistor, et al. (2005). "Human embryonic stem cell-derived oligodendrocyte progenitor cell transplants remyelinate and restore locomotion after spinal cord injury." *J Neurosci* 25(19): 4694-4705.

Kohama, I., K. L. Lankford, et al. (2001). "Transplantation of cryopreserved adult human Schwann cells enhances axonal conduction in demyelinated spinal cord." *J Neurosci* 21(3): 944-950.

Kohm, A. P., P. A. Carpentier, et al. (2002). "Cutting edge: CD4+CD25+ regulatory T cells suppress antigen-specific autoreactive immune responses and central nervous system inflammation during active experimental autoimmune encephalomyelitis." *J Immunol* 169(9): 4712-4716.

Lavdas, A. A., F. Papastefanaki, et al. (2008). "Schwann cell transplantation for CNS repair." *Curr Med Chem* 15(2): 151-160.

Levin, L. I., K. L. Munger, et al. (2010). "Primary infection with the Epstein-Barr virus and risk of multiple sclerosis." *Ann Neurol* 67(6): 824-830.

Li, Y., N. Chu, et al. (2007). "Increased IL-23p19 expression in multiple sclerosis lesions and its induction in microglia." *Brain* 130(Pt 2): 490-501.

Magalon, K., C. Cantarella, et al. (2007). "Enriched environment promotes adult neural progenitor cell mobilization in mouse demyelination models." *Eur J Neurosci* 25(3): 761-771.

Mancardi, G. and R. Saccardi (2008). "Autologous haematopoietic stem-cell transplantation in multiple sclerosis." *Lancet Neurol* 7(7): 626-636.

Markowitz, C. E. (2010). "The current landscape and unmet needs in multiple sclerosis." *Am J Manag Care* 16(8 Suppl): S211-218.

Martino, G., R. J. Franklin, et al. (2010). "Stem cell transplantation in multiple sclerosis: current status and future prospects." *Nat Rev Neurol* 6(5): 247-255.

Muraro, P. A., R. Cassiani Ingoni, et al. (2003). "Hematopoietic stem cell transplantation for multiple sclerosis: current status and future challenges." *Curr Opin Neurol* 16(3): 299-305.

Nistor, G. I., M. O. Totoiu, et al. (2005). "Human embryonic stem cells differentiate into oligodendrocytes in high purity and myelinate after spinal cord transplantation." *Glia* 49(3): 385-396.

Nunes, M. C., N. S. Roy, et al. (2003). "Identification and isolation of multipotential neural progenitor cells from the subcortical white matter of the adult human brain." *Nat Med* 9(4): 439-447.

Okita, K., T. Ichisaka, et al. (2007). "Generation of germline-competent induced pluripotent stem cells." *Nature* 448(7151): 313-317.

Oudega, M. (2007). "Schwann cell and olfactory ensheathing cell implantation for repair of the contused spinal cord." *Acta Physiol (Oxf)* 189(2): 181-189.

Papastefanaki, F., J. Chen, et al. (2007). "Grafts of Schwann cells engineered to express PSA-NCAM promote functional recovery after spinal cord injury." *Brain* 130(Pt 8): 2159-2174.

Pluchino, S., A. Quattrini, et al. (2003). "Injection of adult neurospheres induces recovery in a chronic model of multiple sclerosis." *Nature* 422(6933): 688-694.

Politi, L. S., M. Bacigaluppi, et al. (2007). "Magnetic-resonance-based tracking and quantification of intravenously injected neural stem cell accumulation in the brains of mice with experimental multiple sclerosis." *Stem Cells* 25(10): 2583-2592.

Richter, M. W. and A. J. Roskams (2008). "Olfactory ensheathing cell transplantation following spinal cord injury: hype or hope?" *Exp Neurol* 209(2): 353-367.

Schippling, S., C. Heesen, et al. (2008). "Stem cell transplantation in multiple sclerosis." *J Neurol* 255 Suppl 6: 43-47.

Schwartz, M., A. London, et al. (2009). "Boosting T-cell immunity as a therapeutic approach for neurodegenerative conditions: the role of innate immunity." *Neuroscience* 158(3): 1133-1142.

Schwartz, M. and R. Shechter (2010). "Systemic inflammatory cells fight off neurodegenerative disease." *Nat Rev Neurol* 6(7): 405-410.

Shields, S. A., W. F. Blakemore, et al. (2000). "Schwann cell remyelination is restricted to astrocyte-deficient areas after transplantation into demyelinated adult rat brain." *J Neurosci Res* 60(5): 571-578.

Sospedra, M. and R. Martin (2005). "Immunology of multiple sclerosis." *Annu Rev Immunol* 23: 683-747.

Takahashi, K., K. Tanabe, et al. (2007). "Induction of pluripotent stem cells from adult human fibroblasts by defined factors." *Cell* 131(5): 861-872.

Thomson, J. A., J. Itskovitz-Eldor, et al. (1998). "Embryonic stem cell lines derived from human blastocysts." *Science* 282(5391): 1145-1147.

Viglietta, V., C. Baecher-Allan, et al. (2004). "Loss of functional suppression by CD4+CD25+ regulatory T cells in patients with multiple sclerosis." *J Exp Med* 199(7): 971-979.

Wilby, M. J., E. M. Muir, et al. (1999). "N-Cadherin inhibits Schwann cell migration on astrocytes." *Mol Cell Neurosci* 14(1): 66-84.

Wolswijk, G. (2000). "Oligodendrocyte survival, loss and birth in lesions of chronic-stage multiple sclerosis." *Brain* 123 ( Pt 1): 105-115.

Wolswijk, G. (2002). "Oligodendrocyte precursor cells in the demyelinated multiple sclerosis spinal cord." *Brain* 125(Pt 2): 338-349.

Zawadzka, M. and R. J. Franklin (2007). "Myelin regeneration in demyelinating disorders: new developments in biology and clinical pathology." *Curr Opin Neurol* 20(3): 294-298.

# 19

# Haematopoietic Cell Transplantation and Immunotherapy for Autoimmune Diseases in Children and Adults

Menachem Bitan
*Pediatric Blood and Marrow Transplantation & Immunotherapy Program*
*Department of Pediatric Hematology/Oncology, "Dana" Children's Hospital,*
*Tel-Aviv Sourasky Medical Center, Tel-Aviv,*
*Israel*

## 1. Introduction

### 1.1 Autoimmune diseases

Autoimmune diseases (AD) are individually rare, but together they affect approximately 5-8 percent of the population in Western countries [1-2]. They are usually defined as a clinical syndrome caused by the activation of T cells or B cells, or both, in the absence of an ongoing infection or other discernible cause. In recent years it is well established that low level of autoreactivity is physiologic [3] and crucial to normal immune function. Autoantigen helps to form the repertoire of mature lymphocytes, and the survival of naive T cells [4] and B cells [5]. Thus, the assumption is that lymphocytes evolved not to distinguish self from foreign, but rather to respond to antigen only in certain microenvironments, generally in the presence of inflammatory cytokines [6].
There are several classifications of AD. They may appear to be either systemic (as in the case of systemic lupus erythematosus) or organ-specific (as in the case of type 1 diabetes mellitus). Another classification distinguishes between diseases in which there is a general alteration in the selection, regulation, or death of T cells or B cells and those in which an aberrant response to a particular antigen, self or foreign, causes autoimmunity.
Susceptibility to AD is multifactorial with genetic and enviromental factors being dominant together or alone in each of the syndromes. Infectious-derived antigens are also well known triggers for autoimmunity. Molecular mimicry has clearly been demonstrated in herpes keratoconjunctivitis in mice. T cells that react to the viral protein UL6 cross-react with a peptide derived from a corneal antigen [7]. Rheumatic fever represents an autoimmune response triggered by streptococcal infection and mediated by cross-reactivity between streptococcal and cardiac myosin **[8-10]**. In autoimmune diabetes, T-cells recognize both a peptide derived from the autoantigen glutamic acid decarboxylase and a highly analogous peptide from coxsackievirus P2-C protein **[11]**, and in Guillain–Barr' syndrome antibody cross-reactivity has been demonstrated between human gangliosides and lipopolysaccharides of Campilobacter jejuni **[12]**. Drugs like Procainamide can also alter the immune repertoire. Finally, foreign substances may act as haptens and render autoantigens immunogenic.

### 1.2 Hematopoietic stem cell transplantation

Hematopoietic stem cell transplantation (HSCT) is a well established modality for the treatment of several hematological diseases; however, it can also be used for the treatment of severe forms of immunological diseases.

Conventional AD therapy is effective in most patients, but some patients are resistant to the anti-inflammatory and immunosuppressive agents used or are only capable of responding to high doses of such medicines, which are toxic. In such cases, bone marrow (BM) reconstitution is required. Thus, high doses of immunosuppressants, followed by HSCT, have become an alternative treatment for many diseases involving the immune system. These include multiple sclerosis (MS), systemic sclerosis (SS), rheumatoid arthritis (RA), juvenile idiopathic arthritis (JIA), and systemic lupus erythematosus (SLE) [13-14].

The application of HSCT to the treatment of AD has been studied since the 1970s. The success of this approach has been widely demonstrated in animal models as well as in BM transplant patients who were shown to also have concomitant AD. For example, an allogeneic HSCT which was intended to cure aplastic anemia in 2 patients with concomitant RA, resulted in the complete remission of RA for at least 11 years [14].

The rationale of using HSCT in autoimmune diseases is to achieve the complete ablation of the aberrant immune system and to regenerate a new and antigen-naive immune system. The more widespread use of transplantation is hindered by the risks associated with cytoreductive treatments necessary to create space for the transplanted hematopoietic stem cell population and by the slow kinetics with which immune competence is restored following transplantation. Mild conditioning regimens may be insufficient to create space for donor stem cells. However, fully myeloablative approaches using irradiation and chemotherapy agents may associate with severe side-effects such as the risk of oncogenic DNA damage. Nevertheless, unlike malignancies where any visceral organ impairment is a contraindication to HSCT, disease-related organ dysfunction is often the indication for HSCT of autoimmune disorders. For this reason, the regimen must also avoid further injury to the disease-affected organ. For example, myeloablative agents such as bleomycin, BCNU (carmustine), and radiation that are complicated by pulmonary fibrosis would not be the ideal conditioning agents for a disease such as scleroderma in which a major cause of death is related to pulmonary fibrosis and pulmonary artery hypertension [**15**].

The stem cell graft may be syngeneic (from identical twin), allogeneic (from a donor with identical human leucocyte antigen - HLA - system), or autologous (from the patient). In autologous setting, the goal of regenerating a new, antigen naive immune system, from the patient's own hematopoietic stem cells requires the re-emergence of thymic educated T cells. Therefore, the goal of the conditioning regimen would focus on immune ablation rather than myeloablation [16-17]. Allogeneic grafts are associated with complications such graft versus host disease (GVHD) or graft rejection. GVHD contributes to the elimination of the host's aberrant immune system and thus theorctically, makes allotransplant a better option in the treatment of autoimmune diseases [18]. However, the HSCT treatment related mortality in hematological diseases is higher following allogeneic grafting (15–35%) than following autotransplant (3–10%). Because of these high mortality rates following allotransplants, the autologous method could prove to be a better alternative in autoimmune patients, too [19-20]. On the other hand, in recent years the transplant related mortality (TRM) is extremely low due to better peri-transplant care. Thus, it may shift again for the allo-transplant as the better choice for autoimmune diseases, in the coming years.

## 2. HSCT in specific clinical indications

### 2.1 Multiple sclerosis

Multiple sclerosis (MS) is an organ-specific AD mediated by T cells triggered against structural components of myelin in the central nervous system (CNS). Subsequent to inflammation in the CNS, demyelinization and loss of axons may occur, resulting in interruption of the electrical signal. Most MS patients present episodic relapse and improvement, known as relapsing-remitting MS, followed by a phase called secondary progressive MS. There is yet another form of MS known as primary progressive MS, which is generally resistant to conventional therapies [21].

Available treatments for MS are not curative. They are able to reduce inflammation in the CNS and to delay the advance of the disease, but disease control is frequently unsatisfactory. The use of stem cells in the treatment of MS is based on the immunosuppressor and immunomodulatory effects of HSCT, which may favor the immunological balance [21]. Furthermore, the multi-focal nature of MS makes the injection of stem cells into each affected site impracticable, which means that the cells need to be attracted to the pathological areas. The intravenous administration of stem cells may be an alternative in MS and other neuroinflammatory conditions, in which there is permeability of the hematoencephalic blood brain barrier in the inflammatory areas. Moreover, the discovery that stem cells are capable of reaching the CNS and of transdifferentiating or acquiring oligodendrocyte and possibly neuronal properties, suggests that they may be able to act in re-myelinization and neuron repair.

Intensive immunosuppresion followed by HSCT has been suggested as potential treatment in severe forms of MS. Since 1995, more than 400 patients have been treated with HSCT. Stabilization or improvement occurred in almost 70% of cases at least for 3 years post-transplant. Magnetic resonance revealed the capacity of autologous HSCT to suppress or markedly reduce gadolinium-enhancing lesions. The progression of brain atrophy declined after two years post-HSCT. The profound immunological changes following autologous HSCT may result in restoration of self-tolerance. Relatively young patients with active inflammatory lesions of relatively short duration and rapidly progressive disease, but still low disability scores, unresponsive to conventional therapy seem the best candidates for transplantation. Transplant-related mortality was 6% in the first European Group for Blood and Marrow Transplantation (EBMT) report and 5.3% in the second one. No deaths were reported since 2001. Very high-intensity conditioning regimen is associated with higher risk of toxicity without significant increase in efficacy. The effects of transplantation and transplantation-related morbidity are dependent on patient-selection, time of transplantation and conditioning regimens used [**22**].

### 2.2 Rheumatoid arthritis

Rheumatoid Arthritis (RA) is a systemic AD that, in the long term, can lead to irreversible destruction of the joints, loss of mobility, as well as a reduction in both the quality of life and life span. Cellular and humoral immune responses can contribute to the development of lesions. Rheumatoid factor, an autoantibody specific to the Fc region of human IgG, is found in 80% of patients with RA [23].

In a retrospective analysis summarizing the European experience of the first 78 registered patients, a significant improvement was demonstrated, with 67% achieving an American

College of Rheumatology 50% response (ACR-50) at some time post-transplant [23]. Most of the patients had failed a median of five (range, two to nine) conventional diseasemodifying antirheumatic drugs (DMARDs) before the transplant. Some degree of relapse was seen in 73% of patients post-transplant, but in most cases it was relatively easy to control with drugs that had proven ineffective pre-transplant [24]. A multi-center trial in Australia failed to show any advantage of CD34 selection of the graft after non myeloablative conditioning with cyclophosphamide [25].

### 2.3 Systemic sclerosis

Systemic sclerosis (SSc) is a multi-system autoimmune disease of yet unknown origin, with vasculopathy and progressive fibrosis that is highly variable in its clinical manifestations, but patients with diffuse cutaneous SSc and internal organ involvement have reduced life span [26-29]. Two major clinical subsets are widely accepted, the limited (lcSSc) and the diffuse cutaneous (dcSSc) forms, which can be distinguished by the extent of skin involvement, the autoantibody profile and the pattern of organ involvement. It has an incidence of $1/10^5$, and is responsible for significant morbidity with a 5-year mortality rate of at least 30% of all patients. In patients with rapidly progressive dcSSc, the 5-year mortality is estimated to be 40–50%. Although cyclophosphamide was observed to have a small beneficial effect, more effective therapies for the severe forms of SSc are required to improve outcome [30-34].

HSCT, mostly autologous but also allogeneic in some specific cases, has been employed worldwide since 1996 as a new therapeutic strategy in patients with a poor prognosis. Almost 200 HSCT procedures have been reported in the EBMT data base up to date. Several publication reported significant decrease in the degree of the scleroderma and dermal fibrosis, improved overall function and, in general, stability of internal organ function [35-36] post autologous HSCT. Two ongoing phase III trials have been designed in parallel, the ASTIS and the SCOTT trail aiming to analyze the benefits from autologous HSCT and its effects on survival, skin, and major organ function in patients with severe dcSSc. The backbone of the conditioning regimens focuses on immunoablation rather than myeloablation and uses cyclophosphamide, anti-thymocitic globulin and total body irradiation [37].

### 2.4 Autoimmune cytopenias

Immune thrombocytopenic purpura (ITP) is a disease in which platelets are sensitized by anti-platelet antibodies or circulating immune complexes, provoking the early removal of these cells from the circulation. This process results in thrombocytopenia and bleeding. About one third of patients with ITP do not respond well to conventional therapies. High doses of immunosuppressors may lead to remission of the disease; however, this involves risks related to myelosuppression. HSCT aims to accelerate reestablishment of the hematological parameters and concomitantly reduce the number of autoimmune cells in the organism [38]. Several sporadic case reports of HSCT for autoimmune cytopenias have been published, but only two studies have been reported with moderate numbers of patients. In the US, of 14 patients with chronic refractory ITP submitted to high dose cyclophosphamide (200 mg/kg) followed by autologous HSCT, 6 achieved durable complete responses and 2 obtained durable partial responses [39]. The study concluded that the infusion of hematopoietic stem cells (HSCs) had accelerated the hematological reestablishment. Since clinical improvement was not associated with quantification of anti-GPIb or anti-GPIIIa antibodies, it is likely that other platelet antigens were involved in the ITP. The responses were not associated with the number of CD3+ cells infused into the patients, although the deletion of T lymphocytes may have prevented the re-infusion of auto-reactive T cells [38].

In a recent study presented at the 2011 annual meeting of the EBMT [40], a summary of the updated EBMT registry on HSCT for autoimmune cytopenias was discussed. Twenty-four patients (14 males, 10 females) received 26 transplants. Patients had Evans syndrome (10), autoimmune haemolytic anemia (AIHA) (6), immune thrombocytopenia (5) and autoimmune lymphoproliferative syndrome (3). The median age at diagnosis was 4 yrs. (range 0.3-16) with a median age at transplant of 7.1 yrs (1.5-17). All patients failed multiple second and third line immunesuppressive treatments with median disease duration of 41 months (1 -180 months). Transplants were autologous for 7 and allogeneic for 19 patients. Seven patients died of treatment related mortality, 6 in the allo and 1 in the auto group with a total TRM of 26%. 13 patients had a complete response after a long follow-up (120 months) while 6 patients relapsed, 2 in the allo and 4 in the autologous group. The conclusions of the authors are that allogeneic and autologous HSCT may induce a response in half of patient with severe refractory autoimmune cytopenia. Given the rarity of disease and the low number of transplant per center (1 over 10 years) it is high unlikely that a prospective study can ever be done. At the same time HSCT may be considered for patients with Evans syndrome, AIHA and ITP refractory to 2-3 lines of treatment under the "Clinical Option" criterion. If an HLA identical sibling is available, an allogeneic HSCT may be considered. Alternative donor from a well matched unrelated donor may also be considered in Evans syndrome. In the case that no compatible donor can be identified, autologous HSCT is an option.

### 2.5 Diabetes mellitus

In recent years, there has been a rapid growth in the number of cases of diabetes throughout the world. This epidemic affects approximately 6-8% of the world population and the number of newly diagnosed patients increases yearly **[41]**. Of these, approximately 10% are type 1 diabetes, insulin-dependent diabetes mellitus, an AD caused by the progressive destruction of the insulin-secreting pancreatic ß-cells in the islets of Langerhans **[42-43]** which regulate blood sugar levels by secretion of insulin. Recent clinical data suggest that the disease could be cured if an adequate supply of new ß-cells were made available. Hence, one goal of pancreatic developmental biology is to understand how endogenous ß-cells are made, with the hope of producing them exogenously **[43]**. Pancreatic islet cell transplantation is an attractive treatment of type 1 diabetes **[44]**. Clinical islet transplantation trials based on cadaveric allogeneic islets have demonstrated that it is indeed possible to restore near-physiological insulin secretion capacity in type 1 diabetic patients through transplantation of insulin-producing cells **[45]**.

The immunoablation with immune reconstitution supported by transplantation of autologous hematopoietic stem cells might save pancreatic beta cells from destruction by malfunctioning immune system. This when applied sufficiently early in the course of diabetes type 1 (i.e. prior to destruction of vast majority of these cells) may lead to insulin independence in transplanted patients. In a recently published study **[46]** 15 patients (age 19 - 32) with early diabetes type 1 (no more than 6 weeks from diagnosis, C-peptide positive, Anti GAD - antibodies positive) underwent therapy. With a mean time of observation of 16 months (range 8 - 29 months). No severe complications were observed during the transplantation and in the post transplantation period. Fourteen out of 15 patients became independent of exogenous insulin after the transplantation with median time without exogenous insulin for all these patients of 14 months (range 3 - 29 months). Median day of insulin withdrawal was + 37 (range + 6 to + 103) post transplant. Eleven patients (73%) remain in remission for the median time from transplantation of 16 months. In three patients there was a relapse of requirement for exogenous insulin and the median post-relapse insulin dose for these patients was 0.08 IU/kg of body weight, significantly reduced from pre-transplant dose. The average HbA1c concentration was 11.5 % at diagnosis, 5.88% at 6 months and 5.76% at 12 months after the transplantation. The authors conclude that immunoablation following by autologous HSCT leads to significant reduction for exogenous insulin requirement in all patients and to exogenous insulin independence in early diabetes type 1 in majority of cases.

### 2.6 Crohn's disease

Crohn's disease (CD) is a chronic illness, immunologically mediated, of unknown etiology but probably induced by an exposure to intestinal bacteria or their component antigens leading to an excessive T helper type 1-mediated chronic inflammation of the gastrointestinal (GI) tract in patients with genetic susceptibility **[47-48]**. Some patients remain seriously ill with active disease after all therapeutic options have been exhausted **[49-51]**. Moreover, a distinct excessive mortality from CD exists in this group of patients **[52-55]**. This group of patients may suffer from one or more of the following morbidities: inability to eat, frequent nausea, vomiting, diarrhea, malnutrition, growth retardation in children, fistulas, abdominal pain, extra-intestinal symptoms, psychologic distress from an ileostomy or colostomy bag, iatrogenic addiction to narcotics, toxicities of standard therapies, and multiple surgeries that may lead to short-gut syndrome, chronic total parenteral nutrition, and liver failure.

Appreciating all of the above, it was reasonable to try and use the modality of HSCT in the setup of refractory CD. Thus, 2 main groups, Italian and United States (US), published their data regarding autologous HSCT for refractory CD patients **[56-58]** demonstrating beneficial short- as well as long-term clinical outcome after using the procedure in 4 and 24 patients, respectively, applying nonmyeloablative regimen.

The procedure was safe, without mortality, even in patients heavily pretreated with anti-tumor necrosis factor (TNF) therapy and with ongoing fistulas.

Although relapses have occurred in these series of patients after using a cyclophosphamide/anti-thymocytic globulin (ATG) nonmyeloablative regimen, there has been achievements of treatment-free remissions for as long as 5 years, and remission (CDAI < 150, CSI < 12) rates between 70% to 80% for 5 years. The authors emphasize that because approximately 40% of patients with CD develop intolerable side effects or lose response to anti-TNF **[59]**, further investigation of stem cell therapy including the role of CD34 graft selection and type of conditioning regimen or other methods to maintain remission without surgery for anti-TNF refractory CD appears warranted.

## 3. Important issues related to allogeneic HSCT for autoimmune diseases

Treatment of life-threatening autoimmune diseases in animal models with induced or spontaneous autoimmune diseases can be accomplished by a 2-step procedure involving elimination of self-reactive lymphocytes with an immune ablative conditioning regimen followed by infusion of autologous or allogeneic stem cells, respectively. In animal models it was shown that using such a strategy, autoimmunity could be adequately controlled. It is speculated that de-novo development of the T and B cell repertoire from uncommitted progenitor cells in the presence of the autoantigens may be the best recipe for re-induction of self-tolerance, similarly to the normal ontogeny of the immune system during the induction of self tolerance in fetal stage. Reduced intensity conditioning (RIC) is further applied in recent years aiming to diminish regimen-related toxicity by decreasing conditioning regimen intensity compared to conventional myeloablative transplants.

In the case of allogeneic transplants for malignant disease, instead of using chemoradiotherapy to achieve disease control, relapse is prevented by an immunological graft versus leukemia (GVL) or graft versus tumor (GVT) effect induced by donor lymphocytes, natural killer cells, and/or dendritic cells infused with the allogeneic graft or after HSCT by infusion of peripheral blood donor lymphocytes. For autoimmune diseases this allogeneic effect may also be applied. Unlike autologous HSCT in which the goal is to suppress and restart the immune system from autologous HSCs, the goal of allogeneic stem cells is twofold. First, to change the genetic predisposition to disease by changing the host's susceptible to the donor's resistant stem cell compartment. Second, to introduce donor's lymphocytes with the capacity to eliminate all residual self-reactive host lymphocytes through a process known as graft versus autoimmunity (GVA) effect, in analogy to GVL in leukemia and GVT in some metastatic solid tumors. It is not clear whether a full chimera, in which all HSCs are reconstituted from the donor, or mixed chimerism, with coexistence of both donor and recipient hemato- and immunopoiesis, is sufficient to control disease.

Full donor chimerism in malignancies has been complicated by a high rate of GVHD, an immune-mediated disease in which allogeneic donor lymphocytes are directed against the whole recipient body, resulting in donor T-cell mediated attack against different organs and tissues, causing significant morbidity and mortality. It is assumed that while suffering from GVHD, the patient has the advantage of GVL or GVT, which is the main goal of the transplant. This rational may holds true, at least partially, in the case of autoimmune diseases. Nevertheless, that means swiching one immunological disease by another one with a very similar mechanism. The only difference is the origin of the attacking T-cells. While in the basic autoimmune disease they are autologous T-cells, in GVHD they are donor-derived T-cells.

## 4. Stem cell mobilization from patients with autoimmune diseases

Originally, HSCs were collected directly from the bone marrow donors by repeated aspirations performed under epidural or general anesthesia. Subsequently, to facilitate hematopoietic reconstitution and avoid the discomfort associated with multiple bone punctures, as well as the need for operating room and general anesthesia, the most common method of collecting HSCs has become mobilization from the peripheral blood. Since negligible HSCs are detectable in the peripheral blood during steady state, either a hematopoietic growth factor such as granulocyte colony-stimulating factor (G-CSF) or chemotherapy (usually cyclophosphamide) with or without G-CSF is necessary in order to mobilize HSCs from the marrow to the vasculature where it can be easily collected [60].

Hematopoietic growth factors used to mobilize stem cells also have cytokine immune-modulating effects [61] and, depending on growth factor and autoimmune disease, may either exacerbate or ameliorate disease severity. For example, in experimental autoimmune encephalomyelitis (EAE), an animal model for multiple sclerosis (MS), growth factors such as Flt-3 ligand, stem cell factor (SCF), and G-CSF exacerbate disease, while thrombopoietin (TPO) mobilizes stem cells without affecting disease severity. G-CSF may also cause an exacerbation of MS, sometimes with significant neurological deterioration [60, 62]. In both EAE and MS, simultaneous use of daily corticosteroids or infusion of cyclophosphamide prior to starting G-CSF prevents disease flares [62]. The same may be for RA where G-CSF may cause an increase in joint swelling, tenderness and pain that responds to corticosteroids. On the other hand, G-CSF has not been reported to exacerbate scleroderma. Based on the above, growth factors selected for mobilizing HSCs from patients with autoimmune diseases need to be considered on a disease-specific basis. Hematopoietic growth factors that stimulate production of proinflammatory cytokines or alter trafficking of neutrophils, lymphocytes or dendritic cells may exacerbate some autoimmune diseases. This effect may be prevented by either administration of corticosteroids or mobilization with combined cyclophosphamide and G-CSF. Mobilization with chemotherapy alone or in combination with G-CSF may cause neutropenic fevers and infection-related mortality if prophylactic antibacterial and antifungal antibiotics are not utilized. This can be prevented if only G-CSF will be used. Nevertheless, combined cyclophosphamide with G-CSF for mobilization will sum in higher stem cell yields, an in vivo purge effect by selectively killing lymphocytes in cell cycle, and a disease-ameliorating effect.

## 5. Future directions and therapeutic implications

Future and near-future directions in the area of autoimmune diseases will be influenced by the general role and directions in medicine. Thus, more and more immune biology modulators and therapies directed against specific molecular pathways will become available. This may alter the need for HSCT as the only curative modality or further subject it to those who would fail all the biological treatments.

Individualize or personalized treatment will become the main stream in therapy. This is extremely true for autoimmune diseases where variety of sub-classes and genom-based mapping will give the opportunity to treat each patient in a different, more specific way. On the other hand, it is expected that HSCT would become safer with less treatment-related morbidity and mortality, making transplants more accessible to wider range of patient populations. Thus, we will see more and more allogeneic transplants done for large-scale indications.

## 6. References

[1] Sinha AA, Lopez MT, McDevitt HO. Autoimmune diseases: the failure of self tolerance. *Science* 1990;248:1380-8.

[2] Jacobson DL, Gange SJ, Rose NR, Graham NM. Epidemiology and estimated population burden of selected autoimmune diseases in the United States. *Clin Immunol Immunopathol* 1997;84:223-43.

[3] Dighiero G, Rose NR. Critical self-epitopes are key to the understanding of self-tolerance and autoimmunity. *Immunol Today* 1999;20:423-8.

[4] Goldrath AW, Bevan MJ. Selecting and maintaining a diverse T-cell repertoire. *Nature* 1999;402:255-62.

[5] Gu H, Tarlinton D, Muller W, Rajewsky K, Forster I. Most peripheral B cells in mice are ligand selected. *J Exp Med* 1991;173:1357-71.
[6] Silverstein AM, Rose NR. There is only one immune system! The view from immunopathology. *Semin Immunol* 2000;12:173-8, 257-344.
[7] Zhao ZS, Granucci F, Yeh L, Schaffer PA, Cantor H. Molecular mimicry by herpes simplex virus-type 1: autoimmune disease after viral infection. Science 1998;279:1344-7.
[8] Galvin JE, Hemric ME, Ward K, Cunningham MW. Cytotoxic mAb from rheumatic carditis recognizes heart valves and laminin. *J Clin Invest* 2000;106:217-24.
[9] Guilherme L, Cunha-Neto E, Coelho V, et al. Human heart-infiltrating T-cell clones from rheumatic heart disease patients recognize both streptococcal and cardiac proteins. *Circulation* 1995;92:415-20.
[10] Malkiel S, Liao L, Cunningham MW, Diamond B. T-cell dependent antibody response to the dominant epitope of streptococcal polysaccharide, N-acetyl-glucosamine, is cross-reactive with cardiac myosin. *Infect Immun* 2000;68:5803-8.
[11] Kukreja A, Maclaren NK. Current cases in which epitope mimicry is considered as a component cause of autoimmune disease: immune-mediated (type 1) diabetes. *Cell Moll Life Sci* 2000;57:534-41.
[12] Yuki N. Pathogenesis of Guillain-Barre and Miller Fisher syndromes subsequent to Campylobacter jejuni enteritis. *Jpn J Infect Dis* 1999;52:99-105.
[13] Voltarelli JC, Stracieri ABPL, Oliveira MCB, Paton EJA, Dantas M. Transplante autólogo de células tronco hematopoéticas para nefrite lúpica: resultados brasileiros iniciais. *J Bras Nefrol* 2003; 25: 65-72.
[14] Snowden JA, Kearney P, Kearney A, Cooley HM, Grigg A, Jacobs P, et al. Long-term outcome of autoimmune disease following allogeneic bone marrow transplantation. *Arthritis Rheum* 1998; 41: 453-459.
[15] Abu-Shakra M, Lee P. Exaggerated fibrosis in patients with systemic sclerosis (scleroderma) following radiation therapy. *J Rheumatol* 1993;20:1601-3.
[16] Burt RK, Slavin S, Burns W, Marmont A. Induction of tolerance in autoimmune diseases by hematopoietic stem cell transplantation. *Blood* 2002;99:768-84.
[17] Ikehara S, Good RA, Nakamura T, et al. Rationale for bone marrow transplantation in the treatment of autoimmune diseases. *Proc Natl Acad Sci USA* 1985; 82:2483-7.
[18] Burt RK, Burns W, Hess A. Bone marrow transplantation for multiple sclerosis. *Bone MarrowTransplant*. 1995;16:1-6.
[19] Bombardier C, Gladman DD, Urowitz MB, et al. Derivation of the SLEDAI. A disease activity index for lupus patients. The committee on prognosis studies in SLE. *Arthritis Rheum*. 1992;35:630-40.
[20] Burt RK, Cohen BA, Russell E, et al. Hematopoietic stem cell transplantation for progressive multiple sclerosis: failure of a total body irradiation-based conditioning regimen to prevent disease progression in patients with high disability scores. *Blood* 2003;102:2373-8.
[21] Fassas A, Kimiskidis VK. Stem cell transplantation for multiple sclerosis: what is the evidence? *Blood Rev* 2003; 17: 233-240.
[22] Rogojan C, Frederiksen JL. Hematopoietic stem cell transplantation in multiple sclerosis. *Acta Neurol Scand* 2009: 120: 371–382.

[23] Snowden JA, Passweg J, Moore JJ, Milliken S, Cannell P, Van Laar J, et al. Autologous hemopoietic stem cell transplantation in severe rheumatoid arthritis: a report from the EBMT and ABMTR. *J Rheumatol* 2004; 31: 482-488.

[24] Fassas A, Passweg JR, Anagnostopoulos A, Kazis A, Kozak T, Havrdova E, et al. Hematopoietic stem cell transplantation for multiple sclerosis. A retrospective multicenter study. *J Neurol* 2002;249:1088-1097.

[25] Moore J, Brooks P, Milliken S, Biggs J, Ma D, Handel M, et al: A pilot randomized trial comparing CD34-selected versus unmanipulated hemopoietic stem cell transplantation for severe, refractory rheumatoidarthritis. *Arthritis Rheum* 2002;46:2301-2309.

[26] Steen VD, Medsger TA Jr. Severe organ involvement in systemic sclerosis with diffuse scleroderma. *Arthritis Rheum.* 2000;43:2437-2444.

[27] Bryan C, Knight C, Black CM, Silman AJ. Prediction of five-year survival following presentation with scleroderma: development of a simple model using three disease factors at first visit. *Arthritis Rheum.* 1999;42:2660-2665.

[28] Mayes MD, Lacey JVJ, Beebe-Dimmer J, et al. Prevalence, incidence, survival, and disease characteristics of systemic sclerosis in a large US population. *Arthritis Rheum.* 2003;48:2246-2255.

[29] Furst DE. Rational therapy in the treatment of systemic sclerosis (review). *Curr Opin Rheumatol.* 2000;12:540-544.

[30] Tashkin DP, Elashoff R, Clements PJ, et al. Cyclophosphamide versus placebo in scleroderma lung disease. *N Engl J Med.* 2006;354:2655-2666.

[31] Clements PJ, Furst DE, Wong WK, et al. Highdose versus low-dose D penicillamine in early diffuse systemic sclerosis: analysis of a two-year, double-blind, randomized, controlled clinical trial. *Arthritis Rheum.* 1999;42:1194-1203.

[32] Pope JE, Bellamy N, Seibold JR, et al. A randomized, controlled trial of methotrexate versus placebo in early diffuse scleroderma. *Arthritis Rheum.* 2001;44:1351-1358.

[33] van Bekkum DW. Conditioning regimens for the treatment of experimental arthritis with autologous bone marrow transplantation. *Bone Marrow Transplant.* 2000;25:357-364.

[34] McSweeney PA, Nash RA, Storb R, Furst DE, Gauthier J, Sullivan KM. Autologous stem cell transplantation for autoimmune diseases: issues in protocol development. *J Rheumatol.* 1997; 24(suppl 48):79-84.

[35] McSweeney PA, Nash RA, Sullivan KM, et al. High-dose immunosuppressive therapy for severe systemic sclerosis: initial outcomes. *Blood.* 2002;100:1602-1610.

[36] Nash RA, McSweeney PA, Crofford LJ, et al. High-dose immunosuppressive therapy and autologous hematopoietic cell transplantation for severe systemic sclerosis: long-term follow-up of the US multicenter pilot study. *Blood.* 2007;110:1388-1396.

[37] Binks M, Passweg JR, Furst D, et al. Phase I/II trial of autologous stem cell transplantation in systemic sclerosis: procedure related mortality and impact on skin disease. *Ann Rheum Dis.* 2001;60(6):577-84.

[38] Lim SH, Kell J, al-Sabah A, Bashi W, Bailey-Wood R. Peripheral blood stem-cell transplantation for refractory autoimmune thrombocytopenic purpura. *Lancet* 1997; 349: 475.

[39] Hunh RD, Fogarty PF, Nakamura R, Read EJ, Leitman SF, Rick ME. High-dose cyclophosphamide with autologous lymphocyte-depleted peripheral blood stem

cell (PBSC) support for treatment of refractory chronic autoimmune thrombocytopenia. *Blood* 2003; 101: 71-77.
[40] Rabusin M, Andolina M, Maximova N, et al. Haematopoietic stem cell transplantation in paediatric patients with refractory autoimmune cytopenia: a retrospective analysis from the EBMT registry. EBMT annual meeting 2011.
[41] Meivar-Levy I, Ferber S. Regenerative medicine: using liver to generate pancreas for treating diabetes. *Isr Med Assoc J* 2006; 8: 430-434.
[42] Miszta-Lane H, Mirbolooki M, James Shapiro AM, Lakey JR. Stem cell sources for clinical islet transplantation in type 1 diabetes: embryonic and adult stem cells. *Med Hypotheses* 2006; 67: 909-913.
[43] Murtaugh LC, Melton DA. Genes, signals, and lineages in pancreas development. *Annu Rev Cell Dev Biol* 2003; 19: 71-89.
[44] Balamurugan AN, Bottino R, Giannoukakis N, Smetanka C. Prospective and challenges of islet transplantation for the therapy of autoimmune diabetes. *Pancreas* 2006; 32: 231-243.
[45] Otonkoski T, Gao R, Lundin K. Stem cells in the treatment of diabetes. *Ann Med* 2005; 37: 513-520.
[46] E. Snarski, K. Halaburda, A. Milczarczyk, et al. Immunoablation and haematopoietic stem cell transplantation in early diabetes type 1. EBMT annual meeting 2011.
[47] Bamias G, Nyce MR, DeLaRue SA, et al. New concepts in the pathophysiology of inflammatory bowel disease. *Ann Intern Med*. 2005;143(12): 895-904.
[48] Fiocchi C. Inflammatory bowel disease: etiology and pathogenesis. *Gastroenterology*. 1998;115(1):182-205.
[49] Willoughby JM, Beckett J, Kumar PJ, et.al. Controlled trial of azathioprine in Crohn's disease. *Lancet*. 1971;2(7731):944-947.
[50] Bernstein LH, Frank MS, Brandt LJ, et.al. Healing of perianal Crohn's disease with metronidazole. *Gastroenterology*. 1980;79(2):357-365.
[51] Present DH, Korelitz BI, Wisch N, et al. Treatment of Crohn's disease with 6-mercaptopurine. A longterm, randomized, double-blinded study. *N Engl J Med*. 1980;302(18):981-987.
[52] Farmer RG, Whelan G, Fazio VW. Long-term follow-up of patients with Crohn's disease. Relationship of the clinical pattern and prognosis. *Gastroenterology*. 1985;88(6):1818-1827.
[53] Lapidus A, Bernell O, Hellers G, et al. Clinical course of colorectal Crohn's disease: A 35-year follow up study of 507 patients. *Gastroenterology*. 1998;114(6):1151-1160.
[54] Jess T, Loftus EV Jr, Harmsen WS, et al. Survival and cause specific mortality in patients with inflammatory bowel disease: a long term outcome study in Olmstead County, Minnesota, 1940-2004. *Gut*. 2006;55(9):1248-1254.
[55] Wolters FL, Russel MG, Sijbrandij J, et al. Crohn's disease: increased mortality 10 years after diagnosis in a Europe-wide population based cohort. *Gut*. 2006;55(4):510-518.
[56] Cassinotti A, Annaloro C, Ardizzone S, et al. Autologous haematopoietic stem cell transplantation without CD34+ cell selection in refractory Crohn's disease. *Gut*. 2008;57(2):211-217.
[57] Oyama Y, Craig RM, Traynor AE, et al. Autologous stem cell transplantation in patients with refractory Crohn's disease. *Gastroenterology*. 2005;128(3):552-563.

[58] Burt RK, Craig RM, Milanetti F, et al. Autologous nonmyeloablative hematopoietic stem cell transplantation in patients with severe anti-TNF refractory Crohn disease: long-term follow-up. *Blood.* 2010;116(26):6123-6132.

[59] Reinisch W. How to manage loose of response to anti-TNF in Crohn's disease? *Curr Drug Targets.* 2010;11(2):152-155.

[60] Burt RK, Fassas A, Snowden JA, et al. Collection of hematopoietic stem cells from patients with autoimmune diseases. *Bone Marrow Transplant* 2001; 28:1-12.

[61] Willenborg DO, Staykova MA (2003) Cytokines in the pathogenesis and therapy of autoimmune encephalomyelitis and multiple sclerosis. In: Santamaria P (ed) Cytokines and chemokines in autoimmune disease. Eurekah.com and Kluwer Acad/Plenum Publishers, New York, pp 97–116.

[62] Openshaw H, Stuve O, Antel JP, et al. Multiple sclerosis flares associated with recombinant granulocytes colony-stimulating factor. *Neurology* 2000;54:2147

# 20

# Thionamides-Related Vasculitis in Autoimmune Thyroid Disorders: Review of Current Literature and Case Reports

Elisabetta L. Romeo[1], Giuseppina T. Russo[1], Annalisa Giandalia[1], Provvidenza Villari[1], Angela A. Mirto[1], Mariapaola Cucinotta[2], Giuseppa Perdichizzi[1] and Domenico Cucinotta[1]
[1]*Department of Internal Medicine, University of Messina, Messina,*
[2]*Section of Nuclear Medicine, Department of Radiology, University of Messina, Messina, Italy*

## 1. Introduction

Hyperthyroidism is the consequence of excessive thyroid hormone action (AACE Thyroid Guidelines, 2002). In many cases, it results from excessive activity of the thyroid gland, with a pathologically increased production of thyroid hormones. The causes of hyperthyroidism include several conditions, that are listed in Table 1.

| |
|---|
| • Toxic diffuse goiter (Graves' disease)<br>• Toxic adenoma<br>• Toxic multinodular goiter (Plummer's disease)<br>• Painful subacute thyroiditis<br>• Silent thyroiditis, including lymphocytic and postpartum variations<br>• Iodine-induced hyperthyroidism (for example, related to amiodarone therapy)<br>• Excessive pituitary TSH or trophoblastic disease<br>• Excessive ingestion of thyroid hormone |

Table 1. Causes of hyperthyroidism (AACE Thyroid Guidelines,2002)

Graves' disease is the most common cause of hyperthyroidism. It is an autoimmune disorder, caused by the presence of autoantibodies directed against the thyroid-stimulating hormone (TSH) receptor (TRAb), chronically stimulating thyroid hormone synthesis and secretion, and resulting in an excessive amount of triiodothyronine (T3) and thyroxine (T4) and gland growth. In iodine sufficient areas, this prototypical autoimmune disease is the most common cause of thyrotoxicosis in young women as well as in children and adolescents, and it is characterized by thyrotoxicosis, goitre and typical manifestations such as ophthalmopathy and pretibial myxedema.

According to the American Association of Clinical Endocrinologists guidelines (AACE, 2002), the diagnosis of hyperthyroidism relates on TSH values. Thus, with the exception of the excess of TSH secretion, hyperthyroidism of any cases results in a lower-than-normal or suppressed TSH level, together with an increase of free T4 and free T3 in the case of overt disease.

Once hyperthyroidism has been diagnosed, three main therapeutic options are available, including radioactive iodine, surgical intervention (thyroidectomy) and anti-thyroid drug.

In US, radioactive iodine is currently the treatment of choice for adults with Graves' disease, except for pregnant or breast-feeding women, because of its adverse effects on fetal gland and its appearance in the breast milk. Overall, radioactive iodine is a safe and effective therapy, that can be either administered through an ablative or with a smaller doses regimen in order to render the patient euthyroid. In any case, hypothyroidism requiring a lifelong thyroid replacement therapy is an inevitable consequence with radioiodine therapy.

Thyroidectomy was frequently used in the past, but its use is now limited to pregnant women intolerant to antithyroid drugs, or to patients refusing radioactive iodine as a definitive treatment. Possible complications associated with surgical treatment of Graves' disease include laryngeal nerve damage and vocal cord paralysis, hypoparathyroidism and hypothyroidism.

Anti-thyroid drug treatment is still a widely used approach in the treatment of hyperthyroidism. Since the 1940s, thionamides have been used as anti-thyroid drugs in the management of Grave's disease (Laurberg et al., 2006). This class of drugs includes propylthiouracil (PTU), benzylthiouracil, carbimazole and methimazole (MMI), and all of them have been shown to have comparable efficacy in inducing hyperthyroidism remission (Cooper, 2005).

All these compounds act through the inhibition of thyroid peroxidase, the enzyme responsible for the synthesis of thyroid hormones, thus leading to a reduced hormone secretion (Laurberg et al., 2006). Recently, an alternate mechanism of action has been proposed, relating their efficacy in patients with Graves' disease to a direct immunosuppressive effect (Laurberg et al., 2006).

Despite the similar efficacy, the choice of the anti-thyroid drug is conditioned by other drug characteristics and/or by their pharmacokinetics profile. For instance, MMI has a longer half-life than PTU, and thanks to its once-a-day administration, it represents the best choice when addressing patients compliance. On the other hand, PTU is the drug of choice for treating pregnant and breast-feeding women, because of its limited transfer into the placenta and breast milk (Streetman et al., 2003). PTU is often preferred to MMI also for the additional property of inhibiting the peripheral conversion of T4 to T3.

Although widely used, anti-thyroid drugs have been reported to be associated with a wide range of adverse effects, such as skin eruptions, liver dysfunction and agranulocytosis; fever, arthralgias and arthritis are other common clinical manifestation, usually occurring within the first few months of administration.

The occurrence of these side-effects can be influenced by several factors, such as drug starting dose or treatment duration (Nakamura et al., 2003).

In addition, over the past 2 decades, several cases of thionamides-associated autoimmune vasculitis have been reported, with variable clinical presentation and severity.

Vasculitis are a heterogeneous group of inflammatory disorders of the blood vessels, that occur as a part of several autoimmune disorders. In many cases they are largely mediated by the deposition of immune complexes that precipitate and become trapped within vessel

walls, stimulating an immune response that ultimately leads to vascular injury. This mechanism usually occurs in secondary vasculitis, frequently associated with infections or systemic autoimmune diseases, whereas in the primary vasculitis, immune deposits are generally absent (Kallenberg & Heeringa, 1998).
Clinical manifestations of vasculitis largely depend on the type of vessels and the specific disctrict involved, resulting in a wide-range of signs and symptoms.
The Chapel Hill Consensus Conference nomenclature is one of the most widely used to distinguish different forms of vasculitis, based on vessel size (large, medium, and small), as shown in Table 2 (Jennette & Falk, 2007).

| |
|---|
| Large Vessel Vasculitis |
| • Giant Cell Arteritis<br>• Takayasu Arteritis |
| Medium-Sized Vessel Vasculitis |
| • Polyarteritis Nodosa<br>• Kawasaki Disease |
| Small Vessel Vasculitis |
| • Wegener's Granulomatosis<br>• Churg-Strauss Syndrome<br>• Microscopic Polyangiitis<br>• Henoch-Schönlein Purpura<br>• Cryoglobulinemic Vasculitis<br>• Cutaneous leukocytoclastic angiitis |

Table 2. Classification of vasculitis according to the Chapel Hill Consensus Conference

## 2. Thionamides-related vasculitis in autoimmune thyroid disorders

### 2.1 Autoimmune markers of thionamides-related vasculitis

Overall, vasculitis have been mainly reported in patients treated with PTU, and most of PTU-induced vasculitis are associated with an increase of anti-neutrophil cytoplasmic antibody (ANCA) circulating levels.
ANCA are antibodies directed against myeloid lysosomal enzymes, that can be identified by indirect immunofluorescence (IIF) with human neutrophils. These autoantibodies can have a cytoplasmic (cANCA) or a perinuclear (pANCA) distribution pattern, that can be detected by ELISA (Savige et al., 2000). In particular, cANCA are directed against antiproteinase3 (PR3-ANCA), and they are specific for Wegener's granulomatosis (Van der Wonde et al., 1985), whereas pANCA can be directed against several antigens, the most important being myeloperoxidase (MPO-ANCA). pANCA is a serological marker for microscopic polyangiitis, but it can also be detected in patients with systemic lupus erythematosus, rheumatoid arthritis and drug-induced vasculitis (Jennette & Falk, 1997).
Any of these patterns can occur in patients with drug-induced ANCA-positive vasculitis and atypical ANCA against several antigens, like elastase, azurocin, cathepsine G, lactoferrin and lyzozim have been also reported.
Although the pathogenetic role of these autoantibodies in drug-induced vasculitis has not been fully elucidated yet, several hypotheses have been proposed.

Thus, it has been reported that PTU can selectively accumulate into neutrophils where it can bind to myeloperoxidase, changing or inactivating the heme structure of the enzyme (Lee et al., 1988). It has been suggested that, in susceptible individuals, the enzyme altered by PTU could then stimulate the production of anti-myeloperoxidase antibodies, inducing neutrophils degranulation and vascular damage (D'Cruz et al., 1995). In particular, MPO-ANCA seems to play an important role in the development of tissue damage in vasculitis or glomerulonephritis (Ashizawa et al., 2003; Arimura et al., 1993). It has also been suggested that viral infections could trigger the development of the autoimmune chain reaction.

Overall, ANCA autoantibodies are frequently detected in patients with Graves' disease treated with anti-thyroid drugs, regardless of the presence of clinical manifestations of vasculitis.

Anti-thyroid drugs ANCA-associated vasculitis occurs more frequently in women, consistently with the fact that Graves' disease is more common in female gender.

It has been reported that the prevalence of MPO-ANCA is higher in patients treated with PTU than in those treated with MMI (Wada et al., 2002).

Thus, the prevalence of ANCA positivity has been estimated to average 26% of PTU-treated subjects (Gunton et al., 2000), being even higher in treated children (Hirokazu et al., 2000).

In a study of 117 patients with Graves' disease, Sera et al. reported that MPO-ANCA was negative in all patients treated with MMI as well as in untreated patients, whereas it was detected in 37.5% of patients receiving PTU (Sera et al., 2000). Furthermore, the proportion of patients positive for MPO-ANCA increased with the prolongation of PTU treatment (Sera et al., 2000).

In a retrospective study of 61 patients with Graves' disease, Wada et al. reported that 25% of patients treated with PTU showed positive MPO-ANCA, unlike 3.4% of patients receiving MMI. Moreover, the sole patient MPO-ANCA positive treated with MMI had been taking PTU for six years before starting MMI treatment (Wada et al., 2002).

The annual incidence of MPO-ANCA-associated vasculitis in patients treated with anti-thyroid drugs has been estimated to be between 0.53 and 0.79 patients per 10,000, although several mild cases may not have been reported (Noh et al., 2009).

However, not all ANCA positive patients develop the clinical manifestations of vasculitis, and several factors such as type of drug, ethnicity, timing and dose, treatment duration may concur to the development of overt clinical manifestations.

Overall, the incidence of ANCA positive vasculitis is higher with PTU, being estimated to be 39.2 times the incidence reported with MMI (Noh et al., 2009).

As for ethnicity, the prevalence of ANCA positivity seems to be similar in different ethnical groups, although Gunton et al. suggested that ANCA-positive vasculitis may be more common in patients of Asian origin, being nearly half of the reported cases of PTU-induced ANCA-associated vasculitis from Japan (Gunton et al., 1999).

The timing and doses of thionamides reported in ANCA-associated vasculitis have also been variable. In fact, even if long-term treatment with anti-thyroid drugs seems to have a stronger association with the risk of vasculitis, these complications can also occur within few months after starting the treatment. Furthermore, ANCA-associated vasculitis have been also reported in patients treated with low doses of both MMI and PTU (Noh et al., 2009).

Moreover, it seems that drug dose and duration of anti-thyroid treatment use, together with the titers of antibodies could be related with the clinical course of ANCA-associated vasculitis. Thus, Morita et al. (Morita et al., 2000) reported that anti-thyroid drug-induced ANCA-associated vasculitis was more frequent in patients resistant to drug treatment, who were receiving high doses over a prolonged period of time and with high titers of MPO-ANCA; furthermore, clinical manifestations disappeared according to decreasing values of antibodies. This finding suggests that high titer of MPO-ANCA may be necessary to induce vasculitis.

Beside the role of thionamides in inducing the formation of specific autoantibodies, an alternate hypothesis has to be taken into account.

Thus, given the common autoimmune background, a possible association of ANCA-positivity with the autoimmune disease itself has been suggested.

This hypothesis has been tested in a prospective study, where a group of patients with newly diagnosed Graves' disease were followed up before and during therapy with PTU, and compared to a cross-sectional group of previously diagnosed Graves' patients who had already been treated with PTU, of patients with Hashimoto thyroiditis and those with toxic nodular goiter, as well as to healthy controls. As a result, all untreated newly diagnosed Graves' patients were ANCA negative, but 32.1% became ANCA positive after initiating PTU administration. On the other hand, patients with Hashimoto disease, untreated toxic nodular goiter and euthyroid subjects did not show ANCA positivity. This study suggested that it is PTU treatment, and not hyperthyroidism or autoimmunity, which induces ANCA production (Ozduman Cin et al., 2009). In agreement with this, ANCA prevalence is increased in Graves' disease, but not in patients with other autoimmune thyroid disease, such as Hashimoto thyroiditis (Harper et al., 2004). Furthermore, it has also been demonstrated that PTU administration is associated with ANCA positivity at a similar rate in both patient with Graves' disease and those with toxic multinodular goiter, suggesting that PTU but not Graves' disease itself is the most important factor for ANCA development (Yazisiz et al., 2008).

### 2.2 Clinical manifestations of thionamides-related vasculitis

Clinical presentation and severity of anti-thyroid drug-induced vasculitis are variable, and largely related to the type of vessels and to the anatomical district involved.

Thus, although not all ANCA positive patients develop a clinical disease, a wide-range of clinical symptoms have been reported in patients with thionamides-related vasculitis.

ANCA-associated vasculitis is usually characterized by small vessel inflammation and necrosis, that may involve any system and organ, being arthralgia and fever the most commonly reported clinical manifestations (Morita et al., 2000).

An ANCA-positive vasculitis in association with anti-thyroid drugs was first reported in 1992 by Stankus and Johnson, who described a patient treated with PTU who developed respiratory failure and MPO-ANCA positive test (Stankus & Johnson, 1992).

Since then, several cases of ANCA-associated vasculitis in patients with Graves' disease treated with anti-thyroid drugs have been described, although ANCA-positive vasculitis have also been reported in patients with toxic multi-nodular goiter treated with PTU. Thus, in 1999 a case report of a PTU-induced vasculitis was described in an elderly women with toxic multi-nodular goiter, presenting with haemoptysis and acute renal failure (Gunton et al., 1999).

Overall, drug-induced vasculitis presenting symptoms may include renal involvement (67%), arthralgia (48%), fever (37%), skin manifestations (30%), respiratory tract involvement (27%), myalgia (22%), scleritis (15%) as well as other manifestations (18%) (Gunton et al., 1999).

As for skin manifestations, leukocytoclastic vasculitis, principally affecting the lower limbs, is the most common cutaneous manifestation (Gunton et al., 1999; Day et al., 2003).

In addition, several cases of pulmonary involvement have been reported, including pulmonary infiltrates associated with respiratory failure, eosinophilic pleuritis, interstitial pneumonitis or respiratory distress syndrome and pulmonary harmorrhage (Stankus & Johnson, 1992; Chevrolet et al., 1991).

Renal involvement in drug-induced vasculitis is also common. In 1995, D'Cruz et al. published the first report of renal biopsy-proven vasculitis in two patients treated with anti-thyroid drugs. Both patients developed a crescentic glomerulonephritis and responded to immunosuppressive therapy and dismission of anti-thyroid drugs (D'Cruz et al., 1995).

Recently, Chen YX et al. published a retrospective study of 19 patients with ANCA-positive vasculitis associated with PTU treatment. In this study, renal injury was the most common manifestation, occurring in 94.74% of cases. At renal biopsy, focal proliferative glomerulonephritis and necrotizing glomerulonephritis with crescent formation, minor glomerular abnormalities, IgA nephropathy, membranous nephropathy, focal proliferative glomerulonephritis, granulomatous interstitial nephritis and focal segmental glomerular sclerosis were all described (Chen YX et al., 2007).

Rare fatalities have been also reported in patients with anti-thyroid drugs-associated vasculitis. Batchelor et al. described the case of a 60-year-old man with a history of Graves' disease, treated with PTU, and presenting with rash, pancytopenia, and lymphadenopathy and subsequently developing acute renal failure and diffuse alveolar hemorrhage, who died despite the discontinuation of PTU and an aggressive therapy including immunosuppressive drugs and plasmapheresis (Batchelor & Holley, 2006).

Thus, even if in the majority of cases vasculitis usually resolve after the discontinuation of anti-thyroid drugs, patients can present with more severe or life-threatening manifestations.

In a study evaluating cutaneous and systemic manifestations following thionamides administration, death occurred in 10% of all published cases, with a predominance in patients with involvement of multiple organ systems (ten Holder et al., 2002).

Until 2005, the main case reports of thionamides induced-vasculitis described above all renal, musculoskeletal and cutaneous manifestations. In that period, the first case of thionamides-induced central nervous system (CNS) vasculitis has been also reported (Vanek et al., 2005): a PTU-treated patients presenting with generalized muscle spasms, amnesia and confusion, who showed a complete resolution of CNS symptoms after cessation of drug administration.

Since most of thionamides-related vasculitis have been associated with PTU, MMI treatment has been advocated as safer for the treatment of Graves' disease; however, several cases of vasculitis following MMI administration have been reported.

In 1995, Kawaki et al. reported the first case of ANCA-associated vasculitis caused by MMI: a 24-year-old woman with Graves' disease treated with MMI for 4 years, who developed

recalcitrant ulcers on the lower legs and ANCA positivity, improved after MMI was withdrawn (Kawaki et al., 1995).
Besides skin manifestations, also renal involvement, such as crescentic glomerulonephritis (D'Cruz et al., 1995), and pulmonary involvement, with hemoptysis and hypoxic respiratory failure (Tsai et al., 2001) have been reported in MMI-treated patients.
Furthermore, we recently reported the first case of MMI induced CNS vasculitis in a young woman with Graves' disease, completely recovered after the discontinuation of treatment (Tripodi et al., 2008). CNS vasculitis was suspected on the basis of the clinical features and neurological examination, and confirmed by brain magnetic resonance imaging (RMN) and single-photon emission computed tomography (SPECT). In our patient, ANCA test was negative, supporting the concept that ANCA are not critical for the development of drug-induced vasculitis.
Thus, although less common than with PTU, vasculitis associated with other thionamides-drugs therapy have been also described.
Although more infrequently, carbimazole-associated vasculitis have been reported. Carbimazole has been associated with leukocytoclastic vasculitis and acute renal failure secondary to interstitial nephritis, without any evidence of ANCA positivity (Day et al., 2003), and to ANCA-positive vasculitis with crescentic glomerulonephritis (D'Cruz et al., 1995). Respiratory involvement in carbimazole-treated patients appears to be less common, although a case of MPO-ANCA vasculitis with massive pulmonary hemorrhage and necrotizing glomerulonephritis has been described (Calanas-Continente et al., 2005). Also a case of polyneuropathy, with evidence of microvasculitis in nerve biopsy, was reported as associated to this drug administration (Leger et al., 1984).
In a large cross-sectional study of 407 patients with Graves' disease, Harper et al. reported that both PTU and carbimazole therapy were associated with an increases rate of ANCA-positivity, although the risk in carbimazole-treated patients was smaller than in PTU-treated ones (15.9% and 33.3% respectively vs 4,6% of controls) (Harper et al., 2004). Its administration has also been related to the development of rare side effects, such as those described by Sève et al., who reported the first case of eosinophilic granulomatous vasculitis localized to the stomach in a patient with Graves' disease treated for five months with carbimazole, with complete resolution of clinical manifestations after drug dismission (Sève et al., 2005).
Since there are no evidence that carbimazole can accumulate in neutrophils or to act as a hapten as PTU, the underlying mechanism associated to the development of vasculitis related with other thionamides-drugs has not been yet elucidated.

### 2.3 Anti-thyroid-induced ANCA-associated vasculitis and idiophatic ANCA vasculitis: Comparison of clinical manifestations and outcomes

Clinical and serological characteristics of drug-induced and idiophatic systemic vasculitis are similar; however, the appropriate diagnosis is of great importance since they may have a different treatment and prognosis.
Thus, the removal of anti-thyroid drugs is usually associated with the resolution of the clinical symptoms of vasculitis, whereas patients with idiophatic vasculitis always need to be treated more aggressively with immunosuppressive and anti-inflammatory drugs, or plasmapheresis.

Clinical and serological data from idiophatic and anti-thyroid drug-induced ANCA positive vasculitis were compared in a 11-year retrospective study. In this cohort (Bonaci-Nikolic et al., 2005), both groups of patients showed a similar high frequency of arthralgia and myalgia, whereas skin involvement, especially represented by urticaria and urticaria-like vasculitis, was more common in patients treated with anti-thyroid drugs, with histological evidence of leucocytoclastic vasculitis. Furthermore, patients with idiophatic systemic vasculitis showed more frequently fever, weight loss, renal and respiratory manifestations, pulmonary-renal syndrome, ear/nose and nervous system manifestations.

As for serological profile, patients with drug-induced vasculitis, showed positivity for ANAs and antihistone antibodies, and had high levels of IgM anticardiolipin antibodies cryoglobulinemia and low C4 values (Wiik et al., 2005; Bonaci-Nikolic et al., 2005).

Hence, drug-induced vasculitis seem to have a milder course and a better long-term prognosis, since the withdrawal of anti-thyroid drugs usually leads to the resolution of clinical manifestations in the vast majority of cases.

Thus, the prognosis of anti-thyroid-induced ANCA-associated vasculitis is usually good as long as the drug is discontinued. However, early recognition of clinical symptoms is very important because of the potential risk of life-threatening injury, such as pulmonary-renal syndrome, with pulmonary hemorrhage and renal failure. In these patients, additional treatment with steroids and/or immunosuppressive agents should be recommended.

In a retrospective study of fifteen patients with PTU-induced ANCA-associated vasculitis, Gao et al. investigated treatment protocols and outcomes of patients, suggesting that immunosuppressive therapy should be administrated only in those patients with vital organ involvement, such as lung and kidney vasculitis, in order to prevent progression to irreversible disease.

Interestingly, unlike what is normally found in patients with primary ANCA-associated vasculitis (Hogan et al., 2005), none of the patients with drug-induced vasculitis experienced relapse after the discontinuation of immunosuppressive therapy at follow-up (Gao et al.,2008).

Moreover, immunosuppressive therapy may be administered only for a shorter period of time, usually 6-12 months, than in primary ANCA-associated vasculitis, without any further maintenance therapy (Gao et al., 2008).

## 3. Conclusion

Anti-thyroid drugs are a common and widespread treatment for Graves' disease and the other forms of hyperthyroidism. It is a safe and efficacy treatment, and it is the treatment of choice in patients refusing radioactive iodine as definitive treatment or during pregnancy and breast-feeding.

However, this treatment has been associated with several side effects and among them, vasculitis, with a wide-range of severity and clinical presentations.

Vasculitis are more commonly reported in PTU-treated patients, with a long duration of treatment, and with positivity for ANCA autoantibodies.

Thionamides-related vasculitis usually recover after discontinuation of therapy, although rare cases of fatalities have been also reported.

## 4. References

AACE Thyroid Guidelines. (2002*). Endocrine Practice*, Vol. 8, No. 6, pp. 457-69.

Arimura, Y.; Minoshima, S.; Kamiya, Y.; Tanaka, U.; Nakabayashi, K.; Kitamoto, K.; Nagasawa, T.; Sasaki, T. & Suzuki, K. (1993). Serum myeloperoxidase and serum cytokines in anti-myeloperoxidase antibody-associated glomerulonephritis. *Clinical Nephrology*, Vol. 40, No. 5, pp. 256-2641

Ashizawa, K. & Eguchi, K. (2003). Serum anti-myeloperoxidase antineutrophil cytoplasmic antibodies (MPO-ANCA) in patients with Graves' disease receiving anti-thyroid medication. *Internal Medicine*, Vol. 42, No. 6, pp.463-464

Batchelor, N. & Holley, A. (2006). A fatal case of propylthiouracil-induced ANCA-positive vasculitis. *Medscape General Medicine*, Vol. 8, No.4, p. 10

Bonaci-Nikolic, B.; Nikolic, M.M.; Andrejevic, S.; Zoric, S. & Bukilica, M. (2005). Antineutrophil cytoplasmic antibody (ANCA)-associated autoimmune disease induced by antithyroid drugs: comparison with idiopathic ANCA vasculitides. *Arthritis Research & Therapy*, Vol. 7, No. 5, pp. R1072-1081

Calanas-Continente, A.; Espinosa, M.; Manzano-Garcìa, G.; Santamarìa, R.; Lopez-Rubio, F. & Aljama, P. (2005). Necrotizing glomerulonephritis and pulmonary hemorrhage associated with carbimazole therapy. *Thyroid*, Vol. 15, No. 3

Chen, Y.X.; Yu, H.J.; Ni, L.Y.; Zhang, W.; Xu, Y.W.; Ren, H.; Chen, X.N.; Wang, X.L.; Li, X.; Pan, X.X.; Wang, W.M. & Chen, N. (2007). Propylthiouracil-associated antineutrophil cytoplasmic autoantibody-positive vasculitis: retrospective study of 19 cases. *The Journal of Rheumatology*, Vol. 34, No. 12, pp. 2451-2456

Chevrolet, J.C.; Guelpa, G. & Schifferli, J.A. (1991). Recurrent adult respiratory distress-like syndrome associated with propylthiouracil therapy. *European Respiratory Journal*, Vol. 4, No. 7, pp. 899-901

Cooper, D.S. (2005). Antithyroid drugs. *New England Journal of Medicine*, Vol. 352, No. 9, (March 3), pp. 905-17

D'Cruz, D.; Chesser, A.M.S.; Lightowler, C.; Comer, M.; Hurst, M.J.; Baker, L.R.I. & Raine, A.E.G. (1995). Antineutrophil cytoplasmic antibody-positive crescentic glomerulonephritis associated with anti-thyroid drug treatment. *British Journal of Rheumatology*, Vol. 34, No. 11, pp.1090-1091

Day, C.; Bridger, J.; Rylance, P.; Jackson, M.; Nicholas, J. & Odum, J. (2003). Leukocytoclastic vasculitis and interstitial nephritis with carbimazole treatment. *Nephrology Dialysis Transplantion*, Vol. 18, No. 2, pp. 429-431

Gao, Y.; Chen, M.; Ye, H.; Yu, F.; Guo, X.H. & Zhao, M.H. (2008). Long-term outcomes of patients with propylthiouracil-induced anti-neutrophil cytoplasmic auto-antibody-associated vasculitis. *Rheumatology*, Vol. 47, No. 10 , pp. 1515-1520

Gunton, J.E.; Stiel, J.; Caterson, R.J. & McElduff, A. (1999). Anti-thyroid drugs and antineutrophil cytoplasmic antibody positive vasculitis. A case report and review of the literature. *Journal of Clinical Endocrinology and Metabolism*, Vol. 84, No. 1, pp. 13-16, ISSN 0021-972X

Gunton, J.E.; Stiel, J.; Clifton-Bligh, P.; Wilmshurst, E. & McElduff, A. (2000). Prevalence of positive anti-neutrophil cytoplasmic antibody (ANCA) in patients receiving anti-thyroid medication. *European Journal of Endocrinology*, Vol. 142, No. 6, pp. 587-590, ISSN 0804-4643

Harper, L.; Chin, L.; Daykin, J.; Allahabadia, A.; Heward, J.; Gough, S.C.; Savage, C.O. & Franklyn, J.A. (2004). Propylthiouracil and carbimazole associated-antineutrophil cytoplasmic antibodies (ANCA) in patients with Graves' disease. *Clinical Endocrinology*, Vol. 60, No. 6, pp. 671-675

Hogan, S.L.; Falk, R.J.; Chin, H.; Cai, J.; Jennette, C.E.; Jennette, J.C. & Nachman, P.H. (2005). Predictors of releapse and treatment resistance in antineutrophil cytoplasmic antibody-associated small-vessel vasculitis. *Annals of Internal Medicine*, Vol. 143, No. 9, pp. 621-631

Jennette, J.C. & Falk, R.J. (1997). Small vessel vasculitis. *New England Journal of Medicine*, Vol.337, No. 21, pp. 1512-1523

Jennette, J.C. & Falk, R.J. (2007). The role of pathology in the diagnosis of systemic vasculitis. *Clinical and Experimental Rheumatology*, Vol. 25, No. 1 supp 44, pp. S52-56

Kallenberg, C.G. & Heeringa, P. (1998). Pathogenesis of vasculitis. *Lupus*, Vol. 7, No. 4, pp. 280-284

Kawaki, Y.; Nukaga, H.; Hoshito, M.; Iwata, M. & Otsuka, F. (1995). ANCA associated vasculitis and lupus like syndrome caused by methimazole. *Clinical and Experimental Dermatology*, Vol. 20, No. 4, pp. 345-347

Laurberg, P. (2006). Remission of Graves' disease during anti-thyroid drug therapy. Time to reconsider the mechanism? *European Journal of Endocrinology*, Vol. 155, No. 6, pp. 783-786, ISSN 0804-4643

Laurberg, P.; Andersen, S. & Karmisholt, J. (2006). Antithyroid drug therapy of Graves' hyperthyroidism: realistic goals and focus on evidence. *Expert Review of Endocrinology & Metabolism*, Vol.1, pp. 91-102

Lee, E.; Hirouchi M.; Hosokawa, M.; Sayo, H.; Kohno, M. & Kariya, K. (1988). Inactivation of peroxidase of rat bone marrow by repeated administration of propylthiouracil is accompanied by a change in the heme structure. *Biochemical Pharmacology*, Vol. 37, No. 11, pp.2151-2153

Leger, J.M.; Dancea, S.; Brunet, P. & Hauw, JJ. (1984). Polyneuropathy during treatment with carbimazole. *Revue Neurologique (Paris)*, Vol. 140, No. 11, 652-656

Morita, S.; Ueda, Y. & Eguchi, K. (2000). Anti-thyroid drug-induced ANCA-associated vasculitis: a case report and review of the literature. *Endocrine Journal*, Vol. 47, No. 4, pp. 467-470

Nakamura, H.; Noh, J.Y.; Itoh, K.; Fukata, S.; Miyauchi, A. & Hamada, N. (2007). Comparison of methimazole and propylthiouracil in patients with hyperthyroidism caused by Graves' disease. *Journal of Clinical Endocrinology and Metabolism*, Vol. 92, No. 6, pp. 2157-2162

Ozduman Cin, M.; Morris, Y.; Tiryaki Aydintug, O.; Kamel, N. & Gullu, S. (2007). Prevalence and clinical significance of antineutrophil cytoplasmic antibody in Graves' patients treated with propylthiouracil. *International Journal of Clinical Practice*, Vol. 63, No. 2, pp. 299-302

Sato, H.; Hattori, M.; Fujieda, M.; Sugihara, S.; Inomata, H.; Hoshi, M. & Miyamoto, S. (2000). High prevalence of antineutrophil cytoplasmic antibody positivity in childhood onset Graves' disease treated with propylthiouracil. *Journal of Clinical Endocrinology and Metabolism*, Vol. 85, No. 11, pp. 4270-4273, ISSN 0021-972X

Savige, J.; Davies, D.; Falk, R.J.; Jennette, J.C. & Wiik, A. (2000). Antineutrophil cytoplasmic antibodies and associated disease: a review of the clinical and laboratory features. *Kidney International*, Vol. 57, No. 3, pp. 846-862

Sève, P.; Stankovic, K.; Michalet, V.; Vial, T.; Scoazec, J.Y. & Broussolle, C. (2005). Carbimazole induced eosinophilic granulomatous vasculitis localized to the stomach. *Journal of Internal Medicine*, Vol. 258, No. 2, pp. 191-195

Sera, N.; Ashizawa, K.; Ando, T.; Abe, Y.; Ide, A.; Usa, T.; Tominaga, T.; Ejima, E.; Yokoyama, N. & Eguchi, K. (2000). Treatment with propylthiouracil is associated with appearance of antineutrophil cytoplasmic antibodies in some patients with Graves' disease. *Thyroid*, Vol. 10, No. 7, pp. 595-599

Stankus, S.J. & Johnson, N.T. (1992). Propylthiouracil-induced hypersensitivity vasculitis presenting as respiratory failure. *Chest*, Vol. 102, No. 5, pp. 1595-1596

Streetman, D.D. & Khanderia, U. (2003). Diagnosis and treatment of Graves disease. *Annals of Pharmacotherapy*, Vol. 37, No.7-8, pp. 1100-1109

Ten Holder, S.M.; Joy, M.S. & Falk, R.J. (2002). Cutaneous and systemic manifestation of drug-induced vasculitis. *Annals of Pharmacotherapy*, Vol. 36, No. 1, pp. 130-147

Tripodi, P.F.; Ruggeri, R.M.; Campennì, A.; Cucinotta, M.; Mirto, A.; Lo Gullo, R.; Baldari, S.; Trimarchi, F.; Cucinotta, D. & Russo, G.T. (2008). Central nervous system after starting methimazole in a woman with Graves' disease. *Thyroid,* Vol. 18, No. 9, pp. 1011-1013

Tsai, M.H.; Chang, Y.L.; Wu, V.C.; Chang, C.C. & Huang, T.S. (2001). Methimazole-induced pulmonary haemorrhage associated with antimyeloperoxidase-antineutrophil cytoplasmic antibody: a case report. *Journal of the Formosan Medical Association,* Vol. 100, No. 11, pp. 772-775

Van der Wonde, F.J.; Rasmussen, N.; Lobatto, S.; Wiik, A.; Permin, H.; van Es, L.A.; van der Giessen, M.; van der Hem, G.K. & The, T.H. (1985). Autoantibodies against neutrophils and monocytes: tool for diagnosis and marker of disease activity in Wegener's granulomatosis. *Lancet*, Vol. 1, No. 8426, pp. 425-429

Vanek, C. & Samuels, M.H. (2005). Central nervous system vasculitis caused by propylthiouracil therapy: a case report and literature review. *Thyroid*, Vol. 15, No. 1, pp. 80-84

Wada, N.; Mukai, M.; Kohno, M.; Notoya, A.; Ito, T. & Yoshioka, N. (2002). Prevalence of serum anti-myeloperoxidase antineutrophil cytoplasmic antibodies (MPO-ANCA) in patients with Graves' disease treated with propylthiouracil and thiamazole. *Endocrine Journal*, Vol. 49, No. 3, pp.329-334

Wiik, A. (2005). Clinical and laboratory characteristics of drug-induced vasculitic syndromes. *Arthritis Research & Therapy*, Vol. 7, No. 5, pp. 191-192

Yazisiz, V.; Ongut, G.; Terzioglu, E. & Karayalcin, U. (2010). Clinical importance of antineutrophil cytoplasmic antibody positivity during propylthiouracil treatment. *International Journal of Clinical Practice*, Vol. 41, No. 1, pp. 19-24

# Part 4

# Pathogenesis & Underlying Mechanisms

# 21

# The Ectopic Germinal Centre Response in Autoimmune Disease and Cancer

David I. Stott and Donna McIntyre
*Institute of Infection, Immunity & Inflammation, University of Glasgow, Glasgow, Scotland, U.K.*

## 1. Introduction

### 1.1 The B-cell response in autoimmune disease

The pathological effects of autoimmune diseases on the target tissues can be mediated by autoantibodies, cell-mediated immune responses, or both. It is increasingly evident that some autoimmune diseases previously thought to be essentially T-cell-mediated also have a B-cell component, which may involve direct effects of autoantibody secreted by plasma cells, pro- or anti-inflammatory cytokines secreted by activated effector or regulatory B-cells, or through the highly efficient antigen presentation function of B-cells enabling them to activate $CD4^+$ T-cells and *vice versa.* The number of autoimmune diseases known to be mediated partly or largely through autoantibodies has increased markedly in recent times. Systemic lupus erythematosus (SLE)[1], in which the pathology is mediated via Type II & III hypersensitivity reactions involving anti-DNA autoantibodies, has long been known to fall into this category. Many other autoantibodies are produced by these patients, principally against nuclear antigens, but most are not thought to be involved in pathology. Hashimoto's thyroiditis and Graves' disease patients produce pathogenic autoantibodies against thyroid antigens, the latter being a rare example of an activating autoantibody inducing signalling via the thyroid stimulating hormone receptor. Myasthenia gravis patients produce autoantibodies against the acetylcholine receptor (AChR), present on the motor muscle endplates, thereby inhibiting muscle contraction. Anti-SS-A and anti-SS-B (anti-Ro & anti-La) autoantibodies are implicated in congenital heart block in children born to mothers with Sjögren's Syndrome due to transplacental uptake of IgG autoantibodies; autoantibodies against α-fodrin are also believed to be pathogenic in these patients. Rheumatoid arthritis (RA), one member of the group of systemic rheumatic autoimmune diseases that also includes SLE, psoriatic arthritis and the various forms of myositis, has now gone full cycle in views on its pathological mechanisms.

---

[1] Abbreviations: AChR, Acetylcholine Receptor; AID, Activation Induced Cytidine Deaminase; AMC, Arthrogryposis Multiplex Congenita; ARS, Anti-amino acyl-tRNA Synthetase; Bmem, Memory B-cell; CDR, Complementarity Determining Region; DM, Dermatomyositis; EOMG, Early Onset Myasthenia Gravis; FDC, Follicular Dendritic Cell; G.C., Germinal Centre; IBM, Inclusion Body Myositis; IM, Inflammatory Myopathies; LOMG, Late Onset Myasthenia Gravis; MAA, Myositis-Associated Autoantibodies; MAb, Monoclonal Antibody; MIR, Main Immunogenic Region; MSA, Myositis Specific Autoantibodies; PM, Polymyositis; RA, Rheumatoid Arthritis; SLE, Systemic Lupus Erythematosus; TAA, Tumour-Associated Antigen; TIL, Tumour-Infiltrating Lymphocytes; Tfh, Follicular T helper cell; UNG, Uracil Nucleotidyl Glycosylase.

Initially thought to be caused by the anti-IgG Fc antibody (rheumatoid factor), although approximately 25% of RA patients are rheumatoid factor negative, the evidence then swung in favour of a cell mediated autoimmune response involving effector T-cells and cytokines, principally TNFα. Although these are clearly involved in joint pathology, autoantibodies against cyclic citrullinated proteins are a much better diagnostic marker for RA than rheumatoid factor and there is some limited evidence that they may be pathogenic. It is also now recognised that B-cells play an important role in the pathogenic autoimmune response, as clearly demonstrated by the marked clinical improvement in patients treated with Rituximab®, an anti-CD20 chimaeric (human/mouse) monoclonal antibody that suppresses B-cell responses. Other autoimmune diseases with B-cell involvement include autoimmune haemolytic anaemia, idiopathic thrombocytopaenia, Type I diabetes, and some subtypes of myositis, although the situation is often confused by the presence of non-pathogenic autoantibodies.

### 1.2 The germinal centre response to foreign antigens

Germinal centres (g.c.) are the main sites of generation of high affinity, antibody-secreting plasma cells and Ig class-switched memory B-cells during T-cell-dependent immune responses, extensively reviewed by others (Allen, Okada, & Cyster, 2007; Brink, 2007; Hauser, Shlomchik, & Haberman, 2007; Klein & Dalla-Favera, 2008; Leavy, 2010; Minton, 2011). Here we shall summarise briefly the principal features of the g.c. response. The response is initiated by B-cells binding to their cognate antigen on the surface of antigen presenting cells, such as dendritic cells, in a secondary lymphoid organ (lymph node, spleen, Peyer's patches or human tonsil). The antigen becomes internalised, degraded into peptides which are expressed on the cell surface bound to MHC Class II and presented to a helper T ($T_h$) cell that provides costimulatory activation signals, including binding of the B-cell surface molecule CD40 to its ligand, CD154, on the T-cell membrane.

This interaction takes place at or near the interface between the B-cell follicle and the T-cell area and some activated B-cells proliferate outside the follicle and differentiate into short-lived plasma cells secreting IgM antibodies. Others migrate into the B-cell follicle where they proliferate and differentiate into centroblasts expressing low levels of surface Ig. This region develops into a germinal centre with a dark zone of densely packed, proliferating centroblasts, and a light zone of more loosely packed B-cells (centrocytes) interspersed with the processes of follicular dendritic cells (FDC, Figure 1A). These have distinct stromal origins, unlike the bone marrow derived, extra-follicular dendritic cells; almost uniquely, their C′ and Fc receptors trap immune complexes and retain antigens in their native state for months.

The pre-existing $IgM^+$,$IgD^+$ follicle B-cells are pushed out to form a mantle zone around the developing germinal centre, the whole structure being termed a secondary follicle. Proliferation of the dark zone centroblasts is extremely rapid, with cell cycle times estimated at between 6 and 12 hours. These proliferating clones of B-cells switch on the molecular machinery required for somatic hypermutation of their rearranged, expressed, Ig V-genes, including expression of activation-induced cytidine deaminase (AID). This induces mutations specifically targeted to the Ig V-genes at a frequency of 1 per 1000 base pairs per cell division, although much lower levels of mutation can also occur in some other, non-Ig genes such as Bcl-2 & Bcl-6. AID deaminates cytidine to uracil at C/G base pairs, introducing mismatches in the DNA that can be replaced by T/A base pairs. Uracil nucleotidyl glycosylase (UNG) can remove the uracil leading to insertion of any of the four bases at the abasic site; mismatch repair enzymes also recognise the mismatch and induce single strand breaks which are repaired by error prone DNA polymerases (Di Noia & Neuberger, 2007). The mutations are targeted mainly to the complementarity determining regions (CDRs) which are intimately involved in binding to the epitope and therefore determine specificity and affinity of the antibody. Combined with the rapid proliferation, this results in clones of B-cells expressing receptors with a variety of affinities for the antigen, some high, some low; some will have lost the ability to bind to the antigen altogether and rare B-cells may cross-react with a self-antigen.

Several clones of proliferating, mutating B-cells are usually present within each germinal centre. These cells differentiate into centrocytes expressing mutated antigen receptors and migrate into the light zone. The centrocytes move through the light zone, acquire antigen for a second time from immune complexes on the follicular dendritic cells, which they internalise, process and present to follicular helper T-cells ($T_{fh}$-cells) (Patakas *et al.*, 2011), thereby receiving survival signals, probably via costimulatory molecule interactions including CD40/CD154 and CD80/CD28 binding. These signals, together with $T_{fh}$-cell cytokines (IL-4 and IFNγ) and AID deamination of cytidines, promote induction of class switch recombination (Patakas *et al.*, 2011). Some of these centrocytes differentiate directly into plasmablasts and antibody-secreting plasma cells; others differentiate into Ig class switched memory B-cells, both of which migrate out of the follicle. Competition for limiting availability of antigen results in selection of B-cells expressing high affinity antigen receptors; recent evidence has shown that a broad range of mutations is involved in selection, not only for high affinity receptors but also for stability and expression of the B-cell receptor (Weiser *et al.*, 2011). Cells expressing antigen receptors with low affinity are unable to compete for survival signals and the default response is that they die by apoptosis and are engulfed by macrophages, in which their degenerating nuclei are visible as tingible bodies. Most of this information is derived from studies in mice, in which the germinal centres reach maximum size about two weeks after immunisation and then gradually decline in the absence of further immunisation, disappearing after several weeks. Although the cell composition and structure of secondary follicles appear similar in Man, the kinetics and some of the detailed cellular interactions may differ.

Detailed studies of the kinetics and cellular interactions within germinal centres using multiphoton microscopy of living tissue in combination with B & T-lymphocytes expressing defined antigen receptors from transgenic animals have revealed much more dynamic activity than was previously suspected. It is now recognised that there is less distinction between the dark and light zones than suggested by static immunohistological examination, and there is continual recycling of B-cells both between and within the two zones, although there is net migration from the dark zone to the light zone (Beltman *et al.*, 2011)(Figure 1B). Centrocytes move rapidly through the network of follicular dendritic cell processes, apparently sampling the immune complexes attached to their membranes and some of these cells return to the dark zone for further rounds of proliferation and somatic hypermutation. Migration of B-cells between the zones is controlled by chemokines, possibly secreted by stromal cells within the germinal centre. $T_{fh}$-cells are present mainly in the light zone and recent data suggest that affinity selection of B-cells may involve competition for signals from cognate $T_{fh}$-cells via peptide/MHC Class II binding as well as, or instead of, competition for antigen on the surface of follicular dendritic cells (Victora *et al.*, 2010). Anti-self B-cells that have escaped negative selection in the bone marrow, or have arisen in the germinal centre due to somatic hypermutation, are either eliminated at this stage, suppressed by regulatory T-cells, or alter their antigen specificity by receptor revision, a process similar to V-gene rearrangement in developing B-cells. This involves re-expression of RAG1 and RAG2 and rearrangement of an upstream light chain V-gene to an unused J exon (Nemazee, 2006). Despite the absence of D exons in the rearranged heavy chain locus, we have shown that an upstream heavy chain V-gene can also replace all or part of a rearranged $V_H$-gene, thereby altering the specificity of the receptor away from self antigen (Darlow & Stott, 2005). The architecture, cellular components and processes occurring in a typical germinal centre are summarised in Figure 1.

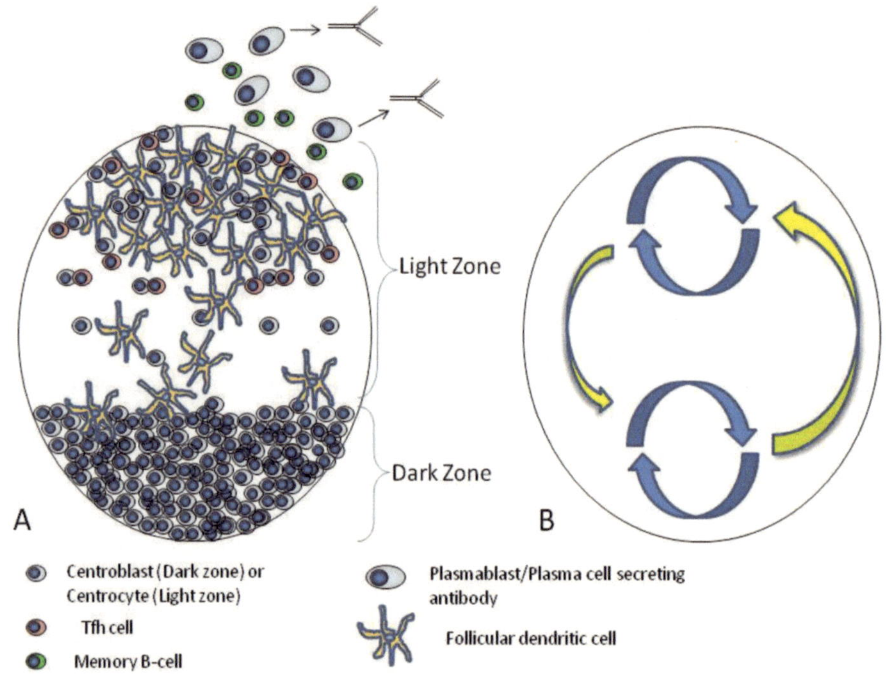


Fig. 1. Diagrammatic representation of a germinal centre in a lymph node.

A: Showing a dark zone containing proliferating clones of mutating centroblasts and a light zone containing centrocytes in contact with follicular dendritic cells and follicular helper T-cells (Tfh cells). Long-lived memory B-cells, plasmablasts and plasma cells secreting antibody molecules migrate out of the g.c. and leave the lymph node via the efferent lymphatic vessel. Apoptotic B-cells, macrophages containing tingible bodies and the mantle zone are not shown.

B: The same germinal centre showing recirculation of B-cells within and between the dark and light zones.

### 1.3 The ectopic germinal centre response in autoimmune disease

It has been known for many years that the target tissues of autoimmune diseases contain infiltrating lymphocytes and other immune cells, including T-cells, B-cells, plasma cells, macrophages, dendritic and follicular dendritic cells. In many cases the infiltrating cells organise themselves into structures resembling germinal centres. Some of these have a mantle zone, suggesting that they were formed from a primary follicle whereas, even when absent, it is often possible to distinguish a dark zone, containing few or no $CD4^+$ T-cells or follicular dendritic cells, and a light zone containing both. Autoantigens have been identified on the finger-like processes of follicular dendritic cells (Shiono *et al.*, 2003) and, in some cases, autoantibodies have been identified in g.c. B-cells. Separate T-cell areas containing dendritic cells and, sometimes, high endothelial venules, can also be seen. The stage of lymphoid neogenesis appears to be directly related to the extent of infiltration of lymphoid and other immune cells (Aloisi & Pujol-Borrell, 2006). Examples of autoimmune diseases in which germinal centre-like structures have been identified in the target, or disease-related tissues are shown in Table 1. It is now apparent that ectopic germinal centres, also known as tertiary lymphoid organs, can also develop in other chronic inflammatory diseases, such as the gut in Crohn's disease and ulcerative colitis patients, in chronic infections (Aloisi & Pujol-Borrell, 2006) and some types of cancer (Table 1). The questions these observations raise are: 1. How do they develop?; 2. How closely do they resemble germinal centres in secondary lymphoid organs?; 3. Are the B-cells within them undergoing a germinal centre response, as described in section 1.2 above?; 4. Are they generating plasma cells secreting pathogenic autoantibodies?; 5. What role do they play in the pathogenesis of autoimmune disease?

| **Autoimmune Diseases** | **Organ containing Germinal Centres** | **Antigen(s) Recognised by GC B-cells** | **Reference** |
|---|---|---|---|
| Hashimoto's thyroiditis | Thyroid | Thyroglobulin, Thyroperoxidase | (Knecht, Saremaslani, & Hedinger, 1981) (Armengol *et al.*, 2001) |
| Graves' disease | Thyroid | Thyroglobulin, Thyroperoxidase | (Armengol *et al.*, 2001) |
| Myasthenia gravis | Thymus | Acetylcholine receptor | (Yoshitake *et al.*, 1994) (SHIONO *et al.*, 2003) |
| Sjögren's syndrome | Salivary glands | SS-A (Ro), SS-B (La) | (Stott *et al.*, 1998) |
| Rheumatoid arthritis | Synovial membranes of joints | IgG Fc, Cyclic citrullinated protein/peptide | (Manzo & Pitzalis, 2007) (Humby *et al.*, 2009) |
| Psoriatic arthritis | Synovial membranes of joints | ? | (Canete *et al.*, 2007) (Gerhard *et al.*, 2002) |
| Cryptogenic fibrosing alveolitis | Lungs | ? | (Wallace *et al.*, 1996) |
| Uveoretinits | Choroid of the eye | ? | (Liversidge *et al.*, 1993) |
| Autoimmune hepatitis | Liver | ? | (Mosnier *et al.*, 1993) |
| Multiple sclerosis | Meninges (?) | ? | (Prineas, 1979) (Serafini *et al.*, 2004) |
| | | | |
| **Chronic Inflammatory Diseases** | | | |
| Crohn's disease | Gastrointestinal tract | ? | (Kaiserling, 2001) |
| Ulcerative colitis | Descending colon | ? | (Kaiserling, 2001) |
| | | | |
| **Infectious Diseases** | | | |
| Chronic hepatitis C infection | Liver | ? | (Mosnier *et al.*, 1993) |
| *Helicobacter pylori* or *Campylobacter* gastritis | Stomach | Bacterial antigens | (Genta, Hamner, & Graham, 1993) (Stolte & Eidt, 1989) |
| Chronic Lyme disease | Synovial membranes of joints | ? | (Ghosh *et al.*, 2005) |
| Oncocerciasis | Skin | ? | (Brattig *et al.*, 2010) |
| | | | |
| **Cancers** | | | |
| Lymphoma of MALT associated with Sjögren's Syndrome | Lymphoma | ? | (Bombardieri *et al.*, 2007a) |
| Ductal breast carcinoma | Breast tumour | Epidermal growth factor receptor family | (Coronella *et al.*, 2002) (Nzula, Going, & Stott, 2003a) (Simsa *et al.*, 2005) and section 5. |
| Medullary breast carcinoma | Breast tumour | Ganglioside | (Coronella *et al.*, 2001) (Kotlan *et al.*, 2005) |

Table 1. Diseases in which ectopic germinal centres have been observed.

It has now been shown by combined immunohistochemistry, identification of antigen specificity of B-cells and plasma cells in and around ectopic germinal centres, and sequence analysis of expressed, rearranged Ig V-genes and their somatic mutations, that germinal centre B-cells in the target tissues of several autoimmune diseases are undergoing clonal expansion, somatic hypermutation and affinity selection, in a similar manner to that seen in the germinal centres of secondary lymphoid organs (Table 1 and section 1.2). This has been demonstrated in Sjögren's syndrome, rheumatoid arthritis, psoriatic arthritis, myasthenia gravis, multiple sclerosis and also in breast cancer. In some of these cases, expression of RAG1 and 2 have been observed (Armengol *et al.*, 2001), indicating that receptor revision also takes place in ectopic germinal centres and therefore the generation and attempted elimination of self-reactive B-cells. The signals involved in tertiary lymphoid organ neogenesis appear to be similar to those in development of secondary lymphoid organs, although the temporal and causal relationship between appearance of these structures in the target tissue and autoimmune pathology-related tissue damage is unclear. One scenario is that an initial event in the tissue, which could, in some cases, include microbial infection, leads to the release of molecules seen by the immune system as "danger signals" (Matzinger, 2007) thereby inducing infiltration of inflammatory cells and subsequent lymphoid neogenesis, causing further tissue damage with concomitant release of self-antigens, more danger signals and a vicious cycle, perpetuating a chronic autoimmune reaction. Alternatively, initial tissue damage may be caused by an autoimmune response commencing in the secondary lymphoid organs, with subsequent events following a similar course to that described above. Lymphotoxins α, β, $\alpha_1\beta_2$ and TNFα have been shown to be required for development of ectopic germinal centres. Growth-factor receptor-bound protein-2 (Grb2) has recently been shown to control orthotopic lymphoid follicle organisation and the germinal centre response by inducing production of lymphotoxin-α via CXCR5 signalling (Jang *et al.*, 2011). These molecules are secreted by infiltrating B and $T_h1$-cells and activated NK cells; on binding to their receptor on stromal cells they induce expression of adhesion molecules and secretion of chemokines which induce further lymphocyte infiltration and segregation into B-cell follicles, formation of a follicular dendritic cell network and T-cell areas. It has also recently been proposed that overexpression of costimulatory molecules on $T_{fh}$-cells may contribute to overcoming B-cell tolerance (Patakas *et al.*, 2011). This may be a contributory factor in ectopic as well as orthotopic germinal centres. Primary B-cell follicles are rarely seen in autoimmune disease target tissues but this may be because chronic antigen stimulation has been in progress for a considerable time before biopsies are taken. For example, in type I diabetes mellitus there is evidence that the autoimmune response develops long before overt disease is diagnosed. Whether ectopic germinal centres are initiated by naïve or memory B-cells is unclear but recent evidence shows that at least some B-cell clones arise *de novo* from naïve B-cells (Sims *et al.*, 2001; Nzula, Going, & Stott, 2003b; Nzula, Going, & Stott, 2003a).

The frequency of ectopic germinal centres varies markedly between autoimmune diseases; as one might expect, the highest incidence is in diseases where pathogenic autoantibodies are most strongly implicated. Thus, they have been identified in thyroid tissues of 100% of Hashimoto's thyroiditis patients and 54 - 63% of Graves' disease cases; in rheumatoid arthritis the figure is 25 - 50% but in Sjögren's syndrome it is only 17%, although variations may to some extent reflect differences in the difficulty of finding the germinal centres. In Sjögren's syndrome, the source is usually biopsies of the small labial salivary glands of which there is a large number; as g.c.s are only present in some of the many small labial salivary glands, they may easily be overlooked. Tissues containing different types of cells respond in a variety of ways to inflammatory signals and this may also determine whether, and to what extent, lymphoid organ neogenesis occurs. The origin of follicular dendritic cells is unclear but it has been proposed that they develop from precursor cells already present in the tissue, either fibroblasts or fibroblast precursor cells (Park & Choi, 2005). Alternatively, the precursor cells may be induced to migrate into the tissue by the same or similar chemokines as those attracting the B and T-lymphocytes. In several autoimmune diseases (Table 1) and animal models of autoimmune diseases (Astorri *et al.*, 2010; Nacionales *et al.*, 2009), it has been demonstrated that ectopic germinal centres are generating plasma cells secreting pathogenic autoantibodies and, almost certainly, memory B-cells bearing anti-self antigen receptors, implying that they aid the diversification of the autoantibody repertoire and contribute to the maintenance of immune pathology. In addition to autoantibody production, self-reactive B-cells generated in ectopic germinal centres may also contribute to autoimmune pathology by secretion of pro-inflammatory cytokines and activation of pathogenic T-cells by presentation of processed self-antigens. B-cells may contribute in this way to immune pathology in autoimmune diseases generally considered to be principally T-cell mediated, and may be one explanation for the efficacy of Rituximab therapy for rheumatoid arthritis.

## 2. Methods

### 2.1 Identification and cellular composition of ectopic germinal centres

The methods we used to identify ectopic germinal centres, characterise their cellular composition, analyse the rearranged Ig V-gene sequences expressed by germinal centre B-cells and identify their antibody specificity have been described in detail in previously published papers (Nzula, Going, & Stott, 2003a; Sims *et al.*, 2001). Briefly, sections were cut from snap frozen tissue biopsies and every tenth section stained for B-cells with anti-CD20. Sections containing germinal centre-like structures or B-cell aggregates were further characterised by staining for T-cells (anti-CD3, CD4, CD8), regulatory T-cells (anti-FoxP3), follicular dendritic cells (anti-FDC (DAKO) or anti-CD35), plasma cells (DAKO), macrophages (anti-CD68) and proliferating cells (anti-Ki67). Double immunofluorescent staining with the above cell subset-specific antibodies and Ki67 was used to identify dividing cells. Acetylcholine receptor-specific B-cells in germinal centres from the thymus of myasthenia gravis patients were identified by $^{125}$I-α-bungarotoxin-labelled acetylcholine receptor and autoradiography (Shiono *et al.*, 2003; Hill *et al.*, 2008); other autoantibody-producing cells were identified by immunofluorescence staining with the relevant antigen.

### 2.2 Cloning and sequence analysis of rearranged Ig V-genes

Ectopic germinal centres and B-cell aggregates were excised by microdissection, digested with proteinase K and the released DNA used as a template for amplification of the rearranged Ig V-genes by nested PCR. Details of the method and the primers are described in Sims *et al.* (2001) and Nzula *et al.* (2003). Amplified DNA was purified by agarose gel electrophoresis, ligated into plasmid DNA and cloned in *E. coli*. Cloned plasmid DNA was purified and the Ig V-genes sequenced in both directions using primers complementary to sequences flanking the cloning site. The best matching germline V, D & J sequences were identified initially by comparison with the VBASE directory of human Ig V-genes and later, after VBASE ceased to be updated, using the Immunogenetics (IMGT) Database of Human

Immunoglobulin Sequences (http://www.imgt.org/). Sequences were analysed using JOINSOLVER (http://joinsolver.niaid.nih.gov/) and IMGTV-QUEST. Silent and replacement somatic mutations were identified by comparison with the germline gene sequence; in early experiments the ratio of replacement to silent mutations was considered to be evidence of affinity selection if significantly higher than 3:1. To correct for the inherent bias towards replacement mutations in CDRs, we have more recently applied the method of Hershberg to determine whether affinity selection has occurred in B-cell clones from ectopic germinal centres (Hershberg *et al.*, 2008). This method employs an algorithm that allows for the effects of microsequences in the complementarity determining regions (CDRs) and the bias towards transition mutations. Clonally related sets of rearranged V-genes were identified by their use of the same germline V, (D) and J exons and shared junctional sequences. Genealogical trees were constructed by analysis of shared and unshared mutations using the parsimony method of phylogenetic analysis (PAUP, (Swofford, 1993)), enabling the assignment of sequences from parent and daughter cells that have been produced during clonal proliferation, thus providing clear evidence of the presence of clonally proliferating, somatically mutating B-cells within the germinal centre.

### 2.3 Cloning antigen-specific autoantibodies from germinal centre B-cells by 'phage display

In order to confirm the antigen specificity of B-cells generated in ectopic germinal centres, and to analyse in detail the relationship between their mutations and antigen specificity, we reconstituted the rearranged Ig V-genes as single chain Fv (scFv) or Fab antibodies by 'phage display. Single chain Fv antibodies comprise the heavy and light chain variable region domains linked by a short peptide. Although linked together by a short additional peptide sequence, the $V_H$ and $V_L$ domains are able to fold into their natural 3-dimensional conformation and pair correctly, as the antibody produced by a B-cell or plasma cell. They contain the antigen binding site, and therefore mimic the antigen specificity of the original antibodies from which they were derived. A caveat that must be born in mind is that the original H and L chain pairings are unknown, except when both genes are cloned from a single cell. The detailed methodology has been described elsewhere (Stott & Sims, 2000; Matthews *et al.*, 2002). Rearranged $V_H$ and $V_L$-genes amplified either from microdissected germinal centres or pooled V-genes from the same B-cell clone, were used to construct scFvs using a $(Gly_4Ser)_3$ linker DNA. The resulting scFv library, comprising a pool of randomly linked $V_H$-$V_L$ genes, was then inserted into the phagemids pCANTAB6 or pHEN2 continuously with the gene encoding the bacteriophage coat protein P3, and grown in *E. coli* in the presence of helper phage. The resulting scFv-P3 fusion protein was expressed on the surface of bacteriophage or as soluble scFv by transfection into a non-permissive, or permissive, strain of *E. coli* respectively. Alternatively, Fab libraries were constructed using whole light chain cDNA and DNA encoding the $V_H$ region and the first constant region domain of the heavy chain by similar techniques (Matthews et al., 2002). An advantage of amplifying directly from genomic DNA is that the distribution of cloned V-genes reflects the usage of those genes by B-cells and plasma cells more accurately than amplification from cDNA, which is biased towards plasma cells. The library of scFvs or Fabs attached to bacteriophage by the P3 'phage coat protein was then panned on plastic plates coated with either a whole extract of the target tissue, or purified recombinant antigen, to identify self-reactive antibodies. Bound 'phage were washed, eluted, re-grown in *E. coli* and panning repeated until the eluate had become enriched with a small number of 'phage clones. These were recloned and their H & L chains sequenced and used to investigate the specificity and properties of their antigen-binding sites.

### 2.4 Statistical analysis

The method of Hershberg *et al.* (2008), described in section 2.2 above, was used to determine the significance of replacement mutations in rearranged Ig V-genes cloned from germinal centre B-cells, as evidence for affinity maturation of the antibodies expressed by them. The distribution of $V_H$ gene families and individual V, D and J exons was assessed using two-tailed $\chi^2$ analysis, corrected for multiple comparisons.

## 3. The ectopic germinal centre response in myasthenia gravis

### 3.1 Pathology of myasthenia gravis

Myasthenia gravis is an organ-specific autoimmune disease characterised by weakness of striated muscles and thymic hyperplasia (Vincent, 2002). Patients are generally divided into subgroups with early-onset (EOMG, pre-40 years) or late onset (LOMG, post-40 years) forms of the disease, or with thymoma in about 10% of patients. It is a classic autoantibody-mediated autoimmune disease, caused by autoantibodies directed against the postsynaptic nicotinic acetylcholine receptor (AChR) at the neuromuscular junction. Many thymoma patients and some late onset patients also have serum antibodies against striated muscle antigens, interferon-α and IL-12. Loss of functional AChRs leads to muscle weakness, usually first evident in weakness of eye movement. This can progress to other striated muscles of the body, causing problems with breathing due to effects on the diaphragm, swallowing difficulties and paralysis. These effects can be life-threatening if untreated. Evidence that the effects are mediated by autoantibodies against the AChR include induction of similar symptoms by: their transfer from mother to baby *in utero*; passive transfer from patients to mice; immunisation of animals with AChR; and marked improvement of symptoms in patients after removal of circulating IgG antibodies by plasmapheresis. Several pathogenic mechanisms are involved (Vincent, 2002; Drachman, 1994): (i) Cross-linking of the receptor by autoantibodies causes loss of AChR by antigenic modulation, leading to internalisation and degradation of the receptors; (ii) The majority of anti-AChR antibodies are of the IgG1 and IgG3 subclasses, which are particularly efficient at complement activation, resulting in lysis and damage to the muscle membrane; (iii) Less commonly, some antibodies cause direct inhibition of the ion channel function of the AChR; (iv) Antibody-dependent cell-mediated cytotoxicity has also been implicated, although there is little direct evidence for this mechanism. The IgG autoantibodies can cross the placenta of pregnant mothers with myasthenia gravis by an active transport mechanism involving the neonatal Fc receptor, FcRn, resulting in transient symptoms of myasthenia gravis in the newborn infant. The symptoms gradually ameliorate as the maternal antibodies are catabolised and replaced by the infant's own antibodies. More rarely, the autoantibodies produced by multiparous mothers can induce severe, often fatal, developmental abnormalities, termed arthrogryposis multiplex congenita, due to paralysis of fetal muscles *in utero* (see section 3.4.5).

### 3.2 Structure and epitopes of the acetylcholine receptor

The AChR is a pentameric transmembrane glycoprotein found almost exclusively at the muscle endplate, comprising two α polypeptide subunits, one β, one δ and, in the adult, one ε subunit; in the fetus there is also one γ subunit, which is gradually replaced by an ε from the third trimester onwards (Fig. 2) (Vincent, 2002). The five subunits are combined into a cylindrical structure with a central cation channel that is closed in the inactive conformation. There are two binding sites for acetylcholine, formed at the interfaces between one α and δ subunit and the second α and ε or γ subunits. Electrical impulses passing down the motor nerve trigger release of acetylcholine molecules at the nerve termini. When these bind to the two receptor binding sites, they cause the central cation channel to open and sodium ions to flood into the muscle resulting in local membrane depolarisation. When this reaches threshold the resulting action potential spreads across the muscle triggering it to contract. Loss of at least 50% of receptors is required to produce overt muscle weakness.

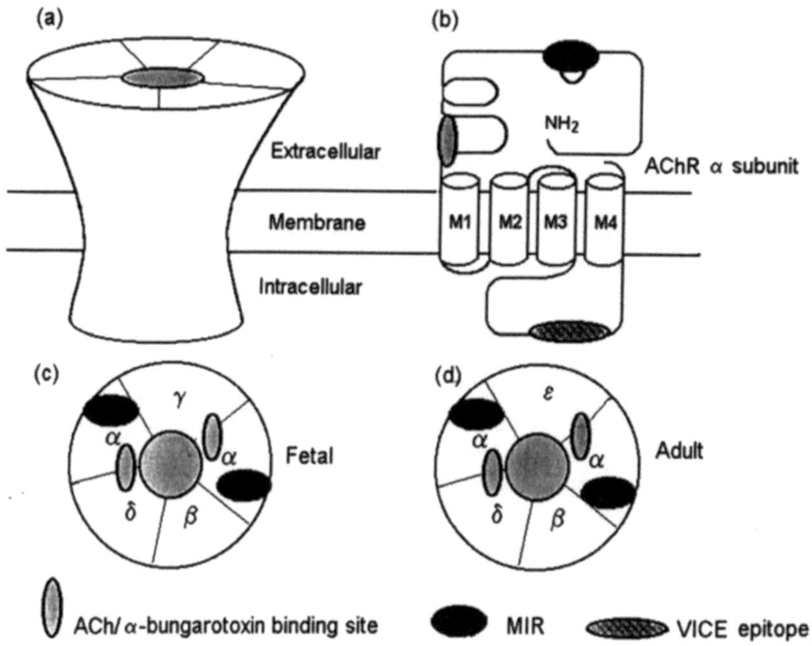


Fig. 2. Diagrammatic representation of the structure of the acetylcholine receptor:

(a) the complete pentameric molecule in the cell membrane; (b) the topology of the subunits, illustrated for the α subunit that contributes to the acetylcholine/α-bungarotoxin binding site, the main immunogenic region (MIR) and the very immunogenic cytoplasmic epitope (VICE); It is doubtful whether the latter plays any significant role in pathogenesis; (c and d) the fetal and adult subtypes of AChR. Reproduced with permission from (Vincent et al., 1997), Plenum Press.

Since the patients' autoantibodies are almost exclusively specific for the complex native conformation of the extracellular AChR subunit domains, and not short peptides or even whole subunit polypeptides, mapping of the autoantibody epitopes has proved to be difficult. The antibodies are mainly IgG1 or IgG3, of high avidity and heterogeneous in their sequences and fine specificity. Disease severity correlates poorly with autoantibody titre, suggesting that pathogenicity may depend upon precise epitope specificity. Many of the antibodies bind to a region of the extracellular domain of the α chain, the main immunogenic region or MIR. Its conformation is affected by the ε ↔ γ interchange, as demonstrated by the observation that some antibodies bind better to the MIR of the fetal AChR than the adult form, even though the $\gamma$ and $\varepsilon$ subunits do not contribute directly to the MIR (Fostieri, Beeson, & Tzartos, 2000). Titres of MIR antibodies vary considerably between patients and other antibodies may play an equally important role in some individuals. Some patients also produce autoantibodies against the acetylcholine binding sites (that also bind α-bungarotoxin); these are the blocking antibodies described above.

### 3.3 Role of the thymus

Early onset myasthenia gravis is associated with thymic hyperplasia characterized by secondary lymphoid organ-like structures in the medulla of >90% of patients. These include T-cell areas containing AChR-specific helper T-cells and large numbers of germinal centres with clearly defined mantle, dark and light zones. Plasmablasts and plasma cells secreting autoantibodies against AChR are also detectable within and around the germinal centres (Hill *et al.*, 2008; SHIONO *et al.*, 2003). Approximately 20% of germinal centres contain plasmablasts positive for antibodies against AChR and AChR is trapped on follicular dendritic cells in c.50% of thymic germinal centres (SHIONO *et al.*, 2003). Anti-AChR-secreting hybridomas and AChR-specific Fabs have been cloned from thymic B-cells and thymectomy results in a reduction in the serum anti-AChR titre and reduced clinical symptoms in some patients, although the benefits of thymectomy have never been rigorously proved (Cardona *et al.*, 1994; Farrar *et al.*, 1997; Graus *et al.*, 1997). The relative contribution of the thymus to production of anti-AChR autoantibodies compared with the secondary lymphoid organs is unknown, but it appears to play a significant role. Therefore, using the methods described in section 2, we tested the hypothesis that thymic germinal centres are sites of ongoing autoimmune responses driven by autoantigen, i.e. sites of activated B-cells, clonally proliferating, somatically mutating their expressed Ig V-genes and undergoing affinity maturation, driven by the acetylcholine receptor.

### 3.4 The thymic germinal centre response in myasthenia gravis

#### 3.4.1 Germinal centres in the thymus

Thymi from 5 EOMG patients were examined by immunohistology. All 5 contained large numbers of germinal centres with typical mantle zones within the thymic medulla, histologically indistinguishable from germinal centres in human tonsil controls. The mantle zones contained densely packed $CD20^{+}$ B-cells surrounding the germinal centre B-cells (Fig. 3A). These were interspersed with a network of follicular dendritic cells extending throughout the dark and light zones (Fig. 3C) and a crescent of T-cells can be seen at the apex of the light zone (Fig. 3B). Proliferating B-cells were distributed throughout the germinal centre but in larger numbers within the dark zone (Fig. 3D). Autoradiography with $^{125}$I-α-bungarotoxin alone, which binds to AChR, diffusely labelled c.50% of germinal centres and appeared to be associated with the follicular dendritic cell processes. No labelling was seen in human tonsils or thymi from two seronegative myasthenia patients and bungarotoxin binding was blocked by the cholinergic drug, carbamyl choline, which is structurally similar to AChR, indicating that the follicular dendritic network contained membrane-bound antigen or immune complexes.

In contrast, $^{125}$I-α-bungarotoxin-labelled AChR bound to individual cells in 20% of germinal centres, including large numbers of moderately labelled centrocytes in the light zone, smaller numbers in the dark zone, and heavily labelled plasmablasts/plasma cells in and around the germinal centres (Fig. 3E & F).

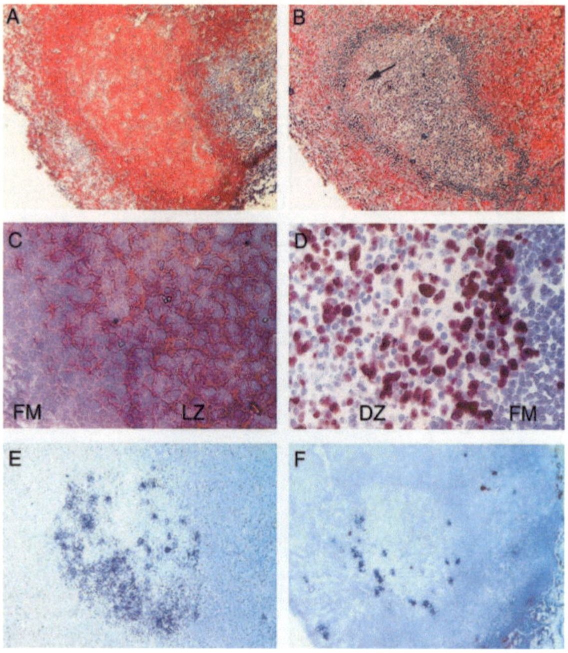


Fig. 3. Immunohistochemically stained serial sections through thymic germinal centres.

A & B: Germinal centres stained (red) with anti-CD20 and anti-CD3 for B and T-cells respectively. The arrow (B) shows a crescent of T-cells in the light zone. C: A network of follicular dendritic cell processes is spread throughout the germinal centre, including both the light and dark zones. D: Germinal centre cells stained with an antibody against proliferating cell nuclear antigen, revealing dividing B-cells in both areas but more concentrated in the dark zone. E & F: $^{125}$I-α-bungarotoxin-labelled AChR reveals individual AChR-specific plasmablasts/plasma cells in and around germinal centres (detected by autoradiography). Diffuse labelling in the light zone probably indicates binding of free $^{125}$I-α-bungarotoxin to AChR trapped on follicular dendritic cells (see text). Reproduced from Sims *et al* (2001).

### 3.4.2 Ig V-gene expression by thymic germinal centre B-cells

In order to determine whether thymic germinal centre B-cells are subjected to antigen-driven clonal proliferation, somatic hypermutation and affinity selection, as seen in the orthotopic germinal centres of secondary lymphoid organs, we cloned and sequenced rearranged Ig heavy chain V-genes from multiple sections through four thymic germinal centres (A – D) and the follicular mantle surrounding one of them (A). 216 rearranged $V_H$-genes, derived from 61 independently rearranged, functional sequences, were obtained from the four germinal centres and 46 $V_H$-genes from the follicular mantle were derived from 24 functional $V_H$-genes. Since the PCR error rate in control experiments was estimated to be less than one base per four $V_H$-genes, only sequences using the same V, D & J exons, the same junctional sequences and a minimum of one base difference per gene, were accepted as mutated members of a clonally related set of B-cells. This conservative assessment almost certainly discards some B-cell clones with low frequencies of somatic mutation and therefore underestimates the true B-cell diversity. When calculating the number of $V_H$-genes used, members of the same B-cell clone were counted only once. However, this reflects the number of individual B-cell clones and non-dividing B-cells rather than the total number of B-cells using a particular gene.

The distribution of $V_H$-gene families was similar in the follicular mantle and all four germinal centres, with predominant use of members of the $V_H3$ gene family compared with the number of germline $V_H$-genes in this family (Fig. 4A). However, since this gene family is also predominantly used by the peripheral blood B-cells of healthy individuals, it was not considered to be significant. No $V_H6$, $V_H7$ or $J_H2$ genes were isolated and $J_H1$ was under-used, but the rarely used $V_H5$-51 gene and the $J_H4$ exon (Fig. 4B) were over-represented, both being used by rearranged V-genes from three different germinal centres in combination with different D exons ($D_H2$-2, $D_H5$-12 and $D_H$-6-19). In many cases the D exon could not be identified due to junctional diversity and removal of bases during recombination. Of those that could be identified, $D_H3$ and $D_H6$ were the most commonly used. These data strongly imply selection for B-cells expressing antigen receptors using particular combinations of V, D and J segments, despite the heterogeneity of the germinal centre B-cells. This would be even more apparent if individual members of the same B-cell clone were counted separately.

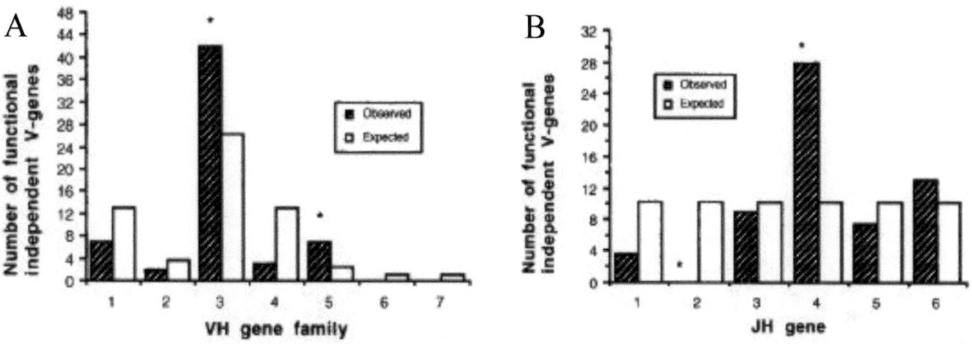


Fig. 4. Frequency of usage of $V_H$ and $J_H$ germline genes by thymic germinal centre B-cells.

A: The frequency of VH gene family usage in all germinal centres analysed differs significantly from predictions from the number of members of each family in the germline. Members of clonally related sets were only counted once. B: The frequency of individual JH exon usage in all germinal centres analysed differs significantly from the number of JH exons in the germline (*$p<0.01$). Reproduced from Sims *et al* (2001).

### 3.4.3 Somatic hypermutation and clonal proliferation of B-cells in thymic germinal centres

All the germinal centres and the follicular mantle contained B-cells expressing both mutated and unmutated Ig V-genes, the latter presumably coming from naïve B-cells. The majority of V-genes from the germinal centres and the follicular mantle were mutated, with considerable variation in the number of mutations, ranging from 0 – 52. Some of the rearranged V-genes in clonally related sets had high ratios of replacement to silent mutations from 4.7:1 to 7.0:1 in the CDRs, which form the antigen-binding site, suggesting affinity selection of mutated antigen receptors is taking place in the germinal centre. Some other sequences had low numbers of replacement mutations, suggesting selection against replacement mutations, as also found by (Zuckerman *et al.*, 2010). 18 different sets of functionally rearranged $V_H$-genes included two or more related sequences sharing the same V, D and J segments and junctional sequences but with significantly more than one mutation per V-gene and, in three cases, they were cloned in separate amplifications from different sections through the same germinal centre and therefore could only be from different B-cells.

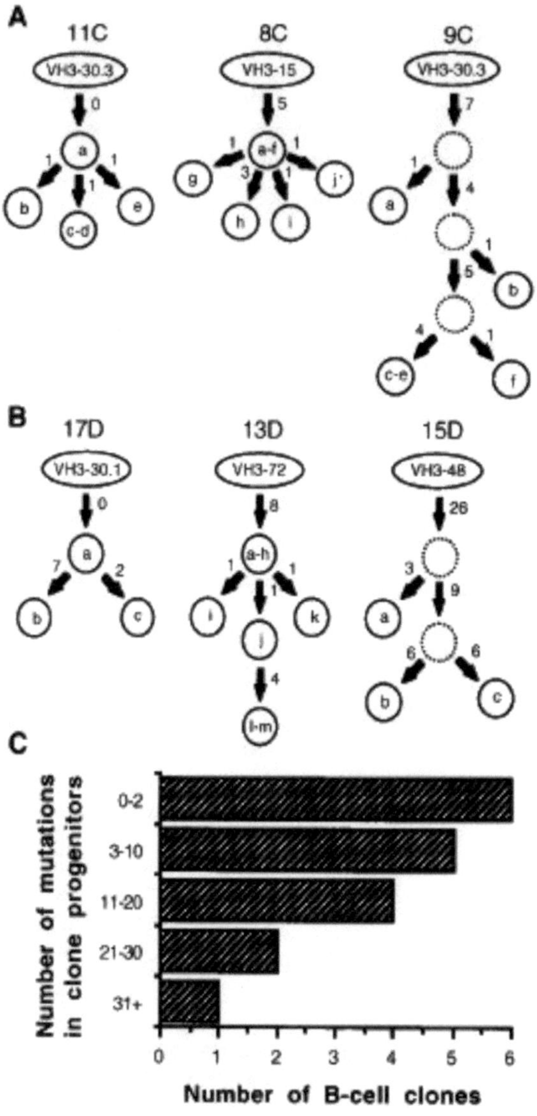


Fig. 5. Examples of clonally related sets of rearranged $V_H$ genes isolated from thymic germinal centres C and D.

The genealogical trees were constructed using the most parsimonious parent-daughter cell relationships of clonally related sets of sequences (section 2.2). The best matching germline gene is depicted as an ellipse. Letters in the circles refer to individual sequences from the same clonally related set. Deduced intermediates are shown as dotted circles. Numbers at the side of the arrows indicate the minimum number of mutations required to generate a daughter cell from the immediate parental cell. The results show that the B-cells from which they were derived are undergoing antigen-driven clonal proliferation and somatic hypermutation from both naïve and memory B-cell precursors. A: B-cell clones from germinal centre C; B: B-cell clones from germinal centre D; C: Frequency of mutations in the $V_H$ genes expressed by the most probable progenitor cells of all 18 B-cell clones analysed. Reproduced from Sims *et al.* (2001).

These related sets of V-genes were therefore derived from members of the same proliferating B-cell clone, showing that antigen-driven B-cell proliferation and somatic hypermutation are taking place within the thymic germinal centres. All of the isolated B-cell clones were small, containing a maximum of five members.

We do not know the total number of clones proliferating within a single germinal centre. We examined every tenth section but may have missed small B-cell clones, so there are likely to be more than we detected. Genealogical trees of related sets of V-genes were constructed by the most parsimonious relationship on the basis of shared and unshared mutations (section 2.5). Six of the 18 clones isolated from two germinal centres containing AChR-specific B-cells were derived from unmutated precursors, i.e. naïve B-cells, whereas the $V_H$-genes of the earliest founder cells isolated from the other 12 clones contained from 5 to >30 mutations. Examples of six of these clones are shown in Fig. 5. Although we cannot rule out the possibility that some of these clones were also derived from unidentified naïve B-cells, it is most probable that the majority were generated from founder memory B-cells. Thus, both memory and naïve B-cells have been stimulated by antigen and are proliferating and mutating their antigen receptors within thymic germinal centres of myasthenia patients.

### 3.4.4 Evidence for selection of AChR-specific B-cell clones in thymic germinal centres

Three B-cell clones from 3 different AChR positive germinal centres expressed the rarely used $V_H$5-51 genes. Furthermore, these three independent sets of V-genes exhibited the same amino acid replacements at three positions. Comparison of our V-gene sequences with those of heavy chains from known AChR-specific hybridomas and Fabs revealed some common features. Germline genes used by four of our B-cell clones also encode anti-AChR antibodies cloned from other EOMG patients, and several of the amino acid substitutions in CDR1 and CDR2 from two B-cell clones were also present in an anti-AChR Fab (Sims *et al.*, 2001; Matthews *et al.*, 2002). It is therefore unlikely that these mutations occurred by chance, suggesting that a common selection process for mutants with high affinity for the AChR is in operation.

### 3.4.5 Evidence for immunisation by the fetal form of acetylcholine receptor

Babies born to mothers with myasthenia gravis can develop transient symptoms due to transplacental transfer of the maternal autoantibodies and, in rare cases, they have severe developmental abnormalities, arthrogryposis multiplex congenita (AMC), caused by maternal anti-AChR antibodies that inhibit the ion channel function of the fetal AChR, causing paralysis during fetal development *in utero*, whereas the adult form of the mother's AChR is relatively unaffected. Fetal AChR-specific antibodies are particularly prevalent in women who have had babies, suggesting that they may be induced by the fetus.

In order to determine the specificity and clonal origins of fetal AChR-specific autoantibodies, combinatorial Fab libraries were constructed from cDNA prepared from thymic cells of two mothers (M2 and M6) of AMC babies. 25 Fab clones were isolated and two clonally related sets were examined in greater detail. All Fabs bound specifically to the $\gamma$ subunit of fetal AChR, except one that recognised the $\beta$ subunit also present in the adult receptor. Sequencing of the fetal-specific Fabs revealed clearly restricted usage of $V_H$, $J_H$, $V_K$ & $J_\kappa$ gene segments and convergent coding mutations. All the Fabs from AMC mother M2 used the $V_H$3-07 gene recombined with $J_H$6b and an unidentified D exon in combination with various $V_\kappa$ genes, suggesting that the heavy chain is the major contributor to AChR binding, at least in this case. The $V_H$3-07 segments were mutated and clonally related. Most of the Fabs from AMC mother M6 used the same combination of mutated $V_H$3-21 and $J_H$5b, with an unidentified D exon, plus a Vκ02-12/$J_\kappa$4 light chain, which was also used in two of the Fabs from M2. In this case, both the $V_H$3-21 and $V_\kappa$02-12 sets of sequences were clonally related, suggesting that they may both be derived from the same B-cell clone. The clonally related sequences from both sets of Fabs from M2 and M6 contained many shared and unshared coding mutations. The apparent founder member of each set of sequences had a large number of base differences from the best matching germline V-gene, suggesting that the clones were derived from mutated memory B-cells (Fig. 6).

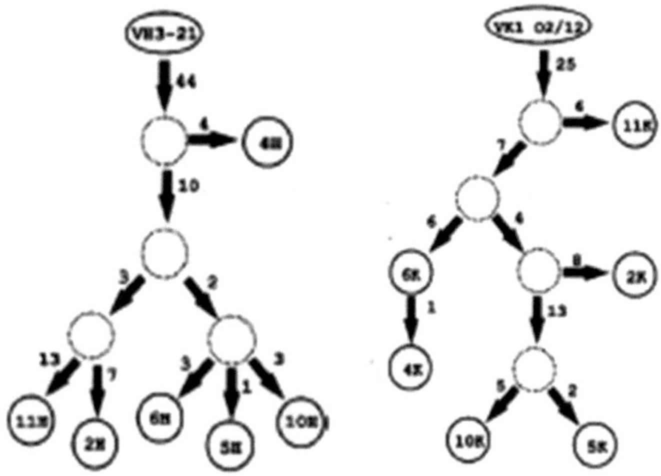


Fig. 6. Clonally related sets of rearranged $V_H$ & $V_\kappa$ genes encoding AChR-binding Fabs cloned from thymic cells from AMC mother M6.

The heavy and light chains were from the same set of Fabs. Genealogical trees were constructed and mutations numbered as described in the legend to figure 5. Fab names are shown in the circles, H referring to the heavy chain and K referring to the κ light chain. Dotted circles represent hypothetical intermediates. Numbers at the side of arrows show the minimum number of mutations required to generate a daughter cell from its immediate parent. Reproduced from Matthews *et al.* (2002).

Several sequences from both clonally related sets of Fabs had many more replacement mutations than expected by chance, indicating affinity selection. There was also clear evidence of convergent mutations. Many independently rearranged sequences from both patients shared consensus mutations. All the Fabs using $V_H$3 genes contained the same 31S→T mutation and most of the Vκ02-12 genes contained a 22SRASET28 motif in CDR1. A search of the GenBank database of all human Ig sequences found only two other κ chains containing this motif, suggesting that it is important in determining the specificity of the anti-AChR autoantibodies.

### 3.5 Conclusions

Since the EOMG thymus contains many typical germinal centres surrounded by mantle zones, including clones of proliferating, AChR-specific B-cells, it is clearly a site of autoantibody diversification. The B-cells are undergoing somatic hypermutation and affinity selection by cognate binding to AChR bound to the membrane processes of follicular dendritic cells, which form a network surrounding B and T-cells in the germinal centres. B-cells expressing high affinity, AChR-specific antigen receptors receive rescue signals from follicular dendritic and helper T-cells inducing them to differentiate into antibody-secreting plasmablasts and plasma cells that migrate out of the follicles and leave the thymus to enter the circulation, in a classical germinal centre type response. The numerous mutations seen in some V-gene sequences suggests that Ig class-switched memory B-cells are also generated and either leave the thymus, or some may recirculate within the germinal centre, undergoing further rounds of somatic hypermutation and affinity selection, consistent with the observations of others that recirculation of centrocytes between the light and dark zones occurs in orthotopic germinal centres. Several of the B-cell clones we identified were derived from highly mutated precursors, which supports this hypothesis. The autoantibodies produced by mothers of AMC babies included antibodies specific for the fetal form of the AChR, directed against the γ subunit.

The reason why large numbers of germinal centres producing AChR-specific B-cells and plasma cells develop in the thymi of myasthenia gravis patients is unclear, but it is possible that the rare thymic myoid cells may be involved. The induction of fetal AChR-specific antibodies in parous women suggests, at least in some cases, that expression of the fetal AChR on thymic epithelial and myoid cells may initiate an immune response, for which the patient's immune system has not been tolerised. Furthermore, generation of thymic germinal centres may be induced by a pre-existing proinflammatory cytokine environment, including IFNγ and TNFα. These molecules have been shown to upregulate expression of AChR subunits in thymic epithelial cells and on the membranes of myoid cells (Poea-Guyon *et al.*, 2005). The chemokines CXCL13 AND CCL21 are produced by endothelial cells of the afferent lymphatic vessels in the thymus, attracting activated T and B-cells, including naïve B-cells, suggesting that this is the mechanism of induction of thymic germinal centres (Berrih-Aknin *et al.*, 2009; Le Panse *et al.*, 2006; Meraouna *et al.*, 2006; Le Panse *et al.*, 2010).

We therefore propose a two step process for initiation of the autoimmune response in myasthenia gravis (SHIONO *et al.*, 2003). In step 1, there is hyperplasia of thymic epithelial cells expressing linear AChR epitopes, including the α and ε subunits, in the context of the MHC Class II antigen HLA-DR52a, a susceptibility factor for EOMG patients. Whereas these peptides would normally induce tolerance, an imbalance in regulatory factors and expression of costimulatory molecules results in activation of thymic $T_h$-cells against AChR epitopes. In step 2, the $T_h$-cells induce an early B-cell response against the linear peptides and some of the resulting antibodies cross-react with conformational epitopes of the native AChR expressed on the thymic myoid cells, leading to myoid cell damage, release of AChR/antibody immune complexes, danger signals, and recruitment of professional antigen presenting cells. These stimulate an enhanced B-cell response accompanied by formation of germinal centres with production of high affinity, class switched, pathogenic autoantibodies. Although some aspects of this hypothesis are conjectural, they are also testable.

## 4. Tissue-infiltrating B-cells in inflammatory myopathies

### 4.1 Introduction

The inflammatory myopathies (IM), collectively called myositis, are classified into three principal subsets, Dermatomyositis (DM), Polymyositis (PM) and Inclusion Body Myositis (IBM) (Bohan & Peter, 1975a; Bohan & Peter, 1975b; Dalakas & Hohlfeld, 2003). Each of these disorders is characterised by moderate to severe muscle weakness and muscle fatigue with inflammatory mononuclear cell infiltration within the muscle, but each disorder has distinct clinical and pathological features. IM can be associated with various autoimmune and connective tissue disorders as well as malignancies, the latter being associated with up to 45% of adult DM patients.

DM, the most common of the inflammatory myopathies, is a multi-organ disease not only affecting skeletal muscle but, often, the skin as well as other tissues and is more commonly found in women than men; it also accounts for up to c.85% of all juvenile IM (Rider, 2007). DM is characterised by a heliotrope rash on the upper eyelid, face or upper trunk accompanying, or more commonly preceding, proximal muscle weakness. Muscle inflammation is predominantly perivascular and/or perimysial or in the interfascicular septae and around, rather than within, the muscle fascicles. Perivascular atrophy is a characteristic feature of DM patients, often in groups at the periphery of the fascicle. In DM, muscle lymphocytic infiltrates consist largely of B-cells and $CD4^+$ T-cells (Arahata & Engel, 1984; Engel & Arahata, 1984) suggesting that DM may be a humorally mediated immune response.

PM and IBM, though separate disorders, are both characterised by scattered necrotic and regenerating muscle fibres and endomysial inflammation with invasion and destruction of non-necrotic muscle fibres. PM generally becomes evident in adulthood and is best defined as a subacute myopathy that evolves over weeks to months and presents with symmetrical weakness of the proximal muscles. Its clinical onset is hard to define with no early recognition signs such as the rash observed in DM. PM is uncommon as a stand-alone disorder and more commonly associates with other autoimmune and connective tissue disorders.

Onset of IBM is usually after the age of 50 and occurs more frequently in men. Muscle weakness can be both proximal and distal and is often asymmetrical. Despite similarities with PM, distinctive features of IBM include: rimmed vacuoles; groups of atrophic fibres; increased lymphocytic invasion of non-necrotic fibres; less frequent myofibre necrosis; and a more slowly progressing clinical course with patients being unresponsive to treatment. In both disorders, inflammatory infiltrates typically consist of $CD8^+$ T-cells and macrophages (Arahata & Engel, 1984; Engel & Arahata, 1984) which invade MHC Class 1 antigen-expressing muscle fibres, a feature absent in normal muscle tissue, leading to fibre necrosis. The muscle fibre invading $CD8^+$ T-cells can be clonally expanded in both PM and IBM (Dalakas, 2004; Fyhr *et al.*, 1997; Hofbauer *et al.*, 2003; Mantegazza *et al.*, 1993; Seitz *et al.*, 2006), which persists over time (Amemiya, Granger, & Dalakas, 2000).

#### 4.1.1 Autoantibodies associated with myositis

As with most autoimmune disorders, different autoantibody specificities have been described in DM and PM; autoantibodies are generally absent from IBM although they have been detected in a small number of cases (Dalakas *et al.*, 1997). They can either be myositis-specific (MSAs) or myositis-associated autoantibodies (MAAs), which can also be associated with other autoimmune diseases. Most bind to protein or ribonucleoprotein complexes involved in protein synthesis, translocation or elongation; MAA target antigens are primarily located in the nucleoplasm or nucleolus. The most prevalent MSAs are directed against amino-acyl-tRNA-synthetases (ARS), and are associated with a distinctive clinical phenotype, anti-synthetase syndrome, characterised by myositis, Raynaud's phenomenon and interstitial lung disease, with a higher mortality. Anti-Jo-1 (anti-histidyl-tRNA synthetase) antibodies are the most prevalent in myositis patients (20-30% of patients), while the other anti-ARS antibodies are only present in 1-3% of IM patients, and are a diagnostic and prognostic marker for disease severity (Mielnik *et al.*, 2006; Zampieri *et al.*, 2005).

#### 4.1.2 Muscle-infiltrating B-cells in myositis

As described above B-cells have been found to be prominent within the muscle infiltrating cell populations of DM patients and are rarely found, or absent, in the inflamed muscle of PM and IBM patients. $CD138^+$ plasma cells have been identified within the infiltrating populations, predominantly in the endomysial areas of muscle tissue of PM and IBM patients (Greenberg *et al.*, 2002; Greenberg *et al.*, 2005). This was confirmed by sequence analysis of immunoglobulin V-genes expressed by laser dissected cells as well as microarray studies which showed an abundance of immunoglobulin transcripts.

The role for B-cells and plasma cells in IM is still currently unresolved, with continuing studies providing further insight into the immune mechanisms. The identification of muscle infiltrating B-cells, plasma cells and autoantibodies suggests that these diseases may be at least partly driven by a loss of B-cell tolerance and, in the case of PM and IBM patients, not solely by the oligoclonal expansion of T-cells. We therefore investigated whether there is clonal expansion of infiltrating, autoantibody producing B-cells *in situ* in IM.

### 4.2 The muscle infiltrating B-cell response in myositis

#### 4.2.1 The cellular composition of infiltrating lymphoid cells in myositis

To determine whether specific, antigen-driven, B-cell adaptive immune responses were occurring *in situ*, we used the methods described in section 2 to study the cellular composition of muscle infiltrating cells in twelve different muscle samples (2 DM, 9 PM, 1 IBM); we also examined their Ig V-gene repertoire and the processes of somatic hypermutation and clonal diversification of the rearranged V-genes. In contrast with other autoimmune diseases (see above), no classical ectopic germinal centre structures were observed within the inflamed muscle; instead, muscle–infiltrating cells were present in cellular aggregations which varied from loose to dense in the appropriate perivascular/perimysial or endomysial locations, as in previous studies. B-cells were a significant component of the inflammatory infiltrate in all samples examined for all three myositis subsets, either as $CD20^+$ B-cells or differentiated plasma cells (Figure 7A-D), although the most significant infiltration of $CD20^+$ B-cells was observed within the muscles of the two DM patients. FDCs were rare, and were seen only in one IBM and three PM samples, and not at all in DM. In addition to these cell phenotypes, $CD3^+$, $CD4^+$, $CD8^+$, $CD68^+$ and $FoxP3^+$ cells were also present. Double immunofluorescence staining of cell phenotypes with the proliferating cell marker Ki67 identified proliferating cells within the infiltrating population. In addition to $CD20^+$ B-cells (Figure 7E & F), proliferating $CD3^+$, $CD4^+$, $CD8^+$ and $CD68^+$ cells were observed, as well as $FoxP3^+$ cells in one DM patient.

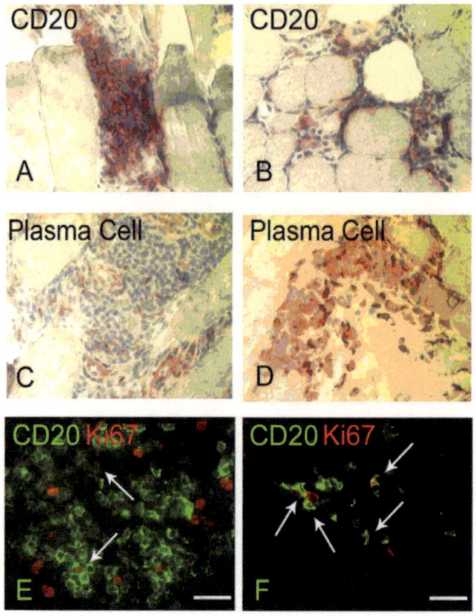


Fig. 7. Immunohistochemical staining of antigen-specific muscle-infiltrating B-cells and plasma cells.

A - D: Infiltrating B-cells and plasma cells (red) within inflamed muscle; E & F: Proliferating B-cells ($CD20^+$ B-cells - Fluorescein-Avidin D (green), $Ki67^+$ - Texas Red-Avidin D (red)). Slides A, B, C & E are from 2 DM patients; D & F are from a PM patient. Original magnification for images A - D: 400x; E & F: 630x. Scale Bar (E & F) represents 15 µm. Arrows indicate double positive staining.

#### 4.2.2 The Ig V-gene repertoire and clonally proliferating, muscle-infiltrating B-cells

Analysis of the repertoire of rearranged Ig V-genes expressed by infiltrating B-cells and plasma cells revealed significant biases for and against individual gene segments and families relative to the normal peripheral blood B-cell and the germline gene repertoires. V-gene usage varied between patients and myositis subsets and, in a few instances, differed significantly between the DM and PM subsets. Interestingly, naïve or unmutated B-cells (0-2 mutations per $V_H$ gene) constituted almost 50% of the B-cells in DM, but <10% in PM, where a large proportion of sequences was highly mutated (c.30% >20 mutations). As expected, mutations were prevalent within CDRs 1 & 2. A total of nine clonally related sequences was found in five of the IM patients studied; 2 DM and 3 PM patients, each with up to four different clones comprising between two and ten clonal variants (Figure 8). These clonally related sequences provide evidence for specific, antigen-driven B-cell immune responses within the inflamed muscle. However, using the method of Hershberg *et al.* (2008), we found no evidence of positive selection in the CDRs of clonally related sequences, nor in any sequences isolated from the DM patients, and only in a small percentage from the PM patients. Finally, using biotinylated recombinant antigens, we identified antigen-specific B and plasma cells in infiltrates from the five out of twelve patients whose autoantibody specificities were known, including Jo-1 (Figure 9).

Parallel studies (Bradshaw *et al.*, 2007) also demonstrated B-cell responses in muscle of 3 DM, 2 PM and 7 IBM patients but very few $CD19^+$ or $CD20^+$ cells were observed, the majority of B-lineage cells being CD138+ plasma cells that had class switched to either IgG or IgA. Clonally related sequences were isolated from whole muscle sections from ten of the twelve myositis patients, with up to four different clonal sets isolated from each muscle sample. Further studies also support the absence of classical ectopic germinal centre structures and the clonal expansion and maturation of B-cells within inflamed muscle (Salajegheh *et al.*, 2010). Collectively this and our work strongly suggest the participation of antigen-specific B-cell immune responses within the muscle.

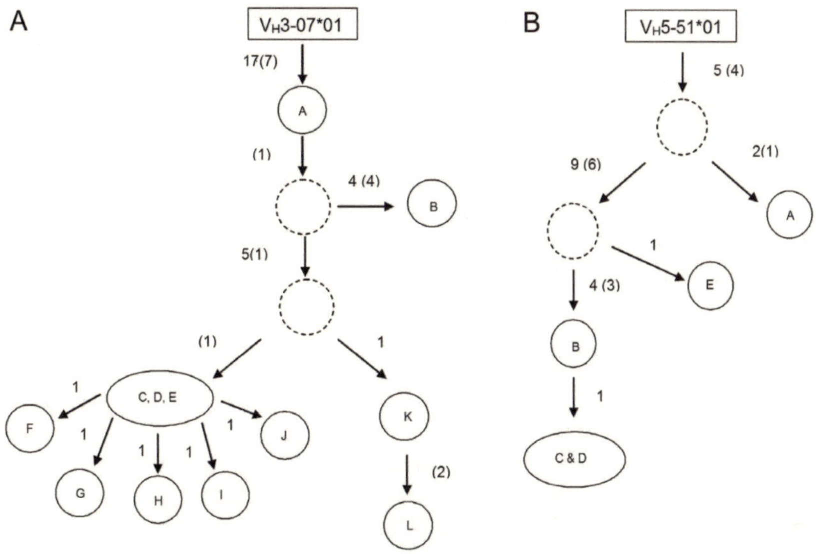


Fig. 8. Oligoclonal expansion of B-cells and plasma cells in inflammatory myopathies

Representative examples of clonal genealogical trees constructed from sequences isolated from muscle-infiltrating B-cells and plasma cells in individual patients, representing the minimum number of cell divisions required to generate each daughter cell. Clone A from a DM patient; clone B from a PM patient. The letters in the circles refer to individual sequences isolated from each B-cell clone. Genealogical trees were constructed and mutations numbered as described in the legend to Figure 5. Bracketed figures representing additional silent mutations. Dashed circles represent hypothetical intermediates whose sequences were not isolated from the muscle-infiltrating population.

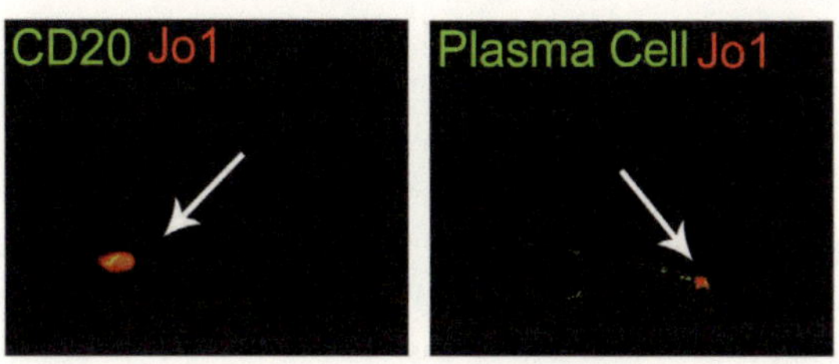


Fig. 9. Infiltrating antigen-specific B-cells and plasma cells in inflammatory myopathies

CD20+ B-cells and antigen-specific cells were visualised by Fluorescein-Avidin D (green) and Texas Red-Avidin D (red) respectively. Original magnification was 630X. Arrows identify antigen-specific cells within the muscle-infiltrating population of polymyositis patients.

### 4.3 Conclusions

As previously described in other autoimmune diseases, a role for B-cells in IM is implied by the clinical improvement in patients administered Rituximab® therapy, including improvements in muscle strength. Some patients relapsed as their B-cell pools repopulated and depletion of autoantibody titres was variable (Chung, Genovese, & Fiorentino, 2007; Cooper et al., 2007; Levine, 2005). The potential of B-cells as therapeutic targets is further supported by the elevations in serum levels and gene expression of B-cell activating factor (BAFF) in IM patients, a cytokine crucial for B-cell maturation and survival, which is also thought to play a role in autoantibody production (Krystufkova *et al.*, 2008; Salajegheh *et al.*, 2010).

Despite all the evidence described here implicating B-cells and loss of B-cell tolerance in the IM, numerous questions still remain to be resolved, including identification of the stimulating antigens and epitopes, sequence characteristics and pathogenicity of high-affinity, antigen-specific antibodies produced *in situ*, and the factors regulating and controlling these autoimmune reactions. The resolution of these questions will enhance our understanding of the immune pathology of IM and facilitate the diagnosis, treatment and management of these diseases.

## 5. The ectopic germinal centre response in breast cancer

In autoimmune diseases there is a failure of immunological tolerance resulting in an immune response to self-antigens, causing pathological damage to the target organ and tissues, the nature of the target tissue depending on the specificity of the response. In malignancy the immune response, if it occurs, is similar in that it is essentially directed against self, i.e. tumour-associated, antigens. These antigens may be mutated, altered by metabolic processes, or merely aberrantly or over-expressed on the tumour. The problem, however, is converse to autoimmune disease in that, whereas in autoimmune disease the aim is to suppress the immune response, preferably specifically against the target organ, in cancer the hope is that it will be possible to boost the immune response which is often too weak to overcome the rapidly growing tumour.

Several autoimmune disorders sometimes associate with certain tumours, most often small cell lung cancer, breast or ovarian carcinomas, ovarian teratomas, neuroblastomas and lymphomas (with Sjögren's syndrome), reviewed by Lang & Vincent and Rosenfeld *et al.* (Lang & Vincent, 2009; Rosenfeld & Dalmau, 2010). In the examples studied, the target autoantigen(s) are expressed on the tumour which seems to autoimmunise against them. Indeed, if the tumour is removed, autoantibody levels often decline (Chalk *et al.*, 1990). In many syndromes, the autoimmune disorder serves as a valuable early warning of the associated tumour, and may even slow its growth (Maddison & Lang, 2008).

### 5.1 Pathology of breast cancer

Breast cancer is the second most common malignancy in women, accounting for 31% of all types of cancer, with a lifetime incidence in the U.K. of 1/8 in women and c.1/1000 in men. Despite advances in screening, diagnosis and therapy, 12,000 women die of breast cancer each year in the U.K. and the global incidence in females is 23%, but there are marked variations between different regions, it being the highest in Western Europe, Australia, New Zealand and North America. The incidence is relatively low in Asian and African countries (figures from Cancer Research UK). There are several different histopathological types of breast cancer, of which the major types are the ductal and lobular carcinomas, either of which can be *in situ* or invasive, the *in situ* type being considered a possible precursor of invasive carcinoma. Ductal and lobular carcinomas *in situ* are confined to the mammary ducts and lobules and have a very high cure rate, approaching 100%. Invasive carcinomas account for the majority of breast cancers and have a much poorer prognosis. Malignant cell growth appears to start in the ducts and lobules and then invades the surrounding tissues and ultimately metastasises to other tissues and organs. A less common type is medullary carcinoma, comprising only c.1 – 5% of breast cancers; this typically has heavy infiltrates of B-lymphocytes and a significantly better prognosis than the invasive ductal and lobular types. Length of disease free survival in breast cancer is unpredictable, with relapse occurring up to ten years post treatment and even beyond; it has been postulated that this may be due to host factors, including the nature and extent of the immune response.

### 5.2 The immune response to breast cancer

Most breast cancers contain infiltrates of lymphoid cells with large numbers of T-cells, including $CD4^+$ and $CD8^+$ T-cells, and variable numbers of B-cells, natural killer cells and macrophages. The degree of infiltration varies between different types of breast cancer with extensive lymphoid cell infiltrates in ductal carcinoma *in situ* and some invasive ductal and lobular carcinomas (Ben Hur *et al.*, 2002). Most studies have focused on the role of cytotoxic T-cells in tumour immunity, with variable success in attempting to suppress tumour growth by boosting the T-cell response to tumour-associated antigens. Relatively few studies have addressed the role of B-cells and humoral immunity in response to cancers, including breast cancer, despite the observation that c.40% of ductal breast carcinomas have significant B-cell infiltration.

There is increasing evidence that B-cells play important dual opposing roles in the immune response to tumours; on the one hand as antigen presenting cells and producers of cytotoxic antibodies effective at killing tumour cells by antibody-dependent cell-mediated cytotoxicity (ADCC) and complement-dependent cell lysis, and as tumour antigen-presenting cells capable of very efficient T-cell activation; on the other hand as promoters of inflammation aiding tumour progression (de Visser, Korets, & Coussens, 2005; de Visser, Eichten, & Coussens, 2006). These seemingly contradictory effects may be due to the difference between a specific, high affinity immune response to antigen versus a low affinity, polyclonal response, or even suppression of the cytotoxic immune response via regulatory B-cells (Mauri, 2010). The importance of antibodies in eliminating tumours is clearly demonstrated by the results of treatment of breast cancer patients with humanised monoclonal antibodies (MAbs) specific for the epidermal growth factor receptor HER-2 (trastuzumab/herceptin and pertuzumab). Not only is herceptin effective in slowing down the progression of established metastatic disease, it has also recently been demonstrated to prevent the emergence of metastases when given as an adjuvant treatment (Hortobagyi, 2005). Pertuzumab has also yielded promising results in clinical trials (Bianco, 2004). Synergistic effects between herceptin and pertuzumab suggest promising new approaches to therapy using cocktails of antibodies (Nahta, Hung, & Esteva, 2004) and elucidation of the molecular structure of the herceptin Fab/HER-2 complex (Cho *et al.*, 2003) allows rational design of therapeutic anti-HER-2 antibodies. MAbs specific for other tumour-associated antigens (TAAs) are needed to work synergistically with trastuzumab and to treat patients who do not overexpress HER-2.

Several molecules have been identified that are either over-expressed, mutated, or structurally modified on tumour cells and are therefore potential targets for immunotherapy, including HER-1, HER-2, MUC-1 and p53 (Taylor-Papadimitriou *et al.*, 2002). Some TAAs appear to overcome tolerance and induce a natural immune response as a result of mutation or altered expression; humoral immune responses to these antigens in breast cancer patients are associated with better early disease stage-specific survival (Angelopoulou *et al.*, 2000;Visco *et al.*, 2000; von Mensdorff-Pouilly *et al.*, 2000) and anti-MUC-1 antibodies are cytotoxic to tumour cells (Snijdewint *et al.*, 2001). TAA-specific tumour infiltrating (TIL) B-lymphocytes and recombinant antibodies have been isolated from both tumour (Kotlan *et al.*, 2000; Kotlan *et al.*, 2005) and lymph nodes (Petrarca *et al.*, 1999; Rothe *et al.*, 2004) of medullary and ductal carcinoma patients, showing that they are responding specifically to the tumour. Evasion of the immune response by the tumour can be overcome by passive immunotherapy or active immunisation regimes. B-cells actively responding in the draining lymph node and tumour are therefore ideal sources to study the immune response to the tumour and provide the most relevant source of potentially therapeutic antibodies.

### 5.3 Ductal carcinoma infiltrating lymphocytes are clustered into germinal centres

We and others found infiltrating lymphocytes in ductal carcinomas were aggregated into clusters containing T-cells, B-cells and follicular dendritic cells with plasmablasts/plasma cells in and around the aggregates (Coronella *et al.*, 2002; Nzula, Going, & Stott, 2003a). These cell clusters appeared to be similar to those seen in the target tissues of autoimmune diseases except that there was no mantle zone (also absent in the salivary glands of patients with Sjögren's syndrome (Stott *et al.*, 1998)), so we examined whether they were responding as germinal centres.

### 5.4 The Ig V-gene repertoire and clonal proliferation of B-cells in ductal carcinoma

We cloned and sequenced 401 rearranged Ig $V_H$-genes from microdissected tumour-infiltrating B-cell foci of 7 patients with invasive ductal carcinoma and 271 $V_H$-genes from paired sentinel lymph nodes of 3 of the patients. 15 sets of $V_H$-genes from clonally related B-cells within individual foci were identified by their shared $V_H$, D, $J_H$ and CDR3 sequences, showing that proliferating, mutating B-cell clones were present in lymphoid foci and that these foci were undergoing a germinal centre response within the tumour, similar to the ectopic germinal centres we have observed in the target tissues of autoimmune diseases (Fig. 10). There was preferential usage of certain $V_H$, D & $J_H$ exons, indicating selection of B-cells expressing antigen receptors encoded by these gene combinations. $V_H$ & $V_L$-genes from proliferating B-cell clones contained numerous mutations, demonstrating that the somatic hypermutation machinery was switched on within the cell cluster, again characteristic of a germinal centre response. Analysis of the pattern of mutations showed that the B-cell clones are undergoing an antigen-driven response accompanied by selection of specific mutations and affinity maturation *in situ*. Clone founder cells were of both naïve and memory B-cell type, showing that a secondary response involving memory B-cells was taking place, but also new B-cells that had not previously encountered antigen moved into cell clusters and were stimulated by antigen. We also cloned rearranged $V_H$-genes from microdissected germinal centres in the paired sentinel lymph node and identified proliferating, hypermutating B-cell clones there too. These also revealed selection for particular $V_H$ & $J_H$-genes showing selection by antigen for B-cells expressing these genes during the immune response but we did not find evidence that members of the same B-cell clones had migrated from the sentinel node to the tumour; this could have been due to insufficient sample sizes (Nzula, Going & Stott, 2003a; Simsa *et al.*, 2005).

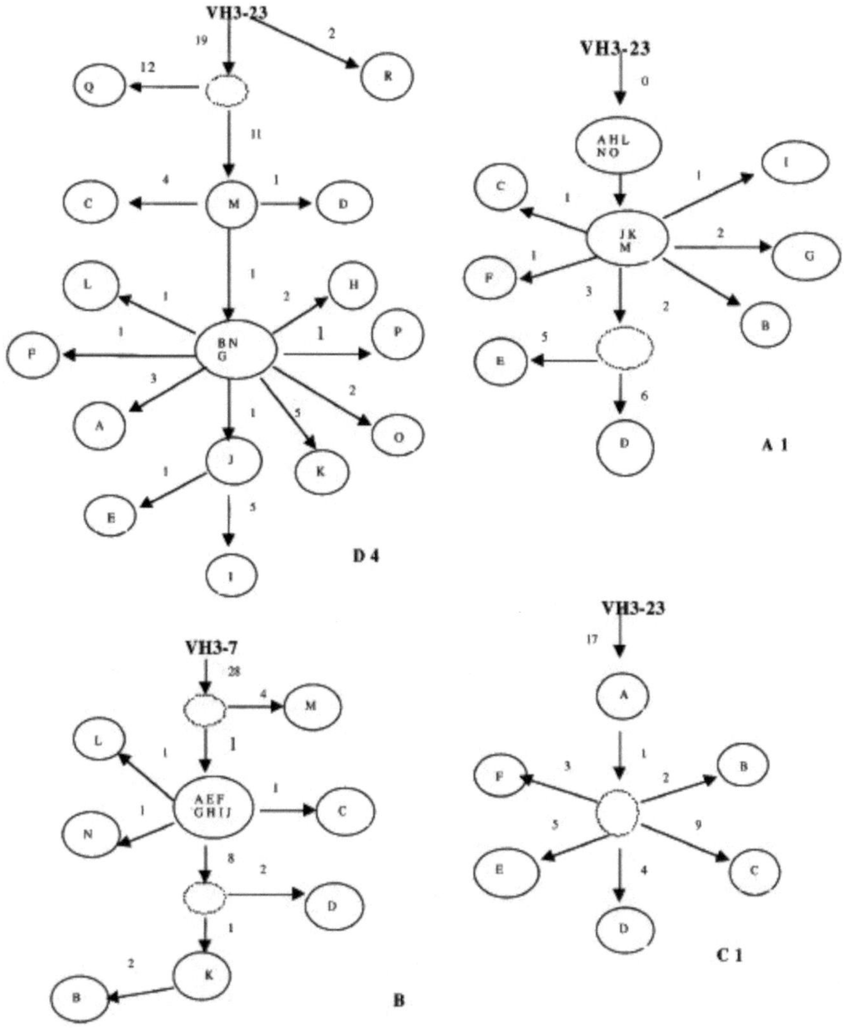


Fig. 10. Examples of proliferating, hypermutating B-cell clones from the breast tumours of four ductal carcinoma patients.

The best matching germline $V_H$-gene is shown at the origin of each tree. The founder rearranged $V_H$-genes of three of these B-cell clones already appear to be mutated, implying that they originated from memory B-cells, whereas clone A1 appears to have been founded by a naïve B-cell. Genealogical trees were constructed and mutations numbered as described in the legend to Figure 5. Reproduced from Nzula *et al.* (2003).

### 5.5 Cloning and characterisation of scFv antibodies

In order to identify the antigens driving the immune response within the tumour, we reconstructed the antigen receptors expressed by germinal centre B-cells as scFv antibodies by cloning $V_H$ and $V_L$-genes into phagemid (pHEN2), as described in section 2.3, to generate scFv-phage libraries expressing randomly assorted combinations of $V_H$ and $V_L$-genes. These "mini-libraries" were made from the B-cells in individual germinal centres within the tumour and are therefore much smaller and more restricted than the very large libraries normally made by random combination of large pools of $V_H$ and $V_L$-genes. Two scFv-phage mini-libraries were constructed from a germinal centre incorporating all the $V_H$-genes pooled from the largest proliferating B-cell clone (D4 in Fig. 10) linked randomly to either the rearranged $V_\kappa$-genes or the rearranged $V_\lambda$-genes amplified from the same germinal centre.

Tumour-binding scFv were selected from the mini-libraries by three or four cycles of panning and elution on a heterologous tumour homogenate pooled from breast tumours of 5 patients. During the panning cycles we observed exponential enrichment of the $V_\lambda$ mini-library, but not the $V_\kappa$ mini-library, indicating that scFv within the $V_\lambda$ mini-library bind specifically to tumour-associated antigens (Fig. 11A). This is consistent with the scFv-libraries being derived from the same B-cell clone, since a single B-cell clone uses either a κ or λ light chain, not both. 13 scFv-phages binding to the tumour extract were cloned and their specificity for tumour tissue confirmed by ELISA. 7 scFv-phage clones that bound to the tumour extract were identified for further characterisation. All 7 used the same combination of $V_H3$-23 with exons D1-26 & $J_H2$, expressed by B-cell clone D4, and the light chain gene $V_\lambda 1c$ with $J_\lambda 3b$.

We also constructed two scFv-phage libraries from DNA extracted from a whole sample of tumour tissue, as described for the mini-libraries. The 2 libraries were panned on the same heterologous tumour homogenate as used with the mini-libraries. After 4 cycles of panning we observed an enrichment of several logs for both libraries, indicating the presence of tumour-specific antibodies (Fig. 11B). The enrichment of both global libraries shows that tumour-specific B-cells derived from independent B-cell clones were present in the tumour, as expected. 19 scFv-phages were cloned from the 2 global libraries and their specificity for tumour tissue confirmed by ELISA using the same tumour homogenate as source of antigen.

### 5.6 Identification of the specificity of proliferating B-cells

Since the scFvs from the $V_H/V_\lambda$ mini-library were derived from proliferating B-cell clone D4, their sequences and antigen specificities reveal the nature of the genes and antigen receptor specificities of the original germinal centre B-cells. We therefore sequenced the scFv clones that showed the strongest binding to the tumour extract and performed a Blast search of the Genbank gene database. The $V_HDJ_H$ heavy chain gene used by all members of B-cell clone D4 exhibited 89% homology with a human anti-HER3 MAb (AF048774) and the $V_\lambda J_\lambda$ light chain gene, also used by the same B-cells, matched a human anti-EGFR antibody (DQ666353.1) with 96% homology. These, and scFvs from the global libraries, were tested for binding to recombinant antigens from the epidermal growth factor receptor family: HER-2, HER-3 and HER-4, kindly provided by Genentech (San Francisco, USA) and Pharmexa A/S (Hørsholm, Denmark) by ELISA. Six scFvs from B-cell clone D4 and one from the global tumour library bound to recombinant HER-2, HER-3 & HER-4, indicating that they recognised a shared epitope expressed by all three members of this EGFR family of receptors (Fig. 12). Specificity for HER-2, HER-3 & HER-4 was confirmed using soluble scFv produced in the non-suppressor strain of *E.coli*.

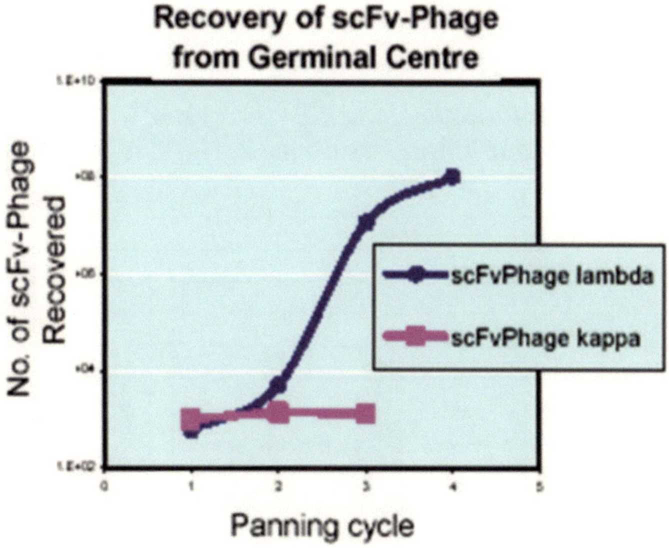


A

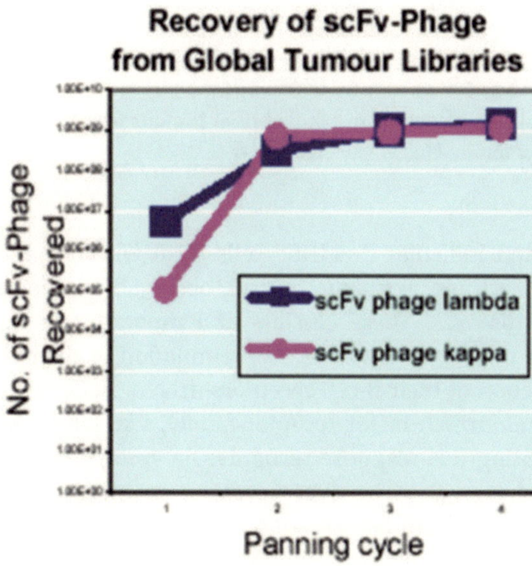


B

Fig. 11. Exponential enrichment of scFv-phage after panning and elution on a breast tumour extract

A. $V_H/V\kappa$ and $V_H/V\lambda$ scFv mini-libraries, using $V_H$-genes from B-cell clone D4, panned on pooled heterologous tumour extract The eluate from each panning was then subjected to further cycles of panning and elution; B. Global $V_H/V\kappa$ and $V_H/V\lambda$ scFv-phage libraries from a human breast tumour, panned on the same heterologous tumour extract as in A.

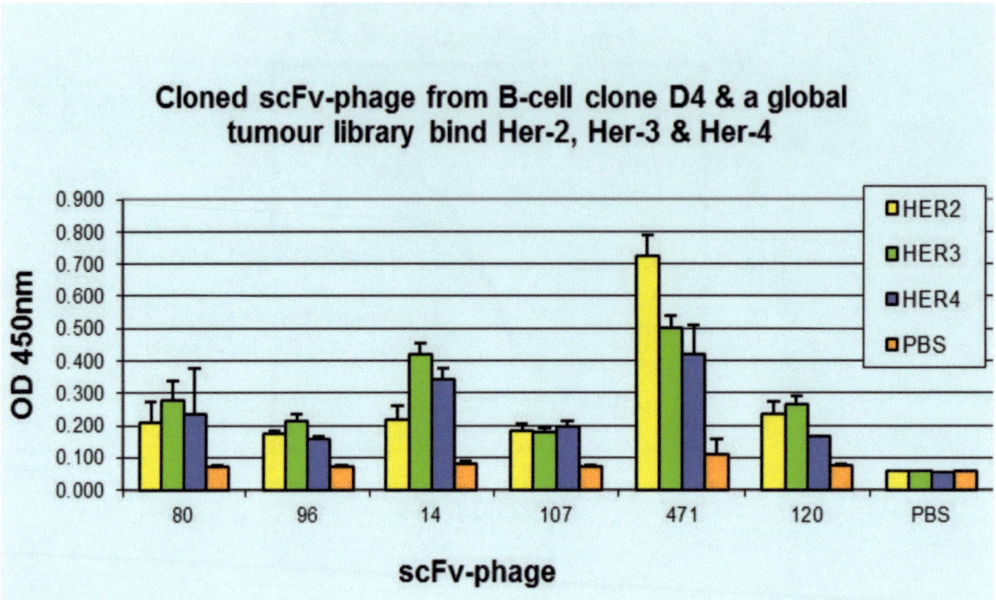


Fig. 12. EGFR family specificity of scFv antibodies cloned from a mammary carcinoma germinal centre.

Individual scFv-phage (80, 96, 14 & 107 & 120) from B-cell clone D4, proliferating and mutating in a breast tumour, and scFv-phage (471), cloned from whole breast tumour tissue, bind to members of the epidermal growth factor receptor family Her-2, Her-3 & Her-4.

### 5.7 Conclusions

Clusters of B-cells, T-cells and follicular dendritic cells form within human ductal breast carcinomas, resembling the ectopic germinal centres observed in the target tissues of patients with autoimmune diseases. These clusters of lymphoid cells contain clones of proliferating B-cells that are undergoing somatic hypermutation of their rearranged, Ig V-(D)-J-genes and affinity selection of their B-cell receptors driven, in the case described here, by members of the epidermal growth factor receptor family, viz. HER2, HER3 and HER4. The antibodies produced during this response recognise an epitope shared by these 3 cell surface receptors, which are known to be overexpressed on breast carcinoma cells and several other types of carcinoma, including ovarian cancer. It is very probable that other tumour associated antigens are also able to stimulate a local B-cell response within the tumour, e.g. antibodies specific for a ganglioside were cloned from medullary carcinoma B-cells, although it is not clear whether these are involved in attacking the tumour (Kotlan *et al.*, 2005).

Single chain Fv antibodies cloned from tumour germinal centre B-cells can readily be converted to complete antibodies by splicing their V-genes on to Ig constant regions of any desired isotype. These fully human antibodies can be produced in large quantities in a protein expression system and are therefore potential candidates for diagnosis, monitoring and therapy of breast and other types of cancer.

## 6. General conclusions

It has become increasingly clear that infiltrating B- and T-lymphocytes organise themselves into ectopic lymphoid follicles and germinal centres within tissues undergoing inflammatory processes. This has been observed in several autoimmune diseases (Table 1), usually within the target organ or tissue, myasthenia gravis being the exception to the rule for reasons discussed in section 3.5. However, ectopic g.c.s are not restricted to autoimmune diseases but can also develop in other chronic inflammatory diseases, such as Crohn's disease and ulcerative colitis; at sites of infection such as the liver during chronic hepatitis C virus infection and the skin of oncocerciasis patients (Brattig *et al.*, 2010); and in neoplasias, including lymphoma of the mucosal-associated lymphoid tissue associated with Sjögren's syndrome (Bombardieri *et al.*, 2007a) and, as shown here, in breast cancer (Table 1).

How these ectopic g.c.s develop, their role in the pathology of autoimmune diseases, and in combating infections and malignancies is still unclear but evidence is beginning to emerge. Cytokines, chemokines and signalling molecules involved in lymphoid neogenesis in the secondary lymphoid organs also appear to be required for ectopic g.c. formation, including lymphotoxins-α, β and $\alpha_1\beta_2$, TNFα, Grb2, the chemokine receptor CXCR5, its ligand CXCL15, and the B-cell attracting chemokines CXCL13 and CCL21, in this case due to release of these molecules within the inflammatory environment, suggesting that g.c. formation may be secondary to inflammation (Aloisi & Pujol-Borrell, 2006).

When reports first emerged of germinal centre-like structures within the target tissues of autoimmune diseases, there was some scepticism regarding whether these structures were involved in true germinal centre reactions. These doubts have now been dispelled. Identification of dark and light zones and a follicular dendritic cell network in intimate contact with B-cells was highly suggestive of a germinal centre reaction, especially when it was shown that autoantigen was trapped on the follicular dendritic cell processes, e.g. (SHIONO *et al.*, 2003). Studies by us and other researchers have shown that the B-cells within ectopic germinal centres are activated to antigen-driven clonal proliferation, somatic hypermutation and class switching, similar to the response in orthotopic g.c.s responding to foreign antigens. That they switch on the somatic hypermutation machinery has been shown in several autoimmune diseases by sequencing studies of the expressed, rearranged Ig V-genes cloned from microdissected g.c.s. This has been confirmed in the salivary gland g.c.s of Sjögren's patients and the synovial g.c.s of rheumatoid arthritis patients by identification of activation induced cytidine deaminase (AID), a key enzyme in somatic hypermutation and class switch recombination (Bombardieri *et al.*, 2007b; Humby *et al.*, 2009). Interestingly, expression of AID has recently been observed in hyperplastic fibroblasts of rheumatoid arthritis patients (Igarashi et al., 2010). Expression correlated with mutations in the *p53* gene and was induced by TNFα *in vitro*. AID is known to induce mutations in non-Ig genes at a lower frequency and it was suggested that the mutations of this tumour suppressor gene may be the cause of the fibroblast hyperplasia. Affinity maturation of B-cell receptors during somatic hypermutation has been demonstrated by analysis of replacement mutations, although early analyses failed to take into account the bias towards replacement mutations in the CDRs resulting from targeting of AID to sequence motifs such as RGYW. Final confirmation requires direct affinity measurements of autoantibodies cloned from germinal centre B-cells and/or by 3-D molecular modelling of the antigen-binding site bound to its epitope, as we have shown for anti-hen egg lysozyme antibodies produced in an orthotopic germinal centre reaction (Adams *et al.*, 2003).

In several cases it has been shown that the autoantibodies generated in ectopic g.c.s have similar specificities to the autoantibodies found in the blood, notably in Hashimoto's thyroiditis, Sjögren's syndrome and rheumatoid arthritis, suggesting that the g.c.s contribute to pathological mechanisms, although whether they are critical in the early stages of development of the disease, or only contribute to its maintenance once the initial tissue damage has commenced, has yet to be established. Production of cytokines and chemokines at sites of damage that attract lymphocytes and contribute to lymphoid neogenesis suggests that the latter may be the more likely scenario. Nevertheless, a detailed understanding of the mechanisms involved in generation of ectopic g.c. structures and maintenance of production of plasma cells and memory B-cells producing potentially pathogenic antibodies is essential for a full understanding of the pathology of autoimmune disease and holds promise for developing new methods of therapy, based on controlling this response or inducing immunological tolerance to the autoantigens.

Even more work needs to be done to determine the role of ectopic g.c.s in other diseases, including sterile and infectious chronic inflammatory diseases and cancer. What other types of cancer, in addition to breast cancer and lymphoma, induce germinal centre reactions within the tumour and the nature of their response in elimination of cancer cells have yet to be determined. The identification of intra-tumour g.c.s producing antibodies and memory B-cells with specificity for members of the epidermal growth factor receptor family holds out hope that therapeutic vaccines can be developed to boost this response for therapy of breast cancer and, potentially other neoplasias, such as ovarian cancer, in which these molecules are overexpressed. Experimental approaches using mouse models of breast cancer support this optimism (Renard *et al.*, 2003; Renard & Leach, 2007; Mukhopadhyay, MS in preparation). Cloning of antibodies against tumour-associated antigens from intra-tumour g.c.s is also a novel way of producing fully human antibodies for passive immunotherapy.

## 7. Acknowledgements

We wish to thank Professors Nick Willcox and Angela Vincent, F.R.S. (Institute for Molecular Medicine, University of Oxford, U.K.), Paul Garside and Iain McInnes (Institute of Infection, Immunity & Inflammation, University of Glasgow, U.K.) for critically reading the manuscript and their helpful suggestions. We also wish to thank all the people who have worked in D.I. Stott's research group and those of his collaborators whose work contributed to the results described here, especially Gary Sims, Michael Matthews, Sazini Nzula and Anne-Sophie Rouziere, whose data on myasthenia gravis and ductal carcinoma are presented in this chapter. Any errors and oversights are entirely our own.

The original research described in this chapter was funded by The Wellcome Trust, the Scottish Executive Health Dept. Chief Scientist Office, Cancer Research UK, the Dr. Robert Mairs Trust and the Medical Research Council.

## 8. References

Adams, C. L., MacLeod, M. K. L., Milner-White, E. J., Aitken, R., Garside, P., & Stott, D. I. 2003, "Complete analysis of the B-cell response to a protein antigen, from *in vivo* germinal centre formation to 3-D modelling of affinity maturation", *Immunology*, vol. 108, pp. 274-287.

Allen, C. D. C., Okada, T., & Cyster, J. G. 2007, "Germinal-Center Organization and Cellular Dynamics", *Immunity*, vol. 27, pp. 190-202.

Aloisi, F. & Pujol-Borrell, R. 2006, "Lymphoid neogenesis in chronic inflammatory diseases", *Nature Reviews Immunology*, vol. 6, pp. 205-217.

Amemiya, K., Granger, R. P., & Dalakas, M. C. 2000, "Clonal restriction of T-cell receptor expression by infiltrating lymphocytes in inclusion body myositis persists over time. Studies in repeated muscle biopsies", *Brain*, vol. 123 ( Pt 10), pp. 2030-2039.

Angelopoulou, K., Yu, H., Bharaj, B., Giai, M., & Diamandis, E. P. 2000, "p53 gene mutation, tumor p53 protein overexpression, and serum p53 autoantibody generation in patients with breast cancer.", *Clin.Biochem.*, vol. 33, pp. 53-62.

Arahata, K. & Engel, A. G. 1984, "Monoclonal antibody analysis of mononuclear cells in myopathies. I: Quantitation of subsets according to diagnosis and sites of accumulation and demonstration and counts of muscle fibers invaded by T cells", *Ann.Neurol.*, vol. 16, no. 2, pp. 193-208.

Armengol, M. P., Juan, M., Lucas-Martin, A., Fernandez-Figueras, M. T., Jaraquemada, D., Gallart, T., & Pujol-Borrell, R. 2001, "Thyroid autoimmune disease: demonstration of thyroid antigen-specific B cells and recombination-activating gene expression in chemokine-containing active intrathyroidal germinal centers", *American Journal of Pathology*, vol. 159, pp. 861-873.

Astorri, E., Bombardieri, M., Gabba, S., Peakman, M., Pozzilli, P., & Pitzalis, C. 2010, "Evolution of Ectopic Lymphoid Neogenesis and In Situ Autoantibody Production in Autoimmune Nonobese Diabetic Mice: Cellular and Molecular Characterization of Tertiary Lymphoid Structures in Pancreatic Islets", *The Journal of Immunology*, vol. 185, pp. 3359-3368.

Beltman, J. B., Allen, C. D. C., Cyster, J. G., & de Boer, R. J. 2011, "B cells within germinal centers migrate preferentially from dark to light zone", *Proceedings of the National Academy of Sciences*, vol. 108, pp. 8755-8760.

Ben Hur, H., Cohen, O., Schneider, D., Gurevich, P., Halperin, R., Bala, U., Mozes, M., & Zusman, I. 2002, "The role of lymphocytes and macrophages in human breast tumorigenesis: an immunohistochemical and morphometric study", *Anticancer Res*, vol. 22, pp. 1231-1238.

Berrih-Aknin, S., Ruhlmann, N., Bismuth, J., Cizeron-Clairac, G., Zelman, E., Shachar, I., Dartevelle, P., De Rosbo, N. K., & Le Panse, R. 2009, "CCL21 overexpressed on lymphatic vessels drives thymic hyperplasia in myasthenia", *Ann.Neurol.*, vol. 66, pp. 521-531.

Bianco, A. R. 2004, "Targeting c-erbB2 and other receptors of the c-erbB family: rationale and clinical applications", *J Chemother.*, vol. 16 Suppl 4, pp. 52-54.

Bohan, A. & Peter, J. B. 1975a, "Polymyositis and dermatomyositis (first of two parts)", *N.Engl.J.Med.*, vol. 292, no. 7, pp. 344-347.

Bohan, A. & Peter, J. B. 1975b, "Polymyositis and dermatomyositis (second of two parts)", *N.Engl.J.Med.*, vol. 292, no. 8, pp. 403-407.

Bombardieri, M., Barone, F., Humby, F., Kelly, S., McGurk, M., Morgan, P., Challacombe, S., De Vita, S., Valesini, G., Spencer, J., & Pitzalis, C. 2007a, "Activation-induced cytidine deaminase expression in follicular dendritic cell networks and interfollicular large B cells supports functionality of ectopic lymphoid neogenesis in autoimmune sialoadenitis and MALT lymphoma in Sjogren's syndrome", *The Journal of Immunology*, vol. 179, pp. 4929-4938.

Bombardieri, M., Barone, F., Humby, F., Kelly, S., McGurk, M., Morgan, P., Challacombe, S., De Vita, S., Valesini, G., Spencer, J., & Pitzalis, C. 2007b, "Activation-Induced Cytidine Deaminase Expression in Follicular Dendritic Cell Networks and Interfollicular Large B Cells Supports Functionality of Ectopic Lymphoid Neogenesis in Autoimmune Sialoadenitis and MALT Lymphoma in Sjogren's Syndrome", *The Journal of Immunology*, vol. 179, pp. 4929-4938.

Bradshaw, E. M., Orihuela, A., McArdel, S. L., Salajegheh, M., Amato, A. A., Hafler, D. A., Greenberg, S. A., & O'Connor, K. C. 2007, "A local antigen-driven humoral response is present in the inflammatory myopathies", *The Journal of Immunology*, vol. 178, no. 1, pp. 547-556.

Brattig, N. W., Tenner-Racz, K., Korten, S., Hoerauf, A., & Buttner, D. W. 2010, "Immunohistology of ectopic secondary lymph follicles in subcutaneous nodules from patients with hyperreactive onchocerciasis (sowda)", *Parasitol.Res*, vol. 107, pp. 657-666.

Brink, R. 2007, "Germinal-Center B Cells in the Zone", *Immunity*, vol. 26, pp. 552-554.

Canete, J. D., Santiago, B., Cantaert, T., Sanmarti, R., Palacin, A., Celis, R., Graell, E., Gil-Torregrosa, B., Baeten, D., & Pablos, J. L. 2007, "Ectopic lymphoid neogenesis in psoriatic arthritis", *Annals Rheumatic Disease*, vol. 66, pp. 720-726.

Cardona, A., Garchon, B., Vernet der Garabedian, E., Morel, P., Gajdos, P., & Bach, J.-F. 1994, "Human IgG monoclonal autoantibodies against muscle acetylcholine receptor: direct evidence for clonal heterogeneity of the anti-self humoral response in myasthenia gravis", *J.Neuroimmunol.*, vol. 53, p. 9.

Chalk, C. H., Murray, N. M., Newsom-Davis, J., O'Neill, J. H., & Spiro, S. G. 1990, "Response of the Lambert-Eaton myasthenic syndrome to treatment of associated small-cell lung carcinoma", *Neurology*, vol. 40, pp. 1552-1556.

Cho, H. S., Mason, K., Ramyar, K. X., Stanley, A. M., Gabelli, S. B., Denney, D. W., Jr., & Leahy, D. J. 2003, "Structure of the extracellular region of HER2 alone and in complex with the Herceptin Fab", *Nature*, vol. 421, pp. 756-760.

Chung, L., Genovese, M. C., & Fiorentino, D. F. 2007, "A pilot trial of rituximab in the treatment of patients with dermatomyositis", *Arch.Dermatol.*, vol. 143, no. 6, pp. 763-767.

Cooper, M. A., Willingham, D. L., Brown, D. E., French, A. R., Shih, F. F., & White, A. J. 2007, "Rituximab for the treatment of juvenile dermatomyositis: a report of four pediatric patients", *Arthritis Rheum.*, vol. 56, no. 9, pp. 3107-3111.

Coronella, J. A., Spier, C., Welch, M., Trevor, K. T., Stopeck, A. T., Villar, H., & Hersh, E. M. 2002, "Antigen-Driven Oligoclonal Expansion of Tumor-Infiltrating B Cells in Infiltrating Ductal Carcinoma of the Breast", *The Journal of Immunology*, vol. 169, pp. 1829-1836.

Coronella, J. A., Telleman, P., Kingsbury, G. A., Truong, T. D., Hays, S., & Junghans, R. P. 2001, "Evidence for an antigen-driven humoral immune response in medullary ductal breast cancer", *Cancer Research*, vol. 61, pp. 7889-7899.

Dalakas, M. C. 2004, "The molecular pathophysiology in inflammatory myopathies", *La Revue de Medecine Interne*, vol. 25, no. Supplement 1, p. S14-S16.

Dalakas, M. C. & Hohlfeld, R. 2003, "Polymyositis and dermatomyositis.", *Lancet.362(9388):971-82.*

Dalakas, M. C., Illa, I., Gallardo, E., & Juarez, C. 1997, "Inclusion body myositis and paraproteinemia: incidence and immunopathologic correlations", *Ann.Neurol.*, vol. 41, no. 1, pp. 100-104.

Darlow, J. M. & Stott, D. I. 2005, "VH replacement in immunoglobulin genes", *Immunology*, vol. 114, pp. 155-165.

de Visser, K. E., Korets, L. V., & Coussens, L. M. 2005, "De novo carcinogenesis promoted by chronic inflammation is B lymphocyte dependent", *Cancer Cell*, vol. 7, pp. 411-423.

de Visser, K. E., Eichten, A., & Coussens, L. M. 2006, "Paradoxical roles of the immune system during cancer development", *Nature Reviews Cancer*, vol. 6, pp. 24-37.

Di Noia, J. M. & Neuberger, M. S. 2007, "Molecular Mechanisms of Antibody Somatic Hypermutation", *Annual Review of Biochemistry*, vol. 76, pp. 1-22.

Drachman, D. B. 1994, "Myasthenia gravis", *New England J.Med.*, vol. 330, pp. 1797-1810.

Engel, A. G. & Arahata, K. 1984, "Monoclonal antibody analysis of mononuclear cells in myopathies. II: Phenotypes of autoinvasive cells in polymyositis and inclusion body myositis", *Ann.Neurol.*, vol. 16, no. 2, pp. 209-215.

Farrar, J., Portolano, S., Willcox, N., Vincent, A., Jacobson, L., Newsom-Davis, J., Rapoport, B., & McLachlan, S. M. 1997, "Diverse Fab specific for acetylcholine receptor epitopes from a myasthenia gravis thymus combinatorial library.", *International Immunology*, vol. 9, pp. 1311-1318.

Fostieri, E., Beeson, D., & Tzartos, S. J. 2000, "The conformation of the main immunogenic region on the alpha-subunit of muscle acetylcholine receptor is affected by neighboring receptor subunits", *FEBS Lett.*, vol. 481, pp. 127-130.

Fyhr, I. M., Moslemi, A. R., Mosavi, A. A., Lindberg, C., Tarkowski, A., & Oldfors, A. 1997, "Oligoclonal expansion of muscle infiltrating T cells in inclusion body myositis", *J.Neuroimmunol.*, vol. 79, no. 2, pp. 185-189.

Genta, R. M., Hamner, H. W., & Graham, D. Y. 1993, "Gastric lymphoid follicles in Helicobacter pylori infection: frequency, distribution, and response to triple therapy", *Hum.Pathol.*, vol. 24, pp. 577-583.

Gerhard, N., Krenn, V., Magalhaes, R., Morawietz, L., Brandlein, S., & Konig, A. 2002, "IgVH-genes analysis from psoriatic arthritis shows involvement of antigen-activated synovial B-lymphocytes", *Z.Rheumatol.*, vol. 61, pp. 718-727.

Ghosh, S., Steere, A. C., Stollar, B. D., & Huber, B. T. 2005, "In situ diversification of the antibody repertoire in chronic Lyme arthritis synovium", *J.Immunol.*, vol. 174, pp. 2860-2869.

Graus, Y. F., de Baets, M. H., Parren, P. W. H. I., Berrih-Aknin, S., Wokke, J., van Breda Vriesman, P. J., & Burton, D. R. 1997, "Human anti-nicotinic acetylcholine receptor recombinant Fab fragments isolated from thymus-derived phage display libraries from myasthenia gravis patients reflect predominant specificities in serum and block the action of pathogenic serum antibodies", *J.Immunol.*, vol. 158, pp. 1919-1929.

Greenberg, S. A., Bradshaw, E. M., Pinkus, J. L., Pinkus, G. S., Burleson, T., Due, B., Bregoli, L., O'Connor, K. C., & Amato, A. A. 2005, "Plasma cells in muscle in inclusion body myositis and polymyositis", *Neurology*, vol. 65, no. 11, pp. 1782-1787.

Greenberg, S. A., Sanoudou, D., Haslett, J. N., Kohane, I. S., Kunkel, L. M., Beggs, A. H., & Amato, A. A. 2002, "Molecular profiles of inflammatory myopathies", *Neurology*, vol. 59, no. 8, pp. 1170-1182.

Hauser, A. E., Shlomchik, M. J., & Haberman, A. M. 2007, "In vivo imaging studies shed light on germinal-centre development", *Nature Reviews Immunology*, vol. 7, pp. 499-504.

Hershberg, U., Uduman, M., Shlomchik, M. J., & Kleinstein, S. H. 2008, "Improved methods for detecting selection by mutation analysis of Ig V region sequences", *International Immunology*, vol. 20, pp. 683-694.

Hill, M. E., SHIONO, H., Newsom-Davis, J., & Willcox, N. 2008, "The myasthenia gravis thymus: a rare source of human autoantibody-secreting plasma cells for testing potential therapeutics", *J.Neuroimmunol.*, vol. 201-202, pp. 50-56.

Hofbauer, M., Wiesener, S., Babbe, H., Roers, A., Wekerle, H., Dornmair, K., Hohlfeld, R., & Goebels, N. 2003, "Clonal tracking of autoaggressive T cells in polymyositis by combining laser microdissection, single-cell PCR, and CDR3-spectratype analysis", *Proc.Natl.Acad.Sci.U.S.A*, vol. 100, no. 7, pp. 4090-4095.

Hortobagyi, G. N. 2005, "Trastuzumab in the Treatment of Breast Cancer", *The New England Journal of Medicine*, vol. 353, pp. 1734-1736.

Humby, F., Bombardieri, M., Manzo, A., Kelly, S., Blades, M. C., Kirkham, B., Spencer, J., & Pitzalis, C. 2009, "Ectopic Lymphoid Structures Support Ongoing Production of Class-Switched Autoantibodies in Rheumatoid Synovium", *PLoS Medicine*, vol. 6, pp. 0001-0017.

Igarashi, H., Hashimoto, J., Tomita, T., YOSHIKAWA, H., & Ishihara, K. 2010, "TP53 mutations coincide with the ectopic expression of activation-induced cytidine deaminase in the fibroblast-like synoviocytes derived from a fraction of patients with rheumatoid arthritis", *Clinical & Experimental Immunology*, vol. 161, pp. 71-80.

Jang, I. K., Cronshaw, D. G., Xie, L. k., Fang, G., Zhang, J., Oh, H., Fu, Y. X., Gu, H., & Zou, Y. 2011, "Growth-factor receptor-bound protein-2 (Grb2) signaling in B cells controls lymphoid follicle organization and germinal center reaction", *Proceedings of the National Academy of Sciences*, vol. 108, pp. 7926-7931.

Kaiserling, E. 2001, "Newly-formed lymph nodes in the submucosa in chronic inflammatory bowel disease", *Lymphology*, vol. 34, pp. 22-29.

Klein, U. & Dalla-Favera, R. 2008, "Germinal centres: role in B-cell physiology and malignancy", *Nature Reviews Immunology*, vol. 8, pp. 22-33.

Knecht, H., Saremaslani, P., & Hedinger, C. 1981, "Immunohistological findings in Hashimoto's thyroiditis, focal lymphocytic thyroiditis and thyroiditis de Quervain. Comparative study", *Virchows Archiv - Abteilung A Pathologische Anatomie*, vol. 393, pp. 215-231.

Kotlan, B., Simsa, P., Gruel, N., Foldi, J., Fridman, W. H., Petranyi, G., & Teillaud, J. L. 2000, "A scFv phage display mini library generated from the immunoglobulin repertoire of breast medullary carcinoma infiltrating B lymphocytes", *Dis.Markers*, vol. 16, pp. 25-27.

Kotlan, B., Simsa, P., Teillaud, J. L., Fridman, W. H., Toth, J., McKnight, M., & Glassy, M. C. 2005, "Novel Ganglioside Antigen Identified by B Cells in Human Medullary Breast Carcinomas: The Proof of Principle Concerning the Tumor-Infiltrating B Lymphocytes", *The Journal of Immunology*, vol. 175, pp. 2278-2285.

Krystufkova, O., Vallerskog, T., Barbasso, H. S., Mann, H., Putova, I., Belacek, J., Malmstrom, V., Trollmo, C., Vencovsky, J., & Lundberg, I. E. 2008, "Increased serum levels of B-cell activating factor (BAFF) in subsets of patients with idiopathic inflammatory myopathies", *Annals of the Rheumatic Diseases.*

Lang, B. & Vincent, A. 2009, "Autoimmune disorders of the neuromuscular junction", *Curr.Opin.Pharmacol.*, vol. 9, pp. 336-340.

Le Panse, R., Bismuth, J., Cizeron-Clairac, G., Weiss, J. M., Cufi, P., Dartevelle, P., De Rosbo, N. K., & Berrih-Aknin, S. 2010, "Thymic remodeling associated with hyperplasia in myasthenia gravis", *Autoimmunity*, vol. 43, pp. 401-412.

Le Panse, R., Cizeron-Clairac, G., Bismuth, J., & Berrih-Aknin, S. 2006, "Microarrays reveal distinct gene signatures in the thymus of seropositive and seronegative myasthenia gravis patients and the role of CC chemokine ligand 21 in thymic hyperplasia", *The Journal of Immunology*, vol. 177, pp. 7868-7879.

Leavy, O. 2010, "B cells: Illuminating the dark zone", *Nature Reviews Immunology*, vol. 11, p. 8.

Levine, T. D. M. 2005, "Rituximab in the Treatment of Dermatomyositis: An Open-Label Pilot Study.", *Arthritis & Rheumatism*, vol. 52, no. 2, pp. 601-607.

Liversidge, J., Dick, A., Cheng, Y.-F., Scott, G. B., & Forrester, J. V. 1993, "Retinal antigen specific lymphocytes, TCR-gamma delta T cells and $CD5^+$ B cells cultured from the vitreous in acute sympathetic ophthalmitis", *Autoimmunity*, vol. 15, pp. 257-266.

Maddison, P. & Lang, B. 2008, "Paraneoplastic neurological autoimmunity and survival in small-cell lung cancer", *J.Neuroimmunol.*, vol. 201-202, pp. 159-162.

Mantegazza, R., Andreetta, F., Bernasconi, P., Baggi, F., Oksenberg, J. R., Simoncini, O., Mora, M., Cornelio, F., & Steinman, L. 1993, "Analysis of T cell receptor repertoire of muscle-infiltrating T lymphocytes in polymyositis. Restricted V alpha/beta rearrangements may indicate antigen-driven selection", *J.Clin.Invest*, vol. 91, no. 6, pp. 2880-2886.

Manzo, A. & Pitzalis, C. 2007, "Lymphoid tissue reactions in rheumatoid arthritis", *Autoimmunity Reviews*, vol. 7, pp. 30-34.

Matthews, I., Sims, G. P., Ledwidge, S., Stott, D. I., Beeson, D., Willcox, N., & Vincent, A. 2002, "Antibodies to Acetylcholine Receptor in Parous Women with Myasthenia: Evidence for Immunization by Fetal Antigen", *Laboratory Investigation*, vol. 82, pp. 1407-1417.

Matzinger, P. 2007, "Friendly and dangerous signals: is the tissue in control?", *Nat Immunol*, vol. 8, pp. 11-13.

Mauri, C. 2010, "Regulation of immunity and autoimmunity by B cells", *Current Opinion in Immunology*, vol. 22, pp. 761-767.

Meraouna, A., Cizeron-Clairac, G., Panse, R. L., Bismuth, J., Truffault, F., Tallaksen, C., & Berrih-Aknin, S. 2006, "The chemokine CXCL13 is a key molecule in autoimmune myasthenia gravis", *Blood*, vol. 108, pp. 432-440.

Mielnik, P., Wiesik-Szewczyk, E., Olesinska, M., Chwalinska-Sadowska, H., & Zabek, J. 2006, "Clinical features and prognosis of patients with idiopathic inflammatory myopathies and anti-Jo-1 antibodies", *Autoimmunity*, vol. 39, no. 3, pp. 243-247.

Minton, K. 2011, "B cells: Short- and long-term memory", *Nature Reviews Immunology*, vol. 11, pp. 160-161.

Mosnier, J.-F., Degott, C., Marcellin, P., Henin, D., Erlinger, S., & Benhamou, J.-P. 1993, "The intraportal lymphoid nodule and its environment in chronic active hepatitis C: An Immunohistochemical study", *Hepatology*, vol. 17, pp. 366-371.

Nacionales, D. C., Weinstein, J. S., Yan, X. J., Albesiano, E., Lee, P. Y., Kelly-Scumpia, K. M., Lyons, R., Satoh, M., Chiorazzi, N., & Reeves, W. H. 2009, "B Cell Proliferation, Somatic Hypermutation, Class Switch Recombination, and Autoantibody Production in Ectopic Lymphoid Tissue in Murine Lupus", *The Journal of Immunology*, vol. 182, pp. 4226-4236.

Nahta, R., Hung, M. C., & Esteva, F. J. 2004, "The HER-2-Targeting Antibodies Trastuzumab and Pertuzumab Synergistically Inhibit the Survival of Breast Cancer Cells", *Cancer Research*, vol. 64, pp. 2343-2346.

Nemazee, D. 2006, "Receptor editing in lymphocyte development and central tolerance", *Nature Reviews Immunology*, vol. 6, pp. 728-740.

Nzula, S., Going, J. J., & Stott, D. I. 2003a, "Antigen-driven clonal proliferation, somatic hypermutation and selection of B-lymphocytes infiltrating human ductal breast carcinoma", *Cancer Res.*, vol. 63, pp. 3275-3280.

Nzula, S., Going, J. J., & Stott, D. I. 2003b, "The role of B lymphocytes in breast cancer: a review and current status", *Cancer Therapy*, vol. 1, pp. 353-362.

Park, C. S. & Choi, Y. S. 2005, "How do follicular dendritic cells interact intimately with B cells in the germinal centre?", *Immunology*, vol. 114, pp. 2-10.

Patakas, A., Platt, A. M., Butcher, J. P., Maffia, P., McInnes, I. B., Brewer, J. M., Garside, P., & Benson, R. A. 2011, "Putative existence of reciprocal dialogue between Tfh and B cells and its impact on infectious and autoimmune disease", *Immunol Lett.*, vol. In press.

Petrarca, C., Casalino, B., Mensdorff-Pouilly, S., Rughetti, A., Rahimi, H., Scambia, G., Hilgers, J., Frati, L., & Nuti, M. 1999, "Isolation of MUC1-primed B lymphocytes from tumour-draining lymph nodes by immunomagnetic beads", *Cancer Immunology, Immunotherapy*, vol. 47, pp. 272-277.

Poea-Guyon, S., Christadoss, P., Le Panse, R., Guyon, T., De Baets, M., Wakkach, A., Bidault, J., Tzartos, S., & Berrih-Aknin, S. 2005, "Effects of cytokines on acetylcholine receptor expression: implications for myasthenia gravis", *The Journal of Immunology*, vol. 174, pp. 5941-5949.

Prineas, J. W. 1979, "Multiple sclerosis: presence of lymphatic capillaries and lymphoid tissue in the brain and spinal cord", *Science*, vol. 203, pp. 1123-1125.

Renard, V. & Leach, D. R. 2007, "Perspectives on the development of a therapeutic HER-2 cancer vaccine", *Vaccine*, vol. 25 Suppl 2, p. B17-B23.

Renard, V., Sonderbye, L., Ebbehoj, K., Rasmussen, P. B., Gregorius, K., Gottschalk, T., Mouritsen, S., Gautam, A., & Leach, D. R. 2003, "HER-2 DNA and Protein Vaccines Containing Potent Th Cell Epitopes Induce Distinct Protective and Therapeutic Antitumor Responses in HER-2 Transgenic Mice", *The Journal of Immunology*, vol. 171, pp. 1588-1595.

Rider, L. G. 2007, "The heterogeneity of juvenile myositis", *Autoimmun.Rev.*, vol. 6, no. 4, pp. 241-247.

Rosenfeld, M. R. & Dalmau, J. 2010, "Update on paraneoplastic and autoimmune disorders of the central nervous system", *Semin.Neurol.*, vol. 30, pp. 320-331.

Rothe, A., Klimka, A., Tur, M. K., Pfitzner, T., Huhn, M., Sasse, S., Mallmann, P., Engert, A., & Barth, S. 2004, "Construction of phage display libraries from reactive lymph nodes of breast carcinoma patients and selection for specifically binding human single chain Fv on cell lines", *Int.J Mol.Med*, vol. 14, pp. 729-735.

Salajegheh, M., Pinkus, J. L., Amato, A. A., Morehouse, C., Jallal, B., Yao, Y., & Greenberg, S. A. 2010, "Permissive environment for B-cell maturation in myositis muscle in the absence of B-cell follicles", *Muscle & Nerve*, vol. 42, no. 4, pp. 576-583.

Seitz, S., Schneider, C. K., Malotka, J., Nong, X., Engel, A. G., Wekerle, H., Hohlfeld, R., & Dornmair, K. 2006, "Reconstitution of paired T cell receptor alpha- and beta-chains from microdissected single cells of human inflammatory tissues", *Proc.Natl.Acad.Sci.U.S.A*, vol. 103, no. 32, pp. 12057-12062.

Serafini, B., Rosicarelli, B., Magliozzi, R., Stigliano, E., & Aloisi, F. 2004, "Detection of ectopic B-cell follicles with germinal centers in the meninges of patients with secondary progressive multiple sclerosis", *Brain Pathol.*, vol. 14, pp. 164-174.

Shiono, H., Roxanis, I., Zhang, W., Sims, G. P., Meager, A., Jacobson, L. W., Liu, J. L., Matthews, I., Wong, Y. L., Bonifati, M., Micklem, K., Stott, D. I., Todd, J. A., Beeson, D., Vincent, A., & Willcox, N. 2003, "Scenarios for autoimmunization of T and B cells in myasthenia gravis", *Ann.N.Y.Acad.Sci.*, vol. 998, pp. 237-256.

Sims, G. P., Hiroyuki, S., Willcox, N., & Stott, D. I. 2001, "Somatic Hypermutation and Selection of B Cells in Thymic Germinal Centers Responding to Acetyl Choline Receptor in Myasthenia Gravis", *J.Immunol.*, vol. 167, pp. 1935-1944.

Simsa, P., Teillaud, J. L., Stott, D. I., Toth, J., & Kotlan, B. 2005, "Tumor-infiltrating B cell immunoglobulin variable region gene usage in invasive ductal breast carcinoma", *Pathol Oncol.Res*, vol. 11, pp. 92-97.

Snijdewint, F. G., Mensdorff-Pouilly, S., Karuntu-Wanamarta, A. H., Verstraeten, A. A., Livingston, P. O., Hilgers, J., & Kenemans, P. 2001, "Antibody-dependent cell-mediated cytotoxicity can be induced by MUC1 peptide vaccination of breast cancer patients", *Int.J Cancer*, vol. 93, pp. 97-106.

Stolte, M. & Eidt, S. 1989, "Lymphoid follicles in antral mucosa: immune response to Campylobacter pylori?", *J Clin.Pathol.*, vol. 42, pp. 1269-1271.

Stott, D. I., Hiepe, F., Hummel, M., Steinhauser, G., & Berek, C. 1998, "Antigen-driven clonal proliferation of B cells within the target tissue of an autoimmune disease . The salivary glands of patients with Sjögren's syndrome.", *J.Clin.Invest.*, vol. 102, pp. 938-946.

Stott, D. I. & Sims, G. P. 2000, "Application of scFv-phage display to analysis of B-cell clones proliferating in the salivary glands of a patient with Sjögren's syndrome", *Disease Markers*, vol. 16, pp. 21-23.

Swofford, D. L. 1993, "PAUP: Phylogenetic analysis using parsimony, version 3.1,".

Taylor-Papadimitriou, J., Burchell, J. M., Plunkett, T., Graham, R., Correa, I., Miles, D., & Smith, M. 2002, "MUC1 and the immunobiology of cancer", *J Mammary.Gland.Biol.Neoplasia.*, vol. 7, pp. 209-221.

Victora, G. D., Schwickert, T. A., Fooksman, D. R., Kamphorst, A. O., Meyer-Hermann, M., Dustin, M. L., & Nussenzweig, M. C. (12-11-2010)Germinal Center Dynamics Revealed by Multiphoton Microscopy witháa Photoactivatable Fluorescent Reporter. Cell 143[4], 592-605.

Vincent, A. 2002, "Unravelling the pathogenesis of myasthenia gravis", *Nature Revs.Immunol.*, vol. 2, pp. 797-804.

Vincent, A. & et al. 1997, "Thymoma and autoimmune neurological disorders," in *Epithelial Tumours of the Thymus*, A. Marx & H. K. Muller-Hermelink, eds., Plenum Press, New York, pp. 195-204.

Visco, V., Bei, R., Moriconi, E., Gianni, W., Kraus, M. H., & Muraro, R. 2000, "ErbB2 immune response in breast cancer patients with soluble receptor ectodomain.", *Am.J.Pathol.*, vol. 156, pp. 1417-1424.

von Mensdorff-Pouilly, S., Verstraeten, A. A., Kenemans, P., Snijdewint, F. G. M., Kok, A., Van Kamp, G. J., Paul, M. A., Van Diest, P. J., Meijer, S., & Hilgers, J. 2000, "Survival in Early Breast Cancer Patients Is Favorably Influenced by a Natural Humoral Immune Response to Polymorphic Epithelial Mucin", *Journal of Clinical Oncology*, vol. 18, p. 574.

Wallace, W. A. H., Howie, S. E. M., Krajewski, A. S., & Lamb, D. 1996, "The immunological architecture of B-lymphocyte aggregates in cryptogenic fibrosing alveolitis", *J.Pathol.*, vol. 178, pp. 323-329.

Weiser, A. A., Wittenbrink, N., Zhang, L., Schmelzer, A. I., Valai, A., & Or-Guil, M. 2011, "Affinity maturation of B cells involves not only a few but a whole spectrum of relevant mutations", *International Immunology*, vol. 23, pp. 345-356.

Yoshitake, T., Masunaga, A., Sugawara, I., Nakamura, H., Itoyama, S., & Oka, T. 1994, "A comparative histological and immunohistochemical study of thymomas with and without myasthenia gravis", *Surgery Today*, vol. 24, pp. 1044-1049.

Zampieri, S., Ghirardello, A., Iaccarino, L., Tarricone, E., Gambari, P. F., & Doria, A. 2005, "Anti-Jo-1 antibodies", *Autoimmunity*, vol. 38, no. 1, pp. 73-78.

Zuckerman, N. S., Howard, W. A., Bismuth, J., Gibson, K., Edelman, H., Berrih-Aknin, S., Dunn-Walters, D., & Mehr, R. 2010, "Ectopic GC in the thymus of myasthenia gravis patients show characteristics of normal GC", *Eur.J Immunol*, vol. 40, pp. 1150-1161.

## 22

# Myasthenia Gravis: New Insights into the Effect of MuSK Antibodies and Acetylcholinesterase Inhibitors

Anna Rostedt Punga
*Uppsala University Hospital, Institute of Neuroscience,*
*Department of Clinical Neurophysiology*
*Sweden*

## 1. Introduction

Myasthenia Gravis (MG) is an autoimmune neuromuscular disorder in which autoantibodies are directed against muscle receptors. MG causes fluctuating muscle weakness, which often involves droopy eyelids, swallowing difficulties and generalized muscle fatigue in the neck and proximal muscles of the legs and arms. The prevalence of MG is two times higher in women than in men. Age is also a prevailing factor, affecting women whom are 20-30 years of age, whereas men are 60-80 years old (Osserman and Genkins 1971). The annual incidence of MG has been reported to be about 3-4 cases per million and the overall prevalence about 60 cases per million; however, higher rates have recently been suggested, indicating a potential prevalence as high as 20 per 100 000 persons. (Kalb, Matell et al. 2002; Phillips 2003). The most common form of MG is associated with antibodies against the nicotinic acetylcholine receptor (AChR), present in about 85% of patients with generalised MG (Vincent and Newsom Davis 1980). In 2001 antibodies against the muscle specific tyrosine kinase (MuSK) were identified in about 40-70% of patients without detectable AChR antibodies (Hoch, McConville et al. 2001). Furthermore, in approximately 5-10% of patients with the generalized disease no antibodies are present in the serum, but these cases all have the features of an autoimmune course. This chapter deals with the clinical phenotype, neurophysiology and consequences at the neuromuscular junction of the autoimmune attack associated with MG as well as treatment options. The focus will be on MuSK antibody seropositive (MuSK+) MG in human patients and the experimental murine model of MuSK+ MG.

## 2. Myasthenia gravis: Targets, consequences and treatment of the autoimmune attack

In 1960, the Scottish neurologist Simpson suggested that MG might be caused by an autoimmune mechanism based on the relatively high incidence of concomitant autoimmune diseases, e.g. rheumatoid arthritis and systemic lupus erytematosus, among the MG patients (Simpson 1960). Abnormalities of the thymus gland were discovered, as well as the presence of lymphorrages in muscles, which further supported Simpson´s hypothesis (Miller 1961). A humoral factor was also implicated in the development of MG after it was found that approximately 20% of babies whose mothers had a diagnosis of MG developed transient neonatal MG (Strickroot 1942). Over the years, the targets of the autoimmune response, the mechanism at the neuromuscular junction (NMJ), clinical and neurophysiological features and treatment options have been outlined and improved.

### 2.1 Targets of the autoimmune attack

The MG autoimmune attack is directed against the receptors and proteins of the neuromuscular junction. Some patients have a thymoma which presents with antibodies against other proteins, seen in the case of thymic pathology. It is not yet clear what triggers the production of autoantibodies but MG is considered to be both a B-and T-cell mediated disorder. The autoimmune attack results in disruption of the postsynaptic endplate morphology and subsequently impaired neuromuscular transmission, which in turn causes the typical symptoms of fatigable skeletal muscle weakness.

#### 2.1.1 Nicotinic acetylcholine receptors

About 80-85% of patients with generalized MG and 55% of patients with ocular MG have autoantibodies directed against the nicotinic AChR (AChR+) (Lindstrom, Seybold et al. 1976; Vincent and Newsom-Davis 1985). The AChR antibodies (Abs) are highly specific for MG and impair the function of the AChRs by three main mechanisms: (1) blocking of the acetylcholine (ACh) binding site (Lefvert, Cuenoud et al. 1981); (2) cross-linking of the AChRs that results in both a functional blockade and accelerated degradation of the AChRs (Drachman, Adams et al. 1981) and (3) complement activation that results in destruction of the postsynaptic muscle membrane (Engel, Lambert et al. 1977). The main immunogenic region (MIR), against which the majority of AChR-Abs in MG or experimental autoimmune MG (EAMG) are directed, is located at the extracellular end of α1 subunits. Pathologically significant autoantibodies must be directed at the extracellular surface of the AChR, where they can bind *in vivo* (Lindstrom, Luo et al. 2008). In MG and chronic EAMG in rats, autoantibodies bound to muscle AChRs target the postsynaptic membrane for complement-binding, which results in focal lysis and reduces the number of AchRs. This chain of events in turn disrupts the architecture of the postsynaptic membrane through an alteration of its normal position next to active zones of ACh release (Lindstrom 2000). The AChR-Abs are of IgG1 type and are typically measured using a standard radioimmunoassay in which the antigen consists of AChR from human muscle labelled with $[^{125}I]$α-bungarotoxin

#### 2.1.2 Muscle specific tyrosine kinase (MuSK)

MuSK is essential in the early development of the NMJ, as well as in the maintenance of the organized structure of the postsynaptic apparatus through clustering of AChRs (Hopf and Hoch 1998; Liyanage, Hoch et al. 2002; Wang, Zhang et al. 2006) (Figure 1). It is further necessary for maintaining the organized structure and integrity of the neuromuscular synapse, as perturbations in MuSK protein expression cause a pronounced disassembly of the NMJ (Kong, Barzaghi et al. 2004; Hesser, Henschel et al. 2006). MuSK mutant mice do not experience successful synaptic differentiation and agrin mutant mice, have small AChR clusters which are scattered abnormally throughout the muscle (DeChiara, Bowen et al. 1996). Other players which are required for synaptogenesis include Dok-7, rapsyn and Lrp4. Dok-7 is a downstream adaptor protein to MuSK, and is important for maintaining the structural integrity of the endplate (Okada, Inoue et al. 2006). Lrp4 was recently identified as the co-receptor for neural agrin and forms a complex which mediates MuSK activation upon agrin-binding (Kim, Stiegler et al. 2008; Zhang, Luo et al. 2008). Rapsyn is a membrane-associated cytoplasmic protein that is concentrated at the NMJ and crucial for the clustering of AChRs (Colledge and Froehner 1998).

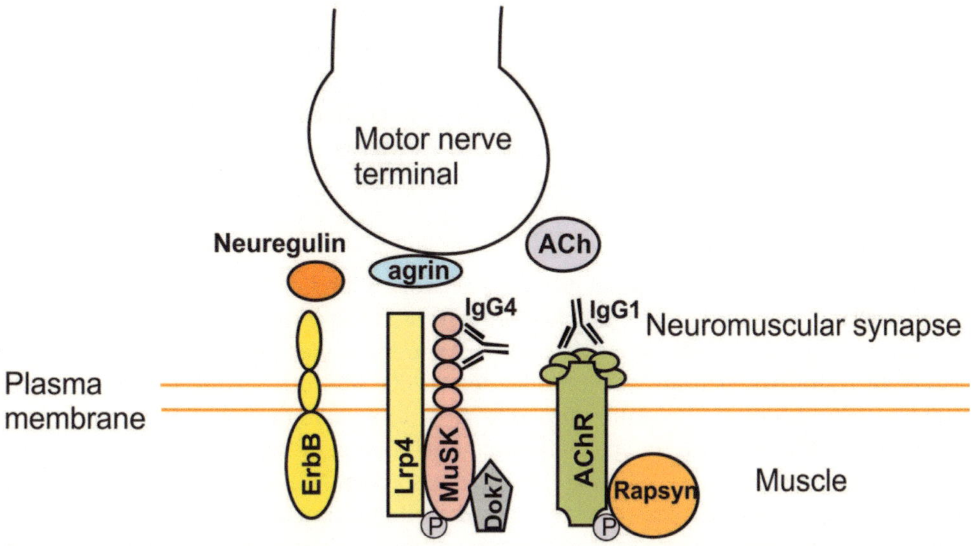


Fig. 1. Agrin-MuSK signalling at the neuromuscular synapse. Neural agrin is released from the motor nerve terminal and attaches to MuSK along with its co-receptor Lrp-4. This binding of agrin induces a cascade of phosphorylation on MuSK and then on other intracellular proteins, such as rapsyn, enabling the clustering of AChR. The autoantibodies in MuSK-antibody seropositive MG are mainly of IgG4-subtype and attach to the IgG-like domains in the extracellular domain of MuSK. The autoantibodies in AChR-antibody seropositive MG are of IgG1 subtype and bind to the main immunogenic region of the AChR, blocking the acetylcholine binding and activating complement pathways which destroy AChRs. Another important pathway at the synapse is ErbB with its neurotransmitter neuregulin.

In 2001, antibodies against the MuSK (MuSK-Ab) were identified and found to be present in about 40-70% of patients who are seronegative for AChR-Abs (Hoch, McConville et al. 2001; Bartoccioni, Marino et al. 2003; Rostedt Punga, Ahlqvist et al. 2006). MuSK-Abs have also been identified in 14% of patients who have been characterized as having low titers of AChR-Abs; thus, MuSK-Abs are not entirely restricted to the AChR-Ab seronegative MG subgroup (Rostedt Punga, Ahlqvist et al. 2006). While MuSK-antibodies are predominantly of IgG4 subclass, up to 30% of the MuSK-antibodies belong to the IgG1 subclass (McConville, Farrugia et al. 2004). Despite the controversial pathogenicity of MuSK-Abs (Lindstrom 2004; Selcen, Fukuda et al. 2004), their role in disrupting the NMJ and development MG has been evidenced in animal studies with MuSK immunization (Shigemoto, Kubo et al. 2006) and passive transfer of sera from MuSK+ patients (Cole, Reddel et al. 2008). Patient-anti MuSK abs have been shown to inhibit neural agrin-mediated formation of AChR clusters in vitro (Hoch, McConville et al. 2001; Cole, Reddel et al. 2008).

### 2.1.3 Thymoma associated antibodies and rapsyn antibodies

MG patients with a tumour of the thymus, thymoma, may have antibodies not only directed to the AChR but also to other components of striated muscle. Two of these components strongly associated with a thymoma are the sarcomeric cytoskeletal protein titin and the calcium release channel of the sarcoplasmic reticulum, the ryanodine receptor (Aarli, Stefansson et al. 1990; Mygland, Tysnes et al. 1992). On the basis of their cross-striational pattern by immunofluorescent staining, they have been named antistriational antibodies.

A fifth antigen is the small postsynaptic AChR-associated protein rapsyn. Antibodies directed against rapsyn have been detected in about 15% of MG-patients, both in patients with and without AChR-Abs. Rapsyn is precisely colocalized with AChRs from the early stages of NMJ formation and similar to MuSK, rapsyn is necessary for the clustering of AChRs (Hall and Sanes 1993; Gautam, Noakes et al. 1995).

### 2.1.4 Seronegative myasthenia

A minority of MG patients is consistently negative for antibodies to the soluble native AChR or MuSK used in standard assays, and is often referred to as seronegative myasthenia gravis (SNMG). There could be antibodies to another neuromuscular junction protein, but given the clinical features which are very similar to AChR+ MG, it is likely that the failure of current assays to detect the antibodies due to a loss of antigenic determinants in the solubilized AChR used in the radioimmunoprecipitation assay, or because the AChR antibodies have only low affinity/avidity for the soluble AChR, is responsible. This was proven in 2008, when a cell-based assay showed that IgG from 66% of SNMG sera, binds to AChRs when they are clustered on the surface of a non-muscle cell line (HEK693 kidney cells) by co-transfecting with rapsyn (Leite, Jacob et al. 2008). This study also confirmed that these Abs are mainly complement activating IgG1, and some were able to induce complement deposition on the AChR clusters. SNMG patients typically behave as AChR+ MG with a similar clinical phenotype and improvement upon immunosuppressive treatment. Patients with symptoms of MG in whom no autoantibodies can be detected are called "seronegative" (AChR-). However, there are strong indicators that AChR- MG also has an autoimmune etiology. In fact a small proportion of AChR- patients were recently found to have autoantibodies to Lrp4, via an in-vitro luciferase-reporter immunoprecipitation method (Higuchi, Hamuro et al. 2011). These antibodies inhibit binding of Lrp4 to its ligand and predominantly belong to the immunoglobulin G1 (IgG1) subclass, a complement activator. Thus, in the future it is anticipated that antibodies in the sera from SNMG patients will be identified.

### 2.2 Clinical picture in different subsets of MG

The clinical hallmark of MG is painless, fatigable weakness, located primarily in the proximal muscle groups of the neck, face, shoulders, arms and legs. The muscle weakness may fluctuate daily, but typically worsens after physical activity and improves with rest. The course of MG is variable, although in most cases the disease is chronic and requires lifelong immunosuppressive medication. Long-lasting remissions are uncommon; however this has been reported in 10–20% of patients (Grob, Brunner et al. 2008). Many patients experience intermittent worsening of symptoms triggered by emotional stress, viral or bacterial infections, due to an upregulation of the immune system, and different medications, including certain antibiotics.

Weakness in the extraocular muscles results in ptosis and diplopia, whereas bulbar muscle weakness causes dysarthria, dysphagia and in worst cases also dyspnea necessitating respirator assistance (myasthenic crisis). Fatigue of the proximal leg and arm muscles causes difficulties in climbing stairs and holding the arms above the head. MG can be subdivided into an ocular and generalized form. In the ocular form, symptoms are restricted to the extraocular muscles resulting in ptosis and diplopia. Most patients, who generalize, i.e. develop symptoms of fatigue in muscles of proximal limbs, facial and bulbar muscles do so within 2 years. Studies have tried to identify factors to help predict prognosis but no such factors have been characterised, including neurophysiological examinations (Rostedt, Sanders et al. 2000). Patients with generalised MG can be divided into early-onset disease (onset <40 years of age) and late-onset disease. Female patients predominate the early-onset group, and often have AChR antibodies and an enlarged hyperplastic thymus gland. Patients with onset after the age of 40 years are more often male and usually have a normal appearance of the thymus. About 10–15% of patients with MG have a thymoma, a tumour of the thymus. MG associated with a thymoma, which is equally common in men and women, can occur at any age and the clinical presentation is often more severe with progressive generalized and oropharyngeal weakness (Evoli, Minisci et al. 2002)

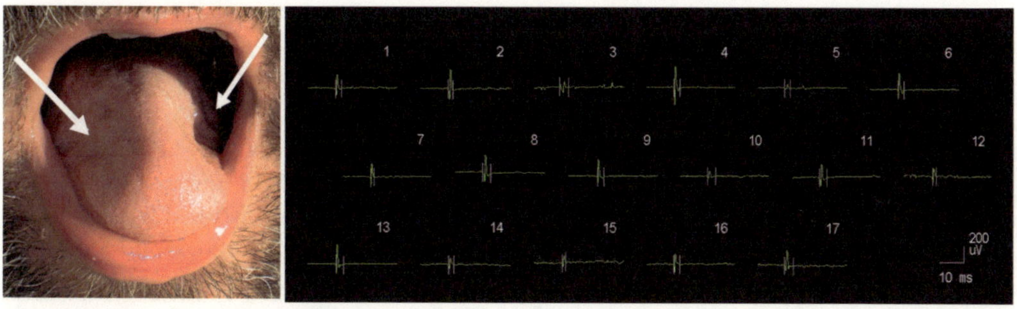


Fig. 2. Clinical and neurophysiological features which can be observed in MuSK+ MG. Left panel: A close-up of the tongue shows pronounced atrophy on the lateral sides of the glossus muscle. Right panel: EMG in these areas of the muscle revealed a myopathic picture.

MuSK+ patients usually differ from the AChR+ patients by having a very focal distribution of the muscle weakness, sometimes being limited to only the neck extensor muscles or to the bulbar muscles. A large Italian cohort of MuSK+ patients revealed a specific pattern of muscle weakness, with prevalent involvement of cranial and bulbar muscles and a high frequency of respiratory crises, and less severe and inconsistent involvement of limb muscles (Evoli, Tonali et al. 2003). This selective muscle weakness of faciobulbar and neck muscles is often very focal, with relative sparing of other muscles. Additionally, muscles which are usually not affected in AChR+ MG, including the paraspinal and esophageal muscles, may be involved (Sanders and Juel 2008). Contrary to conventional AChR+ MG patients, the majority of MuSK+ patients do not experience symptomatic relief from acetylcholine esterase inhibitors (AChEI) (Evoli, Tonali et al. 2003), but may respond with pronounced nicotinic adverse effects, such as muscle fasciculations and cramps (Punga, Flink et al. 2006). Pronounced muscle atrophy of facial muscles has also been described in MuSK+ patients and verified on MRI examinations of the temporalis, masseter and lingual muscles (Farrugia, Robson et al. 2006; Zouvelou, Rentzos et al. 2009). This facial muscle weakness is often seen as a flattening of the forehead and in some patients atrophy of the tongue (Figure 2) is pronounced.

### 2.2.1 Neurophysiology in MG: disturbed neuromuscular transmission

Neurophysiological tests are essential in the diagnosis of MG. There are two different *in vivo* examinations to confirm disturbed neuromuscular transmission: (1) Repetitive nerve stimulation (RNS) and (2) Single-fiber EMG (SFEMG). At low frequency RNS (3 Hz) there is typically a progressive decline in the compound muscle action potential (CMAP) amplitude. This decrement is due to the "run down" of the amplitude of individual end plate potentials (EPP). In MG, a certain proportion of potentials are reduced to a subthreshold level and therefore insufficient to depolarize the muscle fiber. Since the CMAP constitutes the sum of activated muscle fibers, its amplitude is successively reduced with an increasing block of individual muscle fibers. If the amplitude drop, or decrement, exceeds a certain limit, e.g. 5%, the finding is considered significant. RNS is first performed at rest and then after 20 seconds of maximal voluntary muscle contraction, when an improvement of the decrement is typically seen, known as post-exercise facilitation. Additional tests after 1 and 3 minutes explore post-exercise exhaustion.

The amount of ACh released at the NMJ at different times varies minimally, resulting in comparable variations in the rise of EPP and the muscle fiber pair interpotential intervals. This variability is highly sensitive to neuromuscular transmission abnormalities and is increased in MG patients. SFEMG, which is the most sensitive test for MG, measures this variability and can be performed during voluntary muscle contraction or when the nerve is electrically stimulated (Stalberg, Ekstedt et al. 1974). SFEMG reveals deficits of neuromuscular transmission in 95%-99% of MG patients (Sanders 2002) and has proven to be a sensitive marker of early improvement in clinical trials in MG (Meriggioli and Rowin 2003). With an uptake area of about 300 μm the SFEMG electrode selectively records action potentials from a small number (usually 2 or 3) of muscle fibers innervated by a single motor unit and can detect subclinical defects in neuromuscular transmission. The variations in the difference in conduction times taken by impulses from the nerve branching point via the motor end plates along each muscle fiber to the recording site are called jitter. The jitter reflects the safety factor of neuromuscular transmission and in normal conditions the jitter is low. When jitter measurements are made in voluntarily activated muscle, activity from two muscle fibers innervated from the same axon is recorded and one action potential used as a time reference (Figure 3a). Increased jitter indicates a disturbed neuromuscular transmission (Figure 3b). Neuromuscular blockings occur if the jitter if high enough (usually more than 100 μsec), resulting from the failure of transmission of one of the potentials, when one of the muscle fibers fails to transmit an action potential because the EPP does not reach the necessary threshold (Figure 3c). Increased jitter is not pathognomonic for MG and can be seen in other conditions where there is denervation and reinnervation going on simultaneously, such as amyotrophic lateral sclerosis (ALS). Nevertheless, in combination with the clinical picture and immunological analysis of antibodies, the SFEMG is very sensitive for the MG diagnosis. Normal results on SFEMG in a clinically affected muscle basically rule out the diagnosis of MG. In most clinical neurophysiological laboratories, the arm muscle extensor digitorum communis (EDC) and either the facial muscles orbicularis oculi or frontalis are routinely examined.

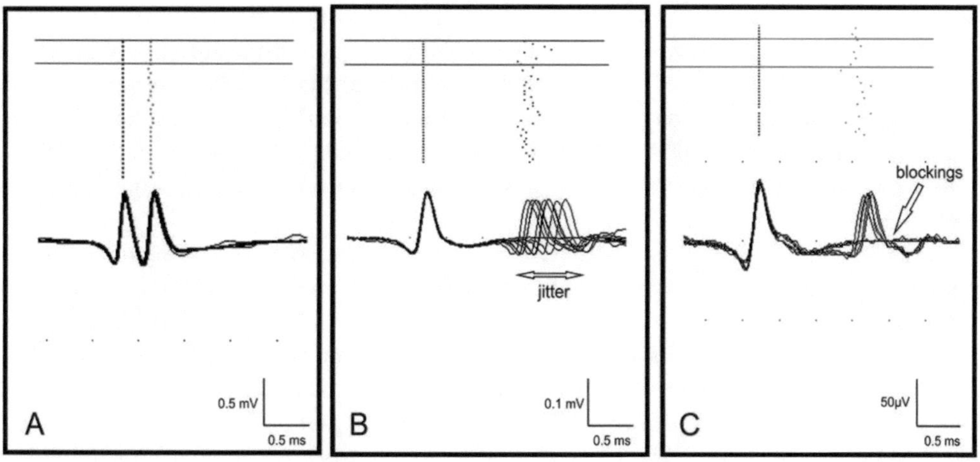


Fig. 3. Single-fiber EMG recording from the orbicularis oculi muscle (A) in a healthy control person and in a patient with MG (B and C). The vertical dotted lines represent the time line of a single muscle fiber and in each box, signals from two muscle fibers belonging to the same motor unit are displayed. A) Normal jitter, i.e. constant time variation in the variability of neuromuscular signaling to fiber 1 and 2. B) Increased jitter, and C) blockings.

### 2.2.2 Focal neurophysiology in MuSK+ MG

In patients with an extremely focal presentation of muscle fatigue and weakness, such as in MuSK+ MG, it may be necessary to specifically examine an involved muscle, such as the neck extensor muscles. Specific examination will help to prevent the oversight of selective defects of neuromuscular transmission (Sanders, El-Salem et al. 2003). In MuSK+ MG, SFEMG has been confirmed as the most sensitive examination in the neurophysiological diagnosis of MuSK+ MG, whereas repetitive nerve stimulation in limb muscles is only diagnostic in about 57% of cases (Evoli, Tonali et al. 2003). One of the standard limb muscles for SFEMG examinations, the EDC muscle, has been reported normal in many cases of MuSK+ MG, unlike AChR+ (Nemoto, Kuwabara et al. 2005; Stickler, Massey et al. 2005), which indicates differences in the distribution of abnormal neuromuscular transmission. In our experience, MuSK+ MG patients have comparable defects of neuromuscular transmission, on SFEMG; as AChR+ MG patients, when proximal muscles such as the deltoid or the orbicularis oculi muscles are examined (Rostedt Punga, Ahlqvist et al. 2006). One study has emphasized that the decrement in facial muscles, such as the orbicularis oculi muscle, is more often abnormal in the MuSK+ patients (Oh, Hatanaka et al. 2006), thus it is also important for RNS to be performed with recording from muscles in the faciobulbar region.

Neurophysiological examinations are also important in MuSK+ MG to detect adverse effects from AChEIs. So-called extra discharges (EDs), which occur after the CMAP on motor nerve stimulation, are sometimes observed in MG patients who are receiving high doses of AChEIs and may signify impending cholinergic crisis (Punga and Stalberg 2009). EDs are more prominent in recordings from distal muscles, such as the abductor digiti minimi (ADM) in the hand (Punga, Sawada et al. 2008). In the same patient different nerves/muscles display different grades of EDs. In some nerves, the discharges are clearly extra components, with increasing intervals from 4 to 12 ms (with a duration of at least 50 ms) and with an amplitude of approximately one third of the CMAP. In other nerves the EDs are seen as irregular discharges of low amplitude (<0.5 mV), with a duration up to 100 ms (Punga, Sawada et al. 2008). EDs may also occur directly after the neostigmine test in MuSK+ patients and then correlate with a worsening in muscle fatigue (Punga, Flink et al. 2006).

Examination using quantitative EMG (QEMG) is characterized by a myopathic pattern in approximately 70% of MuSK+ patients in neck extensor splenius capitis muscle and/or the deltoid muscle, which is considerably more than in the AChR+ group where it is found in approximately 23% of patients (Rostedt Punga, Ahlqvist et al. 2006). None of the above figures include patients treated with high doses of corticosteroids. An additional study using QEMG in MG revealed a myopathic pattern in the facial orbicularis oris muscle in 62% of MuSK+ patients and 50% of AChR+ patients; however, concomitant treatment with corticosteroids confounds pathophysiological conclusion (Farrugia, Kennett et al. 2007). Although denervation is not seen in AChR+ MG and also not in most MuSK+ patients, denervation activity in conjunction with a myopathic picture on QEMG has been observed in the tongue (glossus) muscle (Figure 2) (Punga, unpublished observations).

### 2.3 Treatment

Treatment of MG can be divided into two subclasses: immunosuppressive and symptomatic. Since MG is typically a chronic disorder, long-term immunosuppressive medications is often applied and include corticosteroids, corticosteroid sparing agents such as azathioprine and cyclosporine (which inhibit the T-cells) and antibody treatment with rituximab (which inhibits the B-cell response). Since autoimmune MG patients do not respond similarly to the same treatment, each regimen has to be tailored for each patient. For the acute treatment of exacerbations of weakness it may be necessary to employ plasmapheresis or intravenous immunoglobulins, which result in a prompt reduction of the autoimmune response. Patients with a thymoma or young patients usually undergo a thymectomy, removing the thymus which is hyperplastic, as in the majority of cases of AChR-antibodies. The most commonly used chronic symptomatic treatment consists of nonselective acetylcholinesterase inhibitors. These inhibitors render more acetylcholine available at the NMJ, thus temporarily decreasing fatigue. In general, patients with AChR-abs respond better to both immunosuppressive and symptomatic medication than MuSK+ patients.

#### 2.3.1 Immunosuppressive treatment

##### 2.3.1.1 Corticosteroids

**Corticosteroids** are generally considered to be an effective immunosuppressant for MG patients. Their therapeutic mechanism of action is through inhibition of transcription of inflammatory cytokines (interleukins, IL) and adhesion molecules, and a reduction in trafficking of inflammatory cells such as T-cells, thus reducing the inflammatory response. High doses may also induce apotosis of inflammatory cells (Barnes 2001). Although widely accepted as an appropriate immunosuppressive therapy, the efficacy of glucocorticosteroid treatment in MG has only been tested in a few randomized controlled studies (Howard, Duane et al. 1976; Lindberg, Andersen et al. 1998). Lindberg et al reported significant improvement in muscle function in the group of MG patients who received 2 g i v methylprednisolone on two consecutive days compared to the placebo group, duration of improvement ranged from 4 to 14 weeks. Intriguingly, no change in serum concentration of AChR abs was found after treatment in either of the two groups.

There is also a risk of worsening during the first days of initiation of the high doses, usually lasting less than one week. It appears that gradually increasing the steroid dose over one to two months may significantly reduce this risk. Pascuzzi et al reported improvement in as many as 95% of MG patients receiving long-term treatment with prednisone and remission (defined as no more than minimal eye closure weakness) in 28% of patients (Pascuzzi, Coslett et al. 1984). Additionally, corticosteroids appear to have direct effect on the neuromuscular junction, which may play a role for the early alterations and short-term fluctuations in myasthenic weakness seen in patients being treated with corticosteroids. In one study investigating the rat phrenic nerve-diaphragm, intracellular microelectrode recording of miniature end-plate potentials (MEPPs) was used to investigate the effect of prednisone on neuromuscular transmission. The results indicate that prednisone facilitates spontaneous release of acetylcholine (as manifested by a two- to three-fold increase in MEPP frequency) and decreases MEPP amplitude by about 50% (Wilson, Ward et al. 1974). The side effects, especially with long term treatment, are well known and include glucose intolerance, osteoporosis, weight gain, depression, mood swings, hypokalemia, septic ulcers, cushingoid features, myopathy and hypertension. Alternate day therapy is commonly applied in order to reduce side effects. It is also important to reduce the dose of corticosteroids slowly to a minimum that will maintain the remission or improvement in order to avoid worsening.

#### 2.3.1.2 T-cell inhibiting medications

**Azathioprine** has been used extensively for treatment of MG patients and is considered important as a steroid-sparing agent. Its mechanism of action is to inhibit purine synthesis and hence cell proliferation (Elion 1972). The most rapidly dividing cells, including lymphocytes involved in the autoimmune response, are affected. Prolonged administration of azathioprine prevents the appearance of experimental autoimmune MG (EAMG), for at least four months, in rabbits immunized with AChR (Abramsky, Tarrab-Hazdai et al. 1976). Azathioprine has a delayed onset of effect, on average four to six months, and maximal benefit is reached after a period of approximately 14 months. However, 70-90% of patients have reported a decrease in their myasthenic weakness after some months (Lewis, Selwa et al. 1995). Adverse effects include anorexia, gastrointestinal upset, hepatotoxicity and bone marrow suppression, commonly involving a reduction in white blood cell count. Close monitoring of the blood cell counts, along with liver enzymes, is necessary since a few patients develop a flu-like idiosyncratic reaction which includes fever and malaise and/or a skin rash, requiring discontinuation. Long-term treatment is also associated with an increased risk of developing malignancies (Confavreux, Saddier et al. 1996). Azathioprine is considered important as a steroid-sparing agent in MG treatment, although most studies have described its usefulness in conjunction with corticosteroids. Azathioprine is administered orally with a preferred maintenance dose of 2 to 3 mg/kg per day. The initial dose is 50 mg/d and increases by 50 mg/d every week while monitoring for adverse effects.

**Cyclosporine A** is another steroid-sparing medication which acts through prohibition of the transcription of cytokine genes, including those of IL-2 and IL-4, in activated T cells (Kronke, Leonard et al. 1984) . It is a highly specific inhibitor of T helper cell activation, and also acts to inhibit the phosphatase activity of calcineurin as well as the activation of c-Jun NH2-terminal kinase (JNK) in T lymphocytes and p38 signaling pathways triggered by antigen recognition (Matsuda, Moriguchi et al. 1998). Cyclosporine is widely used to prevent transplant rejection but is used in MG patients not responding to other immunosuppressants. In a therapeutic trial where cyclosporine was compared to placebo, patients in the cyclosporine group had improved strength and a reduction in AChR-Ab titer (Tindall, Phillips et al. 1993). Adverse effects include nephrotoxicity, hypertension and headache; hence, monitoring of blood urea nitrogen and creatinine is necessary. Most patients improve maximally after two to four months of therapy. The usual dose is 3 to 5 mg/kg per day, given orally at 12-hour intervals.

**Mycophenolate mofetil** (MyM) is the 2-morpholinoethyl ester of mycophenolic acid, which inhibits the proliferation of B and T lymphocytes through noncompetitive, reversible inhibition of inosine monophosphate dehydrogenase, a key enzyme in the *de novo* synthetic pathway of guanine nucleotides. Mycophenolic acid blocks inosine monophosphate dehydrogenase, an enzyme that is responsible for conversion of inosine monophosphate to guanosine monophosphate; hence, synthesis of adenosine is enhanced. This results in inhibition of purine synthesis selectively in lymphocytes, thereby inhibiting their proliferation (Allison, Kowalski et al. 1993). In a larger retrospective study, MyM was associated with clinical improvement in approximately 70% of patients after a period of approximately 11 weeks (Meriggioli, Ciafaloni et al. 2003). MyM is also well tolerated in most patients and only discontinued due to the adverse effects in a very small fraction of patients, the most common reason being gastrointestinal intolerance, such as diarrhea. The long-term safety of MyM is not known, but rates of malignancy do not appear to be higher in transplant recipients who receive MyM chronically (Haberal, Karakayali et al. 2002).

#### 2.3.1.3 Other immunosuppressants

**Cyclophosphamide** is a nitrogen mustard with potent immunosuppressant effects and is used to treat MG patients who are resistant to other therapies. It affects the proliferation of B cells and thereby reduces antibody production (Fig 1). The use of cyclophosphamide in MG is limited, but undoubtedly beneficial in severe cases (Perez, Buot et al. 1981). The usual dose range from 1 to 3 mg/kg per day, orally. Nevertheless, adverse effects are prominent and include alopecia, hemorrhagic cystitis, leukopenia and nausea. Long-term treatment brings the risk of infertility and malignancy.

**Etanercept**, a soluble, recombinant human TNF-receptor that competitively blocks the action of TNF-α, has been shown to have steroid-sparing effects in studies on small patient groups. In 54% of patients, with low plasma IL-6 and IFN-γ levels, the clinical scores improved and patients with increased cytokine levels (IL-6, IFN-γ and TNF-α) had worse clinical outcomes (Tuzun, Meriggioli et al. 2005). TNF-α is involved in the generation of AChR-specific T and B cell responses during the development of EAMG and preclinical studies on AChR-immunized mice have shown that etanercept can suppress established EAMG without inducing significant immunosuppression (Christadoss and Goluszko 2002).

**Rituximab (Mabtera®)** Rituximab is a chimeric IgG1 κ monoclonal antibody that targets CD20, a transmembrane phosphoprotein on most B cells. Rituximab depletes B cells by binding to the CD20 molecule and initiating complement-dependent cytolysis or antibody-dependent cell-mediated cytotoxicity (Monson, Cravens et al. 2005). Several case reports have demonstrated the effect of Rituximab in MuSK+ MG patients on the clinical course of bulbar and respiratory symptoms, thus making it an important alternative for the MuSK+ MG patients who are refractory to other immunosuppressive treatment (Hain, Jordan et al. 2006; Baek, Bashey et al. 2007).

#### 2.3.1.4 Thymectomy

The reason for removing the thymus gland in MG patients has historically been due to the presence of hyperplastic germinal centers, mainly in AChR+ patients. Despite the absence of randomized, well-controlled studies, thymectomy in MG patients with and without thymoma is widely practised. Post-operative improvement can take months or years to appear, making it difficult to distinguish thymectomy effects from those of immunosuppressive drugs, which are often used concomitantly (Skeie, Apostolski et al. 2010). Thymectomy is usually performed using a transsternal approach, removing the entire thymus gland, usually in patients less than 60 years of age. In MG patients with a thymoma, the main aim of thymectomy is to preferentially treat the tumour. Once thymoma is diagnosed, thymectomy is indicated irrespective of the severity of MG. One study (Evoli, Tonali et al. 2003) could not prove any effect of thymectomy in 15 MuSK+ patients, whereas MuSK antibodies predicted a poor outcome of thymectomy in another study (Pompeo, Tacconi et al. 2009). Additionally, it has been reported that MuSK+ patients have normal histopathology of the thymus (Leite, Strobel et al. 2005). Thus, current evidence suggests that thymectomy should not be recommended in MuSK+ patients. However, early onset generalized MG without AChR and MuSK antibodies are recommended to have thymectomy in the same way as MG with AChR antibodies.

#### 2.3.1.5 Plasmapheresis and immunoglobulins

Plasma exchange and intravenous immunoglobulin (IvIg) are used for short-term treatment of MG exacerbations and when it is desirable to achieve a rapid clinical response. Plasma exchange temporarily reduces the titer of circulating AChR- and MuSK-abs and usually produces immediate improvement (within days) in most MG patients (Newsom-Davis, Pinching et al. 1978). Circulating anti-AChR pathogenic factors can also be removed using immunoadsorption columns, some of which use immobilised AChR as an immunoadsorbent (Psaridi-Linardaki, Trakas et al. 2005). IvIg is widely used for patients with exacerbating MG. Support for its use comes from randomised controlled trials that show efficacy similar to plasma exchange (Gajdos, Chevret et al. 1997), equal efficacy of two doses (1 g/kg *vs* 2 g/kg) (Gajdos, Tranchant et al. 2005) and a recent double-blind, placebo controlled trial in patients with MG with worsening weakness (Zinman, Ng et al. 2007). The mechanisms by which intravenous immunoglobulins induce improvement are not clear, however studies in murine autoimmune models have implied that competition with autoantibodies and Fc-receptor binding are important factors in reducing the autoimmune response (Samuelsson, Towers et al. 2001).

#### 2.3.2.1 Acetylcholinesterase inhibitors (AChEIs)

AChEIs interfere with the catalytic breakdown of the neurotransmitter ACh, rendering ACh available for a longer period of time at the NMJ and the nicotinic AChRs (nAChRs). The nonselective AChEIs affect both the nAChRs and the muscarinic receptors in exocrine glands. Common adverse effects include muscarinic symptoms, such as increased gut motility, which may lead to stomach pain and diarrhea. Other muscarinic effects are increased gastric acid secretion, hyperhidrosis, increased sweating, salivation, and lacrimation. The presence of daily muscarinic adverse effects correlates with the baseline inhibition of AChE activity in the blood (Punga, Sawada et al. 2008). The most common form of nonselective AChEI is pyridostigmine bromide (PB Mestinon®), which is especially effective at the onset of MG. In some patients, typically those with purely ocular weakness, this treatment may be sufficient to manage the fatigue. Overdose of AChEIs can cause a cholinergic crisis, which is characterized by increasing muscle weakness, which results in dysphagia and respiratory insufficiency in severe cases. The distinction between a cholinergic and a myasthenic crisis, the latter being caused by myasthenic weakness, is important for the medical treatment of the patient. These two conditions have different clinical reactions related to the initial intake of the drug. During incipient overdose in cholinergic crisis, symptoms of weakness increase shortly after ingestion and wane before the next dose, a situation opposite to that seen in myasthenic crisis. This typical pattern may not always be easy to detect; therefore, other markers are useful. For example, the EDs observed on motor nerve stimulation are sometimes observed in MG patients who are receiving high doses of PB and may signify impending cholinergic crisis (Punga and Stalberg 2009).

Recent reports imply that patients with EDs are more prone to have daily nicotinic side effects, including muscle fasciculations and fatigue as a possible sign of overtreatment (Punga, Sawada et al. 2008). In this study, elderly MG patients were more prone to develop cholinergic side effects, as well as EDs. Additionally, MuSK+ MG patients often have a negative edrophonium test and are also reported to clinically benefit less from pyridostigmine bromide (Evoli, Bianchi et al. 2008). Instead, MuSK+ patients may worsen or develop pronounced nicotinic side effects including muscle cramps and fasciculations in response to PB treatment (Evoli, Tonali et al. 2003; Punga, Flink et al. 2006). Based on these observations of hypersensitivity to increased amounts of acetylcholine in MuSK+ patients, the general guidelines do not recommend AChEIs as a form of treatment in this group of patients (Skeie, Apostolski et al. 2010).

EN101 is a selective AChEI, an antisense oligodeoxynucleotide that acts at the mRNA level and selectively reduces the production of the enzymatic isoform of stress-related "read-through" (AChE-R) through destruction of AChE-R mRNA. This compound selectively lowers the levels of AChE-R in both blood and muscle, yet leaves the synaptic variant of AChE-S unaffected. EN101 treatment in rats with EAMG, in which daily oral or intravenous administration of EN101 reduced AChE in blood and muscle and improved survival, muscle strength and disease severity (Brenner, Hamra-Amitay et al. 2003). In this study, stabilization of the CMAP decrement on RNS and muscle strength over the entire course of treatment was also observed. Interestingly, a Phase 1b open-label trial with oral EN101 (Monarsen) was recently conducted in 16 MG patients who were receiving at least 180 mg ofpyridostigmine bromide daily (Argov, McKee et al. 2007). This study reported an overall clinical improvement in approximately 47% of patients, as well as an improvement in the swallowing time component. Further, the effects of EN101 lasted for greater than 24 hours, indicating the possibility of a reduction in multiple dosing through the use of antisense therapy. Further studies are needed to conclude whether EN101 may also have immunomodulatory effects through an effect on the immune cholinergic system and thus mediation of neuroimmune interactions.

### 2.4 Establishment and phenotype of murine models of experimental autoimmune MG (EAMG)

Naturally occurring MG in animals is present in canine MG. This canine form of MG has a natural course of clinical and immunological remission in the majority of dogs, even without initiation of immunosuppressive treatment (Shelton and Lindstrom 2001). Therefore, the use of the canine MG in determining the effect of immunosuppressant medication is limited. EAMG can be induced in rabbits, rats and mice either by passive transfer of human antibodies/sera or by immunization of the antigen in adjuvant. In 1978 it was first shown that active immunization with AChR from Torpedo (ray fish) electric organ, in rabbits leads to flaccid paralysis and an MG-like disease. Since in rabbits the disease has an acute action and shortly leads to death, these animals are not routinely used for EAMG studies. Some studies have used guinea pigs and even primates, but the current most widely used model is EAMG induced in female young mice or rats. The disease in rats has a short acute phase and a chronic phase, which mimics the human disease, excluding the involvement of the thymus (Meinl, Klinkert et al. 1991). In the mice only a chronic phase is induced. EAMG is more difficult to induce in mice and usually requires multiple immunizations and only a fraction of the mice develop disease symptoms. However, the murine model has an advantage of a plethora of mouse-specific reagents and knock-out mouse strains, which enable analyses that cannot be performed in rats. One further advantage of using the mouse is that its immune system is well characterized and the availability of inbred and genetically modified strains permit genetic analysis.

#### 2.4.1 AChR+ EAMG: Clinical phenotype

Immunization with purified denatured *Torpedo* AChR α1, β1, γ, or δ subunits can cause EAMG, but it is inefficient compared to native AChR (Lindstrom, Einarson et al. 1978). Purified α1-subunit is the most potent, as might be expected since its sequence is the most conserved. Also, there are two α1 in an AChR which permit cross-linking by antibodies, which may utilize renaturation to provoke antibodies to the main immunogenic region (MIR) (Lindstrom, Luo et al. 2008). It is of outmost importance to use a mouse strain which possesses IL-6, since mice deficient in IL-6 have been shown to be resistant to the development of EAMG upon immunization (Deng, Goluszko et al. 2002). In the acute phase of active EAMG or EAMG passively transmitted with serum, binding of AChR antibody and its complement target the postsynaptic membrane for attack by macrophages (Lindstrom 2000). Mice immunized with AChR in Complete Freund´s Adjuvant (CFA) develop a flaccid paralysis (Figure 4a), a drooping of the head and tail and weakness primarily of the forelimbs, which may rapidly progress to respiratory failure (Berman and Patrick 1980). The myasthenic phenotype in the AChR+ EAMG mice has been reported to be restored in all cases to nearly normal after treatment with neostigmine intraperitoneally (Berman and Patrick 1980).

#### 2.4.2 MuSK+ EAMG: Clinical phenotype

The antibodies in MuSK+ MG are directed against the extracellular domain of MuSK, which contains IgG-like domains. The first study which proved the pathogenic role of MuSK-antibodies in animals was done in 2006, when New Zealand White rabbits were repeatedly injected with 100-400 μg of purified chimeric protein composed of the MuSK ectodomain

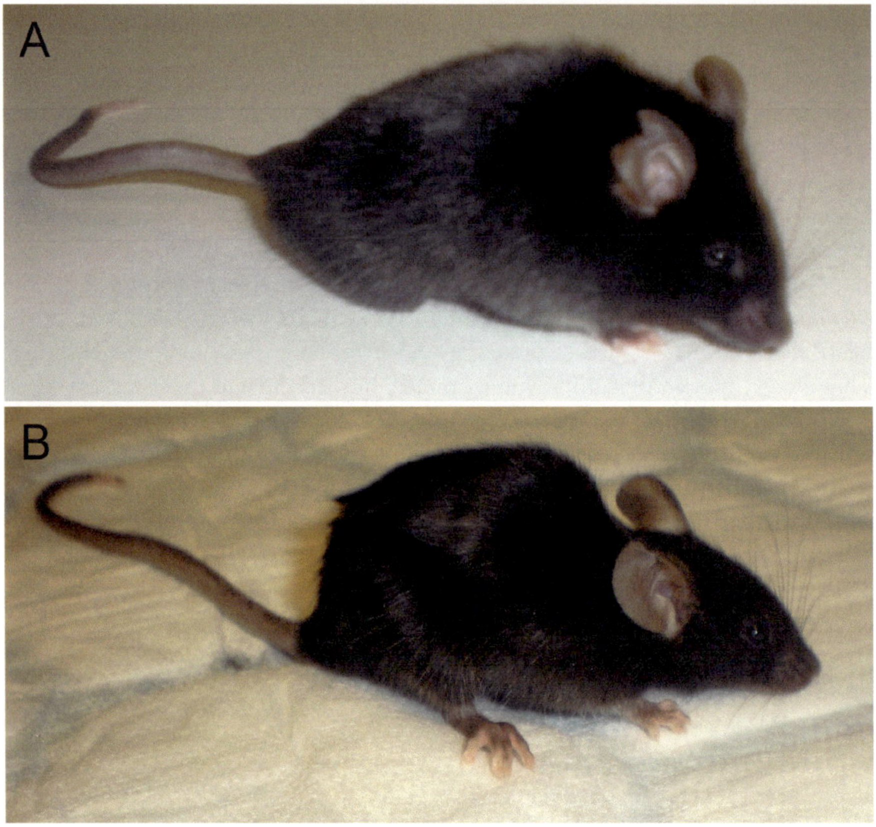


Fig. 4. A) One mouse with typical flaccid paralysis, especially of the limbs, after immunization with torpedo AChR. The clinical course in the AChR+ mice is progessive, however the response to intraperitoneal injection of neostigmine induces an improvement in clinical weakness. B) The phenotype of the mice immunized with rat MuSK shows a severe weakness of the neck extensor muscles, demonstrating a prominent cervical kyphosis and inability to raise the head. The mice are not as affected in the hind limbs as in the forelimbs and faciobulbar area, with difficulties ingesting food and water and subsequent significant weight loss. The MuSK+ mice do not show any clinical improvement from neostigmine injection, on the contrary muscle fasciculations and twitches are seen.

and the Fc region of human IgG1 (MuSK-Fc) (Shigemoto, Kubo et al. 2006). All of the 4 recipient rabbits manifested flaccid weakness after 3 or 4 repeated injections with MuSK-Fc. The actively induced murine model can be produced produced by injection of the extracellular domain of 10 μg of recombinant rat MuSK (aa 21-491) (Jones, Moore et al. 1999) in a mix with CFA in emulsion (Jha, Xu et al. 2006). The prominent features of MuSK+ EAMG in mice resemble the human MuSK+MG phenotype with kyphosis, indicating weakness in the cervical extensor muscles and the thoracic paraspinal muscles (Figure 4b). Additionally, one prominent clinical feature of the MuSK+ mice is the weight loss, which is significant compared to the control mice (Punga, Lin et al, 2011). This finding further supports the involvement of faciobulbar weakness, preventing the MuSK+ EAMG mice to chew and swallow and therefore explaining the irreversible weight loss. Passively induced

MuSK+ EAMG has been accomplished by i.p. injections of plasma (Benveniste, Jacobson et al. 2005) or purified IgG from MuSK+ MG patients (Cole, Reddel et al. 2008) in C57BL6 mice. Cole et al also reported that mice injected with IgG from two of three anti-MuSK-positive patients lost weight, developed myasthenic muscle weakness and a prominent cervicothoracic hump, which may reflect cervical extensor weakness.

### 2.4.3 Morphological changes at the neuromuscular junction and muscle atrophy in EAMG

In experimental mice injected with anti-MuSK-positive patient IgG, postsynaptic AChR staining is reduced to as little as 22% of that seen in control mice in both the tibial and diaphragm muscles (Cole, Reddel et al. 2008). The mice which develop MuSK+ EAMG following this injection show reduced apposition of the nerve terminal and the postsynaptic AChR cluster. In later studies, mice injected with MuSK+ patient IgG have also been found to have reductions in postsynaptic MuSK staining and this loss preceded the impairment of postsynaptic AChRs (Cole, Ghazanfari et al. 2010). In this study, the residual level of MuSK correlated with the degree of impairment of postsynaptic AChR packing. The sera obtained from mice immunized with MuSK inhibit agrin-induced AChR aggregation in C2C12 myotubes (Jha, Xu et al. 2006). Further, disruption of neuromuscular junctions have been observed and it has been proposed that so called delayed synapsing muscles, including the diaphragm, tibalis posterior and sternomastoid are more severely affected than the so called fast-synapsing muscles (Xu, Jha et al. 2006).

In a recent study, morphological changes presynaptically and postsynaptically in whole mount preparations of muscle fibers from the bulbar sternomastoid and omohyoid muscles were examined in control mice and in mice immunized with MuSK (Punga, Lin et al, 2011). In the control mice, the postsynaptic clusters (labeled with α-bungarotoxin) were closely aligned with the presynaptic motor nerve terminal (Figure 5a). However, in the MuSK+ EAMG mice, a severe disruption of the NMJ morphology was observed, especially prominent in the facial and neck muscles (Punga, Lin et al, 2011). The AChR clusters were fragmented and dispersed along the muscle fiber (Figure 5b). Except for disruption of the postsynaptic area with less clustering of AChRs, the nerve terminal area was found to be smaller than in the control mice (Figure 5b), suggesting a secondary presynaptic effect of reduced MuSK signalling. When comparing the morphology of the NMJs in the bulbar omohyoid muscle, the AChR clusters were arranged in the junctional folds in the control mice (Figure 6a). In parallell rounds of mice immunized with MuSK or AChR confocal images revelaled that the AChR clusters were severely fragmented in the MuSK+ mice (Figure 6b), whereas in the AChR+ EAMG mice a similar fragmentation of the AChRs was not observed, although the AChR clusters and the folding of the NMJs were simplified (Figure 6c).

Benveniste et al found increased protein levels of the muscle RING-finger protein 1 (MuRF-1), a marker for skeletal muscle atrophy, in the masseter muscle, but not in the gastrocnemius muscle, of mice injected with plasma from MuSK+ MG patients (Benveniste, Jacobson et al. 2005). Increased mRNA levels of MuRF-1 and atrogin-1 have also been found in the masseter of MuSK+ EAMG mice, but not in the limb muscles, further in support of a atrophy process localized to the facial muscles (Punga, Lin et al, 2011; Punga, unpublished data). There is a difference in the reaction to disturbed or exaggerated agrin-MuSK signalling in different skeletal muscles in the sense that muscles with high MuSK levels have

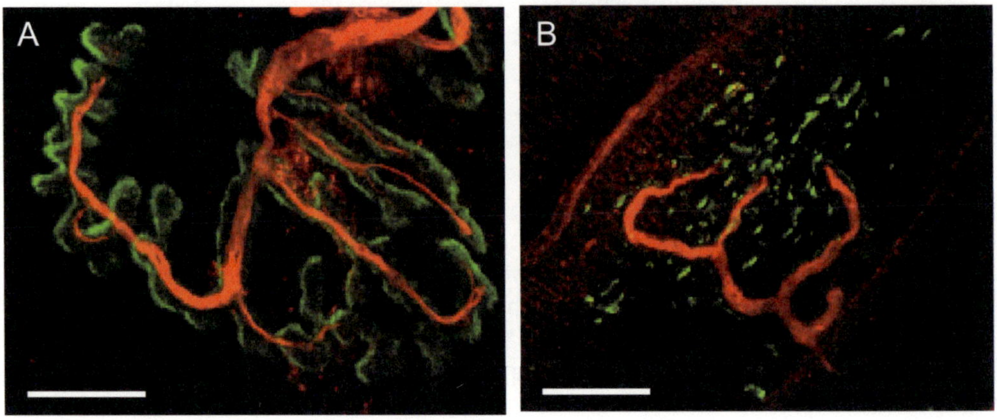


Fig. 5. The effect of MuSK-antibodies at the neuromuscular junction (NMJ) in mice immunized with MuSK. Confocal microscopy images with 100x magnification of immunostained whole mount muscle fibers from the sternomastoid muscle. A) A normal NMJ, where α-bungarotoxin labels the AChR clusters (green) and antibodies against synaptophysin and neurofilament labels the nerve terminal (red). Note the close alignment between the motor nerve terminal and clustered postsynaptic AChRs. B) In MuSK+ MG, the presynaptic nerve terminal area is significantly smaller and the AChR clusters are fragmented and scattered along the muscle fiber. Scale bar is 10 µm.

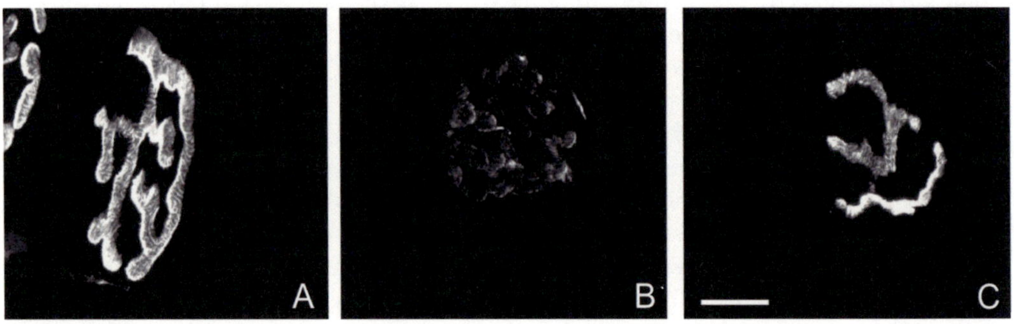


Fig. 6. Immunolabeling of whole mount muscle fibers from the omohyoid muscle, where postsynaptic acetylcholine receptors (AChRs) are labelled with α-bungarotoxin (white). In the control mice (A) a normal pattern with postsynaptic AChR clusters are seen in the junctional folds, adjacent to the motor nerve. In MuSK+ EAMG mice (B), the AChRs are very faint, with a subsequent reduction in postsynaptic AChR cluster area. In AChR+ EAMG mice (C), the staining intensity of the α-bungarotoxin was less reduced than in the MuSK+ EAMG mice, however there is a disruption in AChR cluster morphology with simplification of the postsynaptic morphology and less folding. Scale bar is 10 µm.

an increased plasticity (Punga, Maj et al, 2011). n the contrary, low muscle-intrinsic MuSK levels render some muscles, such as the masseter, more vulnerable to the postsynaptic perturbation of MuSK antibodies with subsequent denervation and atrophy (Punga, Lin et al, 2011). This is hypothesized to play a role for the muscle selectivity also in MuSK+ MG and EAMG.

#### 2.4.4 Cholinergic hyperactivity after AChEIs in EAMG

Evaluation of the response to AChEIs is usually performed by i.p. injection of a mix of neostigmine bromide (0.0375 mg/kg) and atropine sulfate (0.015 mg/kg) in mice with EAMG grade 2 and 3 (Berman and Patrick 1980).

In 3 MuSK+ EAMG mice, the opposite response to the common restoration of weakness in AChR+ EAMG was seen with more pronounced weakness which manifested itself as chin down even more along with nicotinic side effects including muscle fasciculations in the back- and limb muscles and abnormal twitches of the tail (Punga et al, unpublished observations). The observed fragmentation and dispersion of AChR clusters could explain why MuSK+ MG patients do not respond beneficially to AChEIs, since an increased acetylcholine level would not be able to induce a synchronous endplate potential due to the temporal dispersion of AChRs. Additionally, the reason for the cholinergic hyperactivity in MuSK+ MG, here also displayed in the MuSK+ EAMG mice, may be explained by the loss of MuSK at the NMJ, which in turn also diminishes the binding between MuSK-ColQ and AChE. This means that in the MuSK+ EAMG mice where MuSK antibodies disrupt the NMJ and reduce the amount of MuSK, the AChE is also down-regulated (Punga, Lin et al, 2011). Then, when exogenous AChEI is administered, a further blocking of AChE is taking place and consequently this mimics an overdose of AChEIs which causes the nicotinic side effects and in worst cases also cholinergic crisis.

## 3. Conclusion

In summary, studies in the recent years of the murine EAMG model provide further insights regarding the action of MuSK antibodies at the NMJ and give evidence for their pathogenetic role, especially in facial and bulbar muscles. The results of the MuSK antibody attack is fragmentation and dispersion of nicotinic AChRs, postsynaptic perturbation and a subsequent impaired neuromuscular transmission. Since MuSK+ MG is very focal in its clinical manifestations it is very important to examine the clinically weak muscles also neurophysiologically to confirm the diagnosis, and for morphological purpose when examining the NMJ pathophysiology. The findings of dispersion of AChRs may also indicate irreparable changes at the NMJ, explaining muscle atrophies in these patients. It is therefore of importance to identify MG patients as early as possible, and especially MuSK+ MG, since delayed treatment may result in muscle atrophies and even functional denervation due to long time of blocked neuromuscular transmission. Immunosuppressive treatment should always be the main medication in MG and AChEIs is not receommended as symptomatic treatment in MuSK+ patients due to the cholinergic hypsersensitivity and unbeneficial effects.

## 4. Acknowledgment

I thank the group of Professor Markus A Rüegg in the department of Neurobiology/Pharmacology in Basel, Switzerland, for collaboration on the AChR+ and MuSK+ EAMG mouse model, especially professor Rüegg for the scientific discussions, Dr Shuo Lin for the work on the muscle morphology and Filippo Oliveri for production of recombinant rat MuSK. Professor emeritus Erik V Stålberg is acknowledged for guiding and supporting the initial MG studies, for teaching me SFEMG, for the scientific discussions and for the great friendship. I genuinely thank my family for their never-ending love and support.

Financial support was given by a postdoctoral fellowship from the Swedish Association for Medical Research (SSMF), Lars Hiertas memorial foundation and from European Union FP7 project number 242210 "FIGHT-MG".

## 5. References

Aarli, J. A., K. Stefansson, et al. (1990). "Patients with myasthenia gravis and thymoma have in their sera IgG autoantibodies against titin." Clin Exp Immunol 82(2): 284-8.

Abramsky, O., R. Tarrab-Hazdai, et al. (1976). "Immunosuppression of experimental autoimmune myasthenia gravis by hydrocortisone and azathioprine." J Immunol 117(1): 225-8.

Allison, A. C., W. J. Kowalski, et al. (1993). "Mechanisms of action of mycophenolic acid." Ann N Y Acad Sci 696: 63-87.

Argov, Z., D. McKee, et al. (2007). "Treatment of human myasthenia gravis with oral antisense suppression of acetylcholinesterase." Neurology 69(7): 699-700.

Baek, W. S., A. Bashey, et al. (2007). "Complete remission induced by rituximab in refractory, seronegative, muscle-specific, kinase-positive myasthenia gravis." J Neurol Neurosurg Psychiatry 78(7): 771.

Barnes, P. J. (2001). "Molecular mechanisms of corticosteroids in allergic diseases." Allergy 56(10): 928-36.

Bartoccioni, E., M. Marino, et al. (2003). "Identification of disease-specific autoantibodies in seronegative myasthenia gravis." Ann N Y Acad Sci 998: 356-8.

Benveniste, O., L. Jacobson, et al. (2005). "MuSK antibody positive myasthenia gravis plasma modifies MURF-1 expression in C2C12 cultures and mouse muscle in vivo." J Neuroimmunol 170(1-2): 41-8.

Berman, P. W. and J. Patrick (1980). "Experimental myasthenia gravis. A murine system." J Exp Med 151(1): 204-23.

Brenner, T., Y. Hamra-Amitay, et al. (2003). "The role of readthrough acetylcholinesterase in the pathophysiology of myasthenia gravis." Faseb J 17(2): 214-22.

Christadoss, P. and E. Goluszko (2002). "Treatment of experimental autoimmune myasthenia gravis with recombinant human tumor necrosis factor receptor Fc protein." J Neuroimmunol 122(1-2): 186-90.

Cole, R. N., N. Ghazanfari, et al. (2010). "Patient autoantibodies deplete postsynaptic muscle-specific kinase leading to disassembly of the ACh receptor scaffold and myasthenia gravis in mice." J Physiol 588(Pt 17): 3217-29.

Cole, R. N., S. W. Reddel, et al. (2008). "Anti-MuSK patient antibodies disrupt the mouse neuromuscular junction." Ann Neurol 63(6): 782-9.

Colledge, M. and S. C. Froehner (1998). "Signals mediating ion channel clustering at the neuromuscular junction." Curr Opin Neurobiol 8(3): 357-63.

Confavreux, C., P. Saddier, et al. (1996). "Risk of cancer from azathioprine therapy in multiple sclerosis: a case-control study." Neurology 46(6): 1607-12.

DeChiara, T. M., D. C. Bowen, et al. (1996). "The receptor tyrosine kinase MuSK is required for neuromuscular junction formation in vivo." Cell 85(4): 501-12.

Deng, C., E. Goluszko, et al. (2002). "Resistance to experimental autoimmune myasthenia gravis in IL-6-deficient mice is associated with reduced germinal center formation and C3 production." J Immunol 169(2): 1077-83.

Drachman, D. B., R. N. Adams, et al. (1981). "Antibody-mediated mechanisms of ACh receptor loss in myasthenia gravis: clinical relevance." Ann N Y Acad Sci 377: 175-88.

Elion, G. B. (1972). "Significance of azathioprine metabolites." Proc R Soc Med 65(3): 257-60.
Engel, A. G., E. H. Lambert, et al. (1977). "Immune complexes (IgG and C3) at the motor end-plate in myasthenia gravis: ultrastructural and light microscopic localization and electrophysiologic correlations." Mayo Clin Proc 52(5): 267-80.
Evoli, A., M. R. Bianchi, et al. (2008). "Response to therapy in myasthenia gravis with anti-MuSK antibodies." Ann N Y Acad Sci 1132: 76-83.
Evoli, A., C. Minisci, et al. (2002). "Thymoma in patients with MG: characteristics and long-term outcome." Neurology 59(12): 1844-50.
Evoli, A., P. A. Tonali, et al. (2003). "Clinical correlates with anti-MuSK antibodies in generalized seronegative myasthenia gravis." Brain 126(Pt 10): 2304-11.
Farrugia, M. E., R. P. Kennett, et al. (2007). "Quantitative EMG of facial muscles in myasthenia patients with MuSK antibodies." Clin Neurophysiol 118(2): 269-77.
Farrugia, M. E., M. D. Robson, et al. (2006). "MRI and clinical studies of facial and bulbar muscle involvement in MuSK antibody-associated myasthenia gravis." Brain 129(Pt 6): 1481-92.
Gajdos, P., S. Chevret, et al. (1997). "Clinical trial of plasma exchange and high-dose intravenous immunoglobulin in myasthenia gravis. Myasthenia Gravis Clinical Study Group." Ann Neurol 41(6): 789-96.
Gajdos, P., C. Tranchant, et al. (2005). "Treatment of myasthenia gravis exacerbation with intravenous immunoglobulin: a randomized double-blind clinical trial." Arch Neurol 62(11): 1689-93.
Gautam, M., P. G. Noakes, et al. (1995). "Failure of postsynaptic specialization to develop at neuromuscular junctions of rapsyn-deficient mice." Nature 377(6546): 232-6.
Grob, D., N. Brunner, et al. (2008). "Lifetime course of myasthenia gravis." Muscle Nerve 37(2): 141-9.
Haberal, M., H. Karakayali, et al. (2002). "Malignant tumors after renal transplantation." Artif Organs 26(9): 778-81.
Hain, B., K. Jordan, et al. (2006). "Successful treatment of MuSK antibody-positive myasthenia gravis with rituximab." Muscle Nerve 33(4): 575-80.
Hall, Z. W. and J. R. Sanes (1993). "Synaptic structure and development: the neuromuscular junction." Cell 72 Suppl: 99-121.
Hesser, B. A., O. Henschel, et al. (2006). "Synapse disassembly and formation of new synapses in postnatal muscle upon conditional inactivation of MuSK." Mol Cell Neurosci 31(3): 470-80.
Higuchi, O., J. Hamuro, et al. (2011). "Autoantibodies to low-density lipoprotein receptor-related protein 4 in myasthenia gravis." Ann Neurol 69(2): 418-22.
Hoch, W., J. McConville, et al. (2001). "Auto-antibodies to the receptor tyrosine kinase MuSK in patients with myasthenia gravis without acetylcholine receptor antibodies." Nat Med 7(3): 365-8.
Hopf, C. and W. Hoch (1998). "Tyrosine phosphorylation of the muscle-specific kinase is exclusively induced by acetylcholine receptor-aggregating agrin fragments." Eur J Biochem 253(2): 382-9.
Howard, F. M., Jr., D. D. Duane, et al. (1976). "Alternate-day prednisone: preliminary report of a double-blind controlled study." Ann N Y Acad Sci 274: 596-607.
Jha, S., K. Xu, et al. (2006). "Myasthenia gravis induced in mice by immunization with the recombinant extracellular domain of rat muscle-specific kinase (MuSK)." J Neuroimmunol 175(1-2): 107-17.

Jones, G., C. Moore, et al. (1999). "Constitutively active MuSK is clustered in the absence of agrin and induces ectopic postsynaptic-like membranes in skeletal muscle fibers." J Neurosci 19(9): 3376-83.
Kalb, B., G. Matell, et al. (2002). "Epidemiology of myasthenia gravis: a population-based study in Stockholm, Sweden." Neuroepidemiology 21(5): 221-5.
Kim, N., A. L. Stiegler, et al. (2008). "Lrp4 is a receptor for Agrin and forms a complex with MuSK." Cell 135(2): 334-42.
Kong, X. C., P. Barzaghi, et al. (2004). "Inhibition of synapse assembly in mammalian muscle in vivo by RNA interference." EMBO Rep 5(2): 183-8.
Kronke, M., W. J. Leonard, et al. (1984). "Cyclosporin A inhibits T-cell growth factor gene expression at the level of mRNA transcription." Proc Natl Acad Sci U S A 81(16): 5214-8.
Lefvert, A. K., S. Cuenoud, et al. (1981). "Binding properties and subclass distribution of anti-acetylcholine receptor antibodies in myasthenia gravis." J Neuroimmunol 1(1): 125-35.
Leite, M. I., S. Jacob, et al. (2008). "IgG1 antibodies to acetylcholine receptors in 'seronegative' myasthenia gravis." Brain 131(Pt 7): 1940-52.
Leite, M. I., P. Strobel, et al. (2005). "Fewer thymic changes in MuSK antibody-positive than in MuSK antibody-negative MG." Ann Neurol 57(3): 444-8.
Lewis, R. A., J. F. Selwa, et al. (1995). "Myasthenia gravis: immunological mechanisms and immunotherapy." Ann Neurol 37 Suppl 1: S51-62.
Lindberg, C., O. Andersen, et al. (1998). "Treatment of myasthenia gravis with methylprednisolone pulse: a double blind study." Acta Neurol Scand 97(6): 370-3.
Lindstrom, J. (2004). "Is "seronegative" MG explained by autoantibodies to MuSK?" Neurology 62(11): 1920-1.
Lindstrom, J., B. Einarson, et al. (1978). "Immunization of rats with polypeptide chains from torpedo acetylcholine receptor causes an autoimmune response to receptors in rat muscle." Proc Natl Acad Sci U S A 75(2): 769-73.
Lindstrom, J., J. Luo, et al. (2008). "Myasthenia gravis and the tops and bottoms of AChRs: antigenic structure of the MIR and specific immunosuppression of EAMG using AChR cytoplasmic domains." Ann N Y Acad Sci 1132: 29-41.
Lindstrom, J. M. (2000). "Acetylcholine receptors and myasthenia." Muscle Nerve 23(4): 453-77.
Lindstrom, J. M., M. E. Seybold, et al. (1976). "Antibody to acetylcholine receptor in myasthenia gravis. Prevalence, clinical correlates, and diagnostic value." Neurology 26(11): 1054-9.
Liyanage, Y., W. Hoch, et al. (2002). "The agrin/muscle-specific kinase pathway: new targets for autoimmune and genetic disorders at the neuromuscular junction." Muscle Nerve 25(1): 4-16.
Matsuda, S., T. Moriguchi, et al. (1998). "T lymphocyte activation signals for interleukin-2 production involve activation of MKK6-p38 and MKK7-SAPK/JNK signaling pathways sensitive to cyclosporin A." J Biol Chem 273(20): 12378-82.
McConville, J., M. E. Farrugia, et al. (2004). "Detection and characterization of MuSK antibodies in seronegative myasthenia gravis." Ann Neurol 55(4): 580-4.
Meinl, E., W. E. Klinkert, et al. (1991). "The thymus in myasthenia gravis. Changes typical for the human disease are absent in experimental autoimmune myasthenia gravis of the Lewis rat." Am J Pathol 139(5): 995-1008.
Meriggioli, M. N., E. Ciafaloni, et al. (2003). "Mycophenolate mofetil for myasthenia gravis: an analysis of efficacy, safety, and tolerability." Neurology 61(10): 1438-40.

Meriggioli, M. N. and J. Rowin (2003). "Single fiber EMG as an outcome measure in myasthenia gravis: results from a double-blind, placebo-controlled trial." J Clin Neurophysiol 20(5): 382-5.

Miller, J. F. (1961). "Immunological function of the thymus." Lancet 2(7205): 748-9.

Monson, N. L., P. D. Cravens, et al. (2005). "Effect of rituximab on the peripheral blood and cerebrospinal fluid B cells in patients with primary progressive multiple sclerosis." Arch Neurol 62(2): 258-64.

Mygland, A., O. B. Tysnes, et al. (1992). "Ryanodine receptor autoantibodies in myasthenia gravis patients with a thymoma." Ann Neurol 32(4): 589-91.

Nemoto, Y., S. Kuwabara, et al. (2005). "Patterns and severity of neuromuscular transmission failure in seronegative myasthenia gravis." J Neurol Neurosurg Psychiatry 76(5): 714-8.

Newsom-Davis, J., A. J. Pinching, et al. (1978). "Function of circulating antibody to acetylcholine receptor in myasthenia gravis: investigation by plasma exchange." Neurology 28(3): 266-72.

Oh, S. J., Y. Hatanaka, et al. (2006). "Repetitive nerve stimulation of facial muscles in MuSK antibody-positive myasthenia gravis." Muscle Nerve 33(4): 500-4.

Okada, K., A. Inoue, et al. (2006). "The muscle protein Dok-7 is essential for neuromuscular synaptogenesis." Science 312(5781): 1802-5.

Osserman, K. E. and G. Genkins (1971). "Studies in myasthenia gravis: review of a twenty-year experience in over 1200 patients." Mt Sinai J Med 38(6): 497-537.

Pascuzzi, R. M., H. B. Coslett, et al. (1984). "Long-term corticosteroid treatment of myasthenia gravis: report of 116 patients." Ann Neurol 15(3): 291-8.

Perez, M. C., W. L. Buot, et al. (1981). "Stable remissions in myasthenia gravis." Neurology 31(1): 32-7.

Phillips, L. H., 2nd (2003). "The epidemiology of myasthenia gravis." Ann N Y Acad Sci 998: 407-12.

Pompeo, E., F. Tacconi, et al. (2009). "Long-term outcome of thoracoscopic extended thymectomy for nonthymomatous myasthenia gravis." Eur J Cardiothorac Surg 36(1): 164-9.

Psaridi-Linardaki, L., N. Trakas, et al. (2005). "Specific immunoadsorption of the autoantibodies from myasthenic patients using the extracellular domain of the human muscle acetylcholine receptor alpha-subunit. Development of an antigen-specific therapeutic strategy." J Neuroimmunol 159(1-2): 183-91.

Punga, A. R., R. Flink, et al. (2006). "Cholinergic neuromuscular hyperactivity in patients with myasthenia gravis seropositive for MuSK antibody." Muscle Nerve 34(1): 111-5.

Punga A.R., M. Maj, et al. (2011). “MuSK levels differ between adult skeletal muscles and influence postsynaptic plasticity." Eur J Neurosci 33(5):890-8.

Punga A.R., S. Lin, et al (2011). “Muscle-selective synaptic disassembly and reorganization in MuSK antibody positive MG mice.” Exp Neurol, in press.

Punga, A. R., M. Sawada, et al. (2008). "Electrophysiological signs and the prevalence of adverse effects of acetylcholinesterase inhibitors in patients with myasthenia gravis." Muscle Nerve 37(3): 300-7.

Punga, A. R. and E. Stalberg (2009). "Acetylcholinesterase inhibitors in MG: to be or not to be?" Muscle Nerve 39(6): 724-8.

Rostedt, A., L. L. Sanders, et al. (2000). "Predictive value of single-fiber electromyography in the extensor digitorum communis muscle of patients with ocular myasthenia gravis: a retrospective study." J Clin Neuromuscul Dis 2(1): 6-9.

Rostedt Punga, A., K. Ahlqvist, et al. (2006). "Neurophysiological and mitochondrial abnormalities in MuSK antibody seropositive myasthenia gravis compared to other immunological subtypes." Clin Neurophysiol 117(7): 1434-43.

Samuelsson, A., T. L. Towers, et al. (2001). "Anti-inflammatory activity of IVIG mediated through the inhibitory Fc receptor." Science 291(5503): 484-6.

Sanders, D. B. (2002). "Clinical impact of single-fiber electromyography." Muscle Nerve Suppl 11: S15-20.

Sanders, D. B., K. El-Salem, et al. (2003). "Clinical aspects of MuSK antibody positive seronegative MG." Neurology 60(12): 1978-80.

Sanders, D. B. and V. C. Juel (2008). "MuSK-antibody positive myasthenia gravis: questions from the clinic." J Neuroimmunol 201-202: 85-9.

Selcen, D., T. Fukuda, et al. (2004). "Are MuSK antibodies the primary cause of myasthenic symptoms?" Neurology 62(11): 1945-50.

Shelton, G. D. and J. M. Lindstrom (2001). "Spontaneous remission in canine myasthenia gravis: implications for assessing human MG therapies." Neurology 57(11): 2139-41.

Shigemoto, K., S. Kubo, et al. (2006). "Induction of myasthenia by immunization against muscle-specific kinase." J Clin Invest 116(4): 1016-24.

Simpson, J. A. (1960). "Myasthenia Gravis, a new hypothesis. ." Scottish Medical Journal: 419-436.

Skeie, G. O., S. Apostolski, et al. (2010). "Guidelines for treatment of autoimmune neuromuscular transmission disorders." Eur J Neurol 17(7): 893-902.

Stalberg, E., J. Ekstedt, et al. (1974). "Neuromuscular transmission in myasthenia gravis studied with single fibre electromyography." J Neurol Neurosurg Psychiatry 37(5): 540-7.

Stickler, D. E., J. M. Massey, et al. (2005). "MuSK-antibody positive myasthenia gravis: clinical and electrodiagnostic patterns." Clin Neurophysiol 116(9): 2065-8.

Strickroot, F., Schaeffer, RL and Bergo, HE., (1942). "Myasthenia gravis occuring in an infant born of a myasthenic mother." JAMA(120): 1207-1209.

Tindall, R. S., J. T. Phillips, et al. (1993). "A clinical therapeutic trial of cyclosporine in myasthenia gravis." Ann N Y Acad Sci 681: 539-51.

Tuzun, E., M. N. Meriggioli, et al. (2005). "Myasthenia gravis patients with low plasma IL-6 and IFN-gamma benefit from etanercept treatment." J Autoimmun 24(3): 261-8.

Wang, Q., B. Zhang, et al. (2006). "MuSK signaling at the neuromuscular junction." J Mol Neurosci 30(1-2): 223-6.

Wilson, R. W., M. D. Ward, et al. (1974). "Corticosteroids: a direct effect at the neuromuscular junction." Neurology 24(11): 1091-5.

Vincent, A. and J. Newsom-Davis (1985). "Acetylcholine receptor antibody as a diagnostic test for myasthenia gravis: results in 153 validated cases and 2967 diagnostic assays." J Neurol Neurosurg Psychiatry 48(12): 1246-52.

Vincent, A. and J. Newsom Davis (1980). "Anti-acetylcholine receptor antibodies." J Neurol Neurosurg Psychiatry 43(7): 590-600.

Xu, K., S. Jha, et al. (2006). "Delayed synapsing muscles are more severely affected in an experimental model of MuSK-induced myasthenia gravis." Neuroscience 143(3): 655-9.

Zhang, B., S. Luo, et al. (2008). "LRP4 serves as a coreceptor of agrin." Neuron 60(2): 285-97.

Zinman, L., E. Ng, et al. (2007). "IV immunoglobulin in patients with myasthenia gravis: a randomized controlled trial." Neurology 68(11): 837-41.

Zouvelou, V., M. Rentzos, et al. (2009). "MRI Evidence of Early Muscle Atrophy in MuSK Positive Myasthenia Gravis." J Neuroimaging XX, 1-4.

# 23

# Vasoactive Neuropeptides in Autoimmune Diseases

Ekua W. Brenu[1,2], Lotti Tajouri[1,2],
Donald R. Staines[1,3] and Sonya M. Marshall-Gradisnik[1,2]
[1]*Faculty of Health Science and Medicine, Population Health and Neuroimmunology Unit, Bond University, Robina, Queensland,*
[2]*Faculty of Health Science and Medicine, Bond University, Robina, Queensland,*
[3]*Queensland Health, Gold Coast Population Health Unit, Southport, Queensland, Australia*

## 1. Introduction

Neuropeptides are a class of regulatory peptides with effects in nearly all physiological systems and processes. They are important in facilitating neuroendocrine immune interatctions. Bi-directional communication between these two systems in both the central nervous system (CNS) and the periphery are arbitrated by the presence of these peptidergic innervations. These innervations interacting through unique ligand receptor binding complexes have immunomodulatory effects that preserve neuroendocrine and neuroimmune health. A vast majority of neuropeptides are contained within the lymphoid organs and these include calcitonin-gene-related peptide, somatostatin, glanin, neurokinin, substance P, neuropeptide Y and vasoactive neuropeptides (VNs) (Felten et al., 1987; Felten et al., 1992; Fink and Weihe, 1988; Nohr and Weihe, 1991; Weihe et al., 1991). The two most important VNs, associated with most neuro-immune disorders, are vasoactive intestinal peptide (VIP) and pituitary adenylate cyclase activating peptide (PACAP). VNs are widespread throughout the mammalian body including areas such as central nervous system (CNS), peripheral nervous system (PNS) and other organs. They therefore perform a wide spectrum of activities in the body which are required for the regulation of physiological processes. A number of autoimmune disorders with compromises to physiological activities involving the neuroendocrine and immune systems have been shown to be associated with VNs, hence, VNs may have a role in the progression of these autoimmune disorders. Importantly, VIP and PACAP have G-protein coupled receptors (GPCRs) receptors. Binding and ligation of these receptors triggers GPCR reactions resulting in cAMP production. Downstream signalling activities of cAMP can either be advantageous or detrimental to neuroimmune homeostasis especially in diseased states. This chapter therefore examines the vital role of VIP and PACAP in the mechanism and progression of autoimmune disorders including Rheumatoid Arthritis (RA), Multiple Sclerosis (MS), Alzheimer's Disease (AD), and Parkinson's Disease (PD).

## 2. Vasoactive neuropeptides and their receptors

Vasoactive neuropeptides (VNs) similar to other neuropepties are essential and contribute to the maintenance and synchronization of overall physiological processes. Their involvement in almost all physiological processes attests for their unique and critical role in the mammalian body. The two most important VNs reviewed in this chapter have a function in most neuro-immune disorders. These are vasoactive intestinal peptide (VIP) and pituitary adenylate cyclase activating peptide (PACAP). The discovery of VIP was first noticed in the lungs as the name implies, it was shown to regulate vasodilation (Said and Mutt, 1969), PACAP on the other hand was first recognized in the rat anterior pituitary cells (Miyata et al., 1989).

Over the years knowledge of these peptides and their receptor functions have expanded. They are now known to be prevalent in the central nervous system (CNS), endocrine, skeletal, respiratory, cardiac and lymphoid systems specifically in the cortex, thymus, spleen, lymph nodes, hypothalamus, colon, pituitary gland, neurosecretory fibers, gonads, adrenal, germ cells, gastrointestinal tract, ganglia, neurons and muscle fibers (Arimura and Shioda, 1995; Arimura et al., 1991; Bellinger et al., 1996; Bellinger et al., 1990; Dey et al., 1981; Furness and Costa, 1980; Ganea and Delgado, 2002; Hannibal et al., 1998; Kimura et al., 1994; Koves et al., 1993; Shioda et al., 1994). Their presence in these areas can be translated in to the modulation of inflammatory activities (Delgado et al., 2003), apoptosis (Delgado and Ganea, 2000b), hypoxia and nitric oxide (NO) (Cohen et al., 2002; Larocca et al., 2007), co-neurotransmitter functioning of cholinergic and catecholamine transmitters (Hamelink et al., 2002), cerebellar development (Allais et al., 2007) and integrity of the blood brain/blood spinal barrier (BBB/BSB) (Benagiano et al., 1996).

Immune related activities of VIP and PACAP include regulation of chemokine (CCL2, CCL5, CCL9, CXCL1, CXCL2, CXCL3, CXCL8, and CX3CL1) release for the recruitment of monocytes and neutrophils to sites of infections (Delgado et al., 2004a). They also activate anti-inflammatory mechanisms that repress macrophage related activities such as chemotaxis, phagocytosis and induction of respiratory burst, thereby limiting excessive lymphocyte recruitment and secretion of pro-inflammatory factors (Abad et al., 2005; Ganea and Delgado, 2002; Gomariz et al., 2001). VIP and PACAP modulate inflammatory immune equilibrium by decreasing IL-12 and IL-2, IL-12 promotes expansion of $CD4^+$T cells specifically those classified as pro-inflammatory, Th1 cells, while IL-2 is required for the survival and dominance of these cells (Murphy and Reiner, 2002). Antigen induced cell death (AICD) of $CD4^+$ T lymphocytes can also be aborted by VIP and PACAP (Delgado and Ganea, 2000a). This is done where activation of VIP and PACAP produces cAMP which acts as a second messenger to inhibit the transcription of nuclear factor kappa B (NFκB), nuclear factor of activated T cells (NFAT), Egr2 and 3. The outcome of this is a reduction in the expression of Fas ligand (FasL).

An important characteristic of PACAP and VIP is their role as anti-inflammatory effectors. They are able to induce the generation of Th2 type cytokines and chemokines thereby regulating inflammation (Delgado et al., 1999c; Martinez et al., 1996; Wang et al., 1999). This preferential selection enhances Th2 type cytokines and is protective in preventing autoimmunity. In this regard, PACAP and VIP interactions with other cells such as $CD4^+$T lymphocytes has antagonistic effects on Th1 cells through suppression of chemoattractant molecules CXCL10, while enhancing Th2 homing in up-regulating the release of CCL22

from innate immune cells responsible for attracting these cells to sites of infection (Jiang et al., 2002). VPAC1 inhibits excessive production of pro-inflammatory markers from macrophages and microglia cells while VPAC2 sustains Th2 survival and endorses anti-inflammatory effectors (Feldmann et al., 1996). These anti-inflammatory effectors include IL-10, IL-4, IL-5 and IL-1Ra (Delgado et al., 1999a; Delgado et al., 2004b; Feldmann et al., 1996). Anti-inflammatory responses are highly necessary to restore immune balance after an infection or inflammatory episode has been resolved. Usually inflammation initiates a sequence of events that activates pattern recognition receptors, releasing pro-inflammatory molecules (chemokines and cytokines). Thus activating molecules that allow for the recognition and effective elimination of the pathogens. In some instances when recognition of self antigens fails non-specific activation of inflammatory pathways can override or weaken normal immune homeostasis prompting auroreactivity. VIP and PACAP can prevent these reactions occurring in the absence of injury or pathogenic influence. VIP and PACAP also contribute to Treg expansion and suppressive activities in an attempt to maintain homeostasis (Chorny *et al.*, 2006). VIP and PACAP deficits have been recognized in autoimmune diseases such as Rheumatoid Arthritis, Multiple Sclerosis and Parkinson's Disease (Gomariz et al., 2006), where compromises in their function lead to disequilibrium in the Th1/Th2 effector responses (Staines, 2004). However, in therapeutic instances, cells generated as a consequence of VNs therapy, are more likely to be vigilant and highly antigen specific thus ensuring effective targeting of autoreactive immune responses.
VIP and PACAP act through G-protein coupled receptors (GPCRs), VPAC1, VPAC2 and PAC1. These are seven transmembrane receptors with a diverse range of ligand receptor binding complexes involving proteases, ions, peptides, glyocoproteins, and amines (Harmar, 2001). The diversity in superfamilies and subfamilies enables these receptors to bind to a range of ligands and therefore have effects in all areas of the body. VIP and PACAP receptors belong to the GPCRs class II, these receptors have moderate levels of amino acid sequences (Nicole et al., 1998). G-proteins can usually form complexes with more than one receptor, hence, VIP binds with high affinity to VPAC1 and VPAC2 but not PAC1, PACAP on the other hand is able to bind to all three receptors (Harmar et al., 1998). In the periphery monocytes, macrophages, T lymphocytes and mast cells secrete VIP and PACAP and express receptors VPAC1, VPAC2 and PAC1 on their cell surfaces (Gomariz et al., 1994). VIP and PACAP communications with these receptors activates $G\alpha_s$ subunit of the GPCR protein this transforms GDP to GTP and the βγ subunit dissociates from the complex (Figure 1). GTPα complex incites adenylate cyclase (AC) to catalyse ATP to produce cAMP. cAMP binds to regulatory protein kinase A (PKA) phosphorylating cAMP-regulatory element and binding proteins (CREB) (Ganea and Delgado, 2002; Leceta et al., 2000) and other signalling pathways. These interactions can also control the action of other second messenger systems including calcium ions, diacyglycerol and inositol phosphates (Harmar, 2001). Phosphorylation of CREBB generates downstream effects that can either be antagaonistic or agonistic to the host (Christophe, 1993; Vaudry et al., 2000). VPAC receptors have one polypeptide chain with an N-terminal and a C-termnial with adenylate cyclase activity (Laburthe et al., 1994). Thus VIP and PACAP acting through their receptors can inhibit pro-inflammatory cytokines specifically IL-6, IL-12, TNF-α and nitric oxide (NO) production in microglias, macrophages and T lymphocytes (Delgado et al., 1999b; Delgado et al., 1999c; Martinez et al., 1998).

## 3. Role of VNs in autoimmune disorders

### 3.1 Rheumatoid arthritis

In healthy individuals, the joints are covered by a bilayer of synovium. This synovium is made up of an intimal synovial fluid filled layer and sublining layers. The synovium envelopes the joint and acts as a source of nutrients and lubricant to the cartilage and surface of joints respectively (Katrib et al., 2002). The synovium is a structure comprised of a series of cells and an extracellular matrix containing collagen fibrils and matrix proteins. These cells can be classified as either macrophage like synovial (MLS) cells or fibroblast like synoviocytes (FLS) (Bartok and Firestein, 2010; Chang et al., 2010). The former are hematopoietic cells and have similar properties to macrophages in other tissues and thus have similar markers which include CD11b, CD68, Cd14, CD163 and FcRγ while the FLS are in many ways similar to fibroblasts as they also express CD90, vimentin, type IV and V collagens (Zimmermann et al., 2001).

Severe inflammation of the synovial tissues with incidences of joint obstruction in the hands and feet, presenting in the form of pain redness or dystrophy results in RA. These symptoms usually ensue when the synovial tissue is overpopulated by excessive migration of immune cells and production of inflammatory factors. Hypercellularity in the joints results in autoimmunity and inflammation. Cells responsible for these events are activated macrophages, neutrophils and MLS of the innate immune system and T cells of the adaptive immune system and FLS. The increase in the concentration of these cells in the synovial tissues stimulates a cascade of events that promote inflammation in the joints. Importantly, the influx of these cells into the joint areas occurs due to the release of chemoattractant molecules such as IL-8 which successively attract more cells to the synovial tissues (Georganas et al., 2000). Under normal physiological conditions a healthy joint contains immune cells that release a balanced amount of both pro and anti-inflammatory factors that assist in maintaining inflammatory homeostasis in the joint. In the synovial tissues of RA patients, the cells emit a plethora of pro-inflammatory cytokines including IFN-γ, TNF-α, IL-1 and IL-6, chemokines and growth factors (Kokkonen et al., 2010). These molecules stimulate the FLS and in succession these cells also secrete IL-6, matrix metallo-proteinases (MMP) and prostanoids (Fiedorczyk et al., 2005). Heightened activation of cells in the joints also prompts skewness in the cytokine balance, mostly favouring a predominant pro-inflammatory immune profile (Boissier et al., 2008; Ruschpler and Stiehl, 2002). These events are cyclical and as these molecules are continuously being produced the extracellular matrix, cartilage and bone are destroyed.

FLS are present in large quantities in the intimal lining (Takemura et al., 2001). The ability of these cells to thrive and cause damage relates to their resilience to apoptosis which has been attributed to the presence of NF-κB and sentrin-1 (Franz et al., 2000; Han et al., 1998). Additionally, although various death receptor pathways are present in the synovium the percentage of synviocytes that undergo apoptosis is minimal. In the RA synovium, p53 protein in the synoviocytes is to some extent functionally unresponsive due to somatic mutations (Firestein et al., 1997; Han et al., 1999; Yamanishi et al., 2002) thus preventing apoptosis and rather increasing proliferation and survival of these cells in the joints. Other inflammatory molecules produced by FLS including cytokines such as IL-6, IL-18, IL-33, IL-32 (Brennan and McInnes, 2008), colony stimulating factors (CSF) and type I interferons (IFNs) (Alvaro-Gracia et al., 1989; Genovese et al., 2004) collectively assist in breaking down the extra cellular matrix (Muller-Ladner et al., 1996).

The severity and prevalence of RA in patients may have an association with VNs. VNs, in particular VIP function has been shown to be downregulated in FLS of patients with RA this consequently encourages persistence increase in inflammation. As previously indicated, VIP exerts anti-inflammatory effects through VPACR2 and VPACR1 (Juarranz et al., 2008). Reduced VPACR1 in immune cells produces a predominant Th1 immune response (Delgado et al., 2008a) suggesting that the Th1 profile noticed in RA may be attributed to compromises to these VPAC receptors. Especially the VPACR1 expression in the periphery and the joint is deficient in RA the outcome of this is a dampening of anti-inflammatory molecules, thus increasing the persistence of Th1 cells and pro-inflammatory molecules in RA (Delagado et al., 2001). These observations were correlated with a decrease in cAMP an important immunosuppressive agent involved in the VPACR activation pathway (Foey et al., 2003). VPACR1 and VPACR2 act together to maintain immune tolerance. These protective mechanisms usually involve a decrease in IL-6, TLR4, CCL2 and CCL5 (Arranz et al., 2008). VIP decreases TLR-4 signalling by inhibiting molecules required for TLR-4 directed effects, these may include Pellino 1 and 2, TRAM, TIRAP and TRIF which VIP suppresses. These effects may also be attributed to the negative regulation of VIP on TLR and MyD88 pathways. Incidentally, VIP reduces the effects of MyD88 by suppressing the phosphorylation process associated with IRAK-TRAF6 signalling complex and thereby preventing interactions between IRAK1 and TRAF6 and as a consequence loss of TLR-4 signalling (Arranz et al. 2000).

Similarly, VIP decrease disease severity especially as observed in the experimental model of RA, that is the collagen induce arthritis (CIA). This mainly occurs through the recruiting and induction of $CD4^{+}CD25^{+}$Tregs while at the same time inhibiting the effects of pro-inflammatory Th17 and Th1 cells (Deng et al. 2010). An increase in $CD4^{+}CD25^{+}$Tregs also correlates with increases in Foxp3 levels (Chen et al., 2008). Similarly, PACAP is also able to reverse predominant Th1 pro-inflammatory reactions in RA towards Th2 anti-inflammatory influences by inhibiting the expression of TNF-α and IL-6 and encouraging the production of IL-10 (Abad et al., 2001; Delgado et al., 1996; Garrido et al., 1996). VIP and PACAP are thus very important in immunoregulation in RA, as they are necessary in reinforcing the Th1/Th2 cytokine balance and ensuring that shifts in cytokines are not skewed predominantly towards Th1 cells. Hence, in RA VNs, VIP and PACAP administration may therefore be both therapeutic and protective against heightened autoreactive inflammatory reactions that can severely damage the joints.

### 3.2 Multiple sclerosis

MS is a heterogeneous and multifactorial disease characterised by severe inflammation to the central nervous system. The reported prevalence rate worldwide in 2002 was said to be between 1.1 and 2.5 million (Pugliatti et al., 2002). MS is both an autoimmune and neurodegenerative disorder which affects the brain and spinal cord and manifests itself in the form of chronic inflammation, axonal degradation, myelin loss, gliosis, breach in the blood brain barrier (BBB) and abnormal immune regulation. MS patients also experience loss in sensory function, vision and motor skills (Mattle, 2005). MS can be subdivided in to three categories based on the clinical progression of the disease, these include relapsing-remitting MS, secondary progressive MS and primary progressive MS (Hauw et al., 1999). There are many theories on the aetiology of MS, although MS has been shown to have both environmental and genetic components. Susceptibility to MS may be associated with genetic variation, environmental factors, intrinsic factors and epistatic factors (Ewing and Bernard, 1998; Granieri, 2000; Hutter and Laing, 1996; Oksenberg and Barcellos, 2000).

The BBB is specialized to protect the CNS against infiltrates such as autoreactive T cells. In MS, BBB destruction occurs as a consequence of infiltration and permeation of the barrier by leukocytes, in particular autoreactive T cells. Increasing the permeability of the BBB enhances autoreactive reactions and destabilises neuroimmunological processes. There are many cells that are affected in MS pathology these include cells of the innate and adaptive immune system. Most of these cells are highly activated, importantly, dendritic cells are highly activated in MS and also contribute to the skewness towards Th1 immune profile in MS. Autoreactive T cells obstruct proteolipid protein, myelin oligodendrocyte glycoproteins and myelin basic proteins (Zhang et al., 2008). Additionally, both Th1 and Th17 cells tend to drive the disease towards pro-inflammation as these cells produce strong secretions of IFN-γ and IL-17. IL-17 promotes inflammation as they are able to invade and move into the CNS, they can also be found in high levels in the peripheral circulation in cases of severe MS symptoms (Kebir et al., 2007). The ability of pro-inflammatory cells to thrive and secrete inflammatory cytokines can be as a result of a decrease in anti-inflammatory cellular functions. In particular, although Treg cell numbers in MS remain relatively unchanged when compared to non-MS individuals, the suppressive nature of these cells are significantly reduced. Foxp3 expression is also decreased in MS especially in those with secondary relapsing MS (Huan et al., 2005). $CD8^+T$ cells despite being functional in MS act to inhibit $CD4^+T$ and glial cells by releasing cytotoxic molecules that suppress the proliferation of these cells.

VIP has important regulatory effects in MS, in animal models of MS such as in Experimental autoimmune encephalomyelitis (EAE), the presence of VIP in circulation reduces pro-inflammation and restores the Th1/Th2 cytokine balance. The anti-inflammatory effects of VIP/PACAP are important in both the adaptive and innate immune system. In MS, VIP and PACAP prevent heightened immune reactions by decreasing pro-inflammatory molecules produced by macrophages, microglia, dendritic cells, Th1 and Th17 cells. VIP when administered acts to decrease the progression of EAE, prevent neurological damage and relapses (Gonzalez-Rey et al., 2006). PACAP on the other hand represses antigen presenting cell activities initiated by macrophages and dendritic cells (Kato et al., 2004). In the CNS these anti-inflammatory reactions induced by VIP and PACAP are protective in the MS environment where anti-inflammatory reactions are minimal (Gozes et al., 1997; Gressens et al., 1997). Additionally damaged neurons of the CNS may release VIP and PACAP perhaps as a restorative mechanism, in an attempt to rescue homeostasis in the CNS and this has been confirmed by down regulation of molecules such as, TNF-a, IL-6, IL-1β and overactive microglia (Delgado et al., 2002). Hence, destructive effects of overactive microglia causing demyelination and axonal loss may be as a consequence of impaired VIP and PACAP activities. RANTES is another chemokine molecule that is implicated in the pathogenesis of EAE as it has the ability to also elevate inflammation in the CNS, however, VIP via the VPAC1 can dampen NF-kB and effectively RANTES (Li et al., 2006). Thus, suppressing leukocyte infiltration and inflammation in the CNS. VIP has been observed in lymphoid organs and in immune cells such as T and B cells where they increase immune related activities (Delgado et al., 2004b; Pozo, 2003) such as acting on APC through the inhibition of IL-12 produced by macrophages while endorsing the expression of B7-2, favouring a predominant Th2 immune cell profile. As previously stated Treg function is reduced in MS patients and VIP induces the development of $CD4^+CD25^+$Tregs, these VIP-Tregs have more efficient suppressive effects owing to the high expression of CTLA-4 (Fernandez-Martin et al., 2006). They suppress autoreactive T cells and decrease the severity of the disease (Chorny et al., 2006).

VIP effects are thought to be either via VPAC1 or VPAC2 receptors. VIP binding to VPAC1 relates to an induction of Tregs while binding or activating of the VPAC2 receptor is associated with Th2 cell activation (Delgado et al., 2005b; Delgado et al., 2004b; Pozo and Delgado, 2004). VIP and PACAP receptors also play an important role in MS. VPACR2 is necessary to ensure balance between the Th1 and Th2 cytokine profiles by promoting the prevalence of Th2 cells. In MS VPACR2 is compromised owing to the limiting number of receptors that are expressed on immune cell surfaces, this increases the dominance of Th1 cells and cytokines. This compromise to VPAC2 in MS patients may also occur at the molecular level where mRNA expression levels of VPACR2 are down regulated. Additionally, the formation of the VIP ligand receptor complex stimulates cAMP/PKA downstream effects which ultimately dampen IFN-γ and stimulates the generation of GATA3 (Sun et al., 2006). This in effect increases the expression of Th2 immune cells. PACAP also acts directly to reduce pro-inflammatory cytokines IFN-γ, TNF-α, IL-1β and IL-12 released from macrophages and microglia cells in areas of neurological breakdown in the CNS, preventing oligodendrocyte death while increasing the expression of CCR4 on Tregs (Kato et al., 2004). T cells in the presence of these VNs produce brain derived neurotrophic factors that allow for the increase in axonal growth remyelination, neuronal regeneration and decreases neuronal degeneration. VIP also induces astrocytes to produce neurotrophic factors. Thus VIP and PACAP confer both anti-inflammatory and neuroprotective effects on neurons and cells of the neuroimmune system. In other animal models of MS such as in the myelin/oligodendrocyte glycoprotein (MOG) deficient mice, PACAP administration prevents elevations in the severity of MS by decreasing the effects of autoreactive microglia and macrophages (Cunningham et al., 2007). VIP also inhibits co-stimulatory molecules such as CD40, CD80 and CD86 required and produced by over stimulated dendritic cells, microglia and macrophages (Delgado et al., 2005a; Gonzalez-Rey et al., 2007).

### 3.3 Alzheimer disease

Dementia is a well known disorder of the CNS and about 50% of all dementia are associated with AD (Pasquier, 2000). AD is a disease of the CNS characterised by progressive loss in memory and cognition. The current prevalence rate is between 2.8 and 56-56.1 enduring for about 8-10 years following diagnosis (Koedam et al., 2010). There are two subtypes of AD defined based on age of onset, that is, early and late onset. 5% of all cases of AD are associated with early onset (Koedam et al., 2010). Most early onset of AD are autosomal dominant and passed on within families. Similar to MS, AD has a genetic component and mutations in a number of genes have been proposed to underlie some cases of AD. Among these are mutations in the presenilin (PSEN) 1 and 2 (Avila-Gomez et al., 2008) and amyloid precursor protein (Miar et al., 2011). The presence of apolipoprotein E (APOE) specifically APOEε2 and APOEε4 alleles on chromosome 19 may potentially predispose an individual to developing late on set AD (Vemuri et al., 2010).

Diagnosis of AD is based on the observation of neurofibrillary tangles and myeloid plaques in various areas of the CNS (Bierer et al., 1995). These plaques also known as senile plaques occurring in various brain regions are caused by deposition of extracellular fibrillar β-amyloid (Aβ) peptides (Selkoe, 1998). Aβ is a derivative of the proteolytic amyloid precursor protein (Maccioni et al., 2001). The presence of Aβ in the brain or fibrils results in the activation of microglia and the secretion of vast amounts of pro-inflammatory cytokines causing neuronal damage and neuronal loss in the temporal and parietal regions (McGeer et al., 1994). Other brain areas that are affected include the hippocampus and neocortex (Scheff et al., 1996; Scheff et al., 1993). These detrimental effects manifest in the form of loss in cognitive function, memory and cognition. The scope of neurofibrillary tangles in most cases of AD is associated with the level of dementia and the length of the disease as these may have severe effects on neurological function (Arriagada et al., 1992; Bierer et al., 1995).

As the CNS is under constant surveillance by these cells health of the CNS is maintained. Importantly, microglias interact with neurons, glia cells, tissues, vessels and synapses, thus they are able to remove unwanted material, dead cells and repair damaged tissues and synapses (Wake et al., 2009). Microglias upon activation induce the release of cytokines, chemokine, free radicals and acute phase proteins which are important in eliminating foreign pathogens. Nonetheless, the regulation of microglia activation may also be important for maintaining neurological homeostasis. Reduced activation of microglia in the normal brain occurs via interactions with chemokine receptors present on the microglia hence as microglias survey the neuro-environment they bind to molecules on the neurons which inhibit their activation (Randsohoff et al. 2007). Similarly, excessive secretion of pro-inflammatory mediators is prevented through ligand binding between CD200L on the microglia and CD200 on the neuronal cells (Biber et al., 2007). In AD microglias function is to some extent impaired. Senescence may play a role here, as it has been observed that aged microglias or microglia from elderly patients tend to be obscured in their function and have reduced motility (meyer-leuhmann et al., 2008; Streit et al., 2008). However, in most instances microglia function is related to their localization in a particular site, hence, they transform their functions to suite their particular location in the CNS. Development of senile plaques in AD induces the development of microglia phenotype that is associated with plaque formation. These microglias are therefore highly activated and more reactive in response to amyloid deposition (Yan et al. 2009; Bornemann et al., 2001).

The most predominant receptors on microglias are the pattern recognition receptors which include Toll-like receptors (TLRs). Using these receptors, microglia recognise damage associated molecular patterns (DAMPs) molecules and pathogen associated molecular patterns (PAMPs) released from damaged tissues and pathogens respectively. Detection of these molecules elicits an inflammatory response from these microglias. TLR2 and TLR4 are the most influential receptors related to AD. They detect fibrillar Aβ and their interactions with these molecules activate the microglia. TLRs also communicate with other receptors that interact with fAβ such as scavenger receptor A, CD36, CD47, α6β1 integrin. Thus this phenotypically different microglia in areas of plaque formation form as a consequence of engaging with fAβ using the TLRs activating pro-inflammatory Th1 immune responses and produce reactive oxygen species (Mantovani et al. 2004). As with other neurological diseases, activation of microglias results in the secretion of high levels of cytokines and pro-inflammatory factors. Thus increasing neurotoxicity in the CNS and further weakening the neuro-immune environment. This is in contrast to their normal function where they interact with other neurons and glia to decrease their activation brought on by the presence of pro-inflammatory factors and also redundant immune activation (Colton, 2009).

Microglias in the AD patients are abundant in the cortex, this has been shown to be associated with a reduced cognitive function in these patients (Edison et al. 2008). However, this may not be present in all patients with AD. Induction of the α-secretase pathway enhances the protective effects of PACAP via the PAC1 receptor and also the production of amyloid precursor protein alpha (APP-α) thus decreasing the prevalence of Aβ in AD. Hence, PACAP and PAC1 prevent apoptosis of neurons enhancing their survival (Dejda et al., 2005; Onoue et al., 2002). Autoreactivity, due to Aβ can also be averted in the presence of PACAP as these neuropeptides are able to modulate the proliferative properties of these cells and induce them to produce gliotransmitters and gliopeptides which are protective against neuronal degradation and death (Masmoudi-Kouki et al., 2007). PACAP is able to enhance memory creation in animal models (Sacchetti et al., 2001). By binding to its receptor PAC1 it encourages the release of α-secretase and stimulates the release of APLP-2. APLP2 in turn induces the growth of neurons (White et al., 1998). VIP also exerts neuroprotective effects in AD as it its able to dampen the effects of migroglai cells that have been activated by Aβ and thus dampening, the secretion of neurotoxins TNF-α, IL-1β and NO and reducing neuronal death. These effects of VIP are enable through the VPAC1 receptor. VIP binding to VPAC1 sets off a cascade of reactions involving the cAMP/PKA pathway which in sequence activates neurotrophic dependent factors to enhance neuroinal survival (Gozes, 2001). VIP also inhibits IKK, p38 and p42 responsible for NFκB activation and pro-inflammaotry cytokine release (Delgado et al., 2008b).

### 3.4 Parkinson's disease

Aggressive loss of neurons of the striato-nigral centres, nucleus basalis, raphe nuclei, locus coeruleus, autonomic ganglia, amygdala, hippocampus, cingulated, temporal cortex and the olfactory bulb are associated with Parkinson's disease (PD). Neurotransmitters also become deficient in PD, and this has been shown to be the single most important factor causing considerable defects in muscle and manifesting in the form of rigidity, akinesia and tremors (Lee, 1989). The symptoms of PD are therefore comprised of loss in attention cognitive and motor function (Lippa, 2010). PD can either be sporadic or familial. The illness starts off later in life and progressively worsens with death occurring a few years after onset of disease (Doudet, 2001). It is an adult onset disease that affects individuals between the ages of 20 to 75 years with a prevalence rate of 13.4 per 100,000 (Van Den Eeden et al., 2003).

In the periphery total lymphocytes especially $CD3^+$ and $CD4^+CD3^+$ and B cells tend to be reduced in PD patients compared to healthy controls, similarly diminished levels of memory T cells have been observed while activated T cells are elevated (Bas et al., 2001; Fiszer et al., 1994; Offen et al., 1996). Patients may also demonstrate reduced $CD8^+$T, $CD4^+$: $CD8^+$ T, cell ratios, $CD4^+CD25^+$T cells and an increase in IFN-γ and IL-4 T cells (Gruden et al.), with shifts in cytokines towards pro-inflammatory cytokine profile thus causing potential heightened inflammation in the brain. Microglia in the neuro-inflammed CNS facilitates the excessive production of cytokines, neurotrophins, reactive oxygen and nitrogen species (ROS and RNS). In PD, the affected CNS regions include dopaminergic, cholinergic, serotonergic and noradrenergic neurons and their neurotransmitters are implicated in the mechanism of PD (Bosboom et al., 2004). Regions of lewy bodies are dispersed throughout the regions of neuronal loss, these contain alpha-synuclein and ubiquitin and are more prominent in the dopamine neurons of the substantia nigra (Kosaka, 2000; Kosaka and Iseki, 2000).

Additionally, microglia are also compromised in PD, they tend to produce high levels of MHCII antigen leukocyte antigen-DR (HLA-DR) and inflammatory molecules including IL-1β, IL-6 and TNF-α and express ICAM-1 and LFA-1 (McGeer and McGeer, 2008; McGeer et al., 2001). The activated microglia portray high levels of ICAM-1 and LFA-1, thus these molecules in SN may also be implicated in the influx of immune cells in the affected areas (Imamura et al., 2003). In the CNS microglia are responsible for, antigen presentation, removal damaged and apoptotic cells and secretion of pro-inflammatory and neurotrophic factors. These factors can either be protective or toxic to the CNS environment (Sawada et al., 2006), thus microglias have two contradictory roles in the CNS, depending on the CNS environment. Microglia become activated when they come into contact with damaged or lingering neuron when this occurs the microglia will assist in repairing and restoring these damaged neurons. These microglia express TNF-α and IL-6, these cytokines have neurotrophic components (Diogenes and Outeiro, 2010; Gash et al., 2007; Reale et al., 2009). Neurotoxic effects of microglias underlie some of the detrimental effects conferred on neurons in the CNS, neurotixic microglia increase the levels of pro-inflammatory cytokines, neurotrophins, reactive oxygen species and reactive nitrogen species (Long-Smith et al., 2009). They can become harmful when they synthesise and secrete molecules that increase synaptic overactivity and thus increase the damage already present. They may also alter excitotoxicity, abort apoptosis and encourage the growth of neurite in the injured CNS (Barger et al., 1995; Berezovskaya et al., 1995; Imamura et al., 1990; Lazarov-Spiegler et al., 1996; Prewitt et al., 1997; Rabchevsky and Streit, 1997; Toku et al., 1998). Activated microglias are present in other areas of the CNS and therefore initiate and promote inflammation in different brain regions including the putamen, substantia nigra and cingulated cortex where they are responsible for the generation of lewy bodies (Li et al., 2010; McKeith and Mosimann, 2004; Varani et al., 2010). TNF-α and IL-1β have similar signalling mechanisms and induce neurodegeneration in the CNS by activating NKFκB, thus facilitating oxidative damage and consequently neuronal damage (Wahner et al., 2007). The toxic effects of IL-1β and TNF-α can also be attributed to their ability to increase the expression of leukocyte adhesion molecules on the surfaces of the endothelial cells. This elevates inflammation in the CNS affecting neuronal survival (Whitton, 2007). At the molecular level mitochondrial and cytoskeletal dysfunction, oxidative damage, neuroinflammation and abnormal protein accumulation contribute to the progression of PD (Winner et al., 2009).

Inducible nitric oxide synthase (iNOS), and NADP-oxidase secreted by activated microglia increase the production of NO and reactive oxygen species causing neurodegeneration. VIP is able to reduce microglial activation thereby preventing the release and damaging effects of these factors (Delgado and Ganea, 2003). Additionally in the CNS, the release of IFN-γ by activated microglia tends to be rather harmful. IFN-γ binds to its receptor sets off a cascade of events involving transphosphorylation of the receptor-associated janus tyrosine kinases (Jak)1 and 2. This facilitates the recruitment and phosphorylation of signal transducer and activator of transcription (STAT1) (Dell'Albani et al., 2001). These sequences of events stimulate IFN-γ, inducible protein 10, iNOS, CD40 and IL-12. VIP and PACAP together reduce microglia pro-inflammatory activities through VIP and PACAP binding to VPAC1 and dampening the phosphorylation and formation of the Jak1-2/STAT1 complex. This prevents the synthesis of IRF-1, and inhibits IFN-γ and iNOS expression from microglia in the striatum and also in the substantia nigra. These inhibitory effects are facilitated by the cAMP pathway (Delgado, 2003).

TNF-α released in the CNS encourages gliosis, preventing the uptake of glutamate by astrocytes and apoptosis in oligodendrocytes (Kim et al., 2000). When VIP or PACAP is applied to microglia stimulated by LPS from rats in culture it was noticed that VIP and PACAP substantially decreased the expression of TNF-α. These inhibitory effects were facilitated via cAMP pathway (Delgado et al., 1998; Kim et al., 2000). VPAC1 and PAC1 receptors are present on microglial cells therefore they are able to directly act on overactive microglia cells efficiently reducing their neurotoxic effects upon Ligand receptor binding (Kim et al., 2000). Although TNF-α may have detrimemmntal effects on the microglia, in some cases they have been shown to be protective as they release reactive oxygen species that act to protect neurons from harm and stimulate an increase in anti-inflammatory IL-10 (Cheng et al., 1994; Sheng et al., 1995). VIP and PACAP also act to inhibit the presence of macrophage inflammatory protein (MIP-1alpha, 1 beta), macrophage chemoattractant protein (MCP-1) and RANTES, chemokine released by microglia cells (Zhang et al., 2000).

PACAP protects neurons in quinolinic acid- and 6-hydoxydopamine-induced lesions (exprimental model of PD), which correlates with the less severe behavioral symptoms (Tamas et al., 2006). VIP ameliorates dopamine induced cell death and neuronal cell loss of striatal dopaminergic fibers (Offen et al., 2000). These peptides present in the compromised CNS can have important benefits for individuals affected. Although these peptides may not necessarily completely clear the disease, they may prolong the life and function of PD patients.

## 4. Conclusion

In summary, it is apparent that VIP and PACAP are vital for the enhancement of anti-inflammatory reactions in autoimmune diseases with compromises to neuro-endocrine-immune mechanism. These fundamental anti-inflammatory responses assist in decreasing pro-inflammatory reactions observed in most autoimmune diseases including RA, MS, PD and AD. Thus VIP and PACAP are important in suppressing elevated amounts of IFN-γ, TNF-α, IL-6 and IL1β. Modulation of these factors to optimal levels promotes and preserves the survival of cells and tissues affect these diseases. A decrease in their receptors is a common finding in most autoimmune disorders and this is often correlated with decreases in cAMP. Additionally, Th1/Th2/Th17 disequilibrium is noticed in the above mentioned diseases. VIP and PACAP are able to reverse and regulate these shifts in inflammatory cytokines. Their ability to maintain both peripheral and CNS homeostasis highlights their importance in physiological processes.

VIP and PACAP are therefore potential candidates for treating autoimmune disorders. Their administration may substantially reduce symptoms and improve the quality of life of patients with RA, MS, PD and ALS. As VIP and PACAP activate cAMP pathways, therapies that remove inhibitors of cAMP may be important. These inhibitors include Phosphosdiesterase enzymes. Phosphosdiesterase enzymes inhibitors (PDEIs) may have potential advantage in the treatment of autoimmune disorders. PDEIs may also increase the effectiveness of these VNs as they can increase the intracellular cAMP and therefore initiate anti-inflammatory mechanisms. Incidentally, PDEIs are known to prolong life and reduce cytokines, demyelination and inflammation. Hence further studies are required to examine the most effective therapies for these autoimmune disorders.

## 5. References


Abad, C., Juarranz, Y., Martinez, C., Arranz, A., Rosignoli, F., Garcia-Gomez, M., Leceta, J. and Gomariz, R.P. (2005) cDNA array analysis of cytokines, chemokines, and receptors involved in the development of TNBS-induced colitis: homeostatic role of VIP. Inflamm Bowel Dis 11, 674-84.

Abad, C., Martinez, C., Leceta, J., Gomariz, R.P. and Delgado, M. (2001) Pituitary adenylate cyclase-activating polypeptide inhibits collagen-induced arthritis: an experimental immunomodulatory therapy. J Immunol 167, 3182-9.

Allais, A., Burel, D., Isaac, E.R., Gray, S.L., Basille, M., Ravni, A., Sherwood, N.M., Vaudry, H. and Gonzalez, B.J. (2007) Altered cerebellar development in mice lacking pituitary adenylate cyclase-activating polypeptide. Eur J Neurosci 25, 2604-18.

Alvaro-Gracia, J.M., Zvaifler, N.J. and Firestein, G.S. (1989) Cytokines in chronic inflammatory arthritis. IV. Granulocyte/macrophage colony-stimulating factor-mediated induction of class II MHC antigen on human monocytes: a possible role in rheumatoid arthritis. J Exp Med 170, 865-75.

Arimura, A. and Shioda, S. (1995) Pituitary adenylate cyclase activating polypeptide (PACAP) and its receptors: neuroendocrine and endocrine interaction. Front Neuroendocrinol 16, 53-88.

Arimura, A., Somogyvari-Vigh, A., Miyata, A., Mizuno, K., Coy, D.H. and Kitada, C. (1991) Tissue distribution of PACAP as determined by RIA: highly abundant in the rat brain and testes. Endocrinology 129, 2787-9.

Arranz, A., Gutierrez-Canas, I., Carrion, M., Juarranz, Y., Pablos, J.L., Martinez, C. and Gomariz, R.P. (2008) VIP reverses the expression profiling of TLR4-stimulated signaling pathway in rheumatoid arthritis synovial fibroblasts. Mol Immunol 45, 3065-73.

Arriagada, P.V., Growdon, J.H., Hedley-Whyte, E.T. and Hyman, B.T. (1992) Neurofibrillary tangles but not senile plaques parallel duration and severity of Alzheimer's disease. Neurology 42, 631-9.

Avila-Gomez, I.C., Jimenez-Del-Rio, M., Lopera-Restrepo, F. and Velez-Pardo, C. (2008) Association between HFE 187 C>G (H63D) mutation and early-onset familial Alzheimer's disease PSEN-1 839A>C (E280A) mutation. Annals of hematology 87, 671-3.

Barger, S.W., Horster, D., Furukawa, K., Goodman, Y., Krieglstein, J. and Mattson, M.P. (1995) Tumor necrosis factors alpha and beta protect neurons against amyloid beta-peptide toxicity: evidence for involvement of a kappa B-binding factor and attenuation of peroxide and Ca2+ accumulation. Proc Natl Acad Sci U S A 92, 9328-32.

Bartok, B. and Firestein, G.S. (2010) Fibroblast-like synoviocytes: key effector cells in rheumatoid arthritis. Immunological reviews 233, 233-55.

Bas, J., Calopa, M., Mestre, M., Mollevi, D.G., Cutillas, B., Ambrosio, S. and Buendia, E. (2001) Lymphocyte populations in Parkinson's disease and in rat models of parkinsonism. J Neuroimmunol 113, 146-52.

Bellinger, D.L., Lorton, D., Brouxhon, S., Felten, S. and Felten, D.L. (1996) The significance of vasoactive intestinal polypeptide (VIP) in immunomodulation. Adv Neuroimmunol 6, 5-27.

Bellinger, D.L., Lorton, D., Romano, T.D., Olschowka, J.A., Felten, S.Y. and Felten, D.L. (1990) Neuropeptide innervation of lymphoid organs. Ann N Y Acad Sci 594, 17-33.

Benagiano, V., Virgintino, D., Maiorano, E., Rizzi, A., Palombo, S., Roncali, L. and Ambrosi, G. (1996) VIP-like immunoreactivity within neurons and perivascular neuronal processes of the human cerebral cortex. Eur J Histochem 40, 53-6.

Berezovskaya, O., Maysinger, D. and Fedoroff, S. (1995) The hematopoietic cytokine, colony-stimulating factor 1, is also a growth factor in the CNS: congenital absence of CSF-1 in mice results in abnormal microglial response and increased neuron vulnerability to injury. Int J Dev Neurosci 13, 285-99.

Biber, K., Neumann, H., Inoue, K. and Boddeke, H.W. (2007) Neuronal 'On' and 'Off' signals control microglia. Trends Neurosci 30, 596-602.

Bierer, L.M., Hof, P.R., Purohit, D.P., Carlin, L., Schmeidler, J., Davis, K.L. and Perl, D.P. (1995) Neocortical neurofibrillary tangles correlate with dementia severity in Alzheimer's disease. Arch Neurol 52, 81-8.

Boissier, M.C., Assier, E., Falgarone, G. and Bessis, N. (2008) Shifting the imbalance from Th1/Th2 to Th17/treg: the changing rheumatoid arthritis paradigm. Joint, bone, spine : revue du rhumatisme 75, 373-5.

Bosboom, J.L., Stoffers, D. and Wolters, E. (2004) Cognitive dysfunction and dementia in Parkinson's disease. J Neural Transm 111, 1303-15.

Brennan, F.M. and McInnes, I.B. (2008) Evidence that cytokines play a role in rheumatoid arthritis. J Clin Invest 118, 3537-45.

Chang, S.K., Gu, Z. and Brenner, M.B. (2010) Fibroblast-like synoviocytes in inflammatory arthritis pathology: the emerging role of cadherin-11. Immunological reviews 233, 256-66.

Chen, G., Hao, J., Xi, Y., Wang, W., Wang, Z., Li, N. and Li, W. (2008) The therapeutic effect of vasoactive intestinal peptide on experimental arthritis is associated with CD4+CD25+ T regulatory cells. Scand J Immunol 68, 572-8.

Cheng, B., Christakos, S. and Mattson, M.P. (1994) Tumor necrosis factors protect neurons against metabolic-excitotoxic insults and promote maintenance of calcium homeostasis. Neuron 12, 139-53.

Chorny, A., Gonzalez-Rey, E., Ganea, D. and Delgado, M. (2006) Vasoactive intestinal peptide generates CD4+CD25+ regulatory T cells in vivo: therapeutic applications in autoimmunity and transplantation. Ann N Y Acad Sci 1070, 190-5.

Christophe, J. (1993) [The neuropeptide PACAP: its presence, its mode of action and its receptors]. Bull Mem Acad R Med Belg 148, 188-93.

Cohen, G., Gressens, P., Gallego, J. and Gaultier, C. (2002) Depression of hypoxic arousal response in adolescent mice following antenatal vasoactive intestinal polypeptide blockade. J Physiol 540, 691-9.

Cunningham, S., O'Doherty, C., Patterson, C., McDonnell, G., Hawkins, S., Marrosu, M.G. and Vandenbroeck, K. (2007) The neuropeptide genes TAC1, TAC3, TAC4, VIP and PACAP(ADCYAP1), and susceptibility to multiple sclerosis. Journal of neuroimmunology 183, 208-13.

Dejda, A., Sokolowska, P. and Nowak, J.Z. (2005) Neuroprotective potential of three neuropeptides PACAP, VIP and PHI. Pharmacol Rep 57, 307-20.

Delgado, M. (2003) Inhibition of interferon (IFN) gamma-induced Jak-STAT1 activation in microglia by vasoactive intestinal peptide: inhibitory effect on CD40, IFN-induced protein-10, and inducible nitric-oxide synthase expression. J Biol Chem 278, 27620-9.

Delgado, M., Abad, C., Martinez, C., Juarranz, M.G., Leceta, J., Ganea, D. and Gomariz, R.P. (2003) PACAP in immunity and inflammation. Ann N Y Acad Sci 992, 141-57.

Delgado, M. and Ganea, D. (2000a) Vasoactive intestinal peptide and pituitary adenylate cyclase-activating polypeptide inhibit antigen-induced apoptosis of mature T lymphocytes by inhibiting Fas ligand expression. J Immunol 164, 1200-10.

Delgado, M. and Ganea, D. (2000b) VIP and PACAP inhibit activation induced apoptosis in T lymphocytes. Ann N Y Acad Sci 921, 55-67.

Delgado, M. and Ganea, D. (2003) Neuroprotective effect of vasoactive intestinal peptide (VIP) in a mouse model of Parkinson's disease by blocking microglial activation. FASEB J 17, 944-6.

Delgado, M., Gonzalez-Rey, E. and Ganea, D. (2004a) VIP/PACAP preferentially attract Th2 effectors through differential regulation of chemokine production by dendritic cells. FASEB J 18, 1453-5.

Delgado, M., Gonzalez-Rey, E. and Ganea, D. (2005a) The neuropeptide vasoactive intestinal peptide generates tolerogenic dendritic cells. Journal of immunology 175, 7311-24.

Delgado, M., Gonzalez-Rey, E. and Ganea, D. (2005b) The neuropeptide vasoactive intestinal peptide generates tolerogenic dendritic cells. J Immunol 175, 7311-24.

Delgado, M., Leceta, J. and Ganea, D. (2002) Vasoactive intestinal peptide and pituitary adenylate cyclase-activating polypeptide promote in vivo generation of memory Th2 cells. FASEB J 16, 1844-6.

Delgado, M., Leceta, J., Gomariz, R.P. and Ganea, D. (1999a) Vasoactive intestinal peptide and pituitary adenylate cyclase-activating polypeptide stimulate the induction of Th2 responses by up-regulating B7.2 expression. J Immunol 163, 3629-35.

Delgado, M., Martinez, C., Leceta, J., Garrido, E. and Gomariz, R.P. (1996) Differential VIP and VIP1 receptor gene expression in rat thymocyte subsets. Peptides 17, 803-7.

Delgado, M., Munoz-Elias, E.J., Gomariz, R.P. and Ganea, D. (1999b) VIP and PACAP inhibit IL-12 production in LPS-stimulated macrophages. Subsequent effect on IFNgamma synthesis by T cells. J Neuroimmunol 96, 167-81.

Delgado, M., Munoz-Elias, E.J., Kan, Y., Gozes, I., Fridkin, M., Brenneman, D.E., Gomariz, R.P. and Ganea, D. (1998) Vasoactive intestinal peptide and pituitary adenylate cyclase-activating polypeptide inhibit tumor necrosis factor alpha transcriptional activation by regulating nuclear factor-kB and cAMP response element-binding protein/c-Jun. J Biol Chem 273, 31427-36.

Delgado, M., Munoz-Elias, E.J., Martinez, C., Gomariz, R.P. and Ganea, D. (1999c) VIP and PACAP38 modulate cytokine and nitric oxide production in peritoneal macrophages and macrophage cell lines. Ann N Y Acad Sci 897, 401-14.

Delgado, M., Pozo, D. and Ganea, D. (2004b) The significance of vasoactive intestinal peptide in immunomodulation. Pharmacol Rev 56, 249-90.

Delgado, M., Robledo, G., Rueda, B., Varela, N., O'Valle, F., Hernandez-Cortes, P., Caro, M., Orozco, G., Gonzalez-Rey, E. and Martin, J. (2008a) Genetic association of vasoactive intestinal peptide receptor with rheumatoid arthritis: altered expression and signal in immune cells. Arthritis Rheum 58, 1010-9.

Delgado, M., Varela, N. and Gonzalez-Rey, E. (2008b) Vasoactive intestinal peptide protects against beta-amyloid-induced neurodegeneration by inhibiting microglia activation at multiple levels. Glia 56, 1091-103.

Dell'Albani, P., Santangelo, R., Torrisi, L., Nicoletti, V.G., de Vellis, J. and Giuffrida Stella, A.M. (2001) JAK/STAT signaling pathway mediates cytokine-induced iNOS expression in primary astroglial cell cultures. J Neurosci Res 65, 417-24.

Deng, S., Xi, Y., Wang, H., Hao, J., Niu, X., Li, W., Tao, Y. and Chen, G. Regulatory effect of vasoactive intestinal peptide on the balance of Treg and Th17 in collagen-induced arthritis. Cell Immunol 265, 105-10.

Dey, R.D., Shannon, W.A., Jr. and Said, S.I. (1981) Localization of VIP-immunoreactive nerves in airways and pulmonary vessels of dogs, cat, and human subjects. Cell Tissue Res 220, 231-8.

Diogenes, M.J. and Outeiro, T.F. (2010) Neurotrophic factors as a protective strategy in Parkinson's disease. CNS Neurol Disord Drug Targets 9, 754-63.

Doudet, D.J. (2001) Monitoring disease progression in Parkinson's disease. J Clin Pharmacol Suppl, 72S-80S.

Ewing, C. and Bernard, C.C. (1998) Insights into the aetiology and pathogenesis of multiple sclerosis. Immunology and cell biology 76, 47-54.

Feldmann, M., Brennan, F.M. and Maini, R.N. (1996) Role of cytokines in rheumatoid arthritis. Annu Rev Immunol 14, 397-440.

Felten, D.L., Felten, S.Y., Bellinger, D.L., Carlson, S.L., Ackerman, K.D., Madden, K.S., Olschowki, J.A. and Livnat, S. (1987) Noradrenergic sympathetic neural interactions with the immune system: structure and function. Immunol Rev 100, 225-60.

Felten, S.Y., Felten, D.L., Bellinger, D.L. and Olschowka, J.A. (1992) Noradrenergic and peptidergic innervation of lymphoid organs. Chem Immunol 52, 25-48.

Fernandez-Martin, A., Gonzalez-Rey, E., Chorny, A., Ganea, D. and Delgado, M. (2006) Vasoactive intestinal peptide induces regulatory T cells during experimental autoimmune encephalomyelitis. Eur J Immunol 36, 318-26.

Fiedorczyk, M., Klimiuk, P.A., Sierakowski, S., Domyslawska, I. and Chwiecko, J. (2005) [Correlations between serum matrix metalloproteinase (MMP-1, MMP-3, MMP-9, MMP-13) concentrations and markers of disease activity in early rheumatoid arthritis]. Przeglad lekarski 62, 1321-4.

Fink, T. and Weihe, E. (1988) Multiple neuropeptides in nerves supplying mammalian lymph nodes: messenger candidates for sensory and autonomic neuroimmunomodulation? Neurosci Lett 90, 39-44.

Firestein, G.S., Echeverri, F., Yeo, M., Zvaifler, N.J. and Green, D.R. (1997) Somatic mutations in the p53 tumor suppressor gene in rheumatoid arthritis synovium. Proc Natl Acad Sci U S A 94, 10895-900.

Fiszer, U., Mix, E., Fredrikson, S., Kostulas, V. and Link, H. (1994) Parkinson's disease and immunological abnormalities: increase of HLA-DR expression on monocytes in cerebrospinal fluid and of CD45RO+ T cells in peripheral blood. Acta Neurol Scand 90, 160-6.

Foey, A.D., Field, S., Ahmed, S., Jain, A., Feldmann, M., Brennan, F.M. and Williams, R. (2003) Impact of VIP and cAMP on the regulation of TNF-alpha and IL-10 production: implications for rheumatoid arthritis. Arthritis research & therapy 5, R317-28.

Franz, J.K., Pap, T., Hummel, K.M., Nawrath, M., Aicher, W.K., Shigeyama, Y., Muller-Ladner, U., Gay, R.E. and Gay, S. (2000) Expression of sentrin, a novel antiapoptotic molecule, at sites of synovial invasion in rheumatoid arthritis. Arthritis Rheum 43, 599-607.

Furness, J.B. and Costa, M. (1980) Types of nerves in the enteric nervous system. Neuroscience 5, 1-20.

Ganea, D. and Delgado, M. (2002) Vasoactive intestinal peptide (VIP) and pituitary adenylate cyclase-activating polypeptide (PACAP) as modulators of both innate and adaptive immunity. Crit Rev Oral Biol Med 13, 229-37.

Garrido, E., Delgado, M., Martinez, C., Gomariz, R.P. and De la Fuente, M. (1996) Pituitary adenylate cyclase-activating polypeptide (PACAP38) modulates lymphocyte and macrophage functions: stimulation of adherence and opposite effect on mobility. Neuropeptides 30, 583-95.

Gash, D.M., Chen, Y. and Gerhardt, G. (2007) Neurotrophic factors and Parkinson's disease. Handb Clin Neurol 83, 521-33.

Genovese, M.C., Chakravarty, E.F., Krishnan, E. and Moreland, L.W. (2004) A randomized, controlled trial of interferon-beta-1a (Avonex(R)) in patients with rheumatoid arthritis: a pilot study [ISRCTN03626626]. Arthritis Res Ther 6, R73-R77.

Georganas, C., Liu, H., Perlman, H., Hoffmann, A., Thimmapaya, B. and Pope, R.M. (2000) Regulation of IL-6 and IL-8 expression in rheumatoid arthritis synovial fibroblasts: the dominant role for NF-kappa B but not C/EBP beta or c-Jun. Journal of immunology 165, 7199-206.

Gomariz, R.P., Garrido, E., Leceta, J., Martinez, C., Abalo, R. and Delgado, M. (1994) Gene expression of VIP receptor in rat lymphocytes. Biochem Biophys Res Commun 203, 1599-604.

Gomariz, R.P., Juarranz, Y., Abad, C., Arranz, A., Leceta, J. and Martinez, C. (2006) VIP-PACAP system in immunity: new insights for multitarget therapy. Ann N Y Acad Sci 1070, 51-74.

Gomariz, R.P., Martinez, C., Abad, C., Leceta, J. and Delgado, M. (2001) Immunology of VIP: a review and therapeutical perspectives. Curr Pharm Des 7, 89-111.

Gonzalez-Rey, E., Fernandez-Martin, A., Chorny, A., Martin, J., Pozo, D., Ganea, D. and Delgado, M. (2006) Therapeutic effect of vasoactive intestinal peptide on experimental autoimmune encephalomyelitis: down-regulation of inflammatory and autoimmune responses. Am J Pathol 168, 1179-88.

Gonzalez-Rey, E., Varela, N., Chorny, A. and Delgado, M. (2007) Therapeutical approaches of vasoactive intestinal peptide as a pleiotropic immunomodulator. Current pharmaceutical design 13, 1113-39.

Gozes, I. (2001) Neuroprotective peptide drug delivery and development: potential new therapeutics. Trends Neurosci 24, 700-5.

Gozes, I., Bardea, A., Bechar, M., Pearl, O., Reshef, A., Zamostiano, R., Davidson, A., Rubinraut, S., Giladi, E., Fridkin, M. and Brenneman, D.E. (1997) Neuropeptides and neuronal survival: neuroprotective strategy for Alzheimer's disease. Ann N Y Acad Sci 814, 161-6.

Granieri, E. (2000) Exogeneous factors in the aetiology of multiple sclerosis. Journal of neurovirology 6 Suppl 2, S141-6.

Gressens, P., Marret, S., Hill, J.M., Brenneman, D.E., Gozes, I., Fridkin, M. and Evrard, P. (1997) Vasoactive intestinal peptide prevents excitotoxic cell death in the murine developing brain. J Clin Invest 100, 390-7.

Gruden, M.A., Sewell, R.D., Yanamandra, K., Davidova, T.V., Kucheryanu, V.G., Bocharov, E.V., Bocharova, O.R., Polyschuk, V.V., Sherstnev, V.V. and Morozova-Roche, L.A. Immunoprotection against toxic biomarkers is retained during Parkinson's disease progression. J Neuroimmunol.

Hamelink, C., Tjurmina, O., Damadzic, R., Young, W.S., Weihe, E., Lee, H.W. and Eiden, L.E. (2002) Pituitary adenylate cyclase-activating polypeptide is a sympathoadrenal neurotransmitter involved in catecholamine regulation and glucohomeostasis. Proc Natl Acad Sci U S A 99, 461-6.

Han, Z., Boyle, D.L., Manning, A.M. and Firestein, G.S. (1998) AP-1 and NF-kappaB regulation in rheumatoid arthritis and murine collagen-induced arthritis. Autoimmunity 28, 197-208.

Han, Z., Boyle, D.L., Shi, Y., Green, D.R. and Firestein, G.S. (1999) Dominant-negative p53 mutations in rheumatoid arthritis. Arthritis Rheum 42, 1088-92.

Hannibal, J., Ekblad, E., Mulder, H., Sundler, F. and Fahrenkrug, J. (1998) Pituitary adenylate cyclase activating polypeptide (PACAP) in the gastrointestinal tract of the rat: distribution and effects of capsaicin or denervation. Cell Tissue Res 291, 65-79.

Harmar, A.J. (2001) Family-B G-protein-coupled receptors. Genome Biol 2, REVIEWS3013.

Harmar, A.J., Arimura, A., Gozes, I., Journot, L., Laburthe, M., Pisegna, J.R., Rawlings, S.R., Robberecht, P., Said, S.I., Sreedharan, S.P., Wank, S.A. and Waschek, J.A. (1998) International Union of Pharmacology. XVIII. Nomenclature of receptors for vasoactive intestinal peptide and pituitary adenylate cyclase-activating polypeptide. Pharmacol Rev 50, 265-70.

Hauw, J.J., Lubetzki, C. and Tourbah, A. (1999) [Multiple sclerosis: one or several diseases?]. La Revue du praticien 49, 1848-52.

Huan, J., Culbertson, N., Spencer, L., Bartholomew, R., Burrows, G.G., Chou, Y.K., Bourdette, D., Ziegler, S.F., Offner, H. and Vandenbark, A.A. (2005) Decreased FOXP3 levels in multiple sclerosis patients. J Neurosci Res 81, 45-52.

Hutter, C.D. and Laing, P. (1996) Multiple sclerosis: sunlight, diet, immunology and aetiology. Medical hypotheses 46, 67-74.

Imamura, K., Hishikawa, N., Sawada, M., Nagatsu, T., Yoshida, M. and Hashizume, Y. (2003) Distribution of major histocompatibility complex class II-positive microglia and cytokine profile of Parkinson's disease brains. Acta Neuropathol 106, 518-26.

Imamura, K., Ito, M., Suzumura, A., Asai, J. and Takahashi, A. (1990) Generation and characterization of monoclonal antibodies against rat microglia and ontogenic distribution of positive cells. Lab Invest 63, 853-61.

Jiang, X., Jing, H. and Ganea, D. (2002) VIP and PACAP down-regulate CXCL10 (IP-10) and up-regulate CCL22 (MDC) in spleen cells. J Neuroimmunol 133, 81-94.

Juarranz, Y., Gutierrez-Canas, I., Santiago, B., Carrion, M., Pablos, J.L. and Gomariz, R.P. (2008) Differential expression of vasoactive intestinal peptide and its functional receptors in human osteoarthritic and rheumatoid synovial fibroblasts. Arthritis Rheum 58, 1086-95.

Kato, H., Ito, A., Kawanokuchi, J., Jin, S., Mizuno, T., Ojika, K., Ueda, R. and Suzumura, A. (2004) Pituitary adenylate cyclase-activating polypeptide (PACAP) ameliorates experimental autoimmune encephalomyelitis by suppressing the functions of antigen presenting cells. Mult Scler 10, 651-9.

Katrib, A., McNeil, H.P. and Youssef, P.P. (2002) What can we learn from the synovium in early rheumatoid arthritis? Inflammation research : official journal of the European Histamine Research Society ... [et al.] 51, 170-5.

Kebir, H., Kreymborg, K., Ifergan, I., Dodelet-Devillers, A., Cayrol, R., Bernard, M., Giuliani, F., Arbour, N., Becher, B. and Prat, A. (2007) Human TH17 lymphocytes promote blood-brain barrier disruption and central nervous system inflammation. Nature medicine 13, 1173-5.

Kim, W.K., Kan, Y., Ganea, D., Hart, R.P., Gozes, I. and Jonakait, G.M. (2000) Vasoactive intestinal peptide and pituitary adenylyl cyclase-activating polypeptide inhibit tumor necrosis factor-alpha production in injured spinal cord and in activated microglia via a cAMP-dependent pathway. J Neurosci 20, 3622-30.

Kimura, S., Ohshige, Y., Lin, L., Okumura, T., Yanaihara, C., Yanaihara, N. and Shiotani, Y. (1994) Localization of pituitary adenylate cyclase-activating polypeptide (PACAP) in the hypothalamus-pituitary system in rats: light and electron microscopic immunocytochemical studies. J Neuroendocrinol 6, 503-7.

Koedam, E.L., Lauffer, V., van der Vlies, A.E., van der Flier, W.M., Scheltens, P. and Pijnenburg, Y.A. (2010) Early-versus late-onset Alzheimer's disease: more than age alone. Journal of Alzheimer's disease : JAD 19, 1401-8.

Kokkonen, H., Soderstrom, I., Rocklov, J., Hallmans, G., Lejon, K. and Rantapaa Dahlqvist, S. (2010) Up-regulation of cytokines and chemokines predates the onset of rheumatoid arthritis. Arthritis and rheumatism 62, 383-91.

Kosaka, K. (2000) Diffuse Lewy body disease. Neuropathology 20 Suppl, S73-8.

Kosaka, K. and Iseki, E. (2000) Clinicopathological studies on diffuse Lewy body disease. Neuropathology 20, 1-7.

Koves, K., Arimura, A., Vigh, S., Somogyvari-Vigh, A. and Miller, J. (1993) Immunohistochemical localization of PACAP in the ovine digestive system. Peptides 14, 449-55.

Laburthe, M., Couvineau, A., Amiranoff, B. and Voisin, T. (1994) Receptors for gut regulatory peptides. Baillieres Clin Endocrinol Metab 8, 77-110.

Larocca, L., Calafat, M., Roca, V., Franchi, A.M. and Leiros, C.P. (2007) VIP limits LPS-induced nitric oxide production through IL-10 in NOD mice macrophages. Int Immunopharmacol 7, 1343-9.

Lazarov-Spiegler, O., Solomon, A.S., Zeev-Brann, A.B., Hirschberg, D.L., Lavie, V. and Schwartz, M. (1996) Transplantation of activated macrophages overcomes central nervous system regrowth failure. FASEB J 10, 1296-302.

Leceta, J., Gomariz, R.P., Martinez, C., Abad, C., Ganea, D. and Delgado, M. (2000) Receptors and transcriptional factors involved in the anti-inflammatory activity of VIP and PACAP. Ann N Y Acad Sci 921, 92-102.

Lee, R.G. (1989) Pathophysiology of rigidity and akinesia in Parkinson's disease. Eur Neurol 29 Suppl 1, 13-8.

Li, H., Mei, Y., Wang, Y. and Xu, L. (2006) Vasoactive intestinal polypeptide suppressed experimental autoimmune encephalomyelitis by inhibiting T helper 1 responses. J Clin Immunol 26, 430-7.

Li, J.Y., Englund, E., Widner, H., Rehncrona, S., Bjorklund, A., Lindvall, O. and Brundin, P. (2010) Characterization of Lewy body pathology in 12- and 16-year-old intrastriatal mesencephalic grafts surviving in a patient with Parkinson's disease. Mov Disord 25, 1091-6.

Lippa, C.F. (2010) Review of issue: cognitive impairment in Parkinson's disease. Am J Alzheimers Dis Other Demen 25, 387-8.

Long-Smith, C.M., Sullivan, A.M. and Nolan, Y.M. (2009) The influence of microglia on the pathogenesis of Parkinson's disease. Prog Neurobiol 89, 277-87.

Maccioni, R.B., Munoz, J.P. and Barbeito, L. (2001) The molecular bases of Alzheimer's disease and other neurodegenerative disorders. Arch Med Res 32, 367-81.

Martinez, C., Delgado, M., Gomariz, R.P. and Ganea, D. (1996) Vasoactive intestinal peptide and pituitary adenylate cyclase-activating polypeptide-38 inhibit IL-10 production in murine T lymphocytes. J Immunol 156, 4128-36.

Martinez, C., Delgado, M., Pozo, D., Leceta, J., Calvo, J.R., Ganea, D. and Gomariz, R.P. (1998) Vasoactive intestinal peptide and pituitary adenylate cyclase-activating polypeptide modulate endotoxin-induced IL-6 production by murine peritoneal macrophages. J Leukoc Biol 63, 591-601.

Masmoudi-Kouki, O., Gandolfo, P., Castel, H., Leprince, J., Fournier, A., Dejda, A., Vaudry, H. and Tonon, M.C. (2007) Role of PACAP and VIP in astroglial functions. Peptides 28, 1753-60.

Mattle, H.P. (2005) [Multiple sclerosis--update]. Praxis 94, 1167-70.

McGeer, P.L. and McGeer, E.G. (2008) Glial reactions in Parkinson's disease. Mov Disord 23, 474-83.

McGeer, P.L., Rogers, J. and McGeer, E.G. (1994) Neuroimmune mechanisms in Alzheimer disease pathogenesis. Alzheimer Dis Assoc Disord 8, 149-58.

McGeer, P.L., Yasojima, K. and McGeer, E.G. (2001) Inflammation in Parkinson's disease. Adv Neurol 86, 83-9.

McKeith, I.G. and Mosimann, U.P. (2004) Dementia with Lewy bodies and Parkinson's disease. Parkinsonism Relat Disord 10 Suppl 1, S15-8.

Miar, A., Alvarez, V., Corao, A.I., Diaz, M., Alonso, B., Martinez, C., Calatayud, M.T., Menendez, M., Moris, G. and Coto, E. (2011) Amyloid Precursor Protein Gene (APP) Variation in Late-Onset Alzheimer's Disease. Journal of molecular neuroscience : MN.

Miyata, A., Arimura, A., Dahl, R.R., Minamino, N., Uehara, A., Jiang, L., Culler, M.D. and Coy, D.H. (1989) Isolation of a novel 38 residue-hypothalamic polypeptide which stimulates adenylate cyclase in pituitary cells. Biochem Biophys Res Commun 164, 567-74.

Muller-Ladner, U., Kriegsmann, J., Franklin, B.N., Matsumoto, S., Geiler, T., Gay, R.E. and Gay, S. (1996) Synovial fibroblasts of patients with rheumatoid arthritis attach to and invade normal human cartilage when engrafted into SCID mice. Am J Pathol 149, 1607-15.

Murphy, K.M. and Reiner, S.L. (2002) The lineage decisions of helper T cells. Nat Rev Immunol 2, 933-44.

Nicole, P., Du, K., Couvineau, A. and Laburthe, M. (1998) Site-directed mutagenesis of human VIP1 versus VIP2 receptors. Ann N Y Acad Sci 865, 378-81.

Nohr, D. and Weihe, E. (1991) Tachykinin-, calcitonin gene-related peptide-, and protein gene product 9.5-immunoreactive nerve fibers in alveolar walls of mammals. Neurosci Lett 134, 17-20.

Offen, D., Sherki, Y., Melamed, E., Fridkin, M., Brenneman, D.E. and Gozes, I. (2000) Vasoactive intestinal peptide (VIP) prevents neurotoxicity in neuronal cultures: relevance to neuroprotection in Parkinson's disease. Brain research 854, 257-62.

Offen, D., Ziv, I., Sternin, H., Melamed, E. and Hochman, A. (1996) Prevention of dopamine-induced cell death by thiol antioxidants: possible implications for treatment of Parkinson's disease. Exp Neurol 141, 32-9.

Oksenberg, J.R. and Barcellos, L.F. (2000) The complex genetic aetiology of multiple sclerosis. Journal of neurovirology 6 Suppl 2, S10-4.

Onoue, S., Endo, K., Ohshima, K., Yajima, T. and Kashimoto, K. (2002) The neuropeptide PACAP attenuates beta-amyloid (1-42)-induced toxicity in PC12 cells. Peptides 23, 1471-8.

Pasquier, F. (2000) [Alzheimer disease. Diagnosis, progression]. La Revue du praticien 50, 1831-7.

Pozo, D. (2003) VIP- and PACAP-mediated immunomodulation as prospective therapeutic tools. Trends Mol Med 9, 211-7.

Pozo, D. and Delgado, M. (2004) The many faces of VIP in neuroimmunology: a cytokine rather a neuropeptide? FASEB J 18, 1325-34.

Prewitt, C.M., Niesman, I.R., Kane, C.J. and Houle, J.D. (1997) Activated macrophage/microglial cells can promote the regeneration of sensory axons into the injured spinal cord. Exp Neurol 148, 433-43.

Pugliatti, M., Sotgiu, S. and Rosati, G. (2002) The worldwide prevalence of multiple sclerosis. Clin Neurol Neurosurg 104, 182-91.

Rabchevsky, A.G. and Streit, W.J. (1997) Grafting of cultured microglial cells into the lesioned spinal cord of adult rats enhances neurite outgrowth. J Neurosci Res 47, 34-48.

Reale, M., Iarlori, C., Thomas, A., Gambi, D., Perfetti, B., Di Nicola, M. and Onofrj, M. (2009) Peripheral cytokines profile in Parkinson's disease. Brain Behav Immun 23, 55-63.

Ruschpler, P. and Stiehl, P. (2002) Shift in Th1 (IL-2 and IFN-gamma) and Th2 (IL-10 and IL-4) cytokine mRNA balance within two new histological main-types of rheumatoid-arthritis (RA). Cellular and molecular biology 48, 285-93.

Sacchetti, B., Lorenzini, C.A., Baldi, E., Bucherelli, C., Roberto, M., Tassoni, G. and Brunelli, M. (2001) Pituitary adenylate cyclase-activating polypeptide hormone (PACAP) at very low dosages improves memory in the rat. Neurobiol Learn Mem 76, 1-6.

Said, S.I. and Mutt, V. (1969) A peptide fraction from lung tissue with prolonged peripheral vasodilator activity. Scand J Clin Lab Invest Suppl 107, 51-6.

Sawada, M., Imamura, K. and Nagatsu, T. (2006) Role of cytokines in inflammatory process in Parkinson's disease. J Neural Transm Suppl, 373-81.

Scheff, S.W., Sparks, D.L. and Price, D.A. (1996) Quantitative assessment of synaptic density in the outer molecular layer of the hippocampal dentate gyrus in Alzheimer's disease. Dementia 7, 226-32.

Scheff, S.W., Sparks, L. and Price, D.A. (1993) Quantitative assessment of synaptic density in the entorhinal cortex in Alzheimer's disease. Ann Neurol 34, 356-61.

Selkoe, D.J. (1998) The cell biology of beta-amyloid precursor protein and presenilin in Alzheimer's disease. Trends Cell Biol 8, 447-53.

Sheng, W.S., Hu, S., Kravitz, F.H., Peterson, P.K. and Chao, C.C. (1995) Tumor necrosis factor alpha upregulates human microglial cell production of interleukin-10 in vitro. Clin Diagn Lab Immunol 2, 604-8.

Shioda, S., Legradi, G., Leung, W.C., Nakajo, S., Nakaya, K. and Arimura, A. (1994) Localization of pituitary adenylate cyclase-activating polypeptide and its messenger ribonucleic acid in the rat testis by light and electron microscopic immunocytochemistry and in situ hybridization. Endocrinology 135, 818-25.

Staines, D.R. (2004) Is chronic fatigue syndrome an autoimmune disorder of endogenous neuropeptides, exogenous infection and molecular mimicry? Med Hypotheses 62, 646-52.

Sun, W., Hong, J., Zang, Y.C., Liu, X. and Zhang, J.Z. (2006) Altered expression of vasoactive intestinal peptide receptors in T lymphocytes and aberrant Th1 immunity in multiple sclerosis. Int Immunol 18, 1691-700.

Takemura, S., Braun, A., Crowson, C., Kurtin, P.J., Cofield, R.H., O'Fallon, W.M., Goronzy, J.J. and Weyand, C.M. (2001) Lymphoid neogenesis in rheumatoid synovitis. J Immunol 167, 1072-80.

Tamas, A., Lubics, A., Lengvari, I. and Reglodi, D. (2006) Protective effects of PACAP in excitotoxic striatal lesion. Annals of the New York Academy of Sciences 1070, 570-4.

Toku, K., Tanaka, J., Yano, H., Desaki, J., Zhang, B., Yang, L., Ishihara, K., Sakanaka, M. and Maeda, N. (1998) Microglial cells prevent nitric oxide-induced neuronal apoptosis in vitro. J Neurosci Res 53, 415-25.

Van Den Eeden, S.K., Tanner, C.M., Bernstein, A.L., Fross, R.D., Leimpeter, A., Bloch, D.A. and Nelson, L.M. (2003) Incidence of Parkinson's disease: variation by age, gender, and race/ethnicity. Am J Epidemiol 157, 1015-22.

Varani, K., Vincenzi, F., Tosi, A., Gessi, S., Casetta, I., Granieri, G., Fazio, P., Leung, E., MacLennan, S., Granieri, E. and Borea, P.A. (2010) A2A adenosine receptor overexpression and functionality, as well as TNF-alpha levels, correlate with motor symptoms in Parkinson's disease. FASEB J 24, 587-98.

Vaudry, D., Gonzalez, B.J., Basille, M., Yon, L., Fournier, A. and Vaudry, H. (2000) Pituitary adenylate cyclase-activating polypeptide and its receptors: from structure to functions. Pharmacol Rev 52, 269-324.

Vemuri, P., Wiste, H.J., Weigand, S.D., Knopman, D.S., Shaw, L.M., Trojanowski, J.Q., Aisen, P.S., Weiner, M., Petersen, R.C. and Jack, C.R., Jr. (2010) Effect of apolipoprotein E on biomarkers of amyloid load and neuronal pathology in Alzheimer disease. Ann Neurol 67, 308-16.

Wahner, A.D., Sinsheimer, J.S., Bronstein, J.M. and Ritz, B. (2007) Inflammatory cytokine gene polymorphisms and increased risk of Parkinson disease. Arch Neurol 64, 836-40.

Wang, H.Y., Jiang, X., Gozes, I., Fridkin, M., Brenneman, D.E. and Ganea, D. (1999) Vasoactive intestinal peptide inhibits cytokine production in T lymphocytes through cAMP-dependent and cAMP-independent mechanisms. Regul Pept 84, 55-67.

Weihe, E., Nohr, D., Michel, S., Muller, S., Zentel, H.J., Fink, T. and Krekel, J. (1991) Molecular anatomy of the neuro-immune connection. Int J Neurosci 59, 1-23.

White, A.R., Zheng, H., Galatis, D., Maher, F., Hesse, L., Multhaup, G., Beyreuther, K., Masters, C.L. and Cappai, R. (1998) Survival of cultured neurons from amyloid precursor protein knock-out mice against Alzheimer's amyloid-beta toxicity and oxidative stress. J Neurosci 18, 6207-17.

Whitton, P.S. (2007) Inflammation as a causative factor in the aetiology of Parkinson's disease. Br J Pharmacol 150, 963-76.

Winner, B., Vogt-Weisenhorn, D.M., Lie, C.D., Blumcke, I. and Winkler, J. (2009) Cellular repair strategies in Parkinson's disease. Ther Adv Neurol Disord 2, 51-60.

Yamanishi, Y., Boyle, D.L., Rosengren, S., Green, D.R., Zvaifler, N.J. and Firestein, G.S. (2002) Regional analysis of p53 mutations in rheumatoid arthritis synovium. Proc Natl Acad Sci U S A 99, 10025-30.

Zhang, G.X., Baker, C.M., Kolson, D.L. and Rostami, A.M. (2000) Chemokines and chemokine receptors in the pathogenesis of multiple sclerosis. Mult Scler 6, 3-13.

Zhang, X., Tang, Y., Sujkowska, D., Wang, J., Ramgolam, V., Sospedra, M., Adams, J., Martin, R., Pinilla, C. and Markovic-Plese, S. (2008) Degenerate TCR recognition and dual DR2 restriction of autoreactive T cells: implications for the initiation of the autoimmune response in multiple sclerosis. European journal of immunology 38, 1297-309.

Zimmermann, T., Kunisch, E., Pfeiffer, R., Hirth, A., Stahl, H.D., Sack, U., Laube, A., Liesaus, E., Roth, A., Palombo-Kinne, E., Emmrich, F. and Kinne, R.W. (2001) Isolation and characterization of rheumatoid arthritis synovial fibroblasts from primary culture--primary culture cells markedly differ from fourth-passage cells. Arthritis research 3, 72-6.

24

# Antibody-Proteases in the Pathogenesis of Autoimmune Demyelination and Monitoring Patients with Multiple Sclerosis

Dmitry Kostyushev[1], Dmitry Gnatenko[1], Mikhail Paltsev[3], Aleksandr Gabibov[4] and Sergey Suchkov[1,2]
[1]*I.M. Sechenov First Moscow Medical State University*
[2]*Moscow State University of Medicine and Dentistry*
[3]*National Research Center "Kurchatov Institute"*
[4]*M.M. Shemyakin and Yu.A. Ovchinnikov Institute of Bioorganic Chemistry, Russian Academy of Sciences*
*Russia*

## 1. Introduction

Multiple sclerosis (MS) is an autoimmune demyelinating disorder of the central nervous system (CNS) resulting in axon loss and development of disability. (Gabibov et al., 2011) Autoantibodies (autoAbs) are one of the major features and crucial mechanisms in MS pathogenesis known to illustrate this autoagression. The major component in the pathogenesis of MS is primary myelin damage, which is mediated by autoAbs, which trigger the release of separate and pathogenically valuable myelin-associated epitopes into the bloodstream. These molecules acting as a group of sensitizing factors may provoke the immune system and drive disease progression. Being identified at the pre- or early stages or the demyelination, such autoAbs dominate during the whole course of the disease.

Natural catalytic antibodies (*catAbs*) or natural *abzymes* today are one of the principal effectors of the adaptive immune system. In constructive sense, catAbs are multivalent immunoglobulins (Igs), presumably, of IgG and IgM isotypes, endowed with a capacity to hydrolyze an antigenic substrate.

Traditionally, the basic structure of the Ab molecule is essentially *Y*-shaped, with the two tips (*Fab*-fragments) designed to recognize and bind non-self agents or cells. Moreover, the catalytic capacity is also present in *Fab*-fragments of the molecule. In general, the mechanisms of Ab-mediated catalytic action include nucleophilic catalysis, induction of conformational strain, coordination with ions, and stabilization of transition states (TS). Ag-specific or targeted catAbs are preferentially found in the Ig repertoire of patients with a broad scope of diseases to act as pathogenically valuable tools. Since the discovery of catAbs, a wide spectrum of the disease-related abzymes regardless to their natural history or engineering protocols has been described. Moreover, the immune system was shown to express an intrinsic drive to generate natural abzymes in different pathological states in humans. Among them, proteolytic (*Ab-proteases*) and DNA-hydrolyzing (*DNA-abzymes*) autoAbs are of a special practical value.

And today catAbs can be used as either therapeutic tools or as vehicles for delivering therapeutic agents to damaged cells in the human body. Recent applications of abzymes have included a broad scope of medical and allied areas, i.e.,

1. the conversion of drugs to their inactive (non-toxic) forms;
2. the degradation of drugs and harmful substances;
3. the activation of pro-drugs for targeted chemotherapy;
4. the inhibition of infectivity;
5. others.

The aim of this review is to compare data on the medical applications and implementations of disease-associated and engineered abzymes as new tools for treatment of MS, and to specifically focus on their potential value for clinical research and for clinical utility and public health as well.

The mechanisms of catAb action include nucleophilic catalysis, induction of conformational strain, coordination with metal ions, and stabilization of TS. Only Abs that stabilize the Ag TS more than the GS can be catalytic, and such Abs are thus usually identified among those that bind tightly to an analogue of the TS of the relevant reaction. Abs would thus provide a unique opportunity to combine specific Ag recognition with enzymatic turnover.

For Ab-proteases, for instance, a typical mechanism of nucleophilic catalysis has been established. Since the catalytic efficiency of Ab-proteases derives substantially from the ability to recognize the GS with high affinity, proteolytic Abs while demonstrating an exclusive targeted specificity can be used to selectively address a wide range of metabolically and pathogenically valuable protein targets.

In case of DNA-abzymes, Ab-induced conformational strain is proposed to activate phosphodiester bonds and result in DNA hydrolysis, aided by coordination of bivalent cations. As being similar to proteolytic sites, the nuclease activity of DNA-hydrolyzing Abs is described to be encoded by germline variable region genes (*V*-genes).In general, the specific nature of the Ab catalysis was demonstrated by the adherence of those reactions to the well-known Michaelis-Menten equation, the complete inhibition by a proper hapten analogue, and the failure of the Ab to catalyze the hydrolysis of the substrate antagonists.

During the last 10 years, it has been found that Abs contribute to the degradation of a number of autoantigens. These and related "antibody-enzymes", also termed abzymes, were shown to be able to cleave DNA, RNA, carbohydrates, peptides, and proteins Recently, abzyme-dependent catalytic degradation of an autoantigen, MBP (myelin basic protein), was associated with the course of the neurodegenerative disease MS and its rodent model, experimental autoimmune encephalomyelitis (EAE). Autoantibody-mediated degradation of MBP was shown to be site specific, with cleavage sites localized to the immunodominant epitopes of the protein. These findings were supported by studies from others. Interestingly, this reaction was inhibited in vitro by glatiramer acetate (Copaxone), an established treatment for MS. (Belogurov et al., 2008)

There are three groups of autoAbs that are specific for MS: anti-myelin autoAbs (e.g., anti-MBP, anti-MOG (MOG - myelin oligodendrocyte glycoprotein) and anti-neurofilament autoAbs); nonmyelin autoAbs (e.g., anti-HSP autoAbs, among others); and autoAbs demonstrating different levels of specificity and functionality (e.g., catalytic autoAbs [i.e., antibody proteases]). The latter group of anti-myelin antibody proteases is of particular interest in terms of disease monitoring, prognosis and preclinical (pre-early) diagnostics of MS. Catalic antbodies are endowed with a capacity to hydroliyze an antigenic substrate. This has moved antibodies to the level of physiological functionality by providing such antibodies with the ability to mediate direct catalytic and indirect cytotoxic effects on the target. This property is buried in the Fab fragment of the immunoglobulin molecule. Antibody protease were found in most autoimmune conditions, particulary in MS, accomplishing sequence-specific proteolic cleavage of myelin antigens and controlling the degradation of myelin sheath. (Gabibov et al., 2011)

The worldwide median estimated incidence of MS is 2.5 per 100 000 and prevalence is estimated at approximately 1.5 million cases. Usually onset of MS is between age 20 and 40 years. Men are affected approximately twice as rare as women. (Stuve & Oksenberg, 2006 )

Autoantibody mediated tissue destruction is among the main features of organ-specific autoimmunity. Ample data indicate that a significant portion of MS cases is characterized by the presence in the blood of autoantibodies against myelin protein components. Moreover, myelin-specific autoantibodies are detected by highresolution microscopic analysis in the regions of demyelination plaques in human MS and a MS-like disease of marmosets, suggesting their direct contribution to myelin destruction. (Ponomarenko et al., 2006)

Nonetheless, the mechanisms responsible for the induction of autoantibodies and their possible contributions to MS progression are still unknown and are somewhat controversial. Also clonal expansion of B cells and T cells, hallmarks of inflammation in the CNS, are found in MS. The viral mimicry hypothesis was formulated to explain the initiation of this pathology. (Belogurov et al., 2008) But a poor understanding of the etiology of MS has complicated the development of effective therapeutics. (Hafler, 2004)

Despite strong evidence for the contribution of T cell responses to manifestations of autoimmunity in the CNS of patients with MS, recent findings encouraged investigators to search also for B cell-mediated contributions to the MS pathogenesis. (Klawiter & Cross, 2007; Nikbin et al., 2007)

Development of new diagnostics and treating tactics can improve patient life quality and decrease MS treatment cost, as in other autoimmune diseases such as type 1 diabetes. (Hahl et al., 1998)

## 2. Antibodies-mediated demyelination in the pathogenesis of MS

Antibodies can cause demyelination by several effector mechanisms. One of these is the opsonization of myelin for subsequent phagocytosis by macrophages, which has been observed in MS and EAE. Serum anti-myelin antibodies raise macrophage phagocytosis, and the uptake by macrophages of CNS myelin increases after opsonization with complement. Another mechanism of demyelination that involves autoantibodies is through activation of the entire complement cascade leading to membrane attack complex (MAC) deposition and complement-mediated cytolysis.

Antibodies with specificity against minor myelin components have also been detected in MS patients. MOG is the most interesting candidate B-cell autoantigen in MS. Because of its location it is an ideal target for antibody-mediated demyelination. Anti-MOG antibodies are indeed able to cause myelin destruction in EAE models, while other antibodies against major myelin proteins such as MBP or PLP, which are both not located on the myelin surface, do not cause myelin destruction on their own. Anti-MOG Abs mediate a characteristic vesicular transformation of compact myelin in acutely demyelinated lesions that also has been documented in human MS lesions strongly suggesting a role of anti-MOG Abs in MS. The B-cell response to MOG is enhanced in MS also supporting the pathogenic importance of anti-MOG Abs. Interestingly, the presence of serum anti-MOG antibodies, with or without anti-MBP antibodies, in patients presenting with an initial clinical event suggestive of central nervous system demyelination and evidence of multifocal lesions on MRI studies, is predictive of subsequent clinical events that establish the diagnosis of clinically definitive MS. However, the presence of anti-MOG antibodies in patients with nondemyelinating diseases of the CNS, as well as in a substantial number of healthy individuals, has raised important questions about the role of these antibodies in MS, and these need to be addressed in future studies.

### 2.1 Catalysis

The neurodegenerative model of MS is based on the proposition of a primary lesion in myelin followed by myelin breakdown and the release of myelin-compartmentalized proteins, particularly MBP. This is followed by the generation of MBP-derived peptides that become the main sensitizers of T cells. (Hafler, 2004) The hypothesis that interactions between MBP and T cells must occur at sites other than the myelin membrane has been challenged by recent physicochemical studies demonstrating that myelin can become structurally unstable secondary to specific posttranslational modifications of MBP structure. This was shown to result in the increased surface exposure and susceptibility to proteolysis of MBP 83–92. (Husted, 2006) The close association between the proteolytic sensitivity of MBP and the pattern of posttranslational modifications of the molecule may represent one of the key regulatory mechanisms in epitope generation (Lolli et al., 2005). Proteolysis may proceed by any of four distinct pathways that may exert a concerted attack on the MBP molecule, although the mechanisms responsible for the activation and regulation of these potential activities are not known. Thus, epitope generation may occur via:

1. autocatalytic cleavage of the MBP molecule (D'Souza et al., 2005);
2. protease digestion (D'Souza et al., 2006);
3. autoantibody-mediated site-specific cleavage (Ponomarenko et al., 2006);
4. Abdependent oxidative pathway (Wentworth et al., 2001).

The last mechanism, which has been demonstrated in a number of autoimmune pathologies, remains unproven for MS (Wentworth et al., 2001). These pathways are characterized by dramatic differences in reaction velocities and in cleavage site specificity. Obviously the rates of enzymatic reactions are several times higher than those for autocatalysis and Abenzymes (abzymes), perhaps making this pathway the major player in epitope generation. In the case of abzymes, the large excess of the biocatalyst, its high specificity, and its close compartmentalization with the MBP substrate shown in demyelinating lesions are suggestive of its likely effectiveness in vivo. (Ponomarenko et al., 2006; Genain et al., 1999)

Today, the advent of antibody catalysis has demonstrated that antibodies can be programmed to perform complex cell biochemistry, and thus a logical question arises: does the original (nature-gifted) potential for catalysis relate to antibody function? In the sense of the question, it is very interesting to consider the evolution of antibodies, while generally accepting that natural enzymes are primitive molecules compared with antibodies, and that antibodies arose just after the birth of enzymes.

A great deal of evidence has been also adduced to support the medical concept of the *living soul* of abzymes and their significance for utilizing broader autoantibodies properties in the formation of pathogenic patterns and clinical settings at different autoimmune and other conditions. Moreover, the medical concept of abzymes was tested in two ways, clinically and experimentally, i.e., on human and animal models. The progress achieved earlier in designing artificial abzymes initiated the study of biological activities of natural catalytic autoantibodies and their involvement in pathogenesis of major clinical disorders, i.e., evoked the onset of the era of medical abzymology. (Suchkov et al., 2001; Zhou et al., 2002; Tellier, 2002; Nathan, 2002; Kozyr et al., 1998)

Medical abzymology has made a great contribution to the development of general autoimmunity theory: it has put the antibody as a *functional entity* and as the key brick of the theory to the level of *physiological functionality* by providing such antibody with the ability to catalyze and mediate direct and independent cytotoxic effect on cellular and molecular targets.

## 3. Major antigenic targets of the anti-myelin autoAbs

There are extensive information on a significant portion of MS cases, characterized by the presence of autoantibodies against myelin protein components in serum of patients with MS. (Chamczuk et al., 2002; Reindl et al., 1999) Although the mechanism of the autoantibody role in MS pathogenesis is unknown , autoantibodies to MBP and MOG were proposed as biomarkers for clinical prognosis of MS. (Berger et al., 2003) Similar immunoglobulins were also found in mice with induced EAE, which is an animal model of MS. (Fritz et al., 1983)

### 3.1 Myelin basic protein

Myelin basic protein is by far the best studied myelin component in MS. It is the second most abundant myelin protein (approximately 30-40%) after PLP. There are five MBP isoforms with 14-21.5 kDa molecular weights in mammals that result from differential splicing of 11 axons within the Golli-MBP locus. The highly basic MBP is positioned at the intracellular surface of myelin membranes and via interactions with acidic lipid moieties is involved in maintaining the structure of compact myelin. The most abundant 18.5 kDa isoform (170 amino acid length) has been used in most immunological studies.

Different from MOG, and PLP (proteolipid protein), MBP is found in both central and peripheral myelin, and MBP transcripts have also been demonstrated in peripheral lymphoid organs such as lymph nodes and thymus.

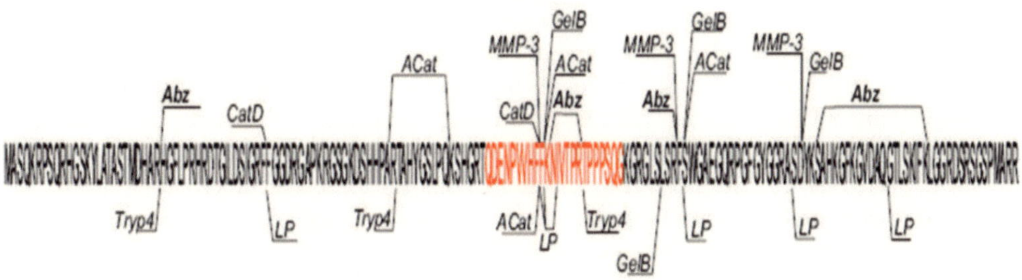


Fig. 1. MBP sites of proteolysis by different enzymes-proteases and Abs-proteases and as a result of spontaneous autocatalytic hydrolysis. The sequence of the encephalitogenic peptide 81–103 is shown in red. Abbrevations: GelB (Gelatinase B), MMP-3 (matrix mettaloproteinase-3), CatD (Cathepsin D), ACat (Autocatalytic cleavage), Abz (Abzyme), LP (Lysosomal Proteases), Tryp4 (Trypsin 4).

### 3.2 Proteolipid protein

Proteolipid protein (PLP) is the most abundant protein in CNS compact myelin (about 50%), highly hydrophobic and evolutionarily conserved across species. There are two main transcripts, the full-length 276 amino acid isoform and DM-20, an isoform that lacks 35 amino acids and is mainly expressed in brain and spinal cord prior to myelination, but also in peripheral lymphoid organs such as the thymus, where full-length PLP is barely found. Interestingly, the major encephalittogenic and immunodominant PLP peptide (139-154) is contained in full-length PLP but not in DM-20. This observation is thought to account for the encephalittogenicity and immunodominance of the PLP (139-154) peptide, since it is essentially not available for thymic negative selection and consequently a high precursor frequency of PLP (139-154)-specific T cells has been observed even in naive unprimed animals.

### 3.3 Myelin oligodendrocyte glycoprotein

Myelin oligodendrocyte glycoprotein, a 218 amino acid trancemembrane glycoprotein of the IG superfamily, is much less abundant (0.01 - 0.05%) than MBP and PLP, and also different from the two major myelin proteins in being located not in compact myelin but exposed on the outermost surface of the oligodendrocyte membrane. Because of this "strategic" location, it is directly accessible to antibodies and believed to be particularly relevant as a target for both cellular and humoral immune responses in MS. MOG, is expressed relatively late during myelination and is only found in the brain/spinal cord and the retina but not in peripheral nerve. Furthermore, MOG expression is either completely or almost completely lacking in peripheral lymphoid tissues, although MOG transcripts have been seen in nonhuman primate peripheral nerve and a few samples of human tonsils and thymus.

## 4. Nonmyelin autoAbs

### 4.1 DNA abzymes and antibody proteases

Catalytic antibodies are endowed with a capacity to hydrolyze an antigenic substrate. (Paul S. 1998; Paul et al., 2005; Friboulet et al., 1999) This has moved antibodies to the level of physiological functionality by providing such antibodies with the ability to mediate direct catalytic and indirect cytotoxic effects on the targets. This property is buried in the Fab fragment of the immunoglobulin molecule. Antibody proteases (antibodies with proteolytic activity) were found in most autoimmune conditions, particularly in MS, accomplishing sequence-specific proteolytic cleavage of the myelin antigens and controlling the degradation of the myelin sheath. The levels of proteolytic activity of the antibody proteases revealed significant correlations with the clinical activity of the course over the disease, and thus with the disability of the patients. The most attractive point is that, in contrast to canonical proteases, for antibody proteases, there is an extra set of cleavage sites in the targeted autoantigens (for sequence-specific proteolytic cleavage) focused predominantly at the immunodominant sites. (Gabibov et al., 2002)

Physiological interaction of autoAb with a living cell is mediated by Fc fragment (Wilkinson et al., 2001). DNA-abzymes are able to realize both cytotoxicity mechanisms-complement-dependent cell lysis and K-cell-mediated lysis. (Fishelson et al., 2001) Fab fragment is not involved in these reactions. This fundamentally distinguishes Ab-mediated classical and DNA-mediated mechanisms of cytotoxicity due to direct involvement of Fab fragment into the catalytic attack on the target cell genome. Catalytic and cytotoxic activities of DNA-abzymes are closely related. This allows to assume on a hypothesis on a new mechanism of the contribution of autoAbs into the pathogenesis of autoimmune disorders. Such mechanism acts independently of complement and cytotoxic T cells; it requires a catalytically active Fab fragment but ignores Fc fragment whose structure is deprived of even buried resources providing direct cytotoxic effect. (Ponomarenko et al., 2000)

Two different mechanisms of DNA-abzymes cytotoxic potential utilization are established-by means of direct cytotoxic effect on a target cell involving the catalytically active Fab fragment and by means of apoptosis due to high affinity of DNA-binding autoAbs for membrane receptors providing the cell with features of possible target. Cross-reactive with such such cells, DNA-abzymes can provoke their degradation resulting in the development of different syndromal manifestations: lupus nephritis in glomerule endothelium cross-reactivity, articular syndrome in synovial cross-reactivity, extracardial manifestations and MCS progression in CM cross-reactivity. (Rekvig et al., February 2004; Raz et al., 1993)

Cross-reactivity of DNA-binding autoAbs with glutamate receptors accumulating at neural cells is of a special interest. Such autoAbs with catalytic and cytotoxic activities can initiate neural cells apoptosis providing the possibility for the development of CNS autoimmune degenerative disorders (Kotzin et al., 2001). The penetration of DNA-binding autoAbs (and DNA-abzymes) into a cell results in activation of cytotoxicity mechanisms, apoptosis induction, etc.

### 4.2 Molecular mechanisms of the involvement of DNA-abzymes in the development of different autoimmunity conditions and pathogenesis of autoimmune disorders

One antigen may generate up to $10^2$-$10^4$ different antibody molecules, a number that may further increase by somatic mutagenesis. Therefore, it seems feasible that different DNA-binding and other non-catalytic antibodies, as well as antibodies with catalytic activities can be synthesized in the course of immune response, either directed against the substrate or as antiidiotypic antibodies to enzymes hydrolyzing nucleic substrates. It is certainly difficult to predict the clinical significance of these catalytic activities, but it is likely that they modify the pathogenesis or clinical process of these autoimmune diseases.

The interest to catalytic (i.e., DNA-hydrolyzing activity) of the autoantibodies is kept on growing up and is strongly supported by the new data including those illustrating cytotoxic activities of the biocatalysts and evidence that abzyme-mediated cytotoxic effects observed in human SLE (system lupus erythematosis) and mouse SLE-like syndromes are caspase-dependent and thus apoptosis-related.

## 5. Prediction of MS

The use of assays for Abs to MBP and MOG for diagnostic and prognostic purposes in patients with a clinically isolated syndrome (CIS), a frequent precursor to clinically definite MS (CDMS), has yielded conflicting results. One study showed that the presence of myelin Abs in the sera of CIS patients was predictive of a shorter time course to the development of CDMS. (Tomassini et al., 2007) Others, however, indicated that positive tests had no prognostic value for progression to CDMS. (Kuhle et al., 2007)

Symbols indicate OD450 values for Abs from individual subjects within each EDSS category for specific MBP peptides or intact MBP and MOG proteins. Lines indicate the relation between EDSS value and the binding activity of specific peptides/proteins: MBP 81-103 (R2 0.332; p 0.005), MBP 130-156 (R2 0.381; p 0.011), MBP 146-170 (R2 0.310; p 0.033), intact MBP

(R2 0.458; p 0.005), intact MOG (R2 0.052; p 0.001), and control Trx carrier protein (R2 0.055; p 0.376)

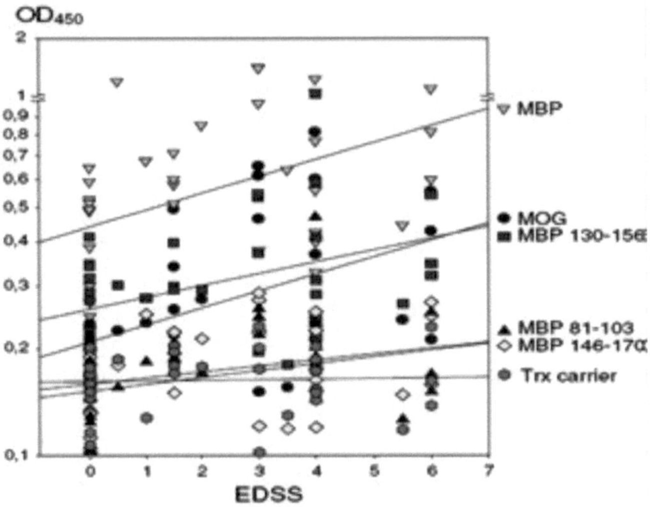


Fig. 2. Correlation of the EDSS of MS patients with the levels of autoantibodies to MBP fragments.

The latter results are in keeping with our demonstration that the binding activities of Abs to intact MBP and MOG proteins were indistinguishable for patients with MS and other neurological diseases (OND). In addition, a screen of MBP peptides showed that the reactivity of Abs from patients with MS and OND could be distinguished only by their differential binding to MBP 43–68 and MBP 146–170. Follow-up studies of patients with MS using assays based on the use of these fragments will be needed to determine whether it provides an improved prognostic tool for patients with CIS.

Interestingly, the parameters of Ab binding associated with disease progression were different from those with potential prognostic value. Disease severity, as determined by Expanded disability status scale (EDSS), correlated with level of autoantibodies to intact MBP and MOG proteins as well as MBP fragments 81–103, 130–156 and 146–170. These findings are in keeping with the demonstrated correlations between levels of anti-MOG and anti-MBP Abs and inflammatory signs revealed by MRI and cerebrospinal fluid analyses. (Kuhle et al., 2007)

### 5.1 Diagnostic protocol

The appearance of Ab-proteases at the pre-early (*preclinical*) stages of demyelination to illustrate myelin degradation has been documented.

The results we had obtained would allow for approaching to a novel generation of diagnostic technologies based on the protocols of clinical and preclinical diagnostics to exploit Ab-proteases and their sequence-specificity.

The protocols would include:

1. isolation of individual Ab-proteases from sera of MS patients or persons to be at risks for suspicious MS (e.g., the relatives);
2. quantification of the proteolytic activity of Ab-proteases;

3. determination of sequence-specificity of the individual Ab-proteases towards MBP as the whole molecule and separate peptides (epitope-bearing) fragmented from the molecule as well;
4. verification of the diagnosis and prediction for the future.

A phenomenon of the *pre-clinical* formation of the abzyme-based armamentarium and Ab-proteases, in particular, would be interpreted as a portion of the proper immune response of the body to the environmental and other shifts. So, a selection of the mode of action for proteolytic antibodies would depend on the metabolic motivation occurring at a particular stage of the disease. Of great interest would be driving motivation to control the mode of action at the *preclinical* stages.

The occurrence of antibody proteases among healthy individuals is due to the development of the pre-early immune imbalances and formation of the preclinical conditions. So, when bursts of the antibody-associated proteolytic activity or the tendency for the latter were evident, the pre-early stages preceding formation of CIS and the exacerbation of the disease could be predicted, even with no observable clinical manifestations. There was definite correlation between the interval before CIS and autoAb (including antibody proteases) status. The occurrence of antibody proteases and the degree of their activity were significantly associated with symptomatology/severity of CIS and clinical course of the disease.

### 5.2 Sequence specificity and clinical implementation

Sequence specificity of Ab-proteases is the capacity to distinguish or not distinguish between particular epitopes in the MBP molecule. Serum anti-MBP auto-Abs obtained from MS patients exhibited sequence-specific proteolytic cleavage of the MBP molecule. Such antibody proteases revealed significant correlations with different manifestations of MS (i.e., progressive and/or remittance phases of the disease), with Expanded Disability Status Scale scores and thus with scales of demyelination and, moreover, with the degree of disability of MS patients. For instance, anti-MBP antibody proteases that are able to recognize 43-68 and 146-170 amino acid sequences within the MBP molecule are predominantly more typical of MS patients, but not of patients with neurodegenerative diseases other than MS. In MS patients with low disease activity (in remission), a family of antibody proteases has been detected with low proteolytic activity that predominantly targets 43-68 and 146-170 amino acid sequences within MBP. Progression of disability in MS patients is accompanied by the bursts of anti-MBP antibody-associated sequence-specific proteolytic activity. Moreover, signs of a trend in the specificity of the activity were found (i.e., specificity of the sequence recognition from 43-68 and 146-170 amino acid sites with low affinity to 81-103 and 82-98 amino acid sites, demonstrating that high-affinity indices are recognized by anti-MBP antibody proteases). (Ponomarenko et al., 2006)

### 5.3 Perspectives in the application of catalytic antibodies for clinical medicine

More than a hundred of abzyme-catalyzed reactions have been described. Catalytic efficacy of some abzymes is comparable with those of enzymes, but the specificity of abzymes is even higher. The practical relevance of abzymes is due to the unique feature drastically distinguishing them from other biocatalysts, i.e., abzymes could be produced for the catalysis of not only all the reactions occuring in the living systems but also be designed for the development of principally new catalysts with no natural counterparts. (Gabibov et al., 2002; Zhou et al., 2002) In this sense, we can anticipate that manmade catalytic antibodies will have considerable practical potential in many different medical applications, i.e., would form the frame of medical abzymology.

Medical abzymology as a novel trend in medical immunology and enzymology, and a new avenue in the clinical practice appears to demonstrate a revolutionary growth today. The antibody catalysis as itself and regardless to a defined field of medical application appears to stress a new area of medical research and a novel field of medical application that provoke considerable interest for medical investigators and clinical practitioners. (Suchkov et al., 2006; Suchkov et al., 2001)

Autoimmune diseases actually represent a challenging frontier in contemporary medical research and clinical practice, and, thus, in areas overlapped with medical abzymology. The proper relation of clinical autoimmunity to the generation of natural catalytic antibody response is absolutely evident, and, in general terms, the phenomenon of autoantibody catalysis can potentially be applied to isolate efficient catalytic domains directed against autoimmune epitopes pathogenically and clinically relevant. This can be done by exposing the autoimmune repertoire to identify autoantigens or their mimicking counterparts capable of recruiting the germ line genes encoding the catalytic site.

## 6. Conclusion

The prospects for progress in developing novel approaches for the diagnosis and treatment of MS have been greatly encouraged by several observations. These include:

1. the identification of a major immunogenic region in MBP, peptide 82–98;
2. the demonstration that both B and T cell responses to MBP are focused on this region, particular for patients who express HLA-DR2;
3. clinical studies suggesting that patients treated with MBP peptide 82–98 can be made tolerant to the protein in association with delayed disease progression or reduced disease activity over time. Autoantibody mediated tissue destruction is among the main features of organ-specific autoimmunity. Since the original discovery of catalytic antibodies, ample data established their contribution to pathological effects in disease as well as their possible biomedical applications. The practical relevance of abzymes is due to the unique characteristic distinguishing them from other biocatalysts: abzymes could be produced for the catalysis of almost all reactions occurring in living systems and catalyzed by appropriate enzymes. Abzymes may also be designed for the development of fundamentally new catalysts without natural analogues. The proved possibility to set a cell on secretion of engineering biocatalysts is intensively discussed. Serum level of proteolytic Abs may provide a clinically important predictive biomarker for demyelination in MS patients and formulating prognosis of the disease. The serum levels of the Ab-mediated catalytic activity as prognostic criteria could also differentiate MS patients with probably favorable or severe disease course or outcome, and outcome criteria are now being designed to assess the overall impact of MS as dependent variables for clinical studies. Ultimately, analysis of autoAb-mediated MBP degradation may provide a supplementary clinical and laboratory tool for assessing the disease progression and disability of MS patients. The possibility of forced stimulation of B-cells to produce proteolytic Abs with a given design is also intensively discussed. Such technology could be widely applied to treat and prevent socially relevant autoimmune disorders.

Achievements in medical abzymology could be a promising basis to design new medicines. The most dynamic trend is related to the synthesis of catalytic Abs that are able to destroy circulating drugs before initiating toxic effects on nervous system and other tissues. Catalytic Abs directly affecting the physiologic reconstruction of tissues and organ systems with complex architectonics including neuroglia are of special value. Neurology is estimated as an interesting area for abzyme application since Abs can be used for the induction of remyelination and the restoration of previously lost glia functions in MS.

List of abbreviations:

MS - Multiple sclerosis
CNS - central nervous system
autoAbs – Autoantibodies
catAbs - catalytic antibodies
Igs – immunoglobulins
TS - transition states
MBP - myelin basic protein
EAE - experimental autoimmune encephalomyelitis
MOG - myelin oligodendrocyte glycoprotein
HSP – heat shock protein
MAC - membrane attack complex
PLP - Proteolipid protein
SLE - system lupus erythematosis
CIS - clinically isolated syndrome
CDMS - clinically definite multiple sclerosis
EDSS - Expanded disability status scale
MRI – magnetic resonance imaging

## 7. References

Abraham S., Guo F., Li L.S., Rader C., Liu C., Barbas C.F. 3rd., Lerner R.A., Sinha S.C. Synthesis of the next-generation therapeutic antibodies that combine cell targeting and antibody-catalyzed prodrug activation. Proc. Natl. Acad. Sci. USA 2007, 104(13):5584-5589

Altmann D. (2005) Evaluating the evidence for multiple sclerosis as an autoimmune disease. Archives of neurology. Vol.62, No.4 (April 2005) ISSN 688-9

Angclucci F, Mirabella M, Frisullo G, Caggiula M, Tonali PA & Batocchi AP, (2005) Scrum levels of anti-myelin antibodies in relapsing— remitting multiple sclerosis patients during different phases of disease activity and immunomodulatory therapy. *Disease markers.* Vol.21, No.2 (2005) ISSN 49-55.]

Belogurov AA, Kurkova IN, Friboulct A et al.' (2008). Recognition and degradation of myelin basic protein peptides by serum autoantibodies: novel biomarker for multiple sclerosis. Journal of immunology. Vol.180, No.2 (January 2008) ISSN 1258-67]

Berger, T., Rubner, P., Schautzer, F., Egg, R., Ulmer, H., Mayringer, I., Dilitz, E., Deisenhammer, F. & Reindl, M. (2003) Anti-myelin antibodies as a predictor of clinically definite multiple sclerosis after a first demyelinating event. The New England journal of medicine Vol.349, No.2 (July 2003) ISSN 139-45

Chamczuk, A. J., Ursell, M., O'Connor, P., Jackowski, G. & Moscarello, M. A. (2002) A rapid ELISA-based serum assay for myelin basic protein in multiple sclerosis. *Journal of immunological methods.* Vol.262, No.1-2 (April 2002) ISSN 21-7.,

D'Souza, C. A., & M. A. Moscarello. (2006). Differences in susceptibility of MBP charge isomers to digestion by stromelysin-1 (MMP-3) and release of an immunodominant epitope. *Neurochemical research..* Vol.31, No.8 (August 2006) ISSN 1045-54.

D'Souza, C. A., D. D. Wood, Y. M. She, & M. A. Moscarello. (2005). Autocatalytic cleavage of myelin basic protein: an alternative to molecular mimicry. *Biochemistry* Vol.44, No.38 (September 2005) ISSN 12905-13.

Fishelson Z, Attali G, Mevorach D. (2001) Complement and apoptosis. Molecular immunology Vol.38, No.2-3 (August 2001) ISSN 207-19

Friboulet A, Avallc B, Dcbat H, Thomas D (1999) A possible role of catalytic antibodies in metabolism. *Immunology today.* Vol.20, No.10 (October 1999) ISSN 474-5

Friboulet A., Avalle B., Debat H., Thomas D. A possible role of catalytic antibodies in metabolism. Immunol. Today 1999, 20(10):474-478

Fritz, R. B., Chou, C. H. & McFarlin, D. E. (1983) Induction of experimental allergic encephalomyelitis in PL/J and (SJL/J x PL/J)F1 mice by myelin basic protein and its peptides: localization of a second encephalitogenic determinant. Journal of immunology Vol.130, No.1 (January 1983) ISSN 191-4

Gabibov A.G., Gololobov G.V., Makarevich O.I., Schourov D.V., Chernova E.A., Yadav R.P. DNA-hydrolyzing autoantibodies. Appl. Biochem. Biotechnol. 1994, 47(2-3):293-302

Gabibov AG, Ponomarcnko NA, Kozyr AV et al *(2002)* Catalytic antibodies and pathology: human and mice models. *Journal of immunological methods.* Vol.269, No.1-2 (November 2002) ISSN 197-211

Genain, C. P., Cannella, B., Hauser, S. L. & Raine, C. S. (1999) Identification of autoantibodies associated with myelin damage in multiple sclerosis., Nature medicine Vol.5, No.2 (February1999) ISSN 170–5.

Hafler, D. A. (2004). Multiple sclerosis. *The Journal of clinical investigation.* Vol.113, No.6 (April 2004) ISSN 788-94.

Husted, C. (2006). Structural insight into the role of myelin basic protein in multiple sclerosis. *Proceedings of the National Academy of Sciences of the United States of America.* Vol.103, No.12 (March 2006) ISSN 4339-40.

Jones LH, Wentworth Jr P. The therapeutic potential for catalytic antibodies: from a concept to a promise. Mini Rev Med Chem 2001;1:125–32

Kotzin BL, Kozora E. (2001) Anti-DNA meets NMDA in neuropsychiatric lupus. Nature medicine Vol.7, No.11 (November 2001) ISSN 1175-6

Kozyr A.V., Kolesnikov A.V., Aleksandrova E.S., Sashchenko L.P., Gnuchev N.V., Favorov P.V., Kotelnikov M.A., Iakhnina E.I., Astsaturov I.A., Prokaeva T.B., Alekberova Z.S., Suchkov S.V., Gabibov A.G. Novel functional activities of anti-DNA autoantibodies from sera of patients with lymphoproliferative and autoimmune diseases. Appl. Biochem. Biotechnol. 1998, 75(1):45-61

Kozyr A.V., Kolesnikov A.V., Zelenova N.A., Sashchenko L.P., Mikhalap S.V., Bulina M.E., Ignatova A.N., Favorov P.V., Gabibov A.G. Autoantibodies to nuclear antigens: correlation between cytotoxicity and DNA-hydrolyzing activity. Appl. Biochem. Biotechnol. 2000, 83(1-3):255-262

Kozyr A.V., Sashchenko L.P., Kolesnikov A.V., Zelenova N.A., Khaidukov S.V., Ignatova A.N., Bobik T.V., Gabibov A.G., Alekberova Z.S., Suchkov S.V., Gnuchev N.V. Anti-DNA autoantibodies reveal toxicity to tumor cell lines. Immunol. Lett. 2002, 80(1):41-49

Kuhle, J., C. Pohl, M. Mehling, G. Edan, M. S. Freedman, H. P. Hartung, C. H. Polman, D. H. Miller, X. Montalban, F. Barkhof, et al. (2007). Lack of association between anti-myelin antibodies and progression to multiple sclerosis. *The New England journal of medicine.* Vol.356, No.4 (January 2007) ISSN 371-8

Kuhle, J., R. L. Lindberg, A. Regeniter, M. Mehling, F. Hoffmann, M. Reindl, T. Berger, E. W. Radue, D. Leppert, and L. Kappos. (2007). Anti-myelin antibodies in clinically isolated syndromes correlate with inflammation in MRI and CSF. *Journal of neurology.* Vol.254, No.2 (February 2007) ISSN 160-8.

Lacroix-Desmazes, S., Bayry, J., Misra, N., Horn, M. P., Villard, S., Pashov, A., Stieltjes, N., d'Oiron, R., Saint-Remy, J. M., Hoebeke, J., *et al.* (2002) *N. Engl. J. Med.* 346, 662–667.

Lerner R.A. Catalytic antibodies: the concept and the promise. Hosp. Pract. (Off. Ed.) 1993, 28(7):53-59

Lolli, F., B. Mulinacci, A. Carotenuto, B. Bonetti, G. Sabatino, B. Mazzanti, A. M. D'Ursi, E. Novellino, M. Pazzagli, L. Lovato, et al. (2005). An N-glucosylated peptide detecting disease-specific autoantibodies, biomarkers of multiple

Matsuura K., Ohara K., Munakata H., Hifumi E., Uda T. Pathogenicity of catalytic antibodies: catalytic activity of Bence Jones proteins from myeloma patients with renal impairment can elicit cytotoxic effects. Biol. Chem. 2006, 387(5):543-548

Mets, B., Winger, G., Cabrera, C., Seo, S., Jamdar, S., Yang, G., Zhao, K., Briscoe, R. J., Almonte, R., Woods, J. H. & Landry, D. W. (1998) *Proc. Natl. Acad. Sci. USA* 95, 10176–10181.

Nathan C. Immunology. Catalytic antibody bridges innate and adaptive immunity. Science 2002, 298(5601):2143-2144

Paul S, Li L, Kalaga R, Wilkins-Stevens P, Stevens FJ, Solomon A. Natural catalytic antibodies: peptide-hydrolyzing activities of Bence Jones proteins and VL fragment. J Biol Chem 1995;270:15257–61.

Paul S, Nishiyama Y, Planque S, Karle S, Taguchi H, Hanson C & Weksler ME. (2005) Antibodies as defensive enzymes. *Springer seminars in immunopathology* Vol.26, No.4 (March 2005) ISSN 485-503. ;

Paul S. (1998) Mechanism and functional role of antibody catalysis. *Applied biochemistry and biotechnology* Vol.75, No.1 (October 1998) ISSN 13-24

Pillet D, PaonM, Vorobiev II, Gabibov AG, Thomas D, Friboulet A. Idiotypic network mimicry and antibody catalysis: lessons for the elicitation of efficient anti-idiotypic protease antibodies. J Immunol Methods 2002;269:5–12.

Ponomarenko NA, Aleksandrova ES, Vorobiev II, Durova OM, Kozyr AV, Kolesnikov AV, et al. (2000) Natural antibody catalytic activities in mice with autoimmune disorders. Doklady biochemistry : proceedings of the Academy of Sciences of the USSR Vol.375 (November 2000) ISSN 224-7

Ponomarenko, N. A., O. M. Durova, I. I. Vorobiev, A. A. Belogurov, Jr., I. N. Kurkova, A. G. Petrenko, G. B. Telegin, S. V. Suchkov, S. L. Kiselev, M. A. Lagarkova, et al. 2006. Autoantibodies to myelin basic protein catalyze site-specific degradation of their antigen. *Proceedings of the National Academy of Sciences of the United States of America.* Vol.103, No.2 (January 2006) ISSN 281-6

Raso, V. & Stollar, B. D. (1975) *Biochemistry* 14, 591–599.

Raz E, Ben-Bassat H, Davidi T, Shlomai Z, Eilat D.(1993) Cross-reactions of anti-DNA autoantibodies with cell surface proteins. European journal of immunology. Vol.23, No.2 (February 1993) ISSN 383-90.

Reindl, M., Linington, C., Brehm, U., Egg, R., Dilitz, E., Deisenhammer, F., Poewe, W. & Berger, T. (1999) Antibodies against the myelin oligodendrocyte glycoprotein and the myelin basic protein in multiple sclerosis and other neurological diseases: a comparative study. Brain Vol.122, No.11 (November 1999) ISSN 2047-56.

Rekvig OP, Kalaaji M, Nossent H. (2004) Anti-DNA antibody subpopulations and lupus nephritis. Autoimmunity reviews. Vol.3, No.2 (February 2004) ISSN 1-6;

Sashchenko L.P., Khaidukov S.V., Kozyr A.V., Luk'yanova T.I., Gabibov A.G., Suchkov S.V., Bobik T.V., Alekberova Z.S., Gnuchev N.V. Caspase-dependent cytotoxicity of anti-DNA autoantibodies. Dokl. Biochem. Biophys. (*in russian*) 2001, 380:313-319

sclerosis. *Proceedings of the National Academy of Sciences of the United States of America* Vol.102, No.29 (July 2005) ISSN 10273-8.

Stcinman L, (1996) Multiple sclerosis: a coordinated immunological attack against myelin in the central nervous system. Cell Vol.85, No.3 (May 1996) ISSN 299-302

Suchkov S.V., Gabibov A.G., Alekberova Z.S., Gnuchev N.V. DNA-abzymes and their clinical significance in systemic lupus erythematosis. Ter. Arkh. (*in russian*) 2001, 73:58-65

Tellier C. Exploiting antibodies as catalysts: potential therapeutic applications. Transfus. Clin. Biol. 2002, 9(1):1-8

Tomassini, V., L. De Giglio, M. Reindl, P. Russo, I. Pestalozza, P. Pantano, T. Berger, and C. Pozzilli. (2007). Anti-myelin antibodies predict the clinical outcome after a first episode suggestive of MS. Multiple sclerosis : clinical and laboratory research Vol.13, No.9 (November 2007) ISSN 1086-94

Tramontano, A., Janda, K. D. & Lerner, R. A. (1986) *Science* 234, 1566–1570.

Viau, M. & Zouali, M. (2005) *Clin. Immunol.* 114, 17–26.

Wentworth P. Jr. Evidence for antibody-catalyzed ozone formation in bacterial killing and inflammation. Science 2002, 296(5576):2247-2249

Wentworth, P., Jr., and K. D. Janda. (2001). Catalytic antibodies: structure and function. *Cell biochemistry and biophysics.* Vol.35, No.1 (2001) ISSN 63-87.

Wentworth, P., Jr., L. H. Jones, A. D. Wentworth, X. Zhu, N. A. Larsen, I. A. Wilson, X. Xu, W. A. Goddard, III, K. D. Janda, A. Eschenmoser, and R. A. Lerner. (2001). Antibody catalysis of the oxidation of water. *Science* Vol.293, No.5536 (September 2001) ISSN 1806-11

Wentworth, P., Jr., McDunn, J. E., Wentworth, A. D., Takeuchi, C., Nieva, J., Jones, T., Bautista, C., Ruedi, J. M., Gutierrez, A., Janda, K. D., *et al.* (2002) *Science* 298, 2195–2199.

Wilkinson RW, Lee-MacAry AE, Davies D, Snary D, Ross EL. (2001) Antibody-dependent cell-mediated cytotoxicity: a flow cytome try-based assay using fluorophores. Journal of immunological methods Vol.258, No.1-2 (December 2001) ISSN 183-91

Zhou Y.X., Karle S., Taguchi H., Planque S., Nishiyama Y., Paul S. Prospects for immunotherapeutic proteolytic antibodies. J. Immunol. Methods 2002, 269:257–268

# 25

# Role of Fatty Acids in the Resolution of Autoimmune and Inflammatory Diseases

Elena Puertollano, María A. Puertollano,
Gerardo Álvarez de Cienfuegos and Manuel A. de Pablo
*University of Jaén, Faculty of Experimental Sciences, Div. of Microbiology Jaén*
*Spain*

## 1. Introduction

The main role of fatty acids is focused on serving as major substrates for energy production; however, fatty acids are also involved in the formation of cellular structures as well as in the transmission of cellular signals. Among the multiple functions attributed to fatty acids are their anti-inflammatory properties. This important characteristic has been applied in the prevention, attenuation or treatment of inflammatory disorders. Based on the previous argument is obvious that several fatty acids (mainly *n*-3 polyunsaturated or *n*-9 monounsaturated fatty acids) are capable of modulating immune system functions. These fatty acids may alter immune response through different mechanisms such as alteration of membrane fluidity, eicosanoid synthesis, oxidative stress, regulation of gene expression, apoptosis or modulation of gastrointestinal microbiota.

Early studies in Greenland Eskimos determined the low prevalence of inflammatory disorders in this population (Kromann et al., 1980). Despite their beneficial effects in the reduction of inflammatory diseases, other studies have demonstrated that the administration of diets containing long-chain *n*-3 polyunsaturated fatty acids may contribute, at least in part, to the reduction of host resistance against infectious agents. In fact, epidemiological investigations described a high incidence of tuberculosis in native Eskimos (Kaplan et al., 1972), who consume a great amount of *n*-3 polyunsaturated fatty acids. These data are clearly illustrative of the potential action of certain fatty acids on the inflammatory response, and of the consequences derived from an excessive immunosuppression.

It is obvious that these fatty acids contained in the diets produce an immune status able to ameliorate inflammatory conditions. Indeed, a growing number of studies using healthy human subjects as well as animal disease models have undoubtedly demonstrated dietary fish oil or olive oil to possess anti-inflammatory properties. For this reason, polyunsaturated or monounsaturated fatty acids have showed beneficial effects in numerous inflammatory diseases characterized by a overactivation of immune system such as asthma (childhood and adult), multiple sclerosis, glomerulonephritis, inflammatory bowel disease (Crohn's disease, ulcerative colitis) and rheumatoid arthritis . Here, we summarize the involvement of fatty acids as anti-inflammatory agents and the action that these fatty acids contained in the human or animal diets exert on the prevention or treatment of autoimmune diseases.

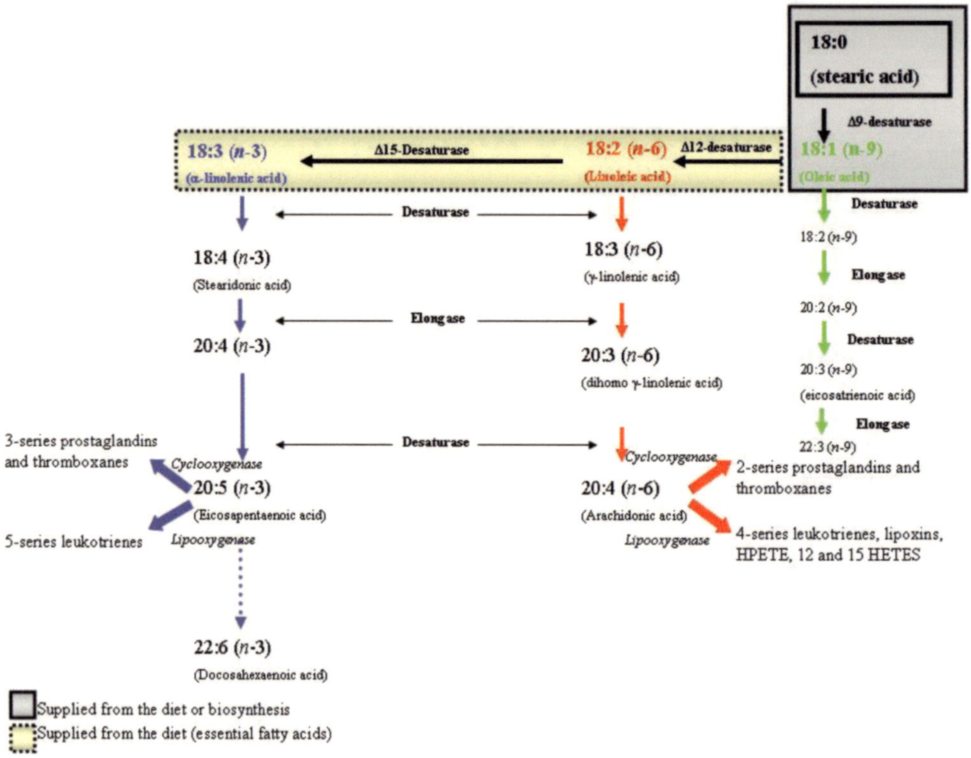


Fig. 1. Different pathways of n-3, n-6 and n-9 fatty acids synthesis. HETEs, hydroxyl-eicosatetraenoic acid; HPETE, hydroperoxy-eicosatetraenoic acids. (Puertollano *et al.*)

## 2. Fatty acids, inflammation and immune system

Polyunsaturated fatty acids (PUFA) are considered essentials to mammalian cells and should be administered in the diet. These essential fatty acids are divided into two great families: *n-3* series derived from linolenic acid (LNA), and *n-6* series derived from linoleic (LA) acid. Different biochemical processes lead to the production of eicosapentanoic acid (EPA) or docohexaenoic acid (DHA) from LNA, as well as arachidonic acid (AA) from linoleic acid. Likewise, another family of non essential fatty acids such as *n-9* series derived from oleic acid, a monounsaturated fatty acid (MUFA), also seems to play an important role in the immunomodulatory process (Yaqoob, 2002) [Figure 1].

In recent years numerous investigations have examined the mechanisms of action responsible for the modulation of immune system by fatty acids and most of them are in agreement that unsaturated fatty acids are potent immunosupressor especially *n-3* PUFA (reviewed in Puertollano et al., 2008). The main mechanisms of action of fatty acids are schematized in figure 2 and include alterations of immune cells membrane fluidity, eicosanoids synthesis modifications, oxidative alteration, regulation of gene expression and apoptosis mechanisms inducement. Table 1 summarized these mechanisms of actions and others recently proposed such as modulation of gastrointestinal microbiota.

All of these mechanisms of action deal to explain the numerous effects of fatty acids on immune system. It is well known that unsaturated fatty acids are involved on the alteration of lymphocyte proliferation. In general, administration of high level of fatty acids, and especially *n-3* series, are related with a reduction on lymphocyte proliferation in both animals and human studies (Meydani et al., 1991; Yaqoob et al., 1994; Moussa et al., 2000). This fact can be especially interesting in the amelioration of diseases characterized by overactivation of immune response like autoimmune disorder. In addition fatty acids can modify another lymphocyte functions like cytokine production.

| |
|---|
| • Eicosanoids production |
| • Membrane fluidity and lipid rafts |
| • Oxidative stress |
| • Signaling transduction |
| • Gene expression |
| • Apoptosis |
| • Ability in antigen presentation |
| • Modulation of gastrointestinal microbiota |

Table 1. Hypothetical mechanisms of dietary lipids on immune functions: factors determining the modulation of immune system.

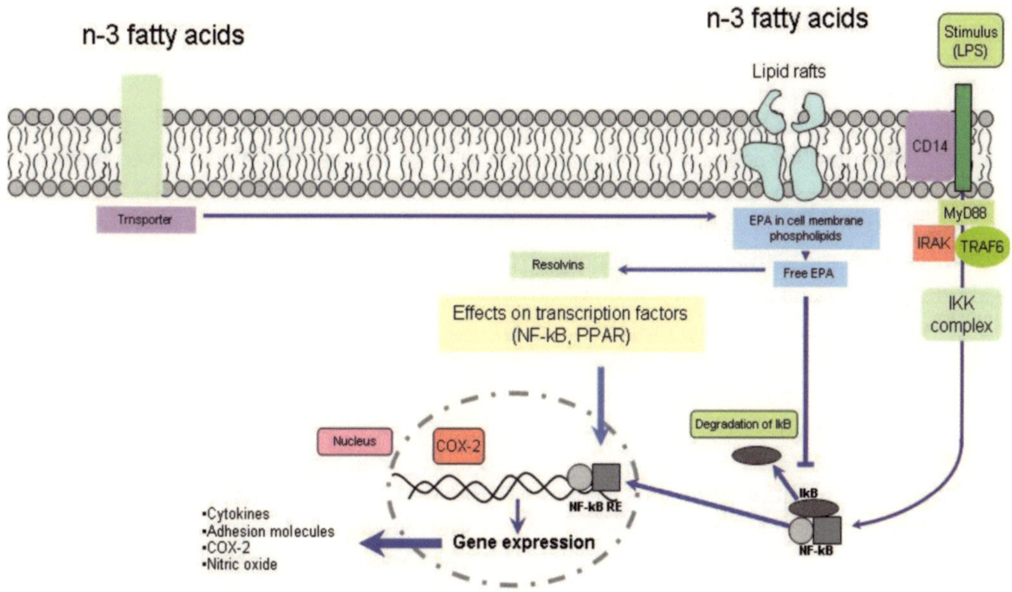


Fig. 2. Schematic diagram of proposed mechanisms of action of *n-3* polyunsaturated fatty acids whereby these fatty acids are involved in the modulation of immune system functions. Abbreviations: CD14, CD14 surface receptor; COX, cyclooxygenase; EPA, eicosapentaenoic acid, IκB, NF-κB inhibitory protein; LPS, lipopolysaccharide; NF-κB, nuclear factor-κB; PPAR, peroxisome proliferator-activated receptor; TLR, Toll-like receptors. (Puertollano *et al.*)

Several studies have demonstrated the immunomodulatory properties of polyunsaturated and monounsaturated fatty acids over reduction of pro and anti-inflammatory cytokines.

In this context interesting investigations indicates that *n-3* PUFA exert a significant inhibition of Th1-type cytokines, whereas they have little effects on Th2-type cytokines (Wallace et al., 2001). In spite of olive oil diets are involved in the reduction of cytokine secretion, their immunosupressant effects are not as potent as those exerted by the administration of a fish oil diet (Puertollano et al., 2004). Fatty acids are able to modify the natural killer (NK) cells activity too. Finally recent studies have proved the action of fatty acids in the expression of adhesion molecules like lymphocyte function antigen-1 (LFA-1) and intercellular adhesion molecule-1 (ICAM-1) (Sanderson et al., 1995; Miles et al., 2001). These facts have been shown in preliminary studies in animal models but it is necessary to confirm it in human studies.

### 2.1 Dietary lipids and inflammatory response

Inflammation is part of immune response and is a complex process affected by different factors, included mediators generated from fatty acids. Eicosanoids from *n-6* series fatty acids (like prostaglandine $E_2$ ($PGE_2$) and leukotriene $B_4$ ($LTB_4$) among others) are considered pro-inflammatory mediators while molecules from *n-3* series (like $PGE_3$ and $LTB_5$) generally are endowed with lower bioactivity. It is necessary to keep an optimal *n-6*/*n-3* balance to achieve a healthy inflammatory state.
Numerous researches have demonstrated that fish oil rich diet promotes a decrease on inflammatory ecoisanoids production from *n-6* PUFA because of the competition between the two metabolic pathways. In this way *n-3* PUFA supplementation of the human diet is able to decrease production of inflammatory eicosanoids like $PGE_2$, $LTB_4$ and thromboxane $B_2$ ($TXB_2$) by inflammatory cells (Meydani et al., 1991; Kelley et al., 1999; Trebble et al., 2003; Rees et al., 2006). In addition *n-3* PUFA have other effects over inflammatory response. One of the most important is the generation of resolvins, a group of mediators derived from EPA and DHA that appear to exert potent anti-inflammatory actions (Calder, 2008a). Decreasing antigen presentation via major histocompatibility complex class II (MHC II), inhibiting T-cell reactivity and diminishing inflammatory cytokine production (Calder et al., 2002; Akhtar Khan, 2010; Kim et al., 2010) are others of the anti-inflammatory effects of *n-3* fatty acids. Autoimmunity can be considered as an exacerbated inflammatory response against self structures; therefore *n-3* long chain fatty acids can be useful in the treatment of these diseases.
Oleic acid is the main fatty acid contained in olive oil. Olive oil has traditionally been used as a placebo in the studies investigating the potential action of other dietary lipids on the modulation of immune functions. Thus, MUFA that constitute olive oil were initially considered as neutral fatty acids. Nevertheless different studies demonstrated that olive oil is clearly involved in anti-inflammatory activities and in the modulation of immune response (reviewed in Puertollano et al., 2010). The anti-inflammatory activity of olive oil appears to be associated with the production of the metabolite eicosatrienoic acid from oleic acid (20:3 *n-9*), which is a potent inhibitor of $LTB_4$ (James et al., 1993). In addition it is possible that beneficial effects of olive oil may be in part due to the presence of natural antioxidants, contributing to an increase in the stability of oil (Linos et al., 1999).
Taken together there is evidence that both *n-3* PUFA and *n-9* MUFA can be useful in treatment of inflammatory disorders associated with autoimmune disease. Table 2 summarizes a list of some of the diseases and conditions with an inflammatory component that could be beneficially affected by *n- 3* and *n-9* series fatty acids.

| |
|---|
| • Acute cardiovascular events |
| • Acute respiratory distress syndrome |
| • Allergic disease |
| • Asthma (childhood and adult) |
| • Atherosclerosis |
| • Cancer cachexia |
| • Chronic obstructive pulmonary disease |
| • Cystic fibrosis |
| • Inflammatory bowel disease (Crohn's disease, ulcerative colitis) |
| • Lupus |
| • Multiple sclerosis |
| • Neurodegenerative disease of ageing |
| • Obesity |
| • Psoriasis |
| • Rheumatoid arthritis |
| • Systemic inflammatory response to surgery, trauma and critical illness |
| • Type 1 diabetes |
| • Type 2 diabetes |

Table 2. Inflammatory disorder where fatty acids could be useful. Diseases are listed in an alphabetical order (Adapted from Calder, 2006).

## 3. Fatty acids and autoimmune disorders

Autoimmunity is the failure of an organism to recognize its own constituent parts as self, which results in immune responses against its own cells and tissues. Autoimmunity involves an inflammatory response against own tissues which are implicated different mechanisms like autoantibodies production, immunocomplex formation and lymphocytes T reactivity. Recently, an important investigation about the implication of fatty acids and dietary lipids in the amelioration of autoimmune diseases has been carried out because of their anti-inflammatory properties (Linos et al., 1999). Below we will summarize the main autoimmune disorder where fatty acids have shown to exert beneficial effects.

### 3.1 Fatty acids and inflammatory bowel disease

Inflammatory bowel disease (IBD) includes Cronh´s disease and ulcerative colitis which are autoimmune disorders characterized by an exacerbated inflammatory response against innocuous stimulus in gastrointestinal tract. Their pathogenesis is considered to include disorders of the immunomodulation of the bowel mucosa which results in lesions of the epithelium tissue layer caused by activated T cells, mononuclear cells and macrophages. In Crohn's disease the mucosa of the whole alimentary tract from the mouth to the anus can be affected, with maximal manifestation in the ileum and colon, while in ulcerative colitis the mucosa of the colon is mainly affected. In both diseases inflammatory cytokines and eicosanoids like $LTB_4$ are actively produced in situ (Sharon et al., 1984).

The gastrointestinal system is subjected to sustained exposure to ingested foods throughout the whole life, and this gives rise to interactions between food components and gastrointestinal mucosal cells. Interactions with transporters and transcription factors contribute to the modulation of various responses, including those of cells involved in inflammatory processes. There are, however, specific chronic diseases of the alimentary tract that are based on inflammatory processes and hence are bound to be susceptible to modulation by dietary FA.

### 3.1.1 Role of dietary lipids on animal models of IBD

Several studies with animal models of IBD, especially chemical induced colitis, have been developed after the recognition of anti-inflammatory properties of *n*-3 PUFA. Generally researches show that fish oil rich diet are involved in the amelioration of the disease comparing with *n-6* fatty acid oil rich diet. In this way different studies have demonstrated convincingly the reduction on colonic damage and ulceration (Vilaseca et al., 1990; Yuceyar et al., 1999), reduction in cell recruitment and activation (Andoh et al., 2003; Whiting et al., 2005) decreasing levels of $LTB_4$ and $PGE_2$ on plasma and gut mucosa (Shoda et al., 1995; Nieto et al., 2002; Hudert et al., 2006) and reduction of pro-inflammatory cytokines (Andoh et al., 2003) in animals fed with *n-3* PUFA rich diet.

The effects of fatty acids on an animal model of Cronh's disease have been proved too. Lately Matsunaga et al. have reported for the first time that *n-3* fatty acids ameliorate the ileum inflammation in a murine model of spontaneous and chronic ileitis that closely resembles human Cronh's disease. Specifically these authors have shown that *n-3* fatty acids diets are capable to decrease the ileum inflammation markers, cells recruitment and infiltration and pro-inflammatory mediators like monocyte chemoattractant protein-1(MCP-1) and IL-6 (Matsunaga et al., 2009).

A number of investigators have studied the effect of olive oil rich diet on animals models of IBD too. In this way Camuesco et al. have reported a lower colonic inflammatory response in rats fed with olive oil-based diet and this anti-inflammatory effect is increased when the olive oil diet is supplemented with a 4% of fish oil (Camuesco et al., 2005). Another study has described a beneficial effect of extra virgin olive oil in colitis associated colon carcinogenesis. A reduction on colonic inflammation, proinflammatory cytokines and less incident and multiplicity of tumours have been reported in rats fed with extra virgin olive oil versus sunflower oil (Sanchez-Fidalgo et al., 2010).

Generally animal models have shown a beneficial effect of *n-3* and *n-9* fatty acids in the development of IBD.

### 3.1.2 Trials in human patients

The established role of AA derived eicsanoids in pathophysiology of inflammatory bowel diet, and especially and inadequate *n*-6/*n*-3 balance, may play an important role in establishing and perpetuating of the disease. Indeed, multivariate analysis suggested that the recently increased consumption of *n*–6 FA in Japan, resulting in an increased ratio of *n*–6 to *n*–3 PUFA and possibly also elevated AA levels, may be responsible for the increased incidence of Crohn's disease in this country (Shoda et al., 1996).

In recent years some pilot studies have been carried out to analyze the effects of fish oil on IBD patients (reviewed by Calder, 2008a). A number of several randomized, placebo-controlled, double-blind studies on the effects of fish oil (2.7–5.6 g/d) in IBD have reported benefits, including improved clinical scores, mucosal histology, sigmoidoscopic score and lower rates of relapse. In this way an interesting study reported a decreased incidence of relapses in patients with Crohn's disease in remission who received a supplemented of enterically coated fish oil for 1 year; there was a significant reduction in the proportion of relapse on fish oil group, 28%, compared with placebo group, 69%, over 12 months. In addition this difference was maintained at 12 months, with an incidence of remission of 59% in fish oil group versus 26% in placebo group (Belluzzi et al., 1996). However another studies have not found beneficial effects of *n-3* fatty acids supplementation in IBD patients (Loeschke et al., 1996; Lorenz-Meyer et al., 1996).

Studies about the effect of olive oil in IBD patients are limited and most of them used the olive oil as a placebo because *n-9* MUFA was considered as a neutral fat. Although preliminary studies of Dr. Gassull research group had demonstrated that *n-9* MUFA might be beneficial inducing remission of Crohn's disease (Gonzalez-Huix et al., 1993; Fernandez-Banares et al., 1994). The first multicentre, randomized and double-blind trial to evaluate the influence of fat composition in enteral nutrition have not been successful. Nevertheless the results are not conclusive because of the small sample size (smaller than was initially estimated). The study was prematurely finished and the source of oleic acid used in this trial was synthetic trioleate and not olive oil as in the other studies (Gonzalez-Huix et al., 1993). Olive oil contains polyphenols, another components with a potent antioxidant activity and this fact may contribute to different effects of vegetables oil and even though olive oil and *n-9* MUFA (Owen et al., 2000).

Studies in which olive oil have been used as a placebo have reported contradictory results. Lorenz et al. have shown an increased activity of disease in patients of ulcerative colitis and Crohn's disease supplemented with olive oil as a placebo versus fish oil group (Lorenz et al., 1989; Romano et al., 2005). However others authors have not founds differences between both groups of supplementation (Greenfield et al., 1993; Trebble et al., 2005).

In spite of several favourable studies about the use of fatty acids, and specially fish oil, in the treatment of IBD the evidence of clinical benefits are limited. The soundest result was the potential of *n-3* PUFA to maintain the patients of Crohn's disease in remission (Belluzzi et al., 1996). However, this observation was not confirmed in a recent larger study using a similar protocol (Feagan et al., 2008). One reason why dietary lipids might be more effective in animal models than in human patients is the different dose of assay. In human trials the dose of fatty acids are lower compared with the dose in animals studies (higher compared with habitual human consumption doses).

### 3.2 Fatty acids and rheumatoid arthritis

Rheumatoid arthritis is a chronic inflammatory autoimmune disease that affects about 1% of adult population and is more frequent in women than men. Rheumatoid arthritis is characterized by joint inflammation, swelling, pain, impaired function, stiffness, osteoporosis, muscle wasting, and the participation of inflammatory cells (macrophages, T lymphocytes, plasma cells infiltrating the synovium). All the mediators of inflammation (cytokines, interleukins and typical pro-inflammatory factors and proteins) are actively produced by synovial cells. COX-2 is over-expressed in the synovium of patients, and its eicosanoid products, in addition to those of the 5-LOX, are found in the synovial fluids (Sano et al., 1992; Sperling, 1995). In addition rheumatoid arthritis is also characterised by signs of systemic inflammation, such as elevated plasma concentrations of some cytokines (e.g. IL-6), acute-phase proteins and rheumatoid factors. The relevance of the pro-inflammatory COX pathway is also underlined by the efficacy of the pharmacological inhibition of this pathway (e.g. by non steroidal anti-inflammatory drugs).

There is evidence that rheumatoid arthritis is less severe in Mediterranean countries where consume of fish oil, fruits and vegetables and olive oil are higher than in other countries (Pattison et al., 2004). This report, joint to the special relevance of COX pathway on the development of the disease, has brought about a great number of studies where the role of dietary lipids in the management of rheumatoid arthritis has been evaluated.

### 3.2.1 Some studies with animal models

Interest in the use of *n-3* fatty acids in rheumatoid arthritis began in the mid-eighties, following the demonstration in several autoimmune strains of mice that *n-3* fatty acids reduced the severity of diffuse proliferative glomerulonephritis (Simopoulos, 2002). Further studies have shown the efficacy of fish oil in the development of the animal disease. For instance in an early study Leslie et al. shown that fish oil increased the time of onset of arthritis and decreased the incidence and severity of this disease in a murine model of type II collagen-induced arthritis(Leslie et al., 1985). Another researchers have reported a mouse model of rheumatoid arthritis fed with fish oil and have shown a significantly lower serum levels of interleukins IL-6, IL-10, IL-12 and in tumour necrosis factor-α (TNF-α), $PGE_2$, $TXB_2$ and $LTB_4$ compared with levels in mice fed corn oil (Venkatraman et al., 1999). Similarly, EPA and DHA incorporation into macrophage phospholipids via oral administration resulted in a reduction of streptococcal cell wall arthritis in Lew/SSN rats (Volker et al., 2000).

On the other hand it is well known that rheumatoid arthritis is characterized by joint and tissue damage and this damage occurs by a variety of mechanisms, many of which involve reactive oxygen species (ROS). ROS can cause destruction of hyaluronic acid and disruption to collagen, proteoglycans, protease inhibitors, and membrane function, the latter via oxidation of membrane fatty acids. The initiation of rheumatoid arthritis is believed to result in an increase in the concentration of macrophages and neutrophils in the synovial fluid and free-radical-producing enzymes. This leads to high levels of ROS in the joints, which increases and prolongs inflammation and damage (Darlington et al., 2001). Olive oil, and especially extra virgin olive oil, is rich in antioxidants compounds. Taking account the role of ROS in joint and tissue damage on development of rheumatoid arthritis, the effect of olive oil can be especially useful in this kind of disease. Indeed Martinez-Dominguez et al. have shown the efficacy of an olive oil supplemented with polyphenols in animal models of arthritis (Martinez-Dominguez et al., 2001).

### 3.2.2 Efficacy of fatty acids on human disease

During the 80s and 90s several studies in patients with rheumatoid arthritis showed the beneficial effects of *n-3* PUFA on the development of the disease. Several authors reported that fish oils reduces the production of inflammatory mediators like LTB 4 by neutrophils and monocytes (Kremer et al., 1985; Kremer et al., 1987; Cleland et al., 1988; Tulleken et al., 1990; van der Tempel et al., 1990) and IL-1β by monocytes (Kremer et al., 1990). There is also evidence of reduction in the plasma concentrations of IL-1 (Espersen et al., 1992)and C-reactive protein (Kremer et al., 1985), and normalized neutrophil function (Sperling et al., 1987).

A number of randomized, placebo-controlled, double-blind studies of fish oil treatments have been reported. In different reviews Calder have summarized the results of studies with a dose of fatty acids between 1.6 and 7.1 g/d (average of 3.5 g/day EPA + DHA) and almost of them reported some benefit (Calder, 2006; Calder, 2008b; Galli et al., 2009). Clinical symptoms were improved, including reduced duration of morning stiffness, number of tender or swollen joints, joint pain, time of fatigue and increased grip strength. Particular relevance has the reduction of the use of anti-inflammatory drugs.

*n*–3 PUFA may act as anti-inflammatory agents by competition whit AA for incorporation in the eicosanoid pathway. This efficacy of *n-3* PUFA may be achieved in rheumatoid arthritis by simultaneously decreasing of *n*-6 PUFA intake, especially AA. Indeed Adam et al. have shown that a diet supplemented with *n-3*-PUFA and AA restricted is able to ameliorate clinical signs of inflammation like tenders and swollen joints and to decrease the formation of eicosanoids such as leukotrienes and prostaglandins (Adam et al., 2003). This study shows also that intakes of preformed AA, in addition to formation from the precursor LA, may be a factor in the modulation of AA levels in the body, and since LA and AA are provided by quite different sources (seed oils vs. lean meat), this should be taken into consideration in the evaluation of strategies for optimal *n–3* FA intakes.

Several reviews about the role of fish oil in rheumatoid arthritis patients have been carried out and most of them conclude that there was strong evidence about benefits of *n-3* PUFA on the management of this disease (Cleland et al., 2000). These reviews have shown that fish oil is able to improve the signs of the disease like number and severity of tender joint, number of swollen joints, physician and patients´ global assessment and use of anti-inflammatory drugs among others effect (Simopoulos, 2002; Stulnig, 2003; Calder, 2006; Calder, 2008a; Galli et al., 2009). Indeed an editorial comment about the use of fish oil in this disease concluded that dietary fish oil supplements should be regarded as part of a standard therapy for rheumatoid arthritis (Cleland et al., 2000).

With reference to olive oil a study by Linos et al. (Linos et al., 1991) has suggested that a beneficial anti-inflammatory effect of olive oil consumption on rheumatoid arthritis may be possible. In fact, this study compared the relative risk of development of rheumatoid arthritis in relation to lifelong consumption of olive oil in a Greek population and demonstrated that high consumers of olive oil (almost every day throughout life) had four times less risk than those who consumed olive oil less than six times per month on average throughout their lives; by contrast the effect of fish consumption was also tested without statistically significant findings (Linos et al., 1991).

A number of studies that examined the benefits of fish oil in rheumatoid arthritis used an olive oil placebo for the control groups. Kremer et al. evaluated the effect of fish oil supplementation on the progression and severity of the disease using olive oil as a placebo. Unexpectedly clinical evaluation and immunologic test showed similar results in both groups. No explanation of the improvements showed by the olive oil groups was given, although changes in immune function may be responsible (Kremer et al., 1990). A more recent research has reported an improvement in beneficial effect of fish oil when is mixed together olive oil versus a supplementation with only fish oil , suggesting a positive action of olive oil in signs and symptoms of rheumatoid arthritis (Berbert et al., 2005).

Taking together all these results and facts revised in this section, it can be concluded that there are strong evidences to justify the positive effects of fish oil in the management of rheumatoid arthritis. On the other hand, although the results are still preliminary, combination of olive oil and fish oil may be more favorable because of the antioxidant effect of olive oil joint to the anti-inflammatory potential of both oils.

### 3.3 Fatty acids in systemic lupus erythematosus

Systemic lupus erythematosus (SLE) is a complex autoimmune disease with heterogeneous clinical manifestations and disease course and most of cases occurring in women of childrenbering age. It is characterized by the deregulated innate and adaptive immune pathways and the development of anti-nuclear antibodies (ANA). Mortality of patients with SLE is significatly correlated wiht development of glomerulonephritis. Binding of autoantibodies, specially IgG anti-DNA, and immunecomplex depositions within the kidneys recruits leukocytes and this infiltration results in an inflammatory response that can lead to irreparale renal parenchymal damage (Pestka, 2010).

#### 3.3.1 Studies with animal models

Several studies with animal models of SLE have been carried out about the role of dietary lipids in the development of the disease and generally most of them concluded a beneficial effect of fish oil (reviewed in Pestka, 2010).
Early studies of Prickett and his research group showed that administration of fish oil to young mice induced a reduction on severity and incidence of renal disease and increased the lifespan of NZB/NZW mice (Prickett et al., 1981; Prickett et al., 1982; Prickett et al., 1983), even fish oil was able to reduce the progression of established renal damage in another mouse model of lupus (Robinson et al., 1986). Other studies have reported a link between increased lifespan and reduced renal damage and reductions of anti-DNA autoantibodies and circulating immunocomplexes in NZB/NZW (Alexander et al., 1987).
Subsequently several studies have demonstrated that the amelioration of disease in these animal models were linked with the action of fish oil over eicosanoids metabolism (Kelley et al., 1985; Spurney et al., 1994; Venkatraman et al., 1999).
Results from Fernandes laboratory have reported that DHA, but not EPA, is the most potent *n-3* fatty acid that suppresses glomerulonephritis and extends life span of systemic lupus erythematosus-prone NZB/NZW mice (Halade et al., 2010). In addition the same authors have proved that the beneficial action of fish oil in lupus animal models is increased by caloric restriction (Jolly et al., 1999; Jolly et al., 2001).

#### 3.3.2 Clinical trials

Numerous studies have evaluated the possible beneficial action of fish oil in lupus patients although the results are not so conclusive like animal studies. Indeed two early clinical trials suggested that fish oil supplementation has little value in management of lupus nephritis when it is compared with olive oil (Westberg et al., 1990; Clark et al., 1993). However two double blind studies have reported a benefit in disease criteria and lupus score (Walton et al., 1991; Duffy et al., 2004). More recently investigations have shown that fish oil, and more specifically EPA, may be useful in the amelioration of lupus disease because of the decreasing oxidative stress, improving endothelial functions and conferring cardiovascular benefits (Nakamura et al., 2005; Wright et al., 2008).
In view of the previous reports we can conclude that, in spite of fish oil supplementation may be useful in the amelioration of lupus and prevention of renal disease, new and larger investigations must be carried out to clarify the role of fatty acids in development of this disease.

### 3.4 Fatty acids and multiple sclerosis

Multiple sclerosis (MS) is a Central Nervous System-specific demyelinating disease and is the most common neurological disorder that occurs in young adults. Although the aetiology of MS remains unknown there is strong evidence for the presence of autoimmune mechanisms in the disease pathogenesis. Pro-inflammatory cytokines from activated T cells and macrophages have been strongly implicated in the pathogenesis of MS, like the up-regulation of adhesion molecules on endothelial cells and the subsequent infiltration of activated T cells into the Central Nervous System.

An association between dietary fat intake and the incidence of multiple sclerosis was first proposed by Swank in 1950 (Swank, 1950). Some epidemiological studies have been carried out later and the most of them indicate that diets rich in saturated fatty acids are detrimentally associated with MS, while PUFA acid rich diets are beneficially associated with MS. Studies from Harbige laboratory have shown that the relationship between linoleic acid (*n-6*) and dihomo-g-linoleic acid (DGLA), and also between DGLA (*n-6*) and AA is clearly disturbed in MS compared with healthy controls. This may indicate a problem with δ6 and δ5 desaturation and / or a greater requirement for these *n-6* fatty acids in many of the MS patients (Harbige et al., 2007).

### 3.4.1 Fatty acids in animal models of multiple sclerosis

Experimental autoimmune encephalomyelitis (EAE) is an experimentally induced CD4+ T cell mediated autoimmune inflammatory and demyelinating disease in rodents often used as a useful animal model of MS.

Administration of PUFA can reduce the clinical severity of EAE. Indeed LA supplementation has been shown to reduce the severity of EAE in guinea pigs when it is administered before EAE induction (Meade et al., 1978; Hughes et al., 1980). Harbige et al. also demonstrated that gamma linoleic acid (GLA) supplementation could reduce the severity of both acute EAE and the relapsing phases of chronic. Further analysis revealed an increase in production of transforming growth factor β-1 and $PGE_2$, both associated with a reduction in the inflammatory response in EAE models (Harbige et al., 1995; Harbige et al., 1997; Harbige et al., 2000).

### 3.4.2 Clinical trials in human patients

Following the preliminary epidemiological studies by Swank, several researches have attempted the role of PUFA in the development of MS. In this way Millar et al. carried out a double-blind study with LA and olive oil during 24 months. These authors reported an improvement in relapse severity and nonsignificant trends towards lower relapse rates but no difference in disability (Millar et al., 1973). Later, Paty et al. did not find such effects in a similar trial with higher doses of oleic acid as a placebo (Paty et al., 1978). No conclusive data have been found in other trials realized with GLA in combination with LNA (Bates et al., 1977).

However more recently Harbige et al. have reported a randomised double-blind placebo controlled trial to determine the effects of supplementation with selected GLA rich borage oil. Data proved that high dose of this oil reduced the relapse rate and disability progression as measured by EDSS (Expanded Disability Status Scale) and compared with a placebo of polyethylene glycol and with low dose of the same oil (Harbige et al., 2007). Although these data are very positive, the number of patients enrolled in the trial is limited (n=36) and no conclusive statements can be made.

The fish oil action in MS has been investigated too but some studies have not been successful. Two double blind controlled clinical trials have been carried out to evaluate the effect of fish oil in the disease without significant findings. In these trials olive oil was used as a placebo again and although nonsignificant trends, toward less disability and certain improvements in quality of life, have been found the results are inconclusive (Bates et al., 1989; Weinstock-Guttman et al., 2005). However others researchers have found beneficial effects of fish oil in MS patients. Shinto et al. have reported that *n-3* fatty acids supplementation significantly decreased matrix metalloproteinase-9 (MMP-9) levels in relapsing-remitting MS. This enzyme is thought to have a significant role in the transmigration of inflammatory cells into the central nervous system by aiding in the disruption of the blood brain barrier. In this way the ability of *n-3* fatty acids to decrease the levels secreted by immune cells may be a significant observation in spite of significant changes in quality of life have not been found (Shinto et al., 2009).

Taken over all epidemiological data, animal data and clinical trial we can confirm that PUFA, particularly *n-6* fatty acids, have a role in the pathogenesis and treatment of multiple sclerosis. However different factors must be better controlled in the clinical trials to achieve convincing results, like trials design, sample size and the choice of an appropriate placebo. This last item is of a great important because of olive oil has been used as a placebo in most of the reviewed clinical trials, however experience of our laboratory and others clearly proved the great immunomodulator potential of this fat, usually considered relatively inert (Puertollano et al., 2004; Puertollano et al., 2010). In this way olive oil may be acting in immune system of MS patients and no significant different with *n-3* and *n-6* PUFA can be found.

### 3.5 Action of dietary lipids in type 1 diabetes mellitus

Type 1 diabetes mellitus (T1DM) is an autoimmune disease characterized by the destruction of insulin-producing beta cells in the pancreatic islets. Dietary factors have been implicated in the aetiology of type 1 diabetes as well as in initiating the autoimmune process that leads to clinical disease. Macrophages and T cells, attracted to the islets, secrete soluble mediators such as oxygen free radicals, nitric oxide (NO), and the cytokines IL-1ß, interferon (IFN)-γ and TNF-α. Increasing evidence suggests that these mediators induce apoptosis, the main mode of ß-cell death in the development of T1DM. Fatty acids, because of their properties as anti-inflamatory compounds as well as cell apoptosis modulators, may be useful in the management of T1DM.

#### 3.5.1 Findings from studies in animal models of type 1 diabetes

Earlier investigations suggested that deficiency of essential fatty acids, including *n-6* and *n-3* PUFA, caused a resistance in development of the diabetes in certain animal models (Lefkowith et al., 1990; Wright et al., 1995).

However, in 2001 Krishna Mohan & Das carried out a study to evaluate the effect of supplementation of various PUFA-rich oils on the incidence of alloxan-induced diabetes in experimental animals (Krishna Mohan et al., 2001). These authors have reported that *n-3* and *n-6* fatty acids may prevent alloxan-induced diabetes in experimental animals administered before of the diabetogenic agent and this preventive action may reside in their ability to enhance antioxidant status, suppress cytokine production, and activate PPARs. These researchers have evaluated also the effect of estearic saturated FA, oleic MUFA and *n-6* AA PUFA in the same model finding that only AA was effective (Suresh et al., 2006).

Recently others authors have evaluated the efficacy of a right balance *n-6/n-3* PUFA in diet of T1DM model NOD mice finding that low *n-6/n-3* ratio delays the onset of diabetes

(Kagohashi et al., 2010b). Other studies from the same laboratory have shown that the most effective strategy in prevention of the disease in the offspring is an adequate dose of *n-6/n-3* PUFA in maternal diet during gestation and lactation (Kagohashi et al., 2010a).

### 3.5.2 Trials with type 1 diabetes mellitus patients

In 2003 an interesting pilot case-study was carried out in Norway to the attempt to test the hypothesis that cod liver oil, taken either by the mother during pregnancy or by the child during the first year of life, is associated with a lower risk of type 1 diabetes among children. A significant association between the use of cod liver oil during the first year of life and a lower risk of type 1 diabetes was found (Stene et al., 2003). In a similar way, an observational longitudinal study was carried out in U.S.A., the Diabetes Autoimmunity Study in the Young (DAISY). During 13 years a total of 1770 children at increased risk for type 1 diabetes were sudied. Th results revealed that dietary intake of *n-3* fatty acids is associated with reduced risk of islet autoimmunity in children at increased genetic risk for type 1 diabetes. This association is further substantiated by the pilot observation of a higher proportion of *n*-3 PUFA in the erythrocyte membranes (Norris et al., 2007). However the same authors later reported that there was a lack of association between *n-3* PUFA intake and conversion to type 1 diabetes in children with islet autoimmunity (Miller et al., 2011).
In spite of certain positive data in animal models and human patients nowadays we can not confirm a justification for the use of fatty acids in preventing the development of type 1 diabetes mellitus.

## 4. Conclusions

In the recent years the immunonutrition area has advanced significantly to elucidate the role of the diet in development and function of immune system and to prevent or ameliorate numerous diseases in which immune system is implicated like infections, cancer, inflammatory disease, allergies and autoimmune disorders. Among the diet components, fatty acids (PUFA in particular), are especially interesting by their immunomodulator and anti-inflammatory role.
Autoimmune disorders are a complex group of disease characterized by an exacerbated immune response against self structures and an elevated inflammatory state. Several investigations have shown that fatty acids and especially *n-3* PUFA act as potent anti-inflammatory molecules and even induce a strong immunosupression. For this reason, the use of fatty acids has been considered a good a therapeutic strategy in prevention and treatment of these diseases.
In spite of convincing data from the several studies with animal model, clinical trials have not achieved similar results. Only clear evidence in management of rheumatoid arthritis and in remission maintenance in Crohn's disease patients justifies the use of fish oil, and perhaps in combination with olive oil. However results from studies with other diseases like ulcerative colitis, lupus and multiple sclerosis are promising. Future studies with a better control of placebo, number of enrolled patients and design are necessary to justify of use of fatty acids in this type of immune disorders.
Finally epidemiological studies report that Mediterranean countries with a traditionall diet rich in fruits and vegetables, fish oil and olive oil and poor in saturated fats, have lower levels of inflammatory disease than countries with other type of diet. In the same way countries like Japan with changes in the habitual diet to "western diet" have increased rates

of inflammatory disease. In our opinion the best strategy recommending to population in general, and autoimmune disease patients in particular, is the maintenance of a healthy diet rich in naturals antioxidants (fruit, vegetables, olive oil), moderate consumption of fats and a well balanced of *n-6/n-3* fatty acids.

## 5. Acknowledgements

To Dr. José Manuel Martínez Martos and Dr. Mª Jesús Ramírez Expósito , from University of Jaén, Div. of Phisiology, for their assistance with the manuscript.

## 6. References

Adam, O., Beringer, C., Kless, T., Lemmen, C., Adam, A., Wiseman, M., Adam, P., Klimmek, R. & Forth, W. (2003). Anti-inflammatory effects of a low arachidonic acid diet and fish oil in patients with rheumatoid arthritis. *Rheumatology international,* Vol 23, No.1, pp 27-36, ISSN/ISBN 0172-8172; 0172-8172.

Akhtar Khan, N. (2010). Polyunsaturated fatty acids in the modulation of T-cell signalling. *Prostaglandins, leukotrienes, and essential fatty acids,* Vol 82, No.4-6, pp 179-187, ISSN/ISBN 1532-2823; 0952-3278.

Alexander, N.J., Smythe, N.L. & Jokinen, M.P. (1987). The type of dietary fat affects the severity of autoimmune disease in NZB/NZW mice. *The American journal of pathology,* Vol 127, No.1, pp 106-121, ISSN/ISBN 0002-9440; 0002-9440.

Andoh, A., Tsujikawa, T., Ishizuka, I., Araki, Y., Sasaki, M., Koyama, S. & Fujiyama, Y. (2003). N-3 fatty acid-rich diet prevents early response of interleukin-6 elevation in trinitrobenzene sulfonic acid-induced enteritis. *International journal of molecular medicine,* Vol 12, No.5, pp 721-725, ISSN/ISBN 1107-3756; 1107-3756.

Bates, D., Cartlidge, N.E., French, J.M., Jackson, M.J., Nightingale, S., Shaw, D.A., Smith, S., Woo, E., Hawkins, S.A. & Millar, J.H. (1989). A double-blind controlled trial of long chain n-3 polyunsaturated fatty acids in the treatment of multiple sclerosis. *Journal of neurology, neurosurgery, and psychiatry,* Vol 52, No.1, pp 18-22, ISSN/ISBN 0022-3050; 0022-3050.

Bates, D., Fawcett, P.R., Shaw, D.A. & Weightman, D. (1977). Trail of polyunsaturated fatty acids in non-relapsing multiple sclerosis. *British medical journal,* Vol 2, No.6092, pp 932-933, ISSN/ISBN 0007-1447; 0007-1447.

Belluzzi, A., Brignola, C., Campieri, M., Pera, A., Boschi, S. & Miglioli, M. (1996). Effect of an enteric-coated fish-oil preparation on relapses in Crohn's disease. *The New England journal of medicine,* Vol 334, No.24, pp 1557-1560, ISSN/ISBN 0028-4793; 0028-4793.

Berbert, A.A., Kondo, C.R., Almendra, C.L., Matsuo, T. & Dichi, I. (2005). Supplementation of fish oil and olive oil in patients with rheumatoid arthritis. *Nutrition (Burbank, Los Angeles County, Calif.),* Vol 21, No.2, pp 131-136, ISSN/ISBN 0899-9007; 0899-9007.

Calder, P.C. (2008a). Polyunsaturated fatty acids, inflammatory processes and inflammatory bowel diseases. *Molecular nutrition & food research,* Vol 52, No.8, pp 885-897, ISSN/ISBN 1613-4133; 1613-4125.

Calder, P.C. (2008b). Session 3: Joint Nutrition Society and Irish Nutrition and Dietetic Institute Symposium on 'Nutrition and autoimmune disease' PUFA, inflammatory processes and rheumatoid arthritis. *The Proceedings of the Nutrition Society,* Vol 67, No.4, pp 409-418, ISSN/ISBN 0029-6651; 0029-6651.

Calder, P.C. (2006). N-3 Polyunsaturated Fatty Acids, Inflammation, and Inflammatory Diseases. *The American Journal of Clinical Nutrition,* Vol 83, No.6 Suppl, pp 1505S-1519S, ISSN/ISBN 0002-9165; 0002-9165.

Calder, P.C., Yaqoob, P., Thies, F., Wallace, F.A. & Miles, E.A. (2002). Fatty acids and lymphocyte functions. *The British journal of nutrition,* Vol 87 Suppl 1, pp S31-48, ISSN/ISBN 0007-1145; 0007-1145.

Camuesco, D., Galvez, J., Nieto, A., Comalada, M., Rodriguez-Cabezas, M.E., Concha, A., Xaus, J. & Zarzuelo, A. (2005). Dietary olive oil supplemented with fish oil, rich in EPA and DHA (n-3) polyunsaturated fatty acids, attenuates colonic inflammation in rats with DSS-induced colitis. *The Journal of nutrition,* Vol 135, No.4, pp 687-694, ISSN/ISBN 0022-3166; 0022-3166.

Clark, W.F., Parbtani, A., Naylor, C.D., Levinton, C.M., Muirhead, N., Spanner, E., Huff, M.W., Philbrick, D.J. & Holub, B.J. (1993). Fish oil in lupus nephritis: clinical findings and methodological implications. *Kidney international,* Vol 44, No.1, pp 75-86, ISSN/ISBN 0085-2538; 0085-2538.

Cleland, L.G. & James, M.J. (2000). Fish oil and rheumatoid arthritis: antiinflammatory and collateral health benefits. *The Journal of rheumatology,* Vol 27, No.10, pp 2305-2307, ISSN/ISBN 0315-162X; 0315-162X.

Cleland, L.G., French, J.K., Betts, W.H., Murphy, G.A. & Elliott, M.J. (1988). Clinical and biochemical effects of dietary fish oil supplements in rheumatoid arthritis. *The Journal of rheumatology,* Vol 15, No.10, pp 1471-1475, ISSN/ISBN 0315-162X; 0315-162X.

Darlington, L.G. & Stone, T.W. (2001). Antioxidants and fatty acids in the amelioration of rheumatoid arthritis and related disorders. *The British journal of nutrition,* Vol 85, No.3, pp 251-269, ISSN/ISBN 0007-1145; 0007-1145.

Duffy, E.M., Meenagh, G.K., McMillan, S.A., Strain, J.J., Hannigan, B.M. & Bell, A.L. (2004). The clinical effect of dietary supplementation with omega-3 fish oils and/or copper in systemic lupus erythematosus. *The Journal of rheumatology,* Vol 31, No.8, pp 1551-1556, ISSN/ISBN 0315-162X; 0315-162X.

Espersen, G.T., Grunnet, N., Lervang, H.H., Nielsen, G.L., Thomsen, B.S., Faarvang, K.L., Dyerberg, J. & Ernst, E. (1992). Decreased interleukin-1 beta levels in plasma from rheumatoid arthritis patients after dietary supplementation with n-3 polyunsaturated fatty acids. *Clinical rheumatology,* Vol 11, No.3, pp 393-395, ISSN/ISBN 0770-3198; 0770-3198.

Feagan, B.G., Sandborn, W.J., Mittmann, U., Bar-Meir, S., D'Haens, G., Bradette, M., Cohen, A., Dallaire, C., Ponich, T.P., McDonald, J.W., Hebuterne, X., Pare, P., Klvana, P., Niv, Y., Ardizzone, S., Alexeeva, O., Rostom, A., Kiudelis, G., Spleiss, J., Gilgen, D., Vandervoort, M.K., Wong, C.J., Zou, G.Y., Donner, A. & Rutgeerts, P. (2008). Omega-3 free fatty acids for the maintenance of remission in Crohn disease: the EPIC Randomized Controlled Trials. *JAMA : the journal of the American Medical Association,* Vol 299, No.14, pp 1690-1697, ISSN/ISBN 1538-3598; 0098-7484.

Fernandez-Banares, F., Cabre, E., Gonzalez-Huix, F. & Gassull, M.A. (1994). Enteral nutrition as primary therapy in Crohn's disease. *Gut,* Vol 35, No.1 Suppl, pp S55-9, ISSN/ISBN 0017-5749; 0017-5749.

Galli, C. & Calder, P.C. (2009). Effects of fat and fatty acid intake on inflammatory and immune responses: a critical review. *Annals of Nutrition & Metabolism,* Vol 55, No.1-3, pp 123-139, ISSN/ISBN 1421-9697; 0250-6807.

Gonzalez-Huix, F., de Leon, R., Fernandez-Banares, F., Esteve, M., Cabre, E., Acero, D., Abad-Lacruz, A., Figa, M., Guilera, M. & Planas, R. (1993). Polymeric enteral diets as primary treatment of active Crohn's disease: a prospective steroid controlled trial. *Gut,* Vol 34, No.6, pp 778-782, ISSN/ISBN 0017-5749; 0017-5749.

Greenfield, S.M., Green, A.T., Teare, J.P., Jenkins, A.P., Punchard, N.A., Ainley, C.C. & Thompson, R.P. (1993). A randomized controlled study of evening primrose oil and fish oil in ulcerative colitis. *Alimentary Pharmacology & Therapeutics,* Vol 7, No.2, pp 159-166, ISSN/ISBN 0269-2813; 0269-2813.

Halade, G.V., Rahman, M.M., Bhattacharya, A., Barnes, J.L., Chandrasekar, B. & Fernandes, G. (2010). Docosahexaenoic acid-enriched fish oil attenuates kidney disease and prolongs median and maximal life span of autoimmune lupus-prone mice. *Journal of immunology (Baltimore, Md.: 1950),* Vol 184, No.9, pp 5280-5286, ISSN/ISBN 1550-6606; 0022-1767.

Harbige, L.S. & Sharief, M.K. (2007). Polyunsaturated fatty acids in the pathogenesis and treatment of multiple sclerosis. *The British journal of nutrition,* Vol 98 Suppl 1, pp S46-53, ISSN/ISBN 0007-1145; 0007-1145.

Harbige, L.S., Layward, L., Morris-Downes, M.M., Dumonde, D.C. & Amor, S. (2000). The protective effects of omega-6 fatty acids in experimental autoimmune encephalomyelitis (EAE) in relation to transforming growth factor-beta 1 (TGF-beta1) up-regulation and increased prostaglandin E2 (PGE2) production. *Clinical and experimental immunology,* Vol 122, No.3, pp 445-452, ISSN/ISBN 0009-9104; 0009-9104.

Harbige, L.S., Layward, L., Morris, M. & Amor, S. (1997). Protective mechanisms by omega-6 lipids in experimental autoimmune encephalomyelitis (EAE) are associated with cytokines and eicosanoids. *Biochemical Society transactions,* Vol 25, No.2, pp 342S, ISSN/ISBN 0300-5127; 0300-5127.

Harbige, L.S., Yeatman, N., Amor, S. & Crawford, M.A. (1995). Prevention of experimental autoimmune encephalomyelitis in Lewis rats by a novel fungal source of gamma-linolenic acid. *The British journal of nutrition,* Vol 74, No.5, pp 701-715, ISSN/ISBN 0007-1145; 0007-1145.

Hudert, C.A., Weylandt, K.H., Lu, Y., Wang, J., Hong, S., Dignass, A., Serhan, C.N. & Kang, J.X. (2006). Transgenic mice rich in endogenous omega-3 fatty acids are protected from colitis. *Proceedings of the National Academy of Sciences of the United States of America,* Vol 103, No.30, pp 11276-11281, ISSN/ISBN 0027-8424; 0027-8424.

Hughes, D., Keith, A.B., Mertin, J. & Caspary, E.A. (1980). Linoleic acid therapy in severe experimental allergic encephalomyelitis in the guinea-pig: suppression by continuous treatment. *Clinical and experimental immunology,* Vol 40, No.3, pp 523-531, ISSN/ISBN 0009-9104; 0009-9104.

James, M.J., Gibson, R.A., Neumann, M.A. & Cleland, L.G. (1993). Effect of dietary supplementation with n-9 eicosatrienoic acid on leukotriene B4 synthesis in rats: a novel approach to inhibition of eicosanoid synthesis. *The Journal of experimental medicine,* Vol 178, No.6, pp 2261-2265, ISSN/ISBN 0022-1007; 0022-1007.

Jolly, C.A., Muthukumar, A., Avula, C.P., Troyer, D. & Fernandes, G. (2001). Life span is prolonged in food-restricted autoimmune-prone (NZB x NZW)F(1) mice fed a diet enriched with (n-3) fatty acids. *The Journal of nutrition,* Vol 131, No.10, pp 2753-2760, ISSN/ISBN 0022-3166; 0022-3166.

Jolly, C.A. & Fernandes, G. (1999). Diet modulates Th-1 and Th-2 cytokine production in the peripheral blood of lupus-prone mice. *Journal of clinical immunology,* Vol 19, No.3, pp 172-178, ISSN/ISBN 0271-9142; 0271-9142.

Kagohashi, Y., Abiru, N., Kobayashi, M., Hashimoto, M., Shido, O. & Otani, H. (2010a). Maternal dietary n-6/n-3 fatty acid ratio affects type 1 diabetes development in the offspring of non-obese diabetic mice. *Congenital anomalies,* Vol 50, No.4, pp 212-220, ISSN/ISBN 1741-4520; 0914-3505.

Kagohashi, Y. & Otani, H. (2010b). Diet with a low n-6/n-3 essential fatty acid ratio when started immediately after the onset of overt diabetes prolongs survival of type 1 diabetes model NOD mice. *Congenital anomalies,* Vol 50, No.4, pp 226-231, ISSN/ISBN 1741-4520; 0914-3505.

Kaplan, G.J., Fraser, R.I. & Comstock, G.W. (1972). Tuberculosis in Alaska, 1970. The continued decline of the tuberculosis epidemic. *The American Review of Respiratory Disease,* Vol 105, No.6, pp 920-926, ISSN/ISBN 0003-0805; 0003-0805.

Kelley, D.S., Taylor, P.C., Nelson, G.J., Schmidt, P.C., Ferretti, A., Erickson, K.L., Yu, R., Chandra, R.K. & Mackey, B.E. (1999). Docosahexaenoic acid ingestion inhibits natural killer cell activity and production of inflammatory mediators in young healthy men. *Lipids,* Vol 34, No.4, pp 317-324, ISSN/ISBN 0024-4201; 0024-4201.

Kelley, V.E., Ferretti, A., Izui, S. & Strom, T.B. (1985). A fish oil diet rich in eicosapentaenoic acid reduces cyclooxygenase metabolites, and suppresses lupus in MRL-lpr mice. *Journal of immunology (Baltimore, Md.: 1950),* Vol 134, No.3, pp 1914-1919, ISSN/ISBN 0022-1767; 0022-1767.

Kim, W., Khan, N.A., McMurray, D.N., Prior, I.A., Wang, N. & Chapkin, R.S. (2010). Regulatory activity of polyunsaturated fatty acids in T-cell signaling. *Progress in lipid research,* Vol 49, No.3, pp 250-261, ISSN/ISBN 1873-2194; 0163-7827.

Kremer, J.M., Lawrence, D.A., Jubiz, W., DiGiacomo, R., Rynes, R., Bartholomew, L.E. & Sherman, M. (1990). Dietary fish oil and olive oil supplementation in patients with rheumatoid arthritis. Clinical and immunologic effects. *Arthritis and Rheumatism,* Vol 33, No.6, pp 810-820, ISSN/ISBN 0004-3591; 0004-3591.

Kremer, J.M., Jubiz, W., Michalek, A., Rynes, R.I., Bartholomew, L.E., Bigaouette, J., Timchalk, M., Beeler, D. & Lininger, L. (1987). Fish-oil fatty acid supplementation in active rheumatoid arthritis. A double-blinded, controlled, crossover study. *Annals of Internal Medicine,* Vol 106, No.4, pp 497-503, ISSN/ISBN 0003-4819; 0003-4819.

Kremer, J.M., Bigauoette, J., Michalek, A.V., Timchalk, M.A., Lininger, L., Rynes, R.I., Huyck, C., Zieminski, J. & Bartholomew, L.E. (1985). Effects of manipulation of dietary fatty acids on clinical manifestations of rheumatoid arthritis. *Lancet,* Vol 1, No.8422, pp 184-187, ISSN/ISBN 0140-6736; 0140-6736.

Krishna Mohan, I. & Das, U.N. (2001). Prevention of chemically induced diabetes mellitus in experimental animals by polyunsaturated fatty acids. *Nutrition (Burbank, Los Angeles County, Calif.),* Vol 17, No.2, pp 126-151, ISSN/ISBN 0899-9007; 0899-9007.

Kromann, N. & Green, A. (1980). Epidemiological studies in the Upernavik district, Greenland. Incidence of some chronic diseases 1950-1974. *Acta Medica Scandinavica,* Vol 208, No.5, pp 401-406, ISSN/ISBN 0001-6101; 0001-6101.

Lefkowith, J., Schreiner, G., Cormier, J., Handler, E.S., Driscoll, H.K., Greiner, D., Mordes, J.P. & Rossini, A.A. (1990). Prevention of diabetes in the BB rat by essential fatty acid deficiency. Relationship between physiological and biochemical changes. *The Journal of experimental medicine,* Vol 171, No.3, pp 729-743, ISSN/ISBN 0022-1007; 0022-1007.

Leslie, C.A., Gonnerman, W.A., Ullman, M.D., Hayes, K.C., Franzblau, C. & Cathcart, E.S. (1985). Dietary fish oil modulates macrophage fatty acids and decreases arthritis susceptibility in mice. *The Journal of experimental medicine,* Vol 162, No.4, pp 1336-1349, ISSN/ISBN 0022-1007; 0022-1007.

Linos, A., Kaklamani, V.G., Kaklamani, E., Koumantaki, Y., Giziaki, E., Papazoglou, S. & Mantzoros, C.S. (1999). Dietary factors in relation to rheumatoid arthritis: a role for olive oil and cooked vegetables? *The American Journal of Clinical Nutrition,* Vol 70, No.6, pp 1077-1082, ISSN/ISBN 0002-9165; 0002-9165.

Linos, A., Kaklamanis, E., Kontomerkos, A., Koumantaki, Y., Gazi, S., Vaiopoulos, G., Tsokos, G.C. & Kaklamanis, P. (1991). The effect of olive oil and fish consumption on rheumatoid arthritis--a case control study. *Scandinavian journal of rheumatology,* Vol 20, No.6, pp 419-426, ISSN/ISBN 0300-9742; 0300-9742.

Loeschke, K., Ueberschaer, B., Pietsch, A., Gruber, E., Ewe, K., Wiebecke, B., Heldwein, W. & Lorenz, R. (1996). N-3 Fatty Acids Only Delay Early Relapse of Ulcerative Colitis in Remission. *Digestive diseases and sciences,* Vol 41, No.10, pp 2087-2094, ISSN/ISBN 0163-2116; 0163-2116.

Lorenz, R., Weber, P.C., Szimnau, P., Heldwein, W., Strasser, T. & Loeschke, K. (1989). Supplementation with n-3 fatty acids from fish oil in chronic inflammatory bowel disease--a randomized, placebo-controlled, double-blind cross-over trial. *Journal of internal medicine.Supplement,* Vol 731, pp 225-232, ISSN/ISBN 0955-7873; 0955-7873.

Lorenz-Meyer, H., Bauer, P., Nicolay, C., Schulz, B., Purrmann, J., Fleig, W.E., Scheurlen, C., Koop, I., Pudel, V. & Carr, L. (1996). Omega-3 fatty acids and low carbohydrate diet for maintenance of remission in Crohn's disease. A randomized controlled multicenter trial. Study Group Members (German Crohn's Disease Study Group). *Scandinavian journal of gastroenterology,* Vol 31, No.8, pp 778-785, ISSN/ISBN 0036-5521; 0036-5521.

Martinez-Dominguez, E., de la Puerta, R. & Ruiz-Gutierrez, V. (2001). Protective effects upon experimental inflammation models of a polyphenol-supplemented virgin olive oil diet. *Inflammation research : official journal of the European Histamine Research Society ...[et al.],* Vol 50, No.2, pp 102-106, ISSN/ISBN 1023-3830; 1023-3830.

Matsunaga, H., Hokari, R., Kurihara, C., Okada, Y., Takebayashi, K., Okudaira, K., Watanabe, C., Komoto, S., Nakamura, M., Tsuzuki, Y., Kawaguchi, A., Nagao, S. & Miura, S. (2009). Omega-3 polyunsaturated fatty acids ameliorate the severity of ileitis in the senescence accelerated mice (SAM)P1/Yit mice model. *Clinical and experimental immunology,* Vol 158, No.3, pp 325-333, ISSN/ISBN 1365-2249; 0009-9104.

Meade, C.J., Mertin, J., Sheena, J. & Hunt, R. (1978). Reduction by linoleic acid of the severity of experimental allergic encephalomyelitis in the guinea pig. *Journal of the neurological sciences,* Vol 35, No.2-3, pp 291-308, ISSN/ISBN 0022-510X; 0022-510X.

Meydani, S.N., Endres, S., Woods, M.M., Goldin, B.R., Soo, C., Morrill-Labrode, A., Dinarello, C.A. & Gorbach, S.L. (1991). Oral (n-3) fatty acid supplementation suppresses cytokine production and lymphocyte proliferation: comparison between young and older women. *The Journal of nutrition,* Vol 121, No.4, pp 547-555, ISSN/ISBN 0022-3166; 0022-3166.

Miles, E.A., Thies, F., Wallace, F.A., Powell, J.R., Hurst, T.L., Newsholme, E.A. & Calder, P.C. (2001). Influence of age and dietary fish oil on plasma soluble adhesion molecule concentrations. *Clinical science (London, England : 1979),* Vol 100, No.1, pp 91-100, ISSN/ISBN 0143-5221; 0143-5221.

Millar, J.H., Zilkha, K.J., Langman, M.J., Wright, H.P., Smith, A.D., Belin, J. & Thompson, R.H. (1973). Double-blind trial of linoleate supplementation of the diet in multiple sclerosis. *British medical journal,* Vol 1, No.5856, pp 765-768, ISSN/ISBN 0007-1447; 0007-1447.

Miller, M.R., Yin, X., Seifert, J., Clare-Salzler, M., Eisenbarth, G.S., Rewers, M. & Norris, J.M. (2011). Erythrocyte membrane omega-3 fatty acid levels and omega-3 fatty acid intake are not associated with conversion to type 1 diabetes in children with islet autoimmunity: The Diabetes Autoimmunity Study in the Young (DAISY). *Pediatric diabetes,* ISSN/ISBN 1399-5448; 1399-543X.

Moussa, M., Le Boucher, J., Garcia, J., Tkaczuk, J., Ragab, J., Dutot, G., Ohayon, E., Ghisolfi, J. & Thouvenot, J.P. (2000). In vivo effects of olive oil-based lipid emulsion on lymphocyte activation in rats. *Clinical nutrition (Edinburgh, Scotland),* Vol 19, No.1, pp 49-54, ISSN/ISBN 0261-5614; 0261-5614.

Nakamura, N., Kumasaka, R., Osawa, H., Yamabe, H., Shirato, K., Fujita, T., Murakami, R., Shimada, M., Nakamura, M., Okumura, K., Hamazaki, K. & Hamazaki, T. (2005). Effects of eicosapentaenoic acids on oxidative stress and plasma fatty acid composition in patients with lupus nephritis. *In vivo (Athens, Greece),* Vol 19, No.5, pp 879-882, ISSN/ISBN 0258-851X; 0258-851X.

Nieto, N., Torres, M.I., Rios, A. & Gil, A. (2002). Dietary polyunsaturated fatty acids improve histological and biochemical alterations in rats with experimental ulcerative colitis. *The Journal of nutrition,* Vol 132, No.1, pp 11-19, ISSN/ISBN 0022-3166; 0022-3166.

Norris, J.M., Yin, X., Lamb, M.M., Barriga, K., Seifert, J., Hoffman, M., Orton, H.D., Baron, A.E., Clare-Salzler, M., Chase, H.P., Szabo, N.J., Erlich, H., Eisenbarth, G.S. & Rewers, M. (2007). Omega-3 polyunsaturated fatty acid intake and islet autoimmunity in children at increased risk for type 1 diabetes. *JAMA : the journal of the American Medical Association,* Vol 298, No.12, pp 1420-1428, ISSN/ISBN 1538-3598; 0098-7484.

Owen, R.W., Mier, W., Giacosa, A., Hull, W.E., Spiegelhalder, B. & Bartsch, H. (2000). Phenolic compounds and squalene in olive oils: the concentration and antioxidant potential of total phenols, simple phenols, secoiridoids, lignansand squalene. *Food and chemical toxicology : an international journal published for the British Industrial Biological Research Association,* Vol 38, No.8, pp 647-659, ISSN/ISBN 0278-6915; 0278-6915.

Pattison, D.J., Symmons, D.P. & Young, A. (2004). Does diet have a role in the aetiology of rheumatoid arthritis? *The Proceedings of the Nutrition Society,* Vol 63, No.1, pp 137-143, ISSN/ISBN 0029-6651; 0029-6651.

Paty, D.W., Cousin, H.K., Read, S. & Adlakha, K. (1978). Linoleic acid in multiple sclerosis: failure to show any therapeutic benefit. *Acta Neurologica Scandinavica,* Vol 58, No.1, pp 53-58, ISSN/ISBN 0001-6314; 0001-6314.

Pestka, J.J. (2010). N-3 Polyunsaturated Fatty Acids and Autoimmune-Mediated Glomerulonephritis. *Prostaglandins, leukotrienes, and essential fatty acids,* Vol 82, No.4-6, pp 251-258, ISSN/ISBN 1532-2823; 0952-3278.

Prickett, J.D., Robinson, D.R. & Steinberg, A.D. (1983). Effects of dietary enrichment with eicosapentaenoic acid upon autoimmune nephritis in female NZB X NZW/F1 mice. *Arthritis and Rheumatism,* Vol 26, No.2, pp 133-139, ISSN/ISBN 0004-3591; 0004-3591.

Prickett, J.D., Robinson, D.R. & Steinberg, A.D. (1982). A diet enriched with eicosapentaenoic acid suppresses autoimmune nephritis in female (NZB x NZW) F1 mice. *Transactions of the Association of American Physicians,* Vol 95, pp 145-154, ISSN/ISBN 0066-9458; 0066-9458.

Prickett, J.D., Robinson, D.R. & Steinberg, A.D. (1981). Dietary enrichment with the polyunsaturated fatty acid eicosapentaenoic acid prevents proteinuria and prolongs survival in NZB x NZW F1 mice. *The Journal of clinical investigation,* Vol 68, No.2, pp 556-559, ISSN/ISBN 0021-9738; 0021-9738.

Puertollano, M.A., Puertollano, E. & de Pablo, M.A. (2010). Host Immune Resistance and Dietary Lipids, In: *Dietary Components and Immune Function* Watson, Zibadi & Preedy (Ed.), pp. 131-153, Humana Press Springer, NY.

Puertollano, M.A., Puertollano, E., Alvarez de Cienfuegos, G. & de Pablo, M.A. (2008). Dietary lipids, modulation of immune functions and susceptibility to infection. *Nutritional Therapy and Metabolism,* Vol 26, No.3, pp 97-108.

Puertollano, M.A., de Pablo, M.A. & Alvarez de Cienfuegos, G. (2004). Olive oil and immune system functions: potential involvement in immunonutrition. *Grasas y aceites,* No.55, pp 42-51.

Rees, D., Miles, E.A., Banerjee, T., Wells, S.J., Roynette, C.E., Wahle, K.W. & Calder, P.C. (2006). Dose-related effects of eicosapentaenoic acid on innate immune function in healthy humans: a comparison of young and older men. *The American Journal of Clinical Nutrition,* Vol 83, No.2, pp 331-342, ISSN/ISBN 0002-9165; 0002-9165.

Robinson, D.R., Prickett, J.D., Makoul, G.T., Steinberg, A.D. & Colvin, R.B. (1986). Dietary fish oil reduces progression of established renal disease in (NZB x NZW)F1 mice and delays renal disease in BXSB and MRL/1 strains. *Arthritis and Rheumatism,* Vol 29, No.4, pp 539-546, ISSN/ISBN 0004-3591; 0004-3591.

Romano, C., Cucchiara, S., Barabino, A., Annese, V. & Sferlazzas, C. (2005). Usefulness of omega-3 fatty acid supplementation in addition to mesalazine in maintaining remission in pediatric Crohn's disease: a double-blind, randomized, placebo-controlled study. *World journal of gastroenterology : WJG,* Vol 11, No.45, pp 7118-7121, ISSN/ISBN 1007-9327; 1007-9327.

Sanchez-Fidalgo, S., Villegas, I., Cardeno, A., Talero, E., Sanchez-Hidalgo, M., Motilva, V. & Alarcon de la Lastra, C. (2010). Extra-virgin olive oil-enriched diet modulates DSS-colitis-associated colon carcinogenesis in mice. *Clinical nutrition (Edinburgh, Scotland),* Vol 29, No.5, pp 663-673, ISSN/ISBN 1532-1983; 0261-5614.

Sanderson, P., Yaqoob, P. & Calder, P.C. (1995). Effects of dietary lipid manipulation upon graft vs host and host vs graft responses in the rat. *Cellular immunology,* Vol 164, No.2, pp 240-247, ISSN/ISBN 0008-8749; 0008-8749.

Sano, H., Hla, T., Maier, J.A., Crofford, L.J., Case, J.P., Maciag, T. & Wilder, R.L. (1992). In vivo cyclooxygenase expression in synovial tissues of patients with rheumatoid arthritis and osteoarthritis and rats with adjuvant and streptococcal cell wall arthritis. *The Journal of clinical investigation,* Vol 89, No.1, pp 97-108, ISSN/ISBN 0021-9738; 0021-9738.

Sharon, P. & Stenson, W.F. (1984). Enhanced synthesis of leukotriene B4 by colonic mucosa in inflammatory bowel disease. *Gastroenterology,* Vol 86, No.3, pp 453-460, ISSN/ISBN 0016-5085; 0016-5085.

Shinto, L., Marracci, G., Baldauf-Wagner, S., Strehlow, A., Yadav, V., Stuber, L. & Bourdette, D. (2009). Omega-3 fatty acid supplementation decreases matrix metalloproteinase-9 production in relapsing-remitting multiple sclerosis. *Prostaglandins, leukotrienes, and essential fatty acids,* Vol 80, No.2-3, pp 131-136, ISSN/ISBN 0952-3278; 0952-3278.

Shoda, R., Matsueda, K., Yamato, S. & Umeda, N. (1996). Epidemiologic analysis of Crohn disease in Japan: increased dietary intake of n-6 polyunsaturated fatty acids and animal protein relates to the increased incidence of Crohn disease in Japan. *The American Journal of Clinical Nutrition,* Vol 63, No.5, pp 741-745, ISSN/ISBN 0002-9165; 0002-9165.

Shoda, R., Matsueda, K., Yamato, S. & Umeda, N. (1995). Therapeutic efficacy of N-3 polyunsaturated fatty acid in experimental Crohn's disease. *Journal of gastroenterology,* Vol 30 Suppl 8, pp 98-101, ISSN/ISBN 0944-1174; 0944-1174.

Simopoulos, A.P. (2002). Omega-3 fatty acids in inflammation and autoimmune diseases. *Journal of the American College of Nutrition,* Vol 21, No.6, pp 495-505, ISSN/ISBN 0731-5724; 0731-5724.

Sperling, R.I. (1995). Eicosanoids in rheumatoid arthritis. *Rheumatic diseases clinics of North America,* Vol 21, No.3, pp 741-758, ISSN/ISBN 0889-857X; 0889-857X.

Sperling, R.I., Weinblatt, M., Robin, J.L., Ravalese, J.,3rd, Hoover, R.L., House, F., Coblyn, J.S., Fraser, P.A., Spur, B.W. & Robinson, D.R. (1987). Effects of dietary supplementation with marine fish oil on leukocyte lipid mediator generation and function in rheumatoid arthritis. *Arthritis and Rheumatism,* Vol 30, No.9, pp 988-997, ISSN/ISBN 0004-3591; 0004-3591.

Spurney, R.F., Ruiz, P., Albrightson, C.R., Pisetsky, D.S. & Coffman, T.M. (1994). Fish oil feeding modulates leukotriene production in murine lupus nephritis. *Prostaglandins,* Vol 48, No.5, pp 331-348, ISSN/ISBN 0090-6980; 0090-6980.

Stene, L.C., Joner, G. & Norwegian Childhood Diabetes Study Group. (2003). Use of cod liver oil during the first year of life is associated with lower risk of childhood-onset type 1 diabetes: a large, population-based, case-control study. *The American Journal of Clinical Nutrition,* Vol 78, No.6, pp 1128-1134, ISSN/ISBN 0002-9165; 0002-9165.

Stulnig, T.M. (2003). Immunomodulation by polyunsaturated fatty acids: mechanisms and effects. *International archives of allergy and immunology,* Vol 132, No.4, pp 310-321, ISSN/ISBN 1018-2438; 1018-2438.

Suresh, Y. & Das, U.N. (2006). Differential effect of saturated, monounsaturated, and polyunsaturated fatty acids on alloxan-induced diabetes mellitus. *Prostaglandins, leukotrienes, and essential fatty acids,* Vol 74, No.3, pp 199-213, ISSN/ISBN 0952-3278; 0952-3278.

Swank, R.L. (1950). Multiple sclerosis; a correlation of its incidence with dietary fat. *The American Journal of the Medical Sciences,* Vol 220, No.4, pp 421-430, ISSN/ISBN 0002-9629; 0002-9629.

Trebble, T.M., Stroud, M.A., Wootton, S.A., Calder, P.C., Fine, D.R., Mullee, M.A., Moniz, C. & Arden, N.K. (2005). High-dose fish oil and antioxidants in Crohn's disease and the response of bone turnover: a randomised controlled trial. *The British journal of nutrition,* Vol 94, No.2, pp 253-261, ISSN/ISBN 0007-1145; 0007-1145.

Trebble, T.M., Wootton, S.A., Miles, E.A., Mullee, M., Arden, N.K., Ballinger, A.B., Stroud, M.A., Burdge, G.C. & Calder, P.C. (2003). Prostaglandin E2 production and T cell function after fish-oil supplementation: response to antioxidant cosupplementation. *The American Journal of Clinical Nutrition,* Vol 78, No.3, pp 376-382, ISSN/ISBN 0002-9165; 0002-9165.

Tulleken, J.E., Limburg, P.C., Muskiet, F.A. & van Rijswijk, M.H. (1990). Vitamin E status during dietary fish oil supplementation in rheumatoid arthritis. *Arthritis and Rheumatism,* Vol 33, No.9, pp 1416-1419, ISSN/ISBN 0004-3591; 0004-3591.

van der Tempel, H., Tulleken, J.E., Limburg, P.C., Muskiet, F.A. & van Rijswijk, M.H. (1990). Effects of fish oil supplementation in rheumatoid arthritis. *Annals of the Rheumatic Diseases,* Vol 49, No.2, pp 76-80, ISSN/ISBN 0003-4967; 0003-4967.

Venkatraman, J.T. & Chu, W.C. (1999). Effects of dietary omega-3 and omega-6 lipids and vitamin E on serum cytokines, lipid mediators and anti-DNA antibodies in a mouse model for rheumatoid arthritis. *Journal of the American College of Nutrition,* Vol 18, No.6, pp 602-613, ISSN/ISBN 0731-5724; 0731-5724.

Vilaseca, J., Salas, A., Guarner, F., Rodriguez, R., Martinez, M. & Malagelada, J.R. (1990). Dietary fish oil reduces progression of chronic inflammatory lesions in a rat model of granulomatous colitis. *Gut,* Vol 31, No.5, pp 539-544, ISSN/ISBN 0017-5749; 0017-5749.

Volker, D.H., FitzGerald, P.E. & Garg, M.L. (2000). The eicosapentaenoic to docosahexaenoic acid ratio of diets affects the pathogenesis of arthritis in Lew/SSN rats. *The Journal of nutrition,* Vol 130, No.3, pp 559-565, ISSN/ISBN 0022-3166; 0022-3166.

Wallace, F.A., Miles, E.A., Evans, C., Stock, T.E., Yaqoob, P. & Calder, P.C. (2001). Dietary fatty acids influence the production of Th1- but not Th2-type cytokines. *Journal of leukocyte biology,* Vol 69, No.3, pp 449-457, ISSN/ISBN 0741-5400; 0741-5400.

Walton, A.J., Snaith, M.L., Locniskar, M., Cumberland, A.G., Morrow, W.J. & Isenberg, D.A. (1991). Dietary fish oil and the severity of symptoms in patients with systemic lupus erythematosus. *Annals of the Rheumatic Diseases,* Vol 50, No.7, pp 463-466, ISSN/ISBN 0003-4967; 0003-4967.

Weinstock-Guttman, B., Baier, M., Park, Y., Feichter, J., Lee-Kwen, P., Gallagher, E., Venkatraman, J., Meksawan, K., Deinehert, S., Pendergast, D., Awad, A.B., Ramanathan, M., Munschauer, F. & Rudick, R. (2005). Low fat dietary intervention with omega-3 fatty acid supplementation in multiple sclerosis patients. *Prostaglandins, leukotrienes, and essential fatty acids,* Vol 73, No.5, pp 397-404, ISSN/ISBN 0952-3278; 0952-3278.

Westberg, G. & Tarkowski, A. (1990). Effect of MaxEPA in patients with SLE. A double-blind, crossover study. *Scandinavian journal of rheumatology,* Vol 19, No.2, pp 137-143, ISSN/ISBN 0300-9742; 0300-9742.

Whiting, C.V., Bland, P.W. & Tarlton, J.F. (2005). Dietary n-3 polyunsaturated fatty acids reduce disease and colonic proinflammatory cytokines in a mouse model of colitis. *Inflammatory bowel diseases,* Vol 11, No.4, pp 340-349, ISSN/ISBN 1078-0998; 1078-0998.

Wright, J.R.,Jr, Fraser, R.B., Kapoor, S. & Cook, H.W. (1995). Essential fatty acid deficiency prevents multiple low-dose streptozotocin-induced diabetes in naive and cyclosporin-treated low-responder murine strains. *Acta Diabetologica,* Vol 32, No.2, pp 125-130, ISSN/ISBN 0940-5429; 0940-5429.

Wright, S.A., O'Prey, F.M., McHenry, M.T., Leahey, W.J., Devine, A.B., Duffy, E.M., Johnston, D.G., Finch, M.B., Bell, A.L. & McVeigh, G.E. (2008). A randomised interventional trial of omega-3-polyunsaturated fatty acids on endothelial function and disease activity in systemic lupus erythematosus. *Annals of the Rheumatic Diseases,* Vol 67, No.6, pp 841-848, ISSN/ISBN 1468-2060; 0003-4967.

Yaqoob, P. (2002). Monounsaturated fatty acids and immune function. *European journal of clinical nutrition,* Vol 56 Suppl 3, pp S9-S13, ISSN/ISBN 0954-3007; 0954-3007.

Yaqoob, P., Newsholme, E.A. & Calder, P.C. (1994). Inhibition of natural killer cell activity by dietary lipids. *Immunology letters,* Vol 41, No.2-3, pp 241-247, ISSN/ISBN 0165-2478; 0165-2478.

Yuceyar, H., Ozutemiz, O., Huseyinov, A., Saruc, M., Alkanat, M., Bor, S., Coker, I. & Batur, Y. (1999). Is administration of n-3 fatty acids by mucosal enema protective against trinitrobenzene-induced colitis in rats? *Prostaglandins, leukotrienes, and essential fatty acids,* Vol 61, No.6, pp 339-345, ISSN/ISBN 0952-3278; 0952-3278.

# Part 5

# Other Conceptual Advances & New Insights

# 26

# Autoimmune Disorder and Autism

Xiaohong Li and Hua Zou
*New York State Institute for Basic Research in Developmental Disabilities*
*USA*

## 1. Introduction

### 1.1 Diagnosis of ASD

Autism (also known as classic autism or autism disorder) is a common neurodevelopmental disorder. Typically diagnosed before three years old, autistic children usually present with significant language delays, social and communication impairments, as well as abnormal repetitive and restrictive behaviors. Autism spectrum disorders (ASD) however, refers to a boarder definition of autism. Based on the severity of the clinical conditions, ASD is further divided into three subgroups namely autism (the most severe type of ASD), Asperger syndrome and pervasive developmental disorder - not otherwise specified (PDD-NOS; also called atypical autism) [1-3].

Of note, current diagnosis criteria of these disorders are based on behavior tests, no single biomarker has been clinically accepted, which mainly due to the difficulties for studying cellular and molecular etiology of ASD. First, subjects among different researches lack of comparability because of the diagnostic heterogeneity [4]. Second, the prevalence of ASD is relatively low therefore sample sizes are usually too small for statistical analysis. Third, comparing with other diseases, the young ages of the autistic subjects make biological study difficult. Forth, valid control groups require age-, gender-, IQ- and socioeconomic status-matched developmentally normal subjects, which most studies failed to satisfy with [5].

### 1.2 Epidemiology

ASD is reported to occur in all racial, ethnic and socioeconomic groups, and are about four times more likely to occur in boys than in girls probably due to the extremes of typical male neuroanatomy of autism [6, 7]. Studies in Asia, Europe and North America have identified individuals with ASD with an approximate prevalence of 6/1,000 to over 10/1,000 [8]. Chronologically, the prevalence of ASD increased from 0.8/1,000 in 1983 to 4.6/1,000 in 1999 in Western Australia, while this ratio increased from 6.6/1,000 in 2000 to 9/1,000 in 2006 in United States [9-11]. This increase is probably because of changes and broadening of the diagnostic criteria and due to heightened awareness, but may also reflect, in part, a true increase due to environmental factors acting upon a genetically vulnerable background [12, 13].

## 2. Immune disorders and autism

The relationship between immune disorders and ASD has been proposed for decades. Based on the epidemiological data, higher rate of autoimmune conditions, such as rheumatoid arthritis, autoimmune thyroid disease, asthma, ulcerative colitis, exits in parents of autistic children [14-17]. Another line of evidence supporting immune dysfunction at least partly responsible for ASD comes from large population studies, which suggest maternal immune dysfunctions may be related to a later diagnosis of ASD in the offspring [18]. Furthermore, cumulative evidences support the theory that ASD is caused by a loss of self-tolerance to one or more neural antigens during early childhood. Using western blot for the presence of IgG antibodies against protein extracts from human brain or sera, multiple brain-specific autoantibodies are detected [19, 20]. Other groups measured the plasma concentration of immunoglobulins and/or cytokines, autistic subjects exclusively exhibited abnormal immunoglobin and/or cytokine profiles [21-24]. It's not known yet whether immune activation plays an initiating or ongoing role in the pathology of ASD. But investigations of dynamic adaptive cellular immune function suggested dysfunctional immune activation, which may be linked to disturbances in behavior and developmental functioning [25].

### 2.1 Autoimmune diseases

Autoimmune diseases are the most common type of immune disorders. And its relationship with autism has been widely studied. Very early study reported an increased number of autoimmune disorders in some families with autism, suggesting immune dysfunction plays a role in autism pathogenesis [26]. Consistent with this result, Sweeten et al investigated the frequency of autoimmune disorders in families that have probands with pervasive developmental disorders and autism, compared with control groups. Autoimmunity was increased significantly in families with pervasive developmental disorders compared with those of healthy and autoimmune control subjects [27]. More persuasive evidence comes from a multicenter study of 308 children with Autism Spectrum Disorder. Regression was significantly associated with a family history of autoimmune disorders. But the only specific autoimmune disorder found to be associated with regression was autoimmune thyroid disease [28].

### 2.2 Cytokines and chemokines

Cytokines and chemokines are thought to mediate the pathogenesis of autism, although the exact mechanism remains unclear. Jyonouchi group determined innate and adaptive immune responses in children with developmental regression and autism spectrum disorders, developmentally normal siblings, and controls. Their results indicated excessive innate immune responses in a number of ASD children that may be most evident in TNF-alpha production [29]. Similarly, Molloy et al reported children with ASD had increased activation of both Th2 and Th1 arms of the adaptive immune response, with a Th2 predominance, and without the compensatory increase in the regulatory cytokine IL-10 [30]. But Li et al showed that proinflammatory cytokines (TNF-alpha, IL-6 and GM-CSF), Th1 cytokine (IFN-gamma) and chemokine (IL-8) were significantly increased in the brains of ASD patients compared with the controls, but not the Th2 cytokines (IL-4, IL-5 and IL-10). The Th1/Th2 ratio was also significantly increased in ASD patients. Based on these results, the author concluded that ASD patients displayed an increased innate and adaptive immune response through the Th1 pathway, suggesting that localized brain inflammation and autoimmune disorder may be involved in the pathogenesis of ASD [31]. Most recently, Ashwood group used larger number of participants than previous studies and found that significant increases in plasma levels of a number of cytokines, including IL-1beta, IL-6, IL-8 and IL-12p40 in the ASD group compared with typically developing controls [32]. All these findings suggest that inflammatory responses may be related to disturbances in behavior. And the characterization of immunological parameters in ASD has important implications for diagnosis, therefore should be considered when designing therapeutic strategies to treat ASD.

### 2.3 Immunoglobulin

Using human fetal and adult brains as antigenic substrates, maternal serum antibodies transferred through placenta are detected by four independent research groups, suggesting an association between the transfer of IgG autoantibodies during early neurodevelopment and the risk of developing of autism in some children [33-37].

Singh et al provided more confirmative evidence by studying regional distribution of antibodies to rat caudate nucleus, cerebral cortex, cerebellum, brain stem and hippocampus of 30 normal and 68 autistic children. Autistic children, but not normal children, had antibodies to caudate nucleus (49% positive sera), cerebral cortex (18% positive sera) and cerebellum (9% positive sera). Brain stem and hippocampus were negative. Since a significant number of autistic children had antibodies to caudate nucleus, the author proposed that an autoimmune reaction to this brain region may cause neurological impairments in autistic children [38]. Agreed with this result, Trajkovski et al measured plasma concentration of IgA, IgM, IgG classes, and IgG1, IgG2, IgG3, and IgG4 subclasses in children with autism. Plasma concentrations of IgM and IgG in autistic children were significantly higher in comparison with their healthy brothers or sisters. Children with autism had significantly higher plasma concentrations of IgG4 compared to their siblings. Increased plasma concentration of IgG1 was found in autistic males as compared with their healthy brothers. Plasma concentrations of IgG and IgG1 in autistic females were increased in comparison with IgG and IgG1 in their healthy sisters [39]. More recently, Enstrom et al report significantly increased levels of the IgG4 subclass in children with autism compared with typically developing control children and compared with developmental delayed controls [40].

However, No consensus has been reached regarding the immunoglobin levels in autistic subjects. Morris and colleagues failed to find any useful biomarker in a small group of subjects, posing question to the current theory [41]. Stern et al found in their study most of the autistic children had normal immune function, suggesting that routine immunologic investigation is unlikely to be of benefit in most autistic children [42].

### 2.4 Gastrointestinal disorders

The report regarding the relationship between autism and gastrointestinal disorders was seen as early as 1971, when Goodwin et al described 6 of 15 randomly selected autistic children with symptoms of malabsorption [43]. Later Horvath et al investigated 412 autistic children, of which 84.1% had at least one of the eight abnormal gastrointestinal symptoms, comparing with 31.2% of the healthy siblings [44]. However, disagreements exit. Kuddo group and Molloy group failed to find any association between chronic gastrointestinal symptoms and autism based on the literature search or their own sample [45, 46]. Fernell et al tested two independent biomarkers of inflammatory reactions (faecal calprotectin and rectal nitric oxide) in 24 autistic children, but didn't find clear link between active intestinal inflammation and autism [47].

Morphological and histological studies provided consistent results with the clinical manifestations. Ileocolonoscopic examinations in 60 children with autism and other developmental disorders revealed that 8% (4/51) affected children but none in controls presented with active ileitis. Chronic colitis was identified in 88% (53/60) affected children compared with 4.5% (1/22) controls [48]. Similarly, another group conducted upper gastrointestinal endoscopy in 36 autistic subjects. 69.4% (25/36) of whom presented with grade I or II reflux esophagitis, 41.7% (15/36) with chronic gastritis, and 66.7% with chronic duodenitis [49].

In addition, biochemical researches reported evidences of abnormal intestinal cytokine profiles. Ashwood et al found enhanced pro-inflammatory cytokine production present in 21 ASD children compared with 65 controls [50]. Furthermore, they investigated the peripheral blood and mucosal CD3+ lymphocyte cytokine profiles in 18 autistic children with gastrointestinal symptoms. In both peripheral blood and mucosa, CD3+ TNFalpha+ and CD3+ IFNgamma+ were increased, while CD3+ IL-10+ were markedly lower in ASD children. And mucosal CD3+ IL-4+ cells were increased in ASD compared with NIC [51]. Similarly, Jyonouchi et al provided evidence that intrinsic defects of innate immune responses in ASD children with gastrointestinal symptoms, suggesting a possible link between GI and behavioral symptoms mediated by innate immune abnormalities [52]. However, DeFelice et al assessed levels of proinflammatory cytokines, interleukin (IL)-6, IL-8, and IL-1beta, produced by intestinal biopsies of children with pervasive developmental disorders but failed to find significant difference between autistic and control groups [53].

How do the gastrointestinal disorders affect brain functions? Currently available pathophysiological studies provided partial explanations. D'Eufemia et al investigated the occurrence of gut mucosal damage using the intestinal permeability test in 21 autistic children without known intestinal disorders. They found increased intestinal permeability in 43% (9/21) autistic patients, but in none of the 40 controls, which suggested an altered intestinal permeability could represent a possible mechanism for the increased passage through the gut mucosa of peptides derived from foods with subsequent behavioral abnormalities [54].

## 3. Genetics of autism

Similar to several other complex diseases, autism was not widely considered to have a strong genetic component until the 1980s. But increasing numbers of epidemiological and genetic studies are deepening our understanding of the genetic contribution autism. First, it is estimated that about 10% of children with ASD have an identifiable co-occuring genetic, neurologic or metabolic disorder, such as the fragile X syndrome and tuberous sclerosis [55]. Second, the relative risk of a newborn child to have autism, if he or she has an affected sibling, increases at least 25 folds comparing with general population [56]. Third, independent twin studies have suggested identical twins have a 60-90% chance to be concordantly diagnosed with autism, and this risk decreases sharply to the sibling risk of 0-24% in non-identical twins [57, 58]. However, based on a large scale study of 503 ASD twins in California, Liu *et al* suggest the heritability has been largely overestimated [59]. They found the concordance rate for monozygotic male twins was 57% and for females 67%, while for same sex dizygotic twins the rate was 33%. Fourth, cumulative reports have confirmed mutations or structural variations of a number of specific genes significantly increase the risk of ASD [56].

### 3.1 Genetic methodology

However, unlike monogenic Mendelian disorders, the genetic and clinical heterogeneity of ASD poses a difficult challenge to precisely define the underlying genetics. This complexity has been blamed for the lack of replicability of the many reported chromosomal susceptibility regions. Therefore, multiple parallel approaches are needed for the exploration of the potential loci underlying the etiology of ASD. In general, there are a number of methods available for genetic studies of ASD, with each having different advantages as well as limitations. The most widely used methods include cytogenetic analysis, linkage and association studies, copy number variation and DNA micro-array analysis.

A cytogenetic study is the most "classic" of genetic methods. Based on the assumption that ASD is a result of unique rare mutations that present sporadically or "de novo" in the population and are not usually inherited, cytogenetics helps to determine the contribution of chromosomal abnormalities in childhood diseases. Cytogenetics has transitioned from light microscopy to molecular cytogenetics to DNA-based microarray detections of structural variations [60]. Copy number variation (CNV) analysis is a newer molecular cytogenetic approach, aiming to detect the insertion or deletion of DNA fragments typically larger than 50 kb [61]. However, extreme caution must be paid when interpreting CNV analysis since it is very dependent on the specific methods employed, which may partly account for the low replicability among studies [62].

Differing from cytogenetics, linkage studies trace genetic loci that are transmitted with autism in the families of affected individuals. Parametric and non-parametric linkage studies are two typical designs. While parametric analysis requires a model for the disease (i.e. frequency of disease alleles and penetrance for each genotype), and therefore is typically employed for single gene disorders and Mendelian forms of complex disorders, "model-free" non-parametric linkage analysis evaluates whether segregation at specific locations is "not-random". Given the uncertainty of the mode of inheritance in ASD, non-parametric linkage is more widely used, providing suggestive evidence of linkage on almost all of the chromosomes [63]. However, linkage studies are unable to identify mutations in critical genes in highly heterogeneous disorders involving many different genes and chromosomal loci [64].

Genetic association studies, including case-control and family-based studies, examine differences in allele or genotype frequencies between two groups [63]. Typically, several microsatellite markers or SNPs are chosen based on linkage studies or biological evidence. The seemingly countless potential candidates make it hard to determine the causative relations between genes and ASD [61]. In addition, although association studies are suitable to identify common susceptibility alleles present in large numbers of patients compared to controls, they usually fail to identify rare, causal mutations [63, 64].

Rapid advances in micro-array technologies have substantially improved our ability to detect submicroscopic chromosomal abnormalities. These tools have allowed for high-output and high-resolution detection of rare and de novo changes in a genome-wide manner. Moreover, newly developed, commercially available whole-exome arrays are increasingly being employed to detect de novo mutations in complex disorders. Based on the fact that the protein coding regions of genes (i.e. exons) habor 85% of the mutations of disease-related traits, whole-exome sequencing offers the possibility to identify disease-causing sequence variations in small kindreds for phenotypically complicated, genetically heterogeneous diseases when traditional linkage studies are impossible [65-69]. As such, studies in this realm have been increasing in the past several years and there will surely benefit the etiological diagnosis and genetic counseling of ASD in the near future [70].

### 3.2 Potential loci in autism

#### 3.2.1 Genome wide linkage analysis

Although there is accumulating evidence supporting a genetic component to ASD, the specific genes involved have yet to be totally clarified. Genome-wide screening of autistic subjects and their first-degree relatives offers an attractive means to search for susceptibility genes. However there has been a disappointing lack of replication of many of the reported susceptibility regions. The reason for this could be due to the epistasis of many interacting genes. But it may also be due to the genetic and clinical heterogeneity present in ASD [71]. The noted effects of heterogeneity of the samples on the corresponding results, have led to attempts to decrease sample heterogeneity by various ways which include narrowing inclusion criteria and studies of specific, autism-related endophenotypes.

A substantial body of evidence has resulted from genome-wide screening for the susceptibility genes of ASD (table 1). Significant replicability has been found for several chromosomal loci including 2q, 5, 7q, 15q and 16p. Two studies provided suggestive evidence for linkage to chromosome 2q using a two-stage genome screen [71, 72], while association tests for specific candidate genes in the chromosome 2q31-q33 region led to negative results [73]. Additional support for the presence of susceptibility loci on chromosome 2q is given by overlapping positive linkage findings in four other independent genomic scans [74-77].

There are three reports about gene variants on chromosome 5. Philippi found strong association with autism for allelic variants of "paired-like homeodomain transcription factor 1" (*PITX1*), a key regulator of hormones within the pituitary-hypothalamic axis [78]. Two other groups used genome-wide linkage and association mapping studies to analyze chromosome 5 gene variations finding that SNPs located at 5p14.1 and 5q15 respectively were significantly associated with autism [79, 80].

Chromosome 16 linkage results have been fairly consistent in showing a peak at 16p11-13, which strongly suggested a gene in this region may contribute to the risk of ASD [81, 82]. 15q11-q13 is another frequently identified locus by linkage studies. Several genes located in this region have been intensively studied and some have provided very promising results [83-86]. But in all of these linkage reports there is a certain lack of reproducibility, and therefore they require further validation based on using a combination of several methods.

Besides these "hot spots", there are other reports regarding associations of other loci with ASD [80, 87-90], including some evidence of linkage to the X chromosome [91]. However, there is little overlap of these potential loci involving potential candidate genes, suggesting that the genetic background of ASD is full of complexity.

#### 3.2.2 Copy number variation (CNV)

Rapid advances in genomic DNA microarray technologies have substantially improved our ability to detect submicroscopic chromosomal abnormalities. Novel rare variants have been detected in association with ASD and these can be either *de novo* or inherited. *De novo* or noninherited CNVs are found in 7%–10% of ASD samples from simplex families (having only one child affected, the majority), in 2%–3% from multiplex families, and in ~1% in non-ASD controls. Further, about 10% of ASD subjects with *de novo* CNVs carry two or more CNVs [100-102]. Inherited CNVs reportedly are found in up to 50% of ASD subjects for whom one of the presumably normal parents also has the duplication/deletion. These familial CNVs may include candidate genes relevant to ASD where they are rare in the normal population.

| Chromosome | Loci | Candidate genes | Ref. |
|---|---|---|---|
| 1 | 1p34.2 | Regulating Synaptic Membrane Exocytosis 3(*RIMS3)* | [90] |
| 2 | 2q | | [71, 72] |
| | 2q31-2q33 | *GAD1,STK17B,ABI2,CTLA4,CD28,NEUROD1, PDE1A,HOXD1, DLX2* | [73] |
| | 2q31 | *SLC25A12* | [92] |
| | 2q24-2q33 | *SLC25A12, CMYA3* | [75] |
| | 2q24-2q33 | *SLC25A12, STK39, ITGA4* | [77] |
| | 2q34 | Neuropilin-2 (*NRP2*) | [74] |
| 3 | 3q25-3q27 | HTR3C | [48] |
| 5 | 5q31 | Paired-like homeodomain transcription factor 1(*PITX1*) | [78] |
| | 5p14.1 | | [79] |
| | 5p15 | *SEMA5A* | [80] |
| 6 | 6q | Abelson's Helper Integration 1 (*AHI1*) | [88] |
| | 6q27 | | [80] |
| 7 | 7q22.1-7q31 | | [93] |
| | 7q31 | Laminin Beta-1 (*LAMB1*),<br>Neuronal cell adhesion molecule (*NRCAM*) | [94, 95][96] |
| | 7q32 | NADH-ubiquinone oxidoreductase 1 alpha subcomplex 5 *(NDUFA5)* | [48] |
| | 7q31-7q33 | wingless-type MMTV integration site family member 2 (*WNT2*) | [97] |
| 11 | 11p12-p13 | | [76] |
| 12 | 12q14 | | [87] |
| 15 | 15q11-q13 | Angelman syndrome gene (*UBE3A*) | [85] |
| | 15q11-q13 | | [83] |
| | 15q13 | Amyloid precursor protein-binding protein A2 (*APBA2* ) | [84] |
| 16 | 16p11-13 | 4-Aminobutyrate Aminotransferase (*ABAT),*<br>CREB-binding protein *(CREBBP),*<br>Glutamate receptor, ionotropic, NMDA 2A *(GRIN2A)* | [98] |
| | 16p11.2 | | [81, 82, 90] |
| 17 | 17q11.2 | | [99] |
| 19 | 19p13 | | [99] |
| 20 | 20q13 | | [80] |
| 22 | 22q13 | *SHANK3* | [89] |
| X | Xp22.11 | *PTCHD1* | [91] |

Table 1. Loci identified by genome wide linkage analysis

Array comparative genomic hybridization (aCGH) is the most widely used method for detection of CNVs. A seminal early report used aCGH, with a mean resolution of one probe every 35 kb, to study a sample of 264 ASD families. After validation by higher-resolution microarray scans, G-banded karyotype, FISH, and microsatellite genotyping, 17 *de novo*

CNVs were confirmed [102]. A Korean group recently reported deletion CNVs at 8p23.1 and 17p11.2 using whole-genome aCGH [103]. Using aCGH with a mean 19 kb resolution, 51 autism-specific CNV were identified in 397 unrelated ASD subjects [100]. Similarly, Qiao and colleagues performed aCGH on 100 autistic subjects and identified 9 CNVs, three of which were unique to their cohort [104]. A Spanish group recently reported the identification of 13 CNVs containing 24 different genes in their sample of 96 ASD subjects [105].

Single-nucleotide polymorphism (SNP) array analysis, primarily developed to determine linkage, now is also employed to determine genomic CNVs [106]. Marshall performed a genome-wide assessment via SNP array analysis. They genotyped proximately 500,000 SNPs for each sample and detected 13 loci with recurrent or overlapping CNVs in a sample of 427 ASD cases [101]. Using SNP markers, another group identified 6 CNVs within a 2.2-megabase (Mb) intergenic Chr 2 region between cadherin 10 (CDH10) and cadherin 9 (CDH9) in a combined sample set of 1,984 ASD probands of European ancestry [107]. In addition, SNP array analysis offers some special advantages in the exploration of potentially relevant gene networks. Two recent reports have provided strong evidence for the involvement of certain genes in important gene networks including neuronal cell-adhesion, ubiquitin degradation and GTPase/Ras signaling [108, 109].

Currently available aCGH methods for identifying CNV typically assay the genome in the 40-kb to several Mb range. Methodological improvements that employ oligonucleotides are providing a high potential resolution down to approximately the 5-kb resolution level for aCGH with genome-wide detection of CNVs [106]. Thus, SNP or oligonucleotide aCGH analysis can detect a CNV as small as a few kilobases. Therefore, it is clear that the higher-density oligonucleotide or SNP arrays offer the higher resolution for analysis of CNVs in the future.

### 3.3 Selected candidate genes

As it is becoming apparent, a genetic predisposition to ASD may involve one or more interconnected genetic networks involving neurogenesis, neuronal migration, synaptogenesis, axon pathfinding and neuronal or glial structure regionalization [110]. Function-targeted studies, mainly by association that focus exclusively on the candidate genes, including some of the most widely studied will be reviewed in the following section (table 2).

Reelin is an extracellular matrix glycoprotein responsible for guiding the migration of several neural cell types and the establishment of neural connection. In the 1980s, it was discovered that reelin plays important roles in the positioning of neuronal cells in the inferior olivery complex, cerebral cortex and cerebellum early in embryonic development [203-205]. Further research has confirmed and further extended our knowledge about the widespread functions reelin plays in laminated regions of the brain, both embryonically and postnatally [206-208].

Given the critical functions of reelin in brain development, and knowing there are neuroanatomical abnormities in autism [209], the reelin gene (*RELN*) was a plausible candidate to investigate in ASDs. Significantly reduced levels of reelin in the human cortex, cerebellum and peripheral blood were confirmed in ASD at both the protein and mRNA levels [210-212]. Genome-wide scans also identified 7q22 as an autism critical region, where *RELN* is located [213].

| Genes | Loci | Positive results | Negative/Unconfirmed results |
|---|---|---|---|
| *RELN* | 7q22 | [111-120] | |
| *SLC6A4* | 17q11.1-17q12 | [121-127] | [128-140] |
| *GABR* | 15q11-15q13 | [141-154] | [155-157] |
| *NLGN* | 3q26(*NLGN1*), 17p13 (*NLGN2*), Xq13 (*NLGN3*), Xp22.3 (*NLGN4*), Yq11.2 (*NLGN4Y*) | [158-163] | [164-169] |
| *OXTR* | 3p24-3p25 | [170-174] | |
| *MET* | 7q31.2 | [175-179] | |
| *SLC25A12* | 2q31 | [180-183] | [184-186] |
| *GluR6* | 6q21 | [187-189] | [190] |
| *CNTNAP2* | 7q35 | [191-196] | |
| *GLO1* | 6p21.3-6p21.2 | [197, 198] | [199, 200] |
| *TPH2* | 12q21.1 | [201] | [197, 202] |

Table 2. Selected candidate genes

*i. Reelin gene (RELN)*

Additionally, case-control and family-based studies provided further evidence supporting the association of *RELN* and ASD. Persico identified a *RELN*-related polymorphic GGC repeat located immediately 5′ of the ATG initiator codon in Italian and American subjects [120]. Using the similar methods and 126 multiplex ASD families, Zhang *et al* examined the polymorphic CGG-repeat of *RELN* [118]. Family-based association tests showed that larger *RELN* alleles (≥11 repeats) were transmitted more often than expected to autistic children. Independant studies regarding the CGG-repeat of *RELN* have also supported its contribution to the genetic risk of autism [112, 113, 115]. Others have also reported significant differences in the transmission of the reelin alleles of exon 22 and intron 59 SNPs to autistic subjects [114]. However, results have not been uniformly positive. Krebs *et al* performed a transmission disequilibrium test (TDT) analysis of the CGG-repeat polymorphism in 167 Caucasian families and found no evidence of linkage or association [119]. Similarly, another two groups failed to find a significant association of *RELN* CGG repeat polymorphisms with liability to autism [116, 117].

The association between *RELN* and ASD were also found in other ethnic groups besides Caucasian populations. Recently, a significant genetic association between the *RELN* SNP2 (located in intron 59) and ASD was reported in a Chinese Han population, and the combination of *RELN* SNP1/SNP2/SNP3/SNP4, all in strong linkage disequilibrium, were reported to have a significant association with ASD [111].

*ii. Human serotonin transporter gene (SLC6A4)*

The human serotonin transporter, encoded by *SLC6A4,* localizes to chromosome 17q11.1-q12 and consists of 15 exons [214]. *SLC6A4* was considered as a candidate gene for autism primarily based on the elevated blood serotonin levels found in a number of autistic probands, as well as the efficacy of potent serotonin transporter inhibitors in reducing rituals and routines [215, 216]. Using the TDT, positive associations of a 5-HTTLPR polymorphism found in the promoter region of the *SLC6A4* gene with autism have been identified by 4 family-based studies and 2 case-control studies [121, 123, 125-127]. Other groups have performed both family-based and case-control analysis and found significant associations of the *SLC6A4* polymorphism with autism [122, 124]. In contrast to these positive reports, 9 family-based studies failed to find evidence for associations of the *SLC6A4* polymorphism with autism [130, 132-134, 136-140], as well as a case-control study [128]. An Indian group performed a series of studies but found no persuasive evidence of the association of the *SLC6A4* polymorphisms with autism [129, 135, 217]. In addition, a systematic review and meta-analysis failed to find a significant overall association of the serotonin polymorphisms examined and autism [131].

*iii. Gamma-aminobutyric acid receptor gene (GABR)*

Gamma-aminobutyric acid (GABA) is the chief inhibitory neurotransmitter in the brain, acting by binding to a GABA receptor. The receptor is a multimeric transmembrane receptor that consists of five subunits arranged around a central pore. The GABA receptor subunits are homologous, but are both structurally and functionally diverse [144]. Three of the GABA receptor subunit genes (*GABRB3, GABRA5* and *GABRG3*) are localized to chromosome 15q11-q13, one of the most complex regions in the genome involved with genome instability, gene expression, imprinting and recombination [156].

The region 15q11-q13 was originally associated with ASD based on several studies which reported a common duplication of this region in ASD subjects [147, 148, 152, 154]. A chromosome-engineered mouse model for human 15q11-13 duplication was developed with autistic features [141, 143, 153]. Cook *et al* examined markers across this region for linkage disequilibrium in 140 families with ASD, detecting significant linkage disequilibrium between *GABRB3* and ASD [218]. This finding was confirmed by others as well [145, 146, 151]. Also, two SNPs located within the *GABRG3* gene were associated with ASD using the Pedigree Disequilibrium Test (PDT) [144]. An independent study demonstrated nominally significant associations between six markers across the *GABRB3* and *GABRA5* genes [142]. Moreover, using ordered-subset analysis (OSA) another group provided evidence of increased linkage at the *GABRB3* locus [149]. Other research has also identified significant association and gene-gene interactions of GABA receptor subunit genes in autism [150].

Nonetheless, conflicting evidence has also been reported. Other groups have reported limited or no association between GABA receptor polymorphisms and autism [155, 156]. Similarly, another group conducted a full genome search for autism susceptibility loci including seven microsatellite markers from 15q11-q13, and found no significant evidence of association or linkage [157]. Thus the linkage results are at best inconclusive.

*iv. Neuroligin genes (NLGN)*

The marked difference in sex ratio for ASD justifies the exploration of genes on the sex chromosome, among which the neuroligin genes (*NLGN*) are perhaps the most widely studied. Five *NLGN* have been identified in the human genome, which are localized at 3q26(*NLGN1*), 17p13 (*NLGN2*), Xq13 (*NLGN3*), Xp22.3 (*NLGN4*), and Yq11.2 (*NLGN4Y*) respectively. They encode a family of cell-adhesion molecules, the neuroligans, essential for the formation of functional neural synapses [163, 169].

The earliest report regarding the potential association of *NLGN* genes and ASD came from the study of multiple Swedish families [163]. The authors screened for *NLGN3* mutations in 36 affected sib-pairs and 122 trios with ASD. They found one *de novo* mutation in *NLGN4* in one family. This mutation creates a stop codon leading to premature termination of the protein. In another family, a C to T transition in *NLGN3* was identified that changed a highly conserved arginine residue into cysteine (R451C) within the esterase domain. It was inherited from the mother. Following this report, several other groups studied this gene but found little support for common mutations of the gene. Limited support came from a Portuguese group, who found missense changes in *NLGN4* as well as the protein-truncating mutations in ASD [162]. A Finnish group conducted a molecular genetic analysis of *NLGN1, NLGN3, NLGN4,* and *NLNG4Y*. Their results suggested neuroligin mutations most probably represent rare causes of autism and concluded that it was unlikely that the allelic variants in these genes would be major risk factors for autism [166]. Others have also failed to obtain positive results, casting doubt on the earlier conclusion [164, 165, 167-169].

Other reports about mutations of *NLGN3* or *NLGN4* have identified splice variants in both genes [161]. Three groups recently reported one missense variant and two single substitutions in independent autistic samples, indicating that a defect of synaptogenesis may predispose to autism [158-160].

*v. Human oxytocin receptor gene (OXTR)*

Oxytocin is a nine-amino-acid peptide synthesized in the hypothalamus. Apart from regulating lactation and uterine contraction, oxytocin acts as a neuromodulator in the central nervous system [219, 220]. Both animal experiments and clinical research have confirmed the role oxytocin plays in social and repetitive behaviors [221]. Therefore the oxytocin system might be potentially involved in the pathogenesis of ASD, and the human oxytocin receptor gene (*OXTR*) has been regarded as a most promising candidate gene to study.

Indeed, research pertaining to the potential association between *OXTR* and autism has come to positive conclusions. Using family-based and population-based association tests, SNPs and haplotypes in the *OXTR* have been reported to confer risk for ASD in different ethnic groups [170, 172-174]. They have also been associated with IQ and adaptive behavior scale scores [172]. Furthermore, a recent study identified significant increases in the DNA methylation status of OXTR in peripheral blood cells and temporal cortex, as well as decreased expression of *OXTR* mRNA in the temporal cortex of autism cases, suggesting that epigenetic dysregulation may be involved in the pathogenesis of ASD [171].

*vi. MET*

The human *MET* gene encodes a transmembrane receptor tyrosine kinase of the hepatocyte growth factor/scatter factor (HGF/SF) [222]. Though primarily identified as an oncogene, MET plays crucial roles in neuronal development [222-224]. Moreover, impaired MET signaling causes abnormal interneuron migration and neural growth in the cortex, as well as decreased proliferation of granule cells, which matches many of the features found in autistic brains [223, 225].

Campbell and colleagues have done a series of studies regarding the association between MET signaling and autism. They first reported the genetic association of a common C allele in the promoter region of *MET*, which results in significant decrease in *MET* promoter activity and altered binding of specific transcription factor complexes [179]. Then they found significantly decreased MET protein levels and increased mRNA expression for proteins involved in regulating MET signaling activity [226]. Furthermore, they screened the exons and 5′ promoter regions for variants in the five genes encoding the proteins that regulate *MET* expression, finding that genetic susceptibility impacting multiple components of the MET signaling pathway contributes to ASD risk [178]. Most recently, they found that the *MET* C allele influences two of the behavioral domains of the autism triad [175]. Other groups have also provided supportive evidence that *MET* gene variations may play a role in autism susceptibility [176, 177].

*vii. SLC25A12*

*SLC25A12* locates in the chromosome 2q31 region, encoding the mitochondrial aspartate/glutamate carrier (AGC1), a key protein involved in mitochondrial function and ATP synthesis. Since the physiological function of neurons greatly depends on energy supply, any alteration in mitochondrial function or ATP synthesis could lead to corresponding changes in neurons [227]. Recently mitochondrial hyperproliferation and partial respiratory chain block were found in two autistic patients, suggesting *SLC25A12* could be a promising candidate gene [228].

Following this report, several studies for genetic variants of the gene were performed. Three different ethnic groups reported linkage and association between ASD and two SNPs (i.e. rs2056202 and rs2292813) in *SLC25A12* [180, 182, 183], while another three independent groups failed to reveal significant association [184-186]. Another group associated one SNP (rs2056202) with ASD but not the other [181]. Thus, the findings so far are inconclusive.

*viii. Other candidate genes*

The glutamate receptor 6 gene (*GRIK2* or *GluR6*) is located at chromosome 6q21. Given that glutamate is the principal excitatory neurotransmitter in the brain and it is involved in cognitive functions such as memory and learning, *GRIK2* was proposed as a gene candidate for ASD [229]. Unfortunately, the limited reports have very different results. Genetic studies in a Caucasian population, Chinese Han and Korean trios provided positive evidence, but using different SNPs [187-189]. Another report failed to find any association of *GRIK2* with autism in an Indian population [189].

Contactin associated protein-2 (*CNTNAP2*) belongs to the neurexin family, within which several members have been identified as being related to autism [230]. A recent research report identified a homozygous mutation of *CNTNAP2* in Amish children with pervasive developmental disorders, seizures, and language regression [196]. Five other studies have supported this finding that *CNTNAP2* may be a genetic susceptibility factor in autism [191-195]. Another group found that *CNTNAP2* provided a strong male affection bias in ASD [193].

Glyoxalase 1 is a cytosolic, ubiquitously expressed, zinc metalloenzyme enzyme involved in scavenging toxic α-oxoaldehydes formed during cellular metabolic reactions. Proteomics analysis found glyoxalase 1 increased in autism brains, and subsequent sequencing of its gene (*GLO1*) identified that homozygosity for a polymorphism of the gene, A419 *GLO1*, resulted in decreased enzyme activity and association with autism [198], although this conclusion was not confirmed by other studies [199, 200]. In addition, one group found a protective effect of the A419 allele of *GLO1* [197].

*TPH1* and *TPH2* encode rate-limiting enzymes that control serotonin biosynthesis. TPH1 is primarily expressed peripherally, while TPH2 is found exclusively in brain tissue. However, despite evidence for the potential involvement of the serotonin system in the etiology of autism, only one of three reports to date conservatively has supported the notion that *TPH2* plays a role in autism susceptibility [197, 201, 202].

## 4. Environmental factors

### 4.1 Prenatal factors

The association between prenatal insults and the pathogenesis of autism has been reported recent decades. Early in 2005, Beversdorf *et al.* conducted surveys regarding incidence and timing of prenatal stressors. They found a higher incidence of prenatal stressors in autism at 21-32 weeks gestation, which peaks at 25-28 weeks. Their finding supported the hypothesis of prenatal stressors as a potential contributor to autism, and the timing was consistent with the embryological age suggested by neuroanatomical findings seen in the cerebellum in autism [231]. More specifically, Meyer *et al* demonstrate that the effects of maternal immune challenge between middle and late gestation periods in mice are dissociable in terms of several neuropsychiatric disorders including autism [232]. However, this conclusion was challenged by another group of scientists. Ploeger *et al.* proposed pleiotropic effects during a very early and specific stage of embryonic development, namely early organogenesis (day 20 to day 40 after fertilization) in order to explain the effect of uterine disturbances to the development of autism [233]. They provided ample evidence from literature for the association between autism and many different kinds of physical anomalies such as limb deformities, craniofacial malformations, brain pathology, and anomalies in other organs, which agrees with the hypothesis that pleiotropic effects are involved in the development of autism.

Drugs are the most important prenatal factors affecting embryo and fetal development. Cumulating data support the relationships between maternal medication and fetogeneous diseases including autism. The obnoxious drug thalidomide turned out not only to relate to fetal abnormality but also to autism. Stromland group retrospectively investigated 100 Swedish thalidomide embryopathy cases and found possible association of thalidomide embryopathy with autism [234]. Another example of drug relating to autism is valproate. Williams *et al* reported six cases whose clinical phenotype was compatible with both fetal valproate syndrome (FVS) and autism. Although the sample size is small, the authors claimed the association between this known teratogen and autism had both clinical and research implications [235]. Similarly, Rasalam group provided another line of evidence that prenatal exposure to sodium valproate is a risk factor for the development of an ASD [236].

Another prenatal factor is intrauterine inflammation. Kannan *et al* conducted an animal study to demonstrate intrauterine inflammation results in alterations in cortical serotonin and disruption of serotonin-regulated thalamocortical development in the newborn brain therefore resulting in impairment of the somatosensory system, such as autism [237]. More persuasive evidence comes from Girard's report. According to their results, end of gestation exposure of pregnant rats to systemic microbial product such as lipopolysacharide (LPS) is an independent risk factor for neurodevelopmental diseases such as cerebral palsy, mental deficiency, and autism. And coadministration of IL-1 receptor antagonist with LPS alleviated the detrimental effects caused by LPS [238].

In addition, maternal complications of pregnancies are proved to be associated with autism. One group performed a discriminant analysis to explore perinatal complications as predictors for autism. They found three maternal medical conditions including urinary infection, high temperatures, and depression to be highly significant and contribute to the separation between the autistic and normal subjects [239].

### 4.2 Postnatal factors

Heavy metals have also been generally considered to contribute to the pathogenesis of autism. Mercury is one of the most widely studied heavy metals. Palmer *et al* studied the association between environmentally released mercury, special education and autism rates in Texas using data from the Texas Education Department and the United States Environmental Protection Agency, and found there was a significant increase in the rates of special education students and autism rates associated with increases in environmentally released mercury. They reported a 43% increase in the rate of special education services and a 61% increase in the rate of autism [240]. Windham group included 284 children with ASD and 657 controls from the San Francisco Bay area in order to explore possible associations between autism spectrum disorders (ASD) and environmental exposures. Their results suggested a potential association between autism and estimated metal concentrations including mercury, cadmium, nickel [241]. Consistent with previous results, Geier *et al* conducted a prospective study which provided biochemical/genomic evidence for mercury susceptibility/toxicity in ASDs indicating a causal role for mercury [242, 243], and they further explored the threshold effect of mercury in a recent publication [244]. In spite of these different pieces of evidence, disagreement exists. IP *et al* performed a cross-sectional cohort study to compare the hair and blood mercury levels of autistic children and a group of normal children. There was no difference in the mean mercury levels. Thus, they concluded that there is no causal relationship between mercury as an environmental neurotoxin and autism [245].

In addition of mercury, lead is also associated with autism. Very early evidence came from a case report, which explored the interaction and possible casual relationship of an elevated blood-lead and autism, as well as treatment of the behavioral symptoms [246]. Later, Canfield *et al* concluded that blood lead concentrations, even those below 10 microgram per deciliter, were inversely associated with children's IQ scores at three and five years of age, and associated declines in IQ were greater at these concentrations than at higher concentrations [247]. Supporting these results, Yorbik group reported that autism could be associated with significant decrease in excretion rate of lead [248].

Hazardous air pollutants have long been related to the development of autism and more evidences have begun to emerge in recent years. Kalkbrenner *et al* conducted a case-control study to screen perinatal exposure to 35 hazardous air pollutants using 383 children with autism spectrum disorders and, as controls, 2,829 children with speech and language impairment. Although the results were biased by exposure misclassification of air pollutants and the use of an alternate developmental disorder as the control group, they provided evidence based on their analysis that methylene chloride, quinoline, and styrene were the plausible candidate exposures for autism spectrum disorders [249]. In another study conducted by Windham group, trichloroethylene, and vinyl chloride have also been related to autism [241].

However, one should notice that the currently available data are mainly derived from epidemiological studies. Considering the limited sample sizes and the different populations, the previous results are hardly conclusive. Further research is needed to explore the possible mechanisms underlying these results.

## 5. Mouse models for autism research

Mouse models provide a powerful strategy to explore experimentally candidate genes for autism susceptibility, and to use environmental challenges to induce gene mutations and cell pathology early in development. Mouse models have also been used to investigate the effects of alterations in signaling pathways on neuronal migration, neurotransmission and brain anatomy, which are relevant to findings in autistic subjects [250]. These models have elucidated neuropathology that might underlie the autism phenotype.

There are currently several mouse models for autism research, most of which are primarily developed by knocking out different candidate genes for other neuropsychiatric diseases such as fragile X syndrome [250, 251], Rett syndrome [252], but now are used as autistic models because of their autistic-like behaviors. Other examples include *Engrailed 1&2* and *PTEN* genetic mice [253, 254]. In addition, there is another group of models constructed by surgical or toxic treatments of candidate regions in the brain, in general during development [255]. Some other reports regarding autistic-like behaviors in BALB/c and A/J mice have also been seen [250, 256-258].

Here the author would like to stress an inbred mouse strain for autistic research. BTBR T(+)*tf/J* mouse, also named as BTBR mouse, is an inbred strain with black top coat and blond undercoat. Anatomically BTBR mice get total absence of the corpus callosum, and severely reduced hippocampal commissure, which are also attributed to their phenotypes [259-262]. Although primarily used as type 2 diabetes model [263-268] and phenylketonuria (PKU) model [269-274], BTBR mice were recently found to be a promising mice model for autism research because they exhibited the three core symptoms for diagnosing autism [275-282]. Using this strain, several groups have begun to explore the pathogenesis of autism. It was well documented that circulating corticosterone is higher in the BTBR than in B6. And higher basal glucocorticoid receptor mRNA and higher oxytocin peptide levels were detected in the brains of BTBR as compared to B6, although their relationship to autism remain disputable [283, 284]. In the meanwhile, potential treatments for autism have been proposed based on the experimental results using BTBR mice. Two independent groups confirm the efficacy of the SERT blocker, fluoxetine for enhancement of social interactions [285, 286]. Another experiment reported repetitive self-grooming behavior in the BTBR mouse model of autism was blocked by the mGluR5 antagonist Methyl-6-phenylethynyl-pyridine (MPEP) [287]. Behavioral therapies offer another option for autism treatment, Young group reported social peers rescued autism-relevant sociability deficits in adolescent BTBR mice, but not cross-fostering [288, 289].

However, the tools to analyze these animals are not yet standardized, and an important effort needs to be made. Crawley *et al* proposed three standards to evaluate animal model, namely face validity (i.e. resemblance to the human symptoms), construct validity (i.e. similarity to the underlying causes of the disease) and predictive validity (i.e. expected responses to treatments that are effective in the human disease) [290]. Using these standards, newly developed tests are used to screen more animal models for autism research.

## 6. Summary and conclusions

Autism spectrum disorders (ASD) is a common neurodevelopment disorder. Diagnosed before three years old, autistic children present significant language delays, social and communication challenges, as well as abnormal repetitive and restrictive behaviors. It is reported that ASD occur in all racial, ethnic and socioeconomic groups, yet are about four times more likely to occur in boys than in girls probably due to the extremes of typical male neuroanatomy of autism.

The relationship between immune disorders and ASD has been proposed based on series of evidences.Secondly, genetic predisposition is considered to be involved in the etiology of ASD. Cumulative evidences indicated ASD had a strong genetic background, both gene-gene and gene-environment interactions attribute to the etiology of autism. Also, it's now generally accepted that ASD is a group of multi-genetic diseases, in which environmental factors play an important part. Given the early onset of the symptoms, prenatal exposures to environmental challenges are considered the major risk factors leading to subsequent mortality of ASD. Various factors have been proven to be potentially detrimental to early neurosystem development, including maternal use of pharmaceutical agents with neurotoxic effects, intrauterine exposure to viral infections or maternal stress , as well as exposure to high levels of environmental pollutants such as heavy metals . Similarly, neonatal exposure to such risk factors may also lead to mortality of ASD, which has been proven in animal studies as well as clinical reports.

At last, ASD animal models provide a feasible and relatively easy way to morphologically and functionally study the etiology of ASD in different levels, and to testify the effectiveness of the potential interventions. Recent advances in this field provide both inbred strains such as BTBR *T+ tf/J* mice and mutant lines. Other mice models for fragile X syndrome, Rett syndrome have also been used for autism related studies due to the autistic-like behaviors exhibited in these patients.

In conclusion, data remain inconclusive for the majority of candidate genes tested so far. Still, we have good reason to be optimistic regarding gene discovery in ASD now and in the future. Cytogenetic, linkage, association studies and array analysis have provided promising results. Emerging genetic technologies and analysis tools offer even more powerful approaches for developing insights into the etiology of ASD. In addition, genetic studies facilitate other autism research such as biochemical and neuroimaging studies, which will, in turn, provide evidence and valuable clues to direct future genetic studies.

## 7. References

[1] Lord, C., M. Rutter and A. Le Couteur, *Autism Diagnostic Interview-Revised: a revised version of a diagnostic interview for caregivers of individuals with possible pervasive developmental disorders.* J Autism Dev Disord, 1994. 24(5): p. 659-85.

[2] Lord, C., et al., *Autism diagnostic observation schedule: a standardized observation of communicative and social behavior.* J Autism Dev Disord, 1989. 19(2): p. 185-212.

[3] Van Naarden, B.K., et al., *Evaluation of a methodology for a collaborative multiple source surveillance network for autism spectrum disorders--Autism and Developmental Disabilities Monitoring Network, 14 sites, United States,* 2002. MMWR Surveill Summ, 2007. 56(1): p. 29-40.

[4] Nonkin, A.R., et al., *Evaluation of a Records-Review Surveillance System Used to Determine the Prevalence of Autism Spectrum Disorders.* J Autism Dev Disord, 2010.

[5] Krause, I., et al., *Brief report: immune factors in autism: a critical review.* J Autism Dev Disord, 2002. 32(4): p. 337-45.

[6] Lintas, C. and A.M. Persico, *Autistic phenotypes and genetic testing: state-of-the-art for the clinical geneticist.* J Med Genet, 2009. 46(1): p. 1-8.

[7] Baron-Cohen, S., R.C. Knickmeyer and M.K. Belmonte, *Sex differences in the brain: implications for explaining autism.* Science, 2005. 310(5749): p. 819-23.

[8] Williams, J.G., J.P. Higgins and C.E. Brayne, *Systematic review of prevalence studies of autism spectrum disorders.* Arch Dis Child, 2006. 91(1): p. 8-15.

[9] Prevalence of autism spectrum disorders - *Autism and Developmental Disabilities Monitoring Network, United States, 2006.* MMWR Surveill Summ, 2009. 58(10): p. 1-20.

[10] *Prevalence of autism spectrum disorders--autism and developmental disabilities monitoring network, six sites, United States,* 2000. MMWR Surveill Summ, 2007. 56(1): p. 1-11.

[11] *Prevalence of autism spectrum disorders--autism and developmental disabilities monitoring network, 14 sites, United States,* 2002. MMWR Surveill Summ, 2007. 56(1): p. 12-28.

[12] King, M. and P. Bearman, *Diagnostic change and the increased prevalence of autism.* Int J Epidemiol, 2009. 38(5): p. 1224-34.

[13] Nonkin, A.R., et al., *Evaluation of a Records-Review Surveillance System Used to Determine the Prevalence of Autism Spectrum Disorders.* J Autism Dev Disord, 2010.

[14] Comi, A.M., et al., *Familial clustering of autoimmune disorders and evaluation of medical risk factors in autism.* J Child Neurol, 1999. 14(6): p. 388-94.

[15] Molloy, C.A., et al., *Familial autoimmune thyroid disease as a risk factor for regression in children with Autism Spectrum Disorder:* a CPEA Study. J Autism Dev Disord, 2006. 36(3): p. 317-24.

[16] Mouridsen, S.E., et al., *Autoimmune diseases in parents of children with infantile autism: a case-control study.* Dev Med Child Neurol, 2007. 49(6): p. 429-32.

[17] Sweeten, T.L., et al., *Increased prevalence of familial autoimmunity in probands with pervasive developmental disorders.* Pediatrics, 2003. 112(5): p. e420.

[18] Careaga, M., J. Van de Water and P. Ashwood, *Immune dysfunction in autism: a pathway to treatment.* Neurotherapeutics, 2010. 7(3): p. 283-92.

[19] Cabanlit, M., et al., *Brain-specific autoantibodies in the plasma of subjects with autistic spectrum disorder.* Ann N Y Acad Sci, 2007. 1107: p. 92-103.

[20] Wills, S., et al., *Detection of autoantibodies to neural cells of the cerebellum in the plasma of subjects with autism spectrum disorders.* Brain Behav Immun, 2009. 23(1): p. 64-74.

[21] Ashwood, P., S. Wills and J. Van de Water, *The immune response in autism: a new frontier for autism research.* J Leukoc Biol, 2006. 80(1): p. 1-15.

[22] Enstrom, A., et al., *Increased IgG4 levels in children with autism disorder.* Brain Behav Immun, 2009. 23(3): p. 389-95.

[23] Heuer, L., et al., Reduced levels of immunoglobulin in children with autism correlates with behavioral symptoms. Autism Res, 2008. 1(5): p. 275-83.

[24] Trajkovski, V., L. Ajdinski and M. Spiroski, *Plasma concentration of immunoglobulin classes and subclasses in children with autism in the Republic of Macedonia: retrospective study.* Croat Med J, 2004. 45(6): p. 746-9.

[25] Ashwood, P., et al., *Altered T cell responses in children with autism.* Brain Behav Immun, 2010.

[26] Comi, A.M., et al., *Familial clustering of autoimmune disorders and evaluation of medical risk factors in autism.* J Child Neurol, 1999. 14(6): p. 388-94.

[27] Sweeten, T.L., et al., *Increased prevalence of familial autoimmunity in probands with pervasive developmental disorders.* Pediatrics, 2003. 112(5): p. e420.
[28] Molloy, C.A., et al., *Familial autoimmune thyroid disease as a risk factor for regression in children with Autism Spectrum Disorder: a CPEA Study.* J Autism Dev Disord, 2006. 36(3): p. 317-24.
[29] Jyonouchi, H., S. Sun and ". H", *Proinflammatory and regulatory cytokine production associated with innate and adaptive immune responses in children with autism spectrum disorders and developmental regression.* J Neuroimmunol, 2001. 120(1-2): p. 170-9.
[30] Molloy, C.A., et al., *Elevated cytokine levels in children with autism spectrum disorder.* J Neuroimmunol, 2006. 172(1-2): p. 198-205.
[31] Li, X., et al., *Elevated immune response in the brain of autistic patients.* J Neuroimmunol, 2009. 207(1-2): p. 111-6.
[32] Ashwood, P., et al., *Elevated plasma cytokines in autism spectrum disorders provide evidence of immune dysfunction and are associated with impaired behavioral outcome.* Brain Behav Immun, 2010.
[33] Singer, H.S., et al., *Antibodies against fetal brain in sera of mothers with autistic children.* J Neuroimmunol, 2008. 194(1-2): p. 165-72.
[34] Braunschweig, D., et al., *Autism: maternally derived antibodies specific for fetal brain proteins.* Neurotoxicology, 2008. 29(2): p. 226-31.
[35] Zimmerman, A.W., et al., *Maternal antibrain antibodies in autism.* Brain Behav Immun, 2007. 21(3): p. 351-7.
[36] Croen, L.A., et al., *Maternal mid-pregnancy autoantibodies to fetal brain protein: the early markers for autism study.* Biol Psychiatry, 2008. 64(7): p. 583-8.
[37] Braunschweig, D., et al., *Autism: maternally derived antibodies specific for fetal brain proteins.* Neurotoxicology, 2008. 29(2): p. 226-31.
[38] Singh, V.K. and W.H. Rivas, *Prevalence of serum antibodies to caudate nucleus in autistic children.* Neurosci Lett, 2004. 355(1-2): p. 53-6.
[39] Trajkovski, V., L. Ajdinski and M. Spiroski, *Plasma concentration of immunoglobulin classes and subclasses in children with autism in the Republic of Macedonia: retrospective study.* Croat Med J, 2004. 45(6): p. 746-9.
[40] Enstrom, A., et al., *Increased IgG4 levels in children with autism disorder.* Brain Behav Immun, 2009. 23(3): p. 389-95.
[41] Morris, C.M., A.W. Zimmerman and H.S. Singer, *Childhood serum anti-fetal brain antibodies do not predict autism.* Pediatr Neurol, 2009. 41(4): p. 288-90.
[42] Stern, L., et al., *Immune function in autistic children.* Ann Allergy Asthma Immunol, 2005. 95(6): p. 558-65.
[43] Goodwin, M.S., M.A. Cowen and T.C. Goodwin, *Malabsorption and cerebral dysfunction: a multivariate and comparative study of autistic children.* J Autism Child Schizophr, 1971. 1(1): p. 48-62.
[44] Horvath, K. and J.A. Perman, *Autism and gastrointestinal symptoms.* Curr Gastroenterol Rep, 2002. 4(3): p. 251-8.
[45] Kuddo, T. and K.B. Nelson, *How common are gastrointestinal disorders in children with autism?.* Curr Opin Pediatr, 2003. 15(3): p. 339-43.
[46] Molloy, C.A. and P. Manning-Courtney, *Prevalence of chronic gastrointestinal symptoms in children with autism and autistic spectrum disorders.* Autism, 2003. 7(2): p. 165-71.

[47] Fernell, E., U.L. Fagerberg and P.M. Hellstrom, *No evidence for a clear link between active intestinal inflammation and autism based on analyses of faecal calprotectin and rectal nitric oxide.* Acta Paediatr, 2007. 96(7): p. 1076-9.
[48] Wakefield, A.J., et al., *Enterocolitis in children with developmental disorders.* Am J Gastroenterol, 2000. 95(9): p. 2285-95.
[49] Horvath, K., et al., *Gastrointestinal abnormalities in children with autistic disorder.* J Pediatr, 1999. 135(5): p. 559-63.
[50] Ashwood, P., et al., *Spontaneous mucosal lymphocyte cytokine profiles in children with autism and gastrointestinal symptoms: mucosal immune activation and reduced counter regulatory interleukin-10.* J Clin Immunol, 2004. 24(6): p. 664-73.
[51] Ashwood, P. and A.J. Wakefield, *Immune activation of peripheral blood and mucosal CD3+ lymphocyte cytokine profiles in children with autism and gastrointestinal symptoms.* J Neuroimmunol, 2006. 173(1-2): p. 126-34.
[52] Jyonouchi, H., et al., *Dysregulated innate immune responses in young children with autism spectrum disorders: their relationship to gastrointestinal symptoms and dietary intervention.* Neuropsychobiology, 2005. 51(2): p. 77-85.
[53] DeFelice, M.L., et al., *Intestinal cytokines in children with pervasive developmental disorders.* Am J Gastroenterol, 2003. 98(8): p. 1777-82.
[54] D'Eufemia, P., et al., *Abnormal intestinal permeability in children with autism.* Acta Paediatr, 1996. 85(9): p. 1076-9.
[55] Caglayan, A.O., *Genetic causes of syndromic and non-syndromic autism.* Dev Med Child Neurol, 2010. 52(2): p. 130-8.
[56] Abrahams, B.S. and D.H. Geschwind, *Advances in autism genetics: on the threshold of a new neurobiology.* Nat Rev Genet, 2008. 9(5): p. 341-55.
[57] Bailey, A., et al., *Autism as a strongly genetic disorder: evidence from a British twin study.* Psychol Med, 1995. 25(1): p. 63-77.
[58] Steffenburg, S., et al., *A twin study of autism in Denmark, Finland, Iceland, Norway and Sweden.* J Child Psychol Psychiatry, 1989. 30(3): p. 405-16.
[59] Liu, K., N. Zerubavel and P. Bearman, *Social demographic change and autism.* Demography, 2010. 47(2): p. 327-43.
[60] Hoffman, E.J. and M.W. State, *Progress in cytogenetics: implications for child psychopathology.* J Am Acad Child Adolesc Psychiatry, 2010. 49(8): p. 736-51; quiz 856-7.
[61] Piggot, J., et al., *Neural systems approaches to the neurogenetics of autism spectrum disorders.* Neuroscience, 2009. 164(1): p. 247-56.
[62] Levitt, P. and D.B. Campbell, *The genetic and neurobiologic compass points toward common signaling dysfunctions in autism spectrum disorders.* J Clin Invest, 2009. 119(4): p. 747-54.
[63] Kumar, R.A. and S.L. Christian, *Genetics of autism spectrum disorders.* Curr Neurol Neurosci Rep, 2009. 9(3): p. 188-97.
[64] Betancur, C., T. Sakurai and J.D. Buxbaum, *The emerging role of synaptic cell-adhesion pathways in the pathogenesis of autism spectrum disorders.* Trends Neurosci, 2009. 32(7): p. 402-12.
[65] Vissers, L.E., et al., *A de novo paradigm for mental retardation.* Nat Genet, 2010. 42(12): p. 1109-12.

[66] Choi, M., et al., *Genetic diagnosis by whole exome capture and massively parallel DNA sequencing.* Proc Natl Acad Sci U S A, 2009. 106(45): p. 19096-101.
[67] Robinson, P.N., *Whole-exome sequencing for finding de novo mutations in sporadic mental retardation.* Genome Biol, 2010. 11(12): p. 144.
[68] Bilguvar, K., et al., *Whole-exome sequencing identifies recessive WDR62 mutations in severe brain malformations.* Nature, 2010. 467(7312): p. 207-10.
[69] Sanders, S., *Whole-exome sequencing: a powerful technique for identifying novel genes of complex disorders.* Clin Genet, 2011. 79(2): p. 132-3.
[70] Betancur, C., *Etiological heterogeneity in autism spectrum disorders: More than 100 genetic and genomic disorders and still counting.* Brain Res, 2010.
[71] Buxbaum, J.D., et al., *Evidence for a susceptibility gene for autism on chromosome 2 and for genetic heterogeneity.* Am J Hum Genet, 2001. 68(6): p. 1514-20.
[72] Shao, Y., et al., *Phenotypic homogeneity provides increased support for linkage on chromosome 2 in autistic disorder.* Am J Hum Genet, 2002. 70(4): p. 1058-61.
[73] Rabionet, R., et al., *Analysis of the autism chromosome 2 linkage region: GAD1 and other candidate genes.* Neurosci Lett, 2004. 372(3): p. 209-14.
[74] Wu, S., et al., *Association of the neuropilin-2 (NRP2) gene polymorphisms with autism in Chinese Han population.* Am J Med Genet B Neuropsychiatr Genet, 2007. 144B(4): p. 492-5.
[75] Blasi, F., et al., *SLC25A12 and CMYA3 gene variants are not associated with autism in the IMGSAC multiplex family sample.* Eur J Hum Genet, 2006. 14(1): p. 123-6.
[76] Szatmari, P., et al., *Mapping autism risk loci using genetic linkage and chromosomal rearrangements.* Nat Genet, 2007. 39(3): p. 319-28.
[77] Ramoz, N., et al., *An analysis of candidate autism loci on chromosome 2q24-q33: evidence for association to the STK39 gene.* Am J Med Genet B Neuropsychiatr Genet, 2008. 147B(7): p. 1152-8.
[78] Philippi, A., et al., *Association of autism with polymorphisms in the paired-like homeodomain transcription factor 1 (PITX1) on chromosome 5q31: a candidate gene analysis.* BMC Med Genet, 2007. 8: p. 74.
[79] Ma, D., et al., *A genome-wide association study of autism reveals a common novel risk locus at 5p14.1.* Ann Hum Genet, 2009. 73(Pt 3): p. 263-73.
[80] Weiss, L.A., et al., *A genome-wide linkage and association scan reveals novel loci for autism.* Nature, 2009. 461(7265): p. 802-8.
[81] Shinawi, M., et al., *Recurrent reciprocal 16p11.2 rearrangements associated with global developmental delay, behavioural problems, dysmorphism, epilepsy, and abnormal head size.* J Med Genet, 2010. 47(5): p. 332-41.
[82] Kumar, R.A., et al., *Recurrent 16p11.2 microdeletions in autism.* Hum Mol Genet, 2008. 17(4): p. 628-38.
[83] Kim, S.J., et al., *Transmission disequilibrium testing of the chromosome 15q11-q13 region in autism.* Am J Med Genet B Neuropsychiatr Genet, 2008. 147B(7): p. 1116-25.
[84] Sutcliffe, J.S., et al., *Partial duplication of the APBA2 gene in chromosome 15q13 corresponds to duplicon structures.* BMC Genomics, 2003. 4(1): p. 15.
[85] Nurmi, E.L., et al., *Linkage disequilibrium at the Angelman syndrome gene UBE3A in autism families.* Genomics, 2001. 77(1-2): p. 105-13.
[86] Shen, Y., et al., *Clinical genetic testing for patients with autism spectrum disorders.* Pediatrics, 2010. 125(4): p. e727-35.

[87] Ma, D.Q., et al., *Dissecting the locus heterogeneity of autism: significant linkage to chromosome 12q14.* Mol Psychiatry, 2007. 12(4): p. 376-84.
[88] Alvarez, R.A., et al., *Association of common variants in the Joubert syndrome gene (AHI1) with autism.* Hum Mol Genet, 2008. 17(24): p. 3887-96.
[89] Qin, J., et al., *Association study of SHANK3 gene polymorphisms with autism in Chinese Han population.* BMC Med Genet, 2009. 10: p. 61.
[90] Kumar, R.A., et al., *A de novo 1p34.2 microdeletion identifies the synaptic vesicle gene RIMS3 as a novel candidate for autism.* J Med Genet, 2010. 47(2): p. 81-90.
[91] Noor, A., et al., *Disruption at the PTCHD1 Locus on Xp22.11 in Autism Spectrum Disorder and Intellectual Disability.* Sci Transl Med, 2010. 2(49): p. 49ra68.
[92] Segurado, R., et al., *Confirmation of association between autism and the mitochondrial aspartate/glutamate carrier SLC25A12 gene on chromosome 2q31.* Am J Psychiatry, 2005. 162(11): p. 2182-4.
[93] Cukier, H.N., et al., *Identification of chromosome 7 inversion breakpoints in an autistic family narrows candidate region for autism susceptibility.* Autism Res, 2009. 2(5): p. 258-66.
[94] Sakurai, T., et al., *Association analysis of the NrCAM gene in autism and in subsets of families with severe obsessive-compulsive or self-stimulatory behaviors.* Psychiatr Genet, 2006. 16(6): p. 251-7.
[95] Hutcheson, H.B., et al., *Examination of NRCAM, LRRN3, KIAA0716, and LAMB1 as autism candidate genes.* BMC Med Genet, 2004. 5: p. 12.
[96] Marui, T., et al., *Association of the neuronal cell adhesion molecule (NRCAM) gene variants with autism.* Int J Neuropsychopharmacol, 2009. 12(1): p. 1-10.
[97] Marui, T., et al., *Association between autism and variants in the wingless-type MMTV integration site family member 2 ( WNT2) gene.* Int J Neuropsychopharmacol, 2010. 13(4): p. 443-9.
[98] Barnby, G., et al., *Candidate-gene screening and association analysis at the autism-susceptibility locus on chromosome 16p: evidence of association at GRIN2A and ABAT.* Am J Hum Genet, 2005. 76(6): p. 950-66.
[99] McCauley, J.L., et al., *Genome-wide and Ordered-Subset linkage analyses provide support for autism loci on 17q and 19p with evidence of phenotypic and interlocus genetic correlates.* BMC Med Genet, 2005. 6: p. 1.
[100] Christian, S.L., et al., *Novel submicroscopic chromosomal abnormalities detected in autism spectrum disorder.* Biol Psychiatry, 2008. 63(12): p. 1111-7.
[101] Marshall, C.R., et al., *Structural variation of chromosomes in autism spectrum disorder.* Am J Hum Genet, 2008. 82(2): p. 477-88.
[102] Sebat, J., et al., *Strong association of de novo copy number mutations with autism.* Science, 2007. 316(5823): p. 445-9.
[103] Cho, S.C., et al., *Copy number variations associated with idiopathic autism identified by whole-genome microarray-based comparative genomic hybridization.* Psychiatr Genet, 2009. 19(4): p. 177-85.
[104] Qiao, Y., et al., *Phenomic determinants of genomic variation in autism spectrum disorders.* J Med Genet, 2009. 46(10): p. 680-8.
[105] Cusco, I., et al., *Autism-specific copy number variants further implicate the phosphatidylinositol signaling pathway and the glutamatergic synapse in the etiology of the disorder.* Hum Mol Genet, 2009. 18(10): p. 1795-804.

[106] Babatz, T.D., et al., *Copy number and sequence variants implicate APBA2 as an autism candidate gene.* Autism Res, 2009. 2(6): p. 359-64.

[107] Wang, K., et al., *Common genetic variants on 5p14.1 associate with autism spectrum disorders.* Nature, 2009. 459(7246): p. 528-33.

[108] Pinto, D., et al., *Functional impact of global rare copy number variation in autism spectrum disorders.* Nature, 2010. 466(7304): p. 368-72.

[109] Glessner, J.T., et al., *Autism genome-wide copy number variation reveals ubiquitin and neuronal genes.* Nature, 2009. 459(7246): p. 569-73.

[110] Geschwind, D.H. and P. Levitt, *Autism spectrum disorders: developmental disconnection syndromes.* Curr Opin Neurobiol, 2007. 17(1): p. 103-11.

[111] Li, H., et al., *The association analysis of RELN and GRM8 genes with autistic spectrum disorder in Chinese Han population.* Am J Med Genet B Neuropsychiatr Genet, 2008. 147B(2): p. 194-200.

[112] Ashley-Koch, A.E., et al., *Investigation of potential gene-gene interactions between APOE and RELN contributing to autism risk.* Psychiatr Genet, 2007. 17(4): p. 221-6.

[113] Dutta, S., et al., *Reelin gene polymorphisms in the Indian population: a possible paternal 5'UTR-CGG-repeat-allele effect on autism.* Am J Med Genet B Neuropsychiatr Genet, 2007. 144B(1): p. 106-12.

[114] Serajee, F.J., H. Zhong and H.A. Mahbubul, *Association of Reelin gene polymorphisms with autism.* Genomics, 2006. 87(1): p. 75-83.

[115] Skaar, D.A., et al., *Analysis of the RELN gene as a genetic risk factor for autism.* Mol Psychiatry, 2005. 10(6): p. 563-71.

[116] Devlin, B., et al., *Alleles of a reelin CGG repeat do not convey liability to autism in a sample from the CPEA network.* Am J Med Genet B Neuropsychiatr Genet, 2004. 126B(1): p. 46-50.

[117] Li, J., et al., *Lack of evidence for an association between WNT2 and RELN polymorphisms and autism.* Am J Med Genet B Neuropsychiatr Genet, 2004. 126B(1): p. 51-7.

[118] Zhang, H., et al., *Reelin gene alleles and susceptibility to autism spectrum disorders.* Mol Psychiatry, 2002. 7(9): p. 1012-7.

[119] Krebs, M.O., et al., *Absence of association between a polymorphic GGC repeat in the 5' untranslated region of the reelin gene and autism.* Mol Psychiatry, 2002. 7(7): p. 801-4.

[120] Persico, A.M., et al., *Reelin gene alleles and haplotypes as a factor predisposing to autistic disorder.* Mol Psychiatry, 2001. 6(2): p. 150-9.

[121] Sutcliffe, J.S., et al., *Allelic heterogeneity at the serotonin transporter locus (SLC6A4) confers susceptibility to autism and rigid-compulsive behaviors.* Am J Hum Genet, 2005. 77(2): p. 265-79.

[122] Coutinho, A.M., et al., *Evidence for epistasis between SLC6A4 and ITGB3 in autism etiology and in the determination of platelet serotonin levels.* Hum Genet, 2007. 121(2): p. 243-56.

[123] Jr Cook, E., et al., *Evidence of linkage between the serotonin transporter and autistic disorder.* Mol Psychiatry, 1997. 2(3): p. 247-50.

[124] Anderson, B.M., et al., *Examination of association of genes in the serotonin system to autism.* Neurogenetics, 2009. 10(3): p. 209-16.

[125] Cho, I.H., et al., *Family-based association study of 5-HTTLPR and the 5-HT2A receptor gene polymorphisms with autism spectrum disorder in Korean trios.* Brain Res, 2007. 1139: p. 34-41.

[126] McCauley, J.L., et al., *Linkage and association analysis at the serotonin transporter (SLC6A4) locus in a rigid-compulsive subset of autism.* Am J Med Genet B Neuropsychiatr Genet, 2004. 127B(1): p. 104-12.

[127] Coutinho, A.M., et al., *Variants of the serotonin transporter gene (SLC6A4) significantly contribute to hyperserotonemia in autism.* Mol Psychiatry, 2004. 9(3): p. 264-71.

[128] Zhong, N., et al., *5-HTTLPR variants not associated with autistic spectrum disorders.* Neurogenetics, 1999. 2(2): p. 129-31.

[129] Guhathakurta, S., et al., *Analysis of serotonin receptor 2A gene (HTR2A): association study with autism spectrum disorder in the Indian population and investigation of the gene expression in peripheral blood leukocytes.* Neurochem Int, 2009. 55(8): p. 754-9.

[130] Ma, D.Q., et al., *Association and gene-gene interaction of SLC6A4 and ITGB3 in autism.* Am J Med Genet B Neuropsychiatr Genet, 2010. 153B(2): p. 477-83.

[131] Huang, C.H. and S.L. Santangelo, *Autism and serotonin transporter gene polymorphisms: a systematic review and meta-analysis.* Am J Med Genet B Neuropsychiatr Genet, 2008. 147B(6): p. 903-13.

[132] Persico, A.M., et al., *Lack of association between serotonin transporter gene promoter variants and autistic disorder in two ethnically distinct samples.* Am J Med Genet, 2000. 96(1): p. 123-7.

[133] Wu, S., et al., *Lack of evidence for association between the serotonin transporter gene (SLC6A4) polymorphisms and autism in the Chinese trios.* Neurosci Lett, 2005. 381(1-2): p. 1-5.

[134] Ramoz, N., et al., *Lack of evidence for association of the serotonin transporter gene SLC6A4 with autism.* Biol Psychiatry, 2006. 60(2): p. 186-91.

[135] Guhathakurta, S., et al., *Population-based association study and contrasting linkage disequilibrium pattern reveal genetic association of SLC6A4 with autism in the Indian population from West Bengal.* Brain Res, 2008. 1240: p. 12-21.

[136] Tordjman, S., et al., *Role of the serotonin transporter gene in the behavioral expression of autism.* Mol Psychiatry, 2001. 6(4): p. 434-9.

[137] Maestrini, E., et al., *Serotonin transporter (5-HTT) and gamma-aminobutyric acid receptor subunit beta3 (GABRB3) gene polymorphisms are not associated with autism in the IMGSA families. The International Molecular Genetic Study of Autism Consortium.* Am J Med Genet, 1999. 88(5): p. 492-6.

[138] Klauck, S.M., et al., *Serotonin transporter (5-HTT) gene variants associated with autism?.* Hum Mol Genet, 1997. 6(13): p. 2233-8.

[139] Betancur, C., et al., *Serotonin transporter gene polymorphisms and hyperserotonemia in autistic disorder.* Mol Psychiatry, 2002. 7(1): p. 67-71.

[140] Koishi, S., et al., *Serotonin transporter gene promoter polymorphism and autism: a family-based genetic association study in Japanese population.* Brain Dev, 2006. 28(4): p. 257-60.

[141] Takumi, T., *A humanoid mouse model of autism.* Brain Dev, 2010.

[142] McCauley, J.L., et al., *A linkage disequilibrium map of the 1-Mb 15q12 GABA(A) receptor subunit cluster and association to autism.* Am J Med Genet B Neuropsychiatr Genet, 2004. 131B(1): p. 51-9.

[143] Nakatani, J., et al., *Abnormal behavior in a chromosome-engineered mouse model for human 15q11-13 duplication seen in autism.* Cell, 2009. 137(7): p. 1235-46.

[144] Menold, M.M., et al., *Association analysis of chromosome 15 gabaa receptor subunit genes in autistic disorder.* J Neurogenet, 2001. 15(3-4): p. 245-59.

[145] Buxbaum, J.D., et al., *Association between a GABRB3 polymorphism and autism.* Mol Psychiatry, 2002. 7(3): p. 311-6.
[146] Kim, S.A., et al., *Association of GABRB3 polymorphisms with autism spectrum disorders in Korean trios.* Neuropsychobiology, 2006. 54(3): p. 160-5.
[147] Kwasnicka-Crawford, D.A., W. Roberts and S.W. Scherer, *Characterization of an autism-associated segmental maternal heterodisomy of the chromosome 15q11-13 region.* J Autism Dev Disord, 2007. 37(4): p. 694-702.
[148] Bolton, P.F., et al., *Chromosome 15q11-13 abnormalities and other medical conditions in individuals with autism spectrum disorders.* Psychiatr Genet, 2004. 14(3): p. 131-7.
[149] Shao, Y., et al., *Fine mapping of autistic disorder to chromosome 15q11-q13 by use of phenotypic subtypes.* Am J Hum Genet, 2003. 72(3): p. 539-48.
[150] Ma, D.Q., et al., *Identification of significant association and gene-gene interaction of GABA receptor subunit genes in autism.* Am J Hum Genet, 2005. 77(3): p. 377-88.
[151] Yoo, H.K., et al., *Microsatellite marker in gamma - aminobutyric acid - a receptor beta 3 subunit gene and autism spectrum disorders in Korean trios.* Yonsei Med J, 2009. 50(2): p. 304-6.
[152] Cai, G., et al., *Multiplex ligation-dependent probe amplification for genetic screening in autism spectrum disorders: efficient identification of known microduplications and identification of a novel microduplication in ASMT.* BMC Med Genomics, 2008. 1: p. 50.
[153] Aldinger, K.A. and S. Qiu, *New mouse genetic model duplicates human 15q11-13 autistic phenotypes, or does it?.* Dis Model Mech, 2010. 3(1-2): p. 3-4.
[154] Depienne, C., et al., *Screening for genomic rearrangements and methylation abnormalities of the 15q11-q13 region in autism spectrum disorders.* Biol Psychiatry, 2009. 66(4): p. 349-59.
[155] Curran, S., et al., *An association analysis of microsatellite markers across the Prader-Willi/Angelman critical region on chromosome 15 (q11-13) and autism spectrum disorder.* Am J Med Genet B Neuropsychiatr Genet, 2005. 137B(1): p. 25-8.
[156] Martin, E.R., et al., *Analysis of linkage disequilibrium in gamma-aminobutyric acid receptor subunit genes in autistic disorder.* Am J Med Genet, 2000. 96(1): p. 43-8.
[157] Maestrini, E., et al., *Serotonin transporter (5-HTT) and gamma-aminobutyric acid receptor subunit beta3 (GABRB3) gene polymorphisms are not associated with autism in the IMGSA families. The International Molecular Genetic Study of Autism Consortium.* Am J Med Genet, 1999. 88(5): p. 492-6.
[158] Zhang, C., et al., *A neuroligin-4 missense mutation associated with autism impairs neuroligin-4 folding and endoplasmic reticulum export.* J Neurosci, 2009. 29(35): p. 10843-54.
[159] Pampanos, A., et al., *A substitution involving the NLGN4 gene associated with autistic behavior in the Greek population.* Genet Test Mol Biomarkers, 2009. 13(5): p. 611-5.
[160] Yan, J., et al., *Analysis of the neuroligin 4Y gene in patients with autism.* Psychiatr Genet, 2008. 18(4): p. 204-7.
[161] Talebizadeh, Z., et al., *Novel splice isoforms for NLGN3 and NLGN4 with possible implications in autism.* J Med Genet, 2006. 43(5): p. e21.
[162] Yan, J., et al., *Analysis of the neuroligin 3 and 4 genes in autism and other neuropsychiatric patients.* Mol Psychiatry, 2005. 10(4): p. 329-32.
[163] Jamain, S., et al., *Mutations of the X-linked genes encoding neuroligins NLGN3 and NLGN4 are associated with autism.* Nat Genet, 2003. 34(1): p. 27-9.

[164] Wermter, A.K., et al., *No evidence for involvement of genetic variants in the X-linked neuroligin genes NLGN3 and NLGN4X in probands with autism spectrum disorder on high functioning level.* Am J Med Genet B Neuropsychiatr Genet, 2008. 147B(4): p. 535-7.

[165] Blasi, F., et al., *Absence of coding mutations in the X-linked genes neuroligin 3 and neuroligin 4 in individuals with autism from the IMGSAC collection.* Am J Med Genet B Neuropsychiatr Genet, 2006. 141B(3): p. 220-1.

[166] Ylisaukko-oja, T., et al., *Analysis of four neuroligin genes as candidates for autism.* Eur J Hum Genet, 2005. 13(12): p. 1285-92.

[167] Gauthier, J., et al., *NLGN3/NLGN4 gene mutations are not responsible for autism in the Quebec population.* Am J Med Genet B Neuropsychiatr Genet, 2005. 132B(1): p. 74-5.

[168] Vincent, J.B., et al., *Mutation screening of X-chromosomal neuroligin genes: no mutations in 196 autism probands.* Am J Med Genet B Neuropsychiatr Genet, 2004. 129B(1): p. 82-4.

[169] Talebizadeh, Z., et al., *Do known mutations in neuroligin genes (NLGN3 and NLGN4) cause autism?.* J Autism Dev Disord, 2004. 34(6): p. 735-6.

[170] Liu, X., et al., *Association of the oxytocin receptor (OXTR) gene polymorphisms with autism spectrum disorder (ASD) in the Japanese population.* J Hum Genet, 2010. 55(3): p. 137-41.

[171] Gregory, S.G., et al., *Genomic and epigenetic evidence for oxytocin receptor deficiency in autism.* BMC Med, 2009. 7: p. 62.

[172] Lerer, E., et al., *Association between the oxytocin receptor (OXTR) gene and autism: relationship to Vineland Adaptive Behavior Scales and cognition.* Mol Psychiatry, 2008. 13(10): p. 980-8.

[173] Jacob, S., et al., *Association of the oxytocin receptor gene (OXTR) in Caucasian children and adolescents with autism.* Neurosci Lett, 2007. 417(1): p. 6-9.

[174] Wu, S., et al., *Positive association of the oxytocin receptor gene (OXTR) with autism in the Chinese Han population.* Biol Psychiatry, 2005. 58(1): p. 74-7.

[175] Campbell, D.B., et al., *Association of MET with social and communication phenotypes in individuals with autism spectrum disorder.* Am J Med Genet B Neuropsychiatr Genet, 2010. 153B(2): p. 438-46.

[176] Jackson, P.B., et al., *Further evidence that the rs1858830 C variant in the promoter region of the MET gene is associated with autistic disorder.* Autism Res, 2009. 2(4): p. 232-6.

[177] Sousa, I., et al., *MET and autism susceptibility: family and case-control studies.* Eur J Hum Genet, 2009. 17(6): p. 749-58.

[178] Campbell, D.B., et al., *Genetic evidence implicating multiple genes in the MET receptor tyrosine kinase pathway in autism spectrum disorder.* Autism Res, 2008. 1(3): p. 159-68.

[179] Campbell, D.B., et al., *A genetic variant that disrupts MET transcription is associated with autism.* Proc Natl Acad Sci U S A, 2006. 103(45): p. 16834-9.

[180] Turunen, J.A., et al., *Mitochondrial aspartate/glutamate carrier SLC25A12 gene is associated with autism.* Autism Res, 2008. 1(3): p. 189-92.

[181] Silverman, J.M., et al., *Autism-related routines and rituals associated with a mitochondrial aspartate/glutamate carrier SLC25A12 polymorphism.* Am J Med Genet B Neuropsychiatr Genet, 2008. 147(3): p. 408-10.

[182] Segurado, R., et al., *Confirmation of association between autism and the mitochondrial aspartate/glutamate carrier SLC25A12 gene on chromosome 2q31.* Am J Psychiatry, 2005. 162(11): p. 2182-4.

[183] Ramoz, N., et al., *Linkage and association of the mitochondrial aspartate/glutamate carrier SLC25A12 gene with autism.* Am J Psychiatry, 2004. 161(4): p. 662-9.
[184] Chien, W.H., et al., *Association study of the SLC25A12 gene and autism in Han Chinese in Taiwan.* Prog Neuropsychopharmacol Biol Psychiatry, 2010. 34(1): p. 189-92.
[185] Rabionet, R., et al., *Lack of association between autism and SLC25A12.* Am J Psychiatry, 2006. 163(5): p. 929-31.
[186] Blasi, F., et al., *SLC25A12 and CMYA3 gene variants are not associated with autism in the IMGSAC multiplex family sample.* Eur J Hum Genet, 2006. 14(1): p. 123-6.
[187] Kim, S.A., et al., *Family-based association study between GRIK2 polymorphisms and autism spectrum disorders in the Korean trios.* Neurosci Res, 2007. 58(3): p. 332-5.
[188] Shuang, M., et al., *Family-based association study between autism and glutamate receptor 6 gene in Chinese Han trios.* Am J Med Genet B Neuropsychiatr Genet, 2004. 131B(1): p. 48-50.
[189] Jamain, S., et al., *Linkage and association of the glutamate receptor 6 gene with autism.* Mol Psychiatry, 2002. 7(3): p. 302-10.
[190] Dutta, S., et al., *Glutamate receptor 6 gene (GluR6 or GRIK2) polymorphisms in the Indian population: a genetic association study on autism spectrum disorder.* Cell Mol Neurobiol, 2007. 27(8): p. 1035-47.
[191] Poot, M., et al., *Disruption of CNTNAP2 and additional structural genome changes in a boy with speech delay and autism spectrum disorder.* Neurogenetics, 2010. 11(1): p. 81-9.
[192] Arking, D.E., et al., *A common genetic variant in the neurexin superfamily member CNTNAP2 increases familial risk of autism.* Am J Hum Genet, 2008. 82(1): p. 160-4.
[193] Alarcon, M., et al., *Linkage, association, and gene-expression analyses identify CNTNAP2 as an autism-susceptibility gene.* Am J Hum Genet, 2008. 82(1): p. 150-9.
[194] Bakkaloglu, B., et al., *Molecular cytogenetic analysis and resequencing of contactin associated protein-like 2 in autism spectrum disorders.* Am J Hum Genet, 2008. 82(1): p. 165-73.
[195] Rossi, E., et al., *A 12Mb deletion at 7q33-q35 associated with autism spectrum disorders and primary amenorrhea.* Eur J Med Genet, 2008. 51(6): p. 631-8.
[196] Strauss, K.A., et al., *Recessive symptomatic focal epilepsy and mutant contactin-associated protein-like 2.* N Engl J Med, 2006. 354(13): p. 1370-7.
[197] Sacco, R., et al., *Case-control and family-based association studies of candidate genes in autistic disorder and its endophenotypes: TPH2 and GLO1.* BMC Med Genet, 2007. 8: p. 11.
[198] Junaid, M.A., et al., *Proteomic studies identified a single nucleotide polymorphism in glyoxalase I as autism susceptibility factor.* Am J Med Genet A, 2004. 131(1): p. 11-7.
[199] Wu, Y.Y., et al., *Lack of evidence to support the glyoxalase 1 gene (GLO1) as a risk gene of autism in Han Chinese patients from Taiwan.* Prog Neuropsychopharmacol Biol Psychiatry, 2008. 32(7): p. 1740-4.
[200] Rehnstrom, K., et al., *No association between common variants in glyoxalase 1 and autism spectrum disorders.* Am J Med Genet B Neuropsychiatr Genet, 2008. 147B(1): p. 124-7.
[201] Coon, H., et al., *Possible association between autism and variants in the brain-expressed tryptophan hydroxylase gene (TPH2).* Am J Med Genet B Neuropsychiatr Genet, 2005. 135B(1): p. 42-6.
[202] Ramoz, N., et al., *Family-based association study of TPH1 and TPH2 polymorphisms in autism.* Am J Med Genet B Neuropsychiatr Genet, 2006. 141B(8): p. 861-7.
[203] Goffinet, A.M., *Events governing organization of postmigratory neurons: studies on brain development in normal and reeler mice.* Brain Res, 1984. 319(3): p. 261-96.

[204] Goffinet, A.M., *The embryonic development of the cerebellum in normal and reeler mutant mice.* Anat Embryol (Berl), 1983. 168(1): p. 73-86.
[205] Goffinet, A.M., *The embryonic development of the inferior olivary complex in normal and reeler (rlORL) mutant mice.* J Comp Neurol, 1983. 219(1): p. 10-24.
[206] D'Arcangelo, G., et al., *A protein related to extracellular matrix proteins deleted in the mouse mutant reeler.* Nature, 1995. 374(6524): p. 719-23.
[207] Del, R.J., et al., *A role for Cajal-Retzius cells and reelin in the development of hippocampal connections.* Nature, 1997. 385(6611): p. 70-4.
[208] Curran, T. and G. D'Arcangelo, *Role of reelin in the control of brain development.* Brain Res Brain Res Rev, 1998. 26(2-3): p. 285-94.
[209] Bailey, A., et al., *A clinicopathological study of autism.* Brain, 1998. 121 ( Pt 5): p. 889-905.
[210] Fatemi, S.H., et al., *Dysregulation of Reelin and Bcl-2 proteins in autistic cerebellum.* J Autism Dev Disord, 2001. 31(6): p. 529-35.
[211] Fatemi, S.H., J.M. Stary and E.A. Egan, *Reduced blood levels of reelin as a vulnerability factor in pathophysiology of autistic disorder.* Cell Mol Neurobiol, 2002. 22(2): p. 139-52.
[212] Fatemi, S.H., et al., *Reelin signaling is impaired in autism.* Biol Psychiatry, 2005. 57(7): p. 777-87.
[213] Scherer, S.W., et al., *Human chromosome 7: DNA sequence and biology.* Science, 2003. 300(5620): p. 767-72.
[214] Ramamoorthy, S., et al., *Antidepressant- and cocaine-sensitive human serotonin transporter: molecular cloning, expression, and chromosomal localization.* Proc Natl Acad Sci U S A, 1993. 90(6): p. 2542-6.
[215] Kim, S.J., et al., *Transmission disequilibrium mapping at the serotonin transporter gene (SLC6A4) region in autistic disorder.* Mol Psychiatry, 2002. 7(3): p. 278-88.
[216] McDougle, C.J., et al., *A double-blind, placebo-controlled study of fluvoxamine in adults with autistic disorder.* Arch Gen Psychiatry, 1996. 53(11): p. 1001-8.
[217] Guhathakurta, S., et al., *Serotonin transporter promoter variants: Analysis in Indian autistic and control population.* Brain Res, 2006. 1092(1): p. 28-35.
[218] Jr Cook, E., et al., *Linkage-disequilibrium mapping of autistic disorder, with 15q11-13 markers.* Am J Hum Genet, 1998. 62(5): p. 1077-83.
[219] Lucht, M.J., et al., *Associations between the oxytocin receptor gene (OXTR) and affect, loneliness and intelligence in normal subjects.* Prog Neuropsychopharmacol Biol Psychiatry, 2009. 33(5): p. 860-6.
[220] Yamasue, H., et al., *Oxytocin, sexually dimorphic features of the social brain, and autism.* Psychiatry Clin Neurosci, 2009. 63(2): p. 129-40.
[221] Green, J.J. and E. Hollander, *Autism and oxytocin: new developments in translational approaches to therapeutics.* Neurotherapeutics, 2010. 7(3): p. 250-7.
[222] Powell, E.M., W.M. Mars and P. Levitt, *Hepatocyte growth factor/scatter factor is a motogen for interneurons migrating from the ventral to dorsal telencephalon.* Neuron, 2001. 30(1): p. 79-89.
[223] Streit, A.C. and C.D. Stern, *Competence for neural induction: HGF/SF, HGF1/MSP and the c-Met receptor.* Ciba Found Symp, 1997. 212: p. 155-65; discussion 165-8.
[224] Park, M., et al., *Mechanism of met oncogene activation.* Cell, 1986. 45(6): p. 895-904.
[225] Levitt, P., K.L. Eagleson and E.M. Powell, *Regulation of neocortical interneuron development and the implications for neurodevelopmental disorders.* Trends Neurosci, 2004. 27(7): p. 400-6.
[226] Campbell, D.B., et al., *Disruption of cerebral cortex MET signaling in autism spectrum disorder.* Ann Neurol, 2007. 62(3): p. 243-50.

[227] Del, A.A. and J. Satrustegui, *Molecular cloning of Aralar, a new member of the mitochondrial carrier superfamily that binds calcium and is present in human muscle and brain.* J Biol Chem, 1998. 273(36): p. 23327-34.
[228] Filipek, P.A., et al., *Mitochondrial dysfunction in autistic patients with 15q inverted duplication.* Ann Neurol, 2003. 53(6): p. 801-4.
[229] Shimizu, E., et al., *NMDA receptor-dependent synaptic reinforcement as a crucial process for memory consolidation.* Science, 2000. 290(5494): p. 1170-4.
[230] Burbach, J.P. and B. van der Zwaag, *Contact in the genetics of autism and schizophrenia.* Trends Neurosci, 2009. 32(2): p. 69-72.
[231] Beversdorf, D.Q., et al., *Timing of prenatal stressors and autism.* J Autism Dev Disord, 2005. 35(4): p. 471-8.
[232] Meyer, U., et al., *The time of prenatal immune challenge determines the specificity of inflammation-mediated brain and behavioral pathology.* J Neurosci, 2006. 26(18): p. 4752-62.
[233] Ploeger, A., et al., *The association between autism and errors in early embryogenesis: what is the causal mechanism?.* Biol Psychiatry, 2010. 67(7): p. 602-7.
[234] Stromland, K., et al., *Autism in thalidomide embryopathy: a population study.* Dev Med Child Neurol, 1994. 36(4): p. 351-6.
[235] Williams, G., et al., *Fetal valproate syndrome and autism: additional evidence of an association.* Dev Med Child Neurol, 2001. 43(3): p. 202-6.
[236] Rasalam, A.D., et al., *Characteristics of fetal anticonvulsant syndrome associated autistic disorder.* Dev Med Child Neurol, 2005. 47(8): p. 551-5.
[237] Kannan, S., et al., *Decreased cortical serotonin in neonatal rabbits exposed to endotoxin in utero.* J Cereb Blood Flow Metab, 2010.
[238] Girard, S., et al., *IL-1 receptor antagonist protects against placental and neurodevelopmental defects induced by maternal inflammation.* J Immunol, 2010. 184(7): p. 3997-4005.
[239] Wilkerson, D.S., et al., *Perinatal complications as predictors of infantile autism.* Int J Neurosci, 2002. 112(9): p. 1085-98.
[240] Palmer, R.F., et al., *Environmental mercury release, special education rates, and autism disorder: an ecological study of Texas.* Health Place, 2006. 12(2): p. 203-9.
[241] Windham, G.C., et al., *Autism spectrum disorders in relation to distribution of hazardous air pollutants in the san francisco bay area.* Environ Health Perspect, 2006. 114(9): p. 1438-44.
[242] Geier, D.A. and M.R. Geier, *A prospective study of mercury toxicity biomarkers in autistic spectrum disorders.* J Toxicol Environ Health A, 2007. 70(20): p. 1723-30.
[243] Geier, D.A., et al., *A comprehensive review of mercury provoked autism.* Indian J Med Res, 2008. 128(4): p. 383-411.
[244] Geier, D.A., et al., *Blood mercury levels in autism spectrum disorder: Is there a threshold level?.* Acta Neurobiol Exp (Wars), 2010. 70(2): p. 177-86.
[245] Ip, P., et al., *Mercury exposure in children with autistic spectrum disorder: case-control study.* J Child Neurol, 2004. 19(6): p. 431-4.
[246] Eppright, T.D., J.A. Sanfacon and E.A. Horwitz, *Attention deficit hyperactivity disorder, infantile autism, and elevated blood-lead: a possible relationship.* Mo Med, 1996. 93(3): p. 136-8.
[247] Canfield, R.L., et al., *Intellectual impairment in children with blood lead concentrations below 10 microg per deciliter.* N Engl J Med, 2003. 348(16): p. 1517-26.
[248] Yorbik, O., et al., *Chromium, cadmium, and lead levels in urine of children with autism and typically developing controls.* Biol Trace Elem Res, 2010. 135(1-3): p. 10-5.

[249] Kalkbrenner, A.E., et al., *Perinatal exposure to hazardous air pollutants and autism spectrum disorders at age 8.* Epidemiology, 2010. 21(5): p. 631-41.
[250] Moy, S.S. and J.J. Nadler, *Advances in behavioral genetics: mouse models of autism.* Mol Psychiatry, 2008. 13(1): p. 4-26.
[251] Mineur, Y.S., L.X. Huynh and W.E. Crusio, *Social behavior deficits in the Fmr1 mutant mouse.* Behav Brain Res, 2006. 168(1): p. 172-5.
[252] Zoghbi, H.Y., *MeCP2 dysfunction in humans and mice.* J Child Neurol, 2005. 20(9): p. 736-40.
[253] Kuemerle, B., et al., *The mouse Engrailed genes: a window into autism.* Behav Brain Res, 2007. 176(1): p. 121-32.
[254] Cheh, M.A., et al., *En2 knockout mice display neurobehavioral and neurochemical alterations relevant to autism spectrum disorder.* Brain Res, 2006. 1116(1): p. 166-76.
[255] Andres, C., *Molecular genetics and animal models in autistic disorder.* Brain Res Bull, 2002. 57(1): p. 109-19.
[256] Brodkin, E.S., *BALB/c mice: low sociability and other phenotypes that may be relevant to autism.* Behav Brain Res, 2007. 176(1): p. 53-65.
[257] Brodkin, E.S., et al., *Social approach-avoidance behavior of inbred mouse strains towards DBA/2 mice.* Brain Res, 2004. 1002(1-2): p. 151-7.
[258] Moy, S.S., et al., *Sociability and preference for social novelty in five inbred strains: an approach to assess autistic-like behavior in mice.* Genes Brain Behav, 2004. 3(5): p. 287-302.
[259] Yang, M., A.M. Clarke and J.N. Crawley, *Postnatal lesion evidence against a primary role for the corpus callosum in mouse sociability.* Eur J Neurosci, 2009. 29(8): p. 1663-77.
[260] Wahlsten, D., P. Metten and J.C. Crabbe, *Survey of 21 inbred mouse strains in two laboratories reveals that BTBR T/+ tf/tf has severely reduced hippocampal commissure and absent corpus callosum.* Brain Res, 2003. 971(1): p. 47-54.
[261] Kusek, G.K., et al., *Localization of two new X-linked quantitative trait loci controlling corpus callosum size in the mouse.* Genes Brain Behav, 2007. 6(4): p. 359-63.
[262] MacPherson, P., et al., *Impaired fear memory, altered object memory and modified hippocampal synaptic plasticity in split-brain mice.* Brain Res, 2008. 1210: p. 179-88.
[263] Hudkins, K.L., et al., *BTBR Ob/Ob mutant mice model progressive diabetic nephropathy.* J Am Soc Nephrol, 2010. 21(9): p. 1533-42.
[264] Flowers, J.B., et al., *Abdominal obesity in BTBR male mice is associated with peripheral but not hepatic insulin resistance.* Am J Physiol Endocrinol Metab, 2007. 292(3): p. E936-45.
[265] Lan, H., et al., *Distinguishing covariation from causation in diabetes: a lesson from the protein disulfide isomerase mRNA abundance trait.* Diabetes, 2004. 53(1): p. 240-4.
[266] Nadler, S.T., et al., *Normal Akt/PKB with reduced PI3K activation in insulin-resistant mice.* Am J Physiol Endocrinol Metab, 2001. 281(6): p. E1249-54.
[267] Stoehr, J.P., et al., *Genetic obesity unmasks nonlinear interactions between murine type 2 diabetes susceptibility loci.* Diabetes, 2000. 49(11): p. 1946-54.
[268] Ranheim, T., et al., *Interaction between BTBR and C57BL/6J genomes produces an insulin resistance syndrome in (BTBR x C57BL/6J) F1 mice.* Arterioscler Thromb Vasc Biol, 1997. 17(11): p. 3286-93.
[269] Gersting, S.W., et al., *Pahenu1 is a mouse model for tetrahydrobiopterin-responsive phenylalanine hydroxylase deficiency and promotes analysis of the pharmacological chaperone mechanism in vivo.* Hum Mol Genet, 2010. 19(10): p. 2039-49.

[270] Martynyuk, A.E., et al., *Epilepsy in phenylketonuria: a complex dependence on serum phenylalanine levels.* Epilepsia, 2007. 48(6): p. 1143-50.
[271] Ercal, N., et al., *Oxidative stress in a phenylketonuria animal model.* Free Radic Biol Med, 2002. 32(9): p. 906-11.
[272] McDonald, J.D., *Postnatal growth in a mouse genetic model of classical phenylketonuria.* Contemp Top Lab Anim Sci, 2000. 39(6): p. 54-6.
[273] Sarkissian, C.N., et al., *A heteroallelic mutant mouse model: A new orthologue for human hyperphenylalaninemia.* Mol Genet Metab, 2000. 69(3): p. 188-94.
[274] Zagreda, L., et al., *Cognitive deficits in a genetic mouse model of the most common biochemical cause of human mental retardation.* J Neurosci, 1999. 19(14): p. 6175-82.
[275] Pobbe, R.L., et al., *General and social anxiety in the BTBR T+ tf/J mouse strain.* Behav Brain Res, 2010.
[276] Pobbe, R.L., et al., *Expression of social behaviors of C57BL/6J versus BTBR inbred mouse strains in the visible burrow system.* Behav Brain Res, 2010. 214(2): p. 443-9.
[277] Wohr, M., F.I. Roullet and J.N. Crawley, *Reduced scent marking and ultrasonic vocalizations in the BTBR T+tf/J mouse model of autism.* Genes Brain Behav, 2010.
[278] Roullet, F.I., M. Wohr and J.N. Crawley, *Female urine-induced male mice ultrasonic vocalizations, but not scent-marking, is modulated by social experience.* Behav Brain Res, 2010.
[279] Scattoni, M.L., L. Ricceri and J.N. Crawley, *Unusual repertoire of vocalizations in adult BTBR T+tf/J mice during three types of social encounters.* Genes Brain Behav, 2010.
[280] Pearson, B.L., et al., *Motor and cognitive stereotypies in the BTBR T+tf/J mouse model of autism.* Genes Brain Behav, 2010.
[281] McFarlane, H.G., et al., *Autism-like behavioral phenotypes in BTBR T+tf/J mice.* Genes Brain Behav, 2008. 7(2): p. 152-63.
[282] Moy, S.S., et al., *Mouse behavioral tasks relevant to autism: phenotypes of 10 inbred strains.* Behav Brain Res, 2007. 176(1): p. 4-20.
[283] Silverman, J.L., et al., *Low stress reactivity and neuroendocrine factors in the BTBR T(+)tf/J mouse model of autism.* Neuroscience, 2010.
[284] Frye, C.A. and D.C. Llaneza, *Corticosteroid and neurosteroid dysregulation in an animal model of autism, BTBR mice.* Physiol Behav, 2010. 100(3): p. 264-7.
[285] Chadman, K.K., *Fluoxetine but not risperidone increases sociability in the BTBR mouse model of autism.* Pharmacol Biochem Behav, 2010.
[286] Gould, G.G., et al., *Density and Function of Central Serotonin (5-HT) Transporters, 5-HT(1A) and 5-HT(2A) Receptors, and Effects of their Targeting on BTBR T+tf/J Mouse Social Behavior.* J Neurochem, 2010.
[287] Silverman, J.L., et al., *Repetitive self-grooming behavior in the BTBR mouse model of autism is blocked by the mGluR5 antagonist MPEP.* Neuropsychopharmacology, 2010. 35(4): p. 976-89.
[288] Yang, M., et al., *Social peers rescue autism-relevant sociability deficits in adolescent mice.* Autism Res, 2010.
[289] Yang, M., V. Zhodzishsky and J.N. Crawley, *Social deficits in BTBR T+tf/J mice are unchanged by cross-fostering with C57BL/6J mothers.* Int J Dev Neurosci, 2007. 25(8): p. 515-21.
[290] Crawley, J.N., *Designing mouse behavioral tasks relevant to autistic-like behaviors.* Ment Retard Dev Disabil Res Rev, 2004. 10(4): p. 248-58.

27

# Chronobiology of and Chronotherapy for Rheumatoid Arthritis

Hideto To
*University of Toyama*
*Japan*

## 1. Introduction

Most humans have a relatively regular activity pattern (sleep, labor, and meal etc.). This activity can be roughly classified into the rest phase and active phase, and body temperature, heart rate, blood pressure, and the dominance of the sympathetic and parasympathetic nerves differ in each phase. These variations display daily rhythms, which are known as circadian rhythms.

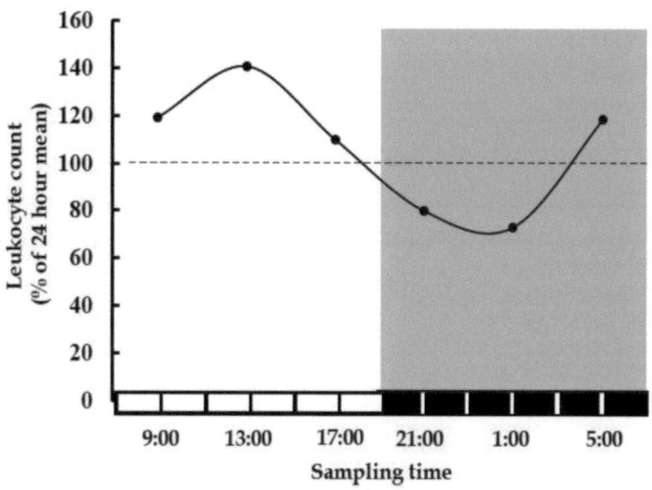


Fig. 1. Circadian rhythm of mouse leukocyte count

For instance, ICR mice, which were housed under standardized light-dark cycle conditions (lights-on and lights-off at 7:00 and 19:00, respectively) at a room temperature of 24 ± 1°C (range) and a relative humidity of 60 ± 10% (range) and were allowed free access to food and water displayed a circadian rhythm in their leukocyte counts with a peak at noon and a trough at midnight (Fig. 1). Many organisms display rhythms in various factors (Table 1). In humans, heart rate and blood pressure decline at night. We spend much of our time in a standing position during the day and sleep in a recumbent position at night. It is thought that the wake-sleep transition and endogenous circadian rhythms are responsible for the circadian rhythms in heart rate and blood pressure. Circadian rhythms also exist for the levels of hormones such as cortisol and melatonin (MLT). The plasma level of cortisol peaks in the morning and that of MLT peaks at midnight. Bone marrow cells, intestinal mucosal cells, and hair matrix cells show relatively active cell division. In the day, there is also a period of time when the number of cells is actively increased by segmentation (DNA synthesis) as well as a period of dormancy. The circadian rhythm of bone marrow cell division involves a peak in the evening and a trough in the midnight, and that of rectal mucosal cell division is higher at 7:00 and lower at 19:00. Thus, various factors in the living body have their own circadian rhythms, and the phases of these cycles vary for each factor.

| No. | Factors | Peak period | Trough period | Ref |
|---|---|---|---|---|
| 1 | Body temperature | 18:00-20:00 | 3:00-6:00 | Lack et al., 2008 |
| 2 | Heart rate | 8:00-18:00 | 4:00-6:00 | Clarke et al., 1976 |
| 3 | Blood pressure | 8:00-20:00 | 0:00-6:00 | Degaute et al., 1991 |
| 4 | Hepatic blood flow | 8:00 | 14:00 | Lemmer et al., 1991 |
| 5 | Glomerular filtration | 16:00 | 4:00 | Koopman et al., 1989 |
| 6 | Lymphocytes | 12:00-17:00 | 7:00 | Miyawaki et al., 1984 |
| 7 | Cortisol<br>Adiponectin<br>Leptin-binding protein | 8:00-13:00<br>8:00-13:00<br>8:00-14:00 | 0:00-4:00<br>2:00-4:00<br>1:00-5:00 | Gavrila et al., 2003 |
| 8 | Melatonin | 2:00-4:00 | 9:00-21:00 | Kennaway et al., 1998 |
| 9 | DNA synthesis in the bone marrow | 16:00 | 0:00 | Smaaland et al., 1991 |
| 10 | DNA synthesis in the rectal mucosa | 7:00 | 19:00 | Buchi et al., 1991 |

Table 1. Circadian rhythms of various factors in humans

| No. | Factors | Peak period | Trough period | Ref |
|---|---|---|---|---|
| 1 | Spontaneous acute dissection and rupture of the thoracic aorta | 7:00-12:00 | 22:00-6:00 | Gallerani et al., 1997 |
| 2 | Myocardial ischemia | 8:00 | 0:00-4:00 | Egstrup et al., 1991 |
| 3 | Ischemic stroke | 8:00 | 18:00-6:00 | Argentino et al., 1990 |
| 4 | Subarachnoid hemorrhage | 6:00-20:00 | 0:00-4:00 | Vermeer et al., 1997 |
| 5 | Asthma | 2:00-5:00 | 7:00-19:00 | Dethlefsen et al., 1985 |
| 6 | Temporal lobe epilepsy | 15:00-21:00 | 0:00-5:00 | Quigg et al., 1998 |
| 7 | Pain sensitivity in teeth | 4:00-7:00 | 11:00-17:00 | Pöllmann et al., 1978 |
| 8 | Migraine | 4:00-10:00 | 21:00-1:00 | Fox et al., 1998 |
| 9 | Stiffness, pain, and functional disability in rheumatoid arthritis | 3:00-7:00 | 13:00-21:00 | Straub et al., 2007 |

Table 2. Circadian rhythms in the risk or frequency of disease occurrence

These circadian rhythms are also associated with the risk or frequency of disease occurrence (Table 2). For example, asthma attacks get worse between midnight and early morning and are seldom observed in the daytime (Fig.2; Dethlefsen et al., 1985). In addition, the risks of spontaneous acute dissection and rupture of the thoracic aorta, myocardial ischemia, ischemic stroke, and subarachnoid hemorrhage are higher during the active phase than during the rest phase. The variations in heart rate, blood pressure, and blood flow, etc., induced by the wake-sleep transition are considered to affect the risk of such problems occurring. Interestingly, pain such as toothache, migraine, and rheumatoid arthritis pain is more acute in the early morning. Collectively, circadian rhythms are recognized in many diseases, and certain time periods are associated with a high risk or frequency of disease occurrence.

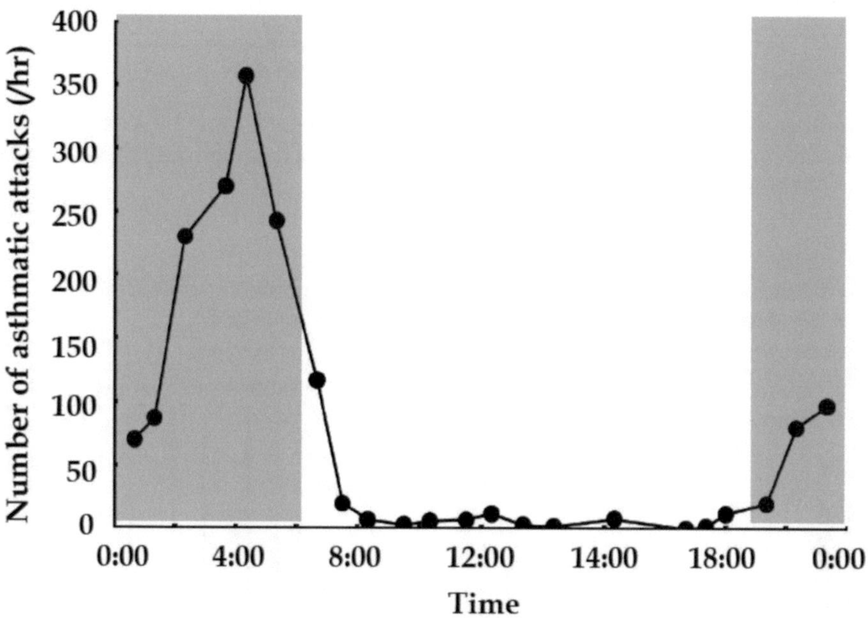


Fig. 2. Circadian rhythm of asthmatic attacks in asthma patients (redrawn from the data of Dethlefsen et al., 1985)

Chronotherapy is defined as the administration of medications in accordance with biological rhythms in order to optimize therapeutic outcomes and/or control adverse effects, and it has been reported that many drugs such as antitumor drugs, antidepressants, and analgesic drugs show rhythm-dependent differences in their effects and pharmacokinetics (Tabuchi et al., 2005; Ushijima et al., 2005; Tampellini et al., 1998). These effects arise from the circadian rhythms found in elements of cellular physiology such as the cell cycle and the expression of receptors, hormones, and enzymes (Iurisci et al., 2006; Matsunaga et al., 2004; Koyanagi et al., 2006). Fig. 3 displays data for the dosing time-dependency of vomiting episodes in urogenital cancer patients treated with cisplatin (Kobayashi et al., 2001). Cisplatin (70 mg/m$^2$) was given to the patients at 5:00 or 17:00. After the cisplatin administration, all episodes of vomiting during a 6-hour period were recorded. Vomiting was markedly decreased in the patients treated at 17:00 compared with that at 5:00 ($P$ = 0.061).

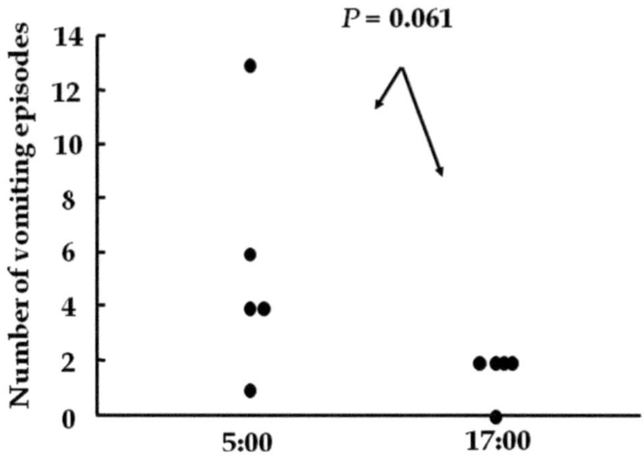


Fig. 3. Number of vomiting episodes according to the time (5:00 vs 17:00) of cisplatin administration in patients with urogenital cancer (redrawn from the data of Kobayashi et al., 2001)

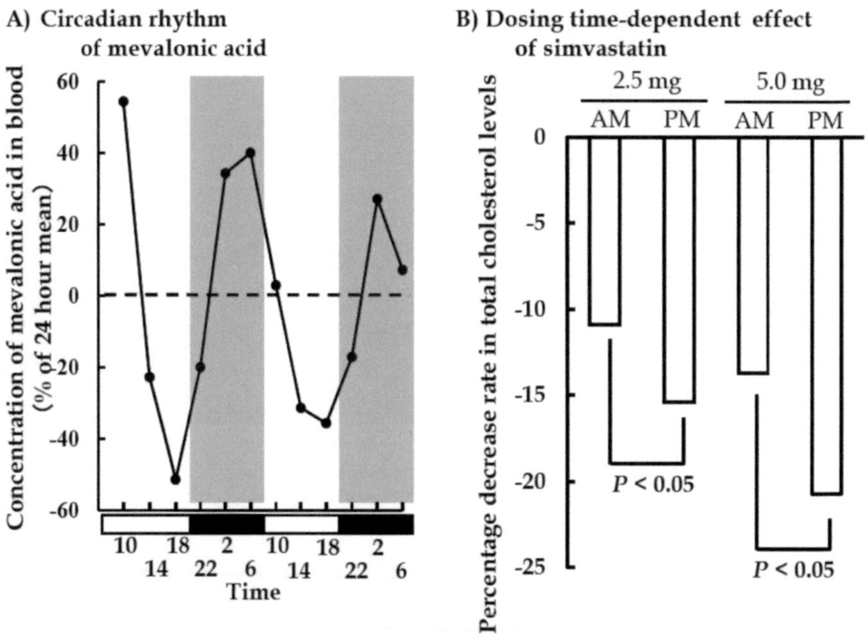


Fig. 4. Circadian rhythm of plasma mevalonic acid levels and the influence of simvastatin dosing time on total cholesterol levels (redrawn from the data of Jones et al., 1992, and Saito et al., 1991)

Moreover, it has been reported that circadian rhythms exist for asthma attacks and cholesterol synthesis, and medicinal treatment based on chronotherapy has been actively applied to the treatment of asthma, hypertension, and hyperlipidemia (D'Alonzo et al., 1995;

Hermida et al., 2010; Haus, 2007; Saito et al., 1991; Smolensky et al., 2007). Hydroxymethyl glutaryl coenzyme A (HMGCoA) reductase participates in the biosynthesis of mevalonic acid and is the rate-limiting enzyme of cholesterol biosynthesis. The plasma mevalonic acid levels in healthy volunteers showed a clear circadian rhythm, with higher levels seen at night and lower levels observed at daytime (Fig. 4A). Simvastatin is an HMGCoA reductase inhibitor. When simvastatin was administered to hyperlipidemic patients once a day in the morning or evening, the evening group displayed a significantly decreased total cholesterol level compared with the morning group (Fig. 4B). Thus, cholesterol biosynthesis may be effectively inhibited when simvastatin is administered in the evening, when the activity of HMGCoA reductase begins to increase.

Taken together, many organisms display circadian rhythms in various factors, and chronotherapy that takes into account circadian rhythms is thought to be a useful therapeutic method.

## 2. Chronobiology of rheumatoid arthritis

Rheumatoid arthritis (RA) is an autoimmune disorder of unknown etiology and a chronic progressive disease that reduces the quality of life of individuals that suffer from the condition (Harris ED Jr., 1990; Gabriel SE., 2001). Although many requirements must be met to establish a diagnosis of RA, morning stiffness is a characteristic feature of RA (Arnett et al., 1988). Tumor necrosis factor-α (TNF-α), interleukin-1β (IL-1β), and interleukin-6 (IL-6), which are inflammatory cytokines, show high concentrations in human blood and synovial fluid, and excess production of these cytokines plays a central role in the pathogenesis of RA (Feldmann et al., 1996; McInnes et al., 2005). Morning stiffness shows a circadian rhythm with a peak in the early morning in RA patients. The IL-6 concentration in blood also shows a circadian rhythm peaking from midnight to early morning, which mirrors the timing of morning stiffness (Crofford et al., 1997).

In this chapter, I would like to introduce the circadian rhythm of rheumatoid arthritis and its mechanism.

### 2.1 Circadian rhythm of rheumatoid arthritis

RA is an autoimmune disorder of unknown etiology, and morning stiffness is a characteristic of the condition (Arnett et al., 1988). Pain, functional disability, and stiffness show circadian rhythms with a peak in the early morning in many RA patients (Fig. 5) (Bellamy et al., 1991; Kowanko et al., 1982), and the circadian rhythms of pain and stiffness may play a role in local and systemic inflammatory responses. Herold and Günther (Herold et al., 1987) reported that plasma C-reactive protein (CRP) levels, an indicator of inflammatory responses, showed a circadian rhythm with a peak in the early morning and a trough in the evening in RA patients, which matches the rhythms of pain and stiffness. Proinflammatory cytokines, such as TNF-α and IL-6, are secreted from activated monocytes, and macrophages increase CRP levels in hepatocytes. There are clear circadian rhythms in the blood concentrations of these cytokines, with higher levels seen in the early morning in RA patients (Crofford et al., 1997; Perry et al., 2009). Since the circadian rhythms of CRP and cytokines are similar, it is considered that cytokine rhythms contribute to the rhythm of CRP levels.

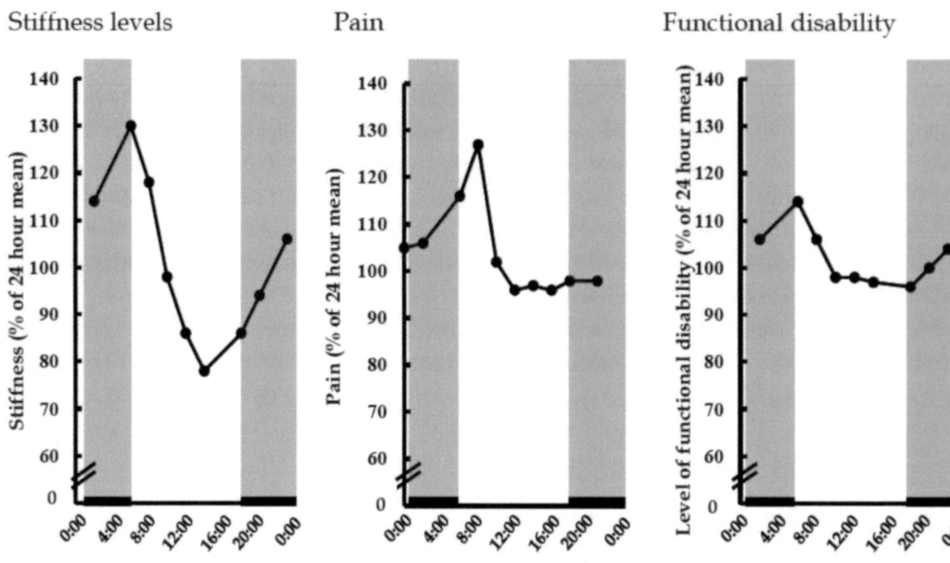


Fig. 5. Circadian rhythms of stiffness, pain, and functional disability in RA patients (redrawn from the data of Strub et al., 2007)

To clarify the relationship between the inflammatory response and cytokines in RA, we studied these circadian rhythms in RA model animals. MRL/lpr mice are an RA model that develop autoimmune disorders that share similarities with human RA and systemic lupus erythematosus (Abe et al., 1980; Koopman et al., 1988). It is difficult to monitor stiffness in RA model animals; however, the circadian rhythm of CRP was found to correspond to that of morning stiffness in RA patients (Herold et al., 1987). Using MRL/lpr mice, we estimated the plasma serum amyloid A (SAA) concentration, which is an acute-phase protein and a sensitive marker of acute inflammatory states, because the CRP level cannot be detected in mice. SAA is also synthesized in the liver upon stimulation by cytokines such as TNF-α and IL-6 (Baumann et al., 1994; Gabay et al., 1999). Before RA onset, there was no significant circadian rhythm in plasma SAA levels (To et al., 2011). However, an obvious circadian rhythm in the plasma SAA concentration involving higher levels in the morning was observed in the MRL/lpr mice that developed RA. There was no significant circadian rhythm in plasma TNF-α levels before RA onset (To et al., 2011). After RA onset, plasma TNF-α levels showed an obvious daily variation, with higher levels in the morning and lower levels at midnight. Collagen-induced arthritis (CIA) represents a true autoimmune reaction against major joint components that is associated with class II major histocompatibility complex genes and pannus formation. CIA model animals display similarities with RA in terms of pathology, immunology, and genetics (Wooley et al., 1984; Holmdahl et al., 1989). It was previously reported that CIA mice showed increased cytokines levels, similar to RA patients (Marinova-Mutafchieva et al., 1997; Mussener et al., 1997). In CIA mice, the SAA level was increased compared with that in the control group and showed a significant circadian rhythm involving higher levels in the morning after RA onset (Fig. 6). The plasma TNF-α concentration also showed a circadian rhythm with a peak in the morning (Fig. 6) (To et al., 2009).

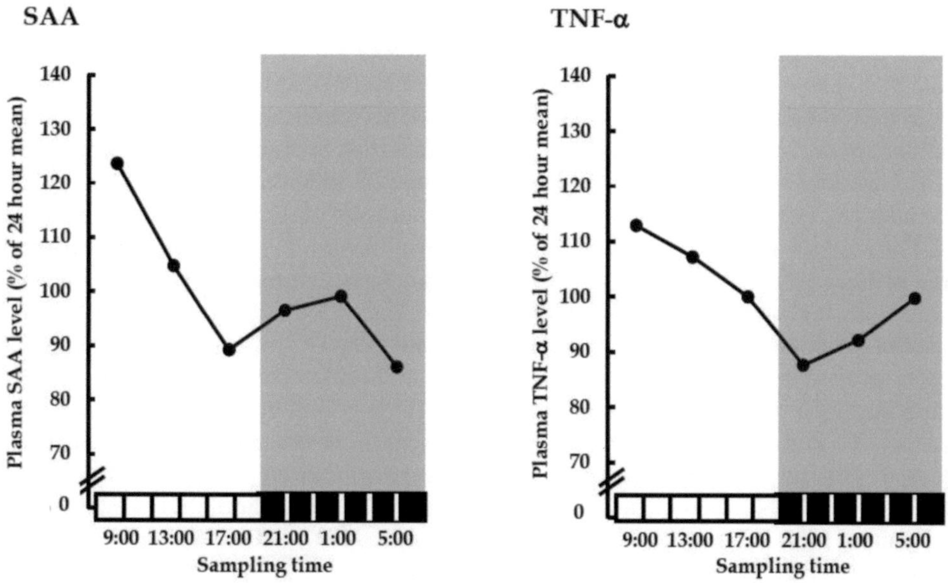


Fig. 6. Circadian rhythm of plasma SAA and TNF-α levels in CIA mice (redrawn from the data of To et al., 2009)

In healthy humans, there is no significant circadian rhythm in plasma IL-6 levels. Moreover, no circadian rhythm is found in patients with various other inflammatory connective tissue diseases. Only RA patients show a clear circadian rhythm in plasma IL-6 concentrations, with higher levels seen from night to early morning and lower levels observed during the daytime (Crofford et al., 1997; Arvidson et al., 1994). Therefore, it is considered that the circadian rhythm in plasma IL-6 levels, which is not present before RA, is a phenomenon peculiar to RA because identical results were obtained in RA patients and RA model animals.

Collectively, the synchronization of the circadian rhythms of the inflammatory response and cytokine levels was also observed in RA patients and RA model animals. It is thought that the inflammatory response contributes to morning stiffness in RA because pain and stiffness develop in the early morning, when the CRP level is higher. Therefore, it is thought that the circadian rhythms of inflammatory cytokines play important roles in the expression of RA symptoms and that these rhythms are important for diagnosing RA.

### 2.2 Factors affecting the circadian rhythm of rheumatoid arthritis

Although the causes of the cytokine circadian rhythms generated by RA onset have not been completely clarified, it is thought that the MLT and cortisol balance and clock genes are involved in the mechanism.

The circadian rhythms of mammals are mediated by the transcriptional/ posttranscriptional machinery regulating the *clock* genes including *Clock, Bmal 1, period,* and *Cryptochrome* (*Cry*) (Sato et al., 2006). Hashiramoto et al. reported that *Cry*, which is one of the *clock* genes, contributes to the induction of arthritis and increases the serum TNF-α level (Hashiramoto et al., 2010). In this study, the number of activated CD3(+) CD69(+) T cells was significantly increased among lymphocytes from *Cry1*$^{-/-}$*Cry2*$^{-}$ mice. *Cry1*$^{-/-}$*Cry2*$^{-}$ mice display aggravated arthritis and increased serum TNF-α concentrations compared with wild type mice. Thus, *Cry* may play an important role in the inducement of RA.

Cutolo et al. proposed that the balance between MLT and cortisol is related to the formation of cytokine circadian rhythms (Straub et al., 2007; Cutolo et al., 2003). MLT has an immunoenhancing effect and induces cytotoxic properties in monocytes etc. (Morrey et al., 1994). Additionally, MLT enhances the expression of inflammatory cytokines (Garcia-Mauriño et al., 1997). In contrast, glucocorticoid suppresses the expression of cytokines such as IL-1, IL-6, and TNF-α. In humans, the MLT level in plasma shows a circadian rhythm with a peak at 3:00 (Kennaway et al., 1998), and the plasma cortisol level shows a circadian rhythm with higher levels seen at 8:00 (Miyatake et al., 1980). The secretion of MLT and cortisol in RA patients differs from that in healthy subjects; i.e., the serum MLT levels of RA patients peak about 2 hours earlier than those in healthy controls (Sulli et al., 2002). Furthermore, the peak cortisol level was found to be lower in RA patients than in the controls (Neeck et al., 1990). These changes in the hormone balance may contribute to the increased cytokine expression seen in RA. It was reported that the serum cytokine and MLT concentrations also showed circadian rhythms with peaks from midnight to early morning, which mirror those of morning stiffness (Arvidson et al., 1997; Sulli et al., 2002). Thus, MLT may be involved in the circadian rhythm of RA symptoms.

We studied the corticosterone concentrations in MRL/lpr mice before/after RA onset. The corticosterone concentration before RA onset showed a significant circadian rhythm with higher levels during the early dark phase and lower levels during the period from the late dark phase to the early light phase (Fig. 7). After RA onset, there was a clear circadian rhythm in the corticosterone level. As rodents are nocturnal animals, the phases of their circadian rhythm for glucocorticoid secretion are shifted by about 12 hours compared with those for humans (Koyanagi et al., 2006). At 21:00, when the corticosterone level peaked, the corticosterone level after RA onset had decreased by 40.9% compared with that before RA onset (Fig. 7). The change in corticosterone secretion in the MRL/lpr mice was similar to that seen in RA patients. On the other hand, the MLT levels in rodents displayed a circadian rhythm with a peak at midnight, as is seen in humans (Conti et al., 1998).

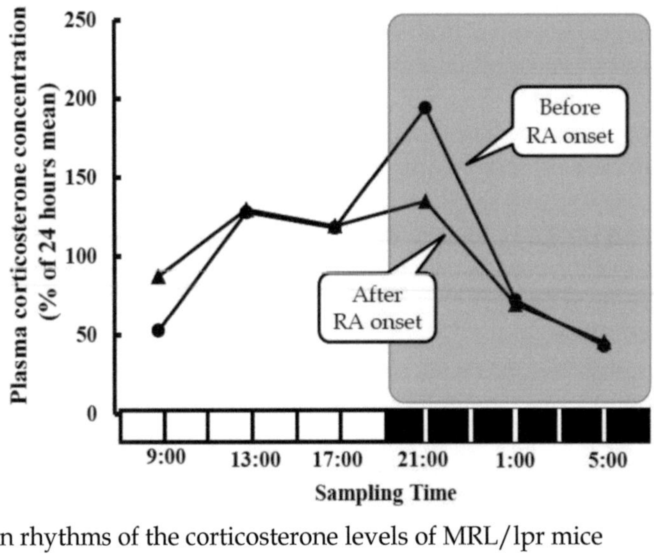


Fig. 7. Circadian rhythms of the corticosterone levels of MRL/lpr mice

Fig.8 shows a hypothesis for the interaction of cytokines and the secretion of MLT and glucocorticoid. Cytokine overexpression is controlled by the secretion balance between the circadian rhythms of MLT and corticosterone. However, the secretion of glucocorticoid declines in RA, and the induction of cytokine expression is increased by MLT. Consequently, the cytokine circadian rhythm follows that of MLT. The phases of the circadian rhythm for glucocorticoid and leukocyte counts, etc., differ by about 12 hours between humans and rodents. However, the phases of the circadian rhythms for the inflammatory response and cytokines are similar between humans and rodents. This may be caused by the similar circadian rhythms for MLT levels between human and rodents. Therefore, it is thought that the circadian rhythm and balance of MLT, which induces the expression of cytokines, and glucocorticoid, which suppresses their expression, participate in the circadian rhythm of RA symptoms.

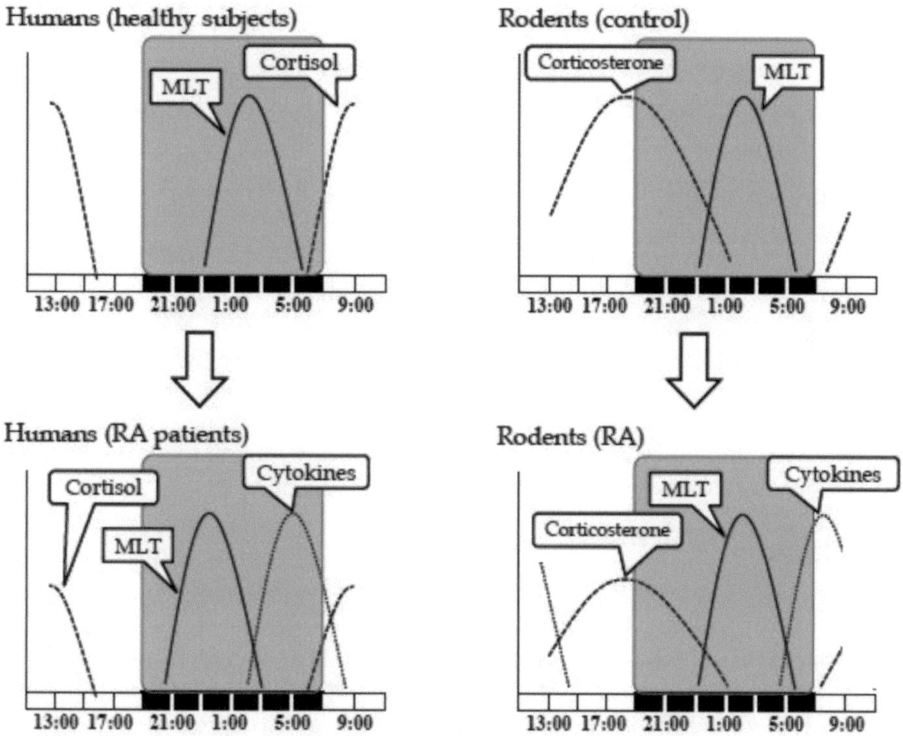


Fig. 8. Interaction of cytokines and the secretion of MLT and glucocorticoid

## 3. Chronotherapy for rheumatoid arthritis

In the treatment of RA, non-steroidal anti-inflammatory drugs (NSAID) are used to decrease pain; steroids are used to reduce pain and inflammation; and disease modifying antirheumatic drugs (DMARD) are used prior to the development of destructive changes in bones, joints, and organ tissues. In addition, biological DMARD can be used to target specific cytokines.

In this Chapter, I summarize the chronopharmacology and chronotherapies of these drugs.

### 3.1 NSAID and glucocorticoids

Arthritis develops in many RA patients. Thus, NSAID such as indomethacin are often used as analgesics. Levi et al. reported on the use of chronotherapy involving indomethacin for osteoarthritis (Levi et al., 1985). The patients with osteoarthritis took an indomethacin sustained-release (ISR) oral preparation once a day at 8:00, noon, or 20:00. The evening dosing protocol showed higher safety than the morning dosing protocol.

Glucocorticoids have been used in RA therapy to treat symptoms such as joint stiffness and joint pain. Generally, glucocorticoids are administered in the morning according to the circadian rhythm of endogenous glucocorticoids. De Silva et al. performed a double-blind cross-over study to determine the effect of the timing of prednisolone administration on morning stiffness (De Silva et al., 1984). The duration of morning stiffness was markedly shorter in the night (22:00- 23:00) dosing group than in the morning (6:00- 7:00) dosing group. Moreover, Arvidson et al. also reported that the 2:00-treated group displayed a markedly decreased duration of morning stiffness and joint pain and reduced serum IL-6 levels compared with the 7:30-treated group (Arvidson et al., 1997). From these results, it is thought that administering glucocorticoids at night is useful for the treatment of RA.

Interesting evidence has been reported for glucocorticoid chronotherapy in recent years. Buttgereit et al. developed a new modified-release formulation of prednisone that releases prednisone about 4 hours after ingestion (Buttgereit et al., 2008). When RA patients were randomly given a modified-release tablet at bedtime or an immediate-release prednisone tablet in the morning, the relative change in the duration of joint morning stiffness was significantly higher with the modified-release tablet than with the immediate-release tablet. Furthermore, administering the modified-release prednisone at night did not change the patients' adrenocortical function over 12 months (Alten et al., 2010). These results show that chronotherapy with a modified-release prednisone tablet is safe and effective as a treatment for RA therapy, even though it was thought that administering glucocorticoids at night would have negative effects upon the circadian rhythm of endogenous cortisol and reduce hypothalamic-pituitary-adrenal axis function. Therefore, chronotherapy using the modified-release prednisone tablet is considered to be a useful RA therapy.

### 3.2 Methotrexate

Methotrexate (MTX) is one of the most commonly used DMARD. It inhibits cytokine production by suppressing lymphocyte proliferation (Williams et al., 2001) and TNF-α transcriptional activity (Becker et al., 1998). MTX induces a high American College of Rheumatology improvement response rate (Choi et al., 2002), inhibits joint inflammation (Kremer et al., 1992; Weinblatt et al., 1992), and conveys a marked survival benefit (Choi et al., 2002) in RA patients although the exact mechanisms underlying its antirheumatic effects are not fully understood (Dolhain et al., 1998; Gerards et al., 2003). Currently, MTX is used as an anchor drug in RA therapy. However, MTX also causes adverse effects, such as myelosuppression and interstitial pneumonitis because it is an anticancer agent. Therefore, it is necessary to design a safe and effective dosing protocol for MTX treatment.

#### 3.2.1 Basic study

In recent years, it has been stated that cytokines are an important factor in the pathogenesis of RA (Chu et al., 1991) and that the levels of proinflammatory cytokines are increased in RA patients. Blood cytokine levels show circadian rhythms in RA patients (Arvidson et al., 1997;

Sulli et al., A, 2002), and these rhythms correspond to those of morning stiffness. We consider that RA therapy associated with cytokine circadian rhythms might be more effective than the RA therapy used commonly in clinical practice.

In previous studies, we revealed that the circadian rhythms of SAA and TNF-α levels, which peak in the light phase, were maintained after RA onset in CIA and MRL/lpr mice (Fig. 6 and 9; To et al., 2009 and 2011). Based on the circadian rhythms of plasma SAA and TNF-α levels in MRL/lpr mice (Fig. 9), MTX was administered three times a week for 2 weeks at 1:00 or 13:00, when the TNF-α level begins to decrease and increase, respectively. The TNF-α levels did not differ between the control and 13:00-treated groups, although they were significantly lower in the 1:00-treated group than in the control group ($P < 0.05$). The SAA concentration in the 1:00-treated group was significantly lower than those in the control and 13:00-treated groups (vs. control: $P < 0.01$, vs. 13:00: $P < 0.05$; Fig. 9) (To et al., 2011).

In the CIA model, clear circadian rhythms in SAA and TNF-α levels were observed, with higher levels seen in the morning and lower levels observed at night (Fig. 6; To et al., 2009), and MTX was intraperitoneally injected at 5:00 or 17:00 every 7 days for 3 weeks. The 5:00-treated group displayed significantly reduced arthritis scores compared with the control and 17:00-treated groups ($P < 0.01$, respectively; Fig. 9). On the other hand, the arthritis scores of the 17:00-treated group did not differ from those of the control group for the entire study period in mice.

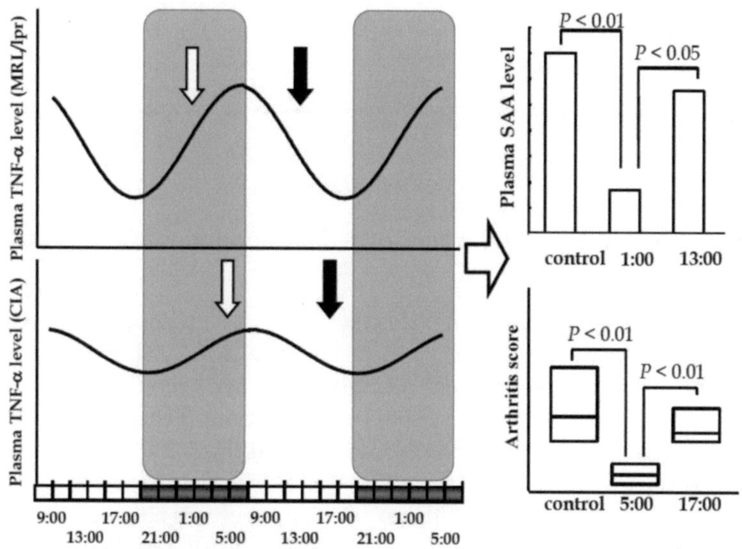


Fig. 9. Influence of MTX dosing time on antirheumatic effects

In these studies, the dosing time-dependent changes in the SAA level corresponded to identical changes in the TNF-α level. It is likely that the SAA level is reduced due to a decrease in the TNF-α concentration after MTX administration from midnight to early morning. In addition, arthritis and inflammation were reduced in the dark phase, when the plasma TNF-α concentration began to increase, in both the CIA model and MRL/lpr mice. These findings reveal that the therapeutic effects of MTX treatment can be improved by administering MTX when the serum TNF-α level begins to increase.

MTX causes myelosuppression and is used as an antitumor drug. It is reported that the toxicity caused by MTX varies significantly in mice depending on the dosing time (Ohdo et al., 1997). In our studies using CIA mice, the MTX dosing groups showed no significant decreases in their leukocyte counts compared with the control group. In RA therapy, MTX is used at very low doses compared with those used in cancer chemotherapy. Its chronotoxicity was studied using 400 mg/kg of MTX to estimate the toxicity of MTX as an antitumor drug (Ohdo et al., 1997). However, no adverse effects were observed in our studies because only 60 mg/kg of MTX was administered to mice. Thus, MTX may reduce plasma TNF-α levels by suppressing transcriptional activity rather than suppressing lymphocyte proliferation.

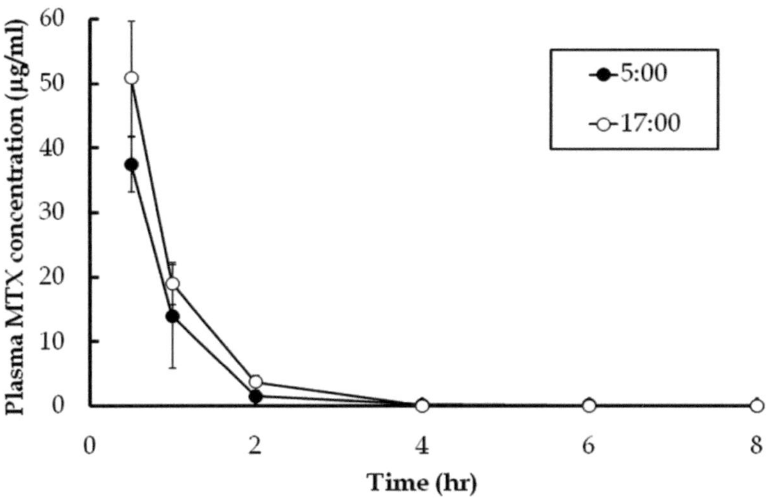


Fig. 10. Plasma concentration of MTX after drug administration at 5:00 or 17:00 (redrawn from the data of To et al., 2009)

To clarify the mechanism underlying dosing time dependency, we investigated the influence of dosing time on the pharmacokinetics of MTX. MTX is largely excreted in urine. Both renal blood flow and the glomerular filtration rate have been found to follow circadian rhythms, with a peak during the active period in animals. The MTX concentration was expected to be higher in the 17:00-treated group than in the 5:00-treated group since MTX was administered during the inactive period. In our study, the plasma MTX concentrations at 0.5 and 2 hour after MTX injection in the 17:00 group were significantly higher than those in the 5:00 group (0.5 hour: $P < 0.05$, 2 hour: $P < 0.01$; Fig. 10). On the other hand, the 5:00 group showed significantly higher plasma MTX levels than the 17:00 group at 4, 6, and 8 hour (4 hour: $P < 0.01$, 6 hour: $P < 0.01$, 8 hour: $P < 0.05$; Fig. 10). However, the area under the plasma-time concentration curve (AUC) was 23,622 μg/ml/hr at 5:00 and 32,305 μg/ml/hr at 17:00. The AUC in the 17:00-treated group, which showed no decrease in the arthritis score, was 1.28-fold higher than that in the 5:00-treated group, which had a significantly arthritis reduced score. Thus, no relationship was detected between the concentration of MTX and its efficacy. It was reported in previous studies that there were no dosing time-dependent changes in MTX pharmacokinetics in patients with cancer (Balis et al., 1989; Robinson et al., 1989). Moreover, no difference was noted in MTX pharmacokinetics according to the injection time when MTX was administered to RA patients intramuscularly at 10:00 or 18:00 (Carpentier et al., 1998).

From the results of our studies and the circadian cycles of cytokines in RA patients, it is thought that MTX has a significant dosing-time-dependent anti-inflammatory action and that this effect might be due to the circadian rhythms of cytokine levels rather than the pharmacokinetics of MTX.

It was shown that there were daily variations in the plasma SAA and TNF-α concentrations in CIA and MRL/lpr mice after the onset of RA and that their arthritis score and SAA and TNF-α levels were relieved after the administration of MTX at specific times in synchronization with the circadian rhythm of TNF-α. Therefore, we consider that choosing an optimal dosing time associated with the circadian rhythm of RA symptoms could lead to effective MTX treatment for RA.

### 3.2.2 Clinical study

From our studies in RA model animals, we anticipated that higher therapeutic effects could be achieved with chronotherapy compared with the current treatment schedule, in which MTX is administered during the night. In RA patients, pain and stiffness are accentuated in the early morning, and proinflammatory cytokines show circadian rhythms that peak from midnight to early morning (Crofford et al., 1997; Perry et al., 2009). Based on our findings in animal studies and the circadian TNF-α rhythms of RA patients, we changed the dosing schedules of RA patients from the standard MTX schedule, in which MTX is administered three times a week (day 1: after breakfast and supper, day 2: after breakfast only), to a chronotherapy schedule, in which the dose and number of doses per week were not changed, but MTX was administered once a day after supper, to examine whether a dosing-time dependency of the therapeutic effects of MTX treatment could be detected in Japanese RA patients. The disease activity score (DAS) 28, modified health assessment questionnaire (MHAQ) score, and adverse effects were assessed. DAS28 is a composite score based on tender and swollen joint counts (28 joints), the patient's global assessment of their disease activity (100 mm Visual Analog Scale (VAS): 0 = no activity, 100 = extreme activity), and the CRP level. DAS28 values were calculated as follows:

$$\text{DAS28 (CRP)} = 0.56 \times \sqrt{(\text{TJC28})} + 0.28 \times \sqrt{(\text{SJC28})} + 0.014 \times \text{GH} + 0.36 \times \ln(\text{CRP}+1) + 0.96,$$

where TJC = tender joint count, SJC = swollen joint count, GH = general health, and CRP = CRP level in mg/l. A score of $\geq 4.1$ indicates high disease activity, a score $> 2.7$ and $\leq 4.1$ indicates moderate disease activity, a score $< 2.7$ indicates low disease activity, and a score $< 2.3$ indicates disease remission (van Gestel et al., 1996). The European league against rheumatism (EULAR) response states were classified as follows: good responders were patients displaying an improvement of $> 1.2$ and a present score of $\leq 2.7$; moderate responders were patients displaying an improvement of $> 0.6$ and $\leq 1.2$ and a present score of $\leq 4.1$, or an improvement of $> 1.2$ and a present score of $> 4.1$; and non-responders were any patients displaying an improvement of $\leq 0.6$ or patients displaying an improvement of $> 0.6$ and $\leq 1.2$ and a present score of $> 4.1$ (Fransen et al., 2005).

The chronotherapy administered MTX after supper proved highly effective despite the dose and the number of doses remaining the same, although many patients did not derive a therapeutic benefit from the therapy. As the half-life of MTX is about 2 hours, the MTX had disappeared from the plasma by 10 hours after its administration. Therefore, it was thought that the plasma concentration produced by administrating MTX after supper was insufficient. We therefore administered MTX before bedtime once a day to a patient in whom MTX was ineffective in the previous study. Consequently, the DAS28 of the patient decreased from 5.45 (4 months) to 3.25 (7 months) over the study (moderate response) (Fig.11). From this result, it was considered that a higher therapeutic effect can be achieved by administrating MTX before bedtime compared with after supper.

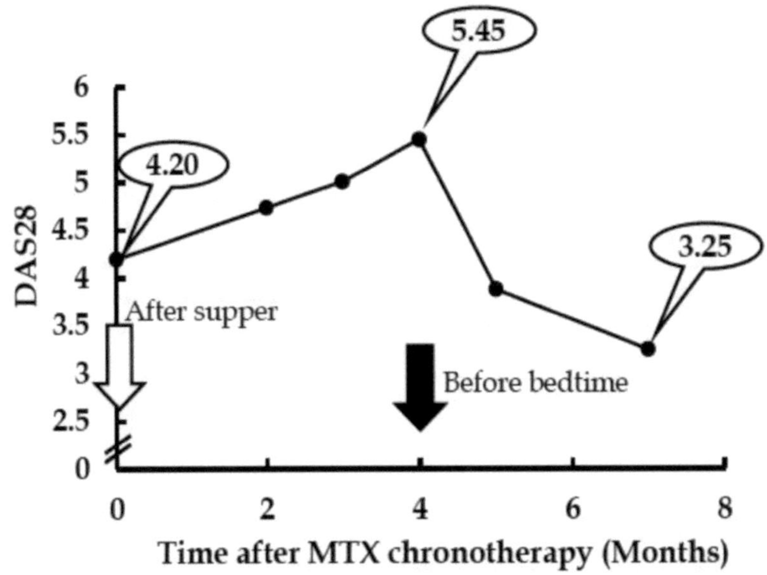


Fig. 11. Influence of MTX chronotherapy on DAS28 score (case data)

We studied the effects of MTX chronotherapy before bedtime, and the dose and the number of doses per week were not changed. Twenty-two rheumatoid arthritis patients between 41 and 78 years of age were enrolled, and 77% received MTX chronotherapy for the entire 3 months of the study. Fig. 12 shows the change in DAS28 in a female RA patient to whom MTX was administered at bedtime. After the start of the chronotherapy, her DAS28 value was markedly decreased by 1.5 at only one month, and the effect was maintained throughout the 3 months of the study. In particular, all of her joint swelling disappeared, and the tenderness in many of her joints was relieved after the chronotherapy.

The chronotherapy improved the DAS28 score in 14 of 17 patients (82.4%), and the mean DAS28 value was significantly decreased by 0.460 at one month, 0.506 at two months, and 0.521 at three months after the start of the chronotherapy ($P < 0.05$ and $P < 0.01$, respectively) (Fig. 13; To et al., 2011). In particular, despite the dose and the number of doses remaining the same, 23.5% of patients attained clinical remission. DAS28 is calculated from the following 4 parameters: the tender and swollen joint counts, the patient's global assessment of disease activity, and the CRP concentration. The median tender joint count changed little throughout the study. On the other hand, the swollen joint count was markedly decreased in all patients after 3 months chronotherapy. The CRP level continued to improve throughout the 3 month study period and had improved by 64.2% after the chronotherapy compared with the baseline. The patient's global assessment of disease activity is susceptible to patient bias because each patient evaluates their own degree of illness. In this study, the patients understood that the method of MTX administration had changed. The patient's global assessment of disease activity did not show definite changes, even though a placebo effect of the chronotherapy was anticipated. Therefore, it was considered that the placebo effect did not contribute to the observed significant decrease in the DAS28 score.

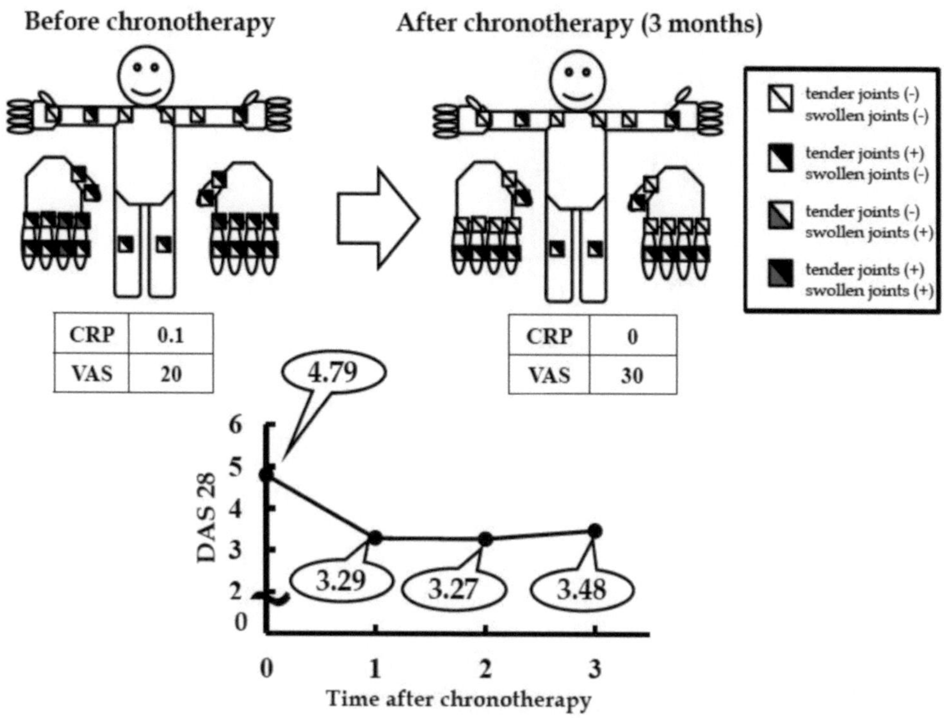


Fig. 12. Influence of MTX chronotherapy (before bedtime) on DAS28 score (case data)

The MHAQ is used to estimate the functional capacity of RA patients. It assesses the ability of patients to perform daily activities using eight questions. The final MHAQ score is the mean score of the eight questions and ranges from 0 to 3, with higher levels reflecting greater disability (Pincus et al., 1983). It was revealed that chronotherapy improved the functional capacity of the RA patients although we could not clarify the factors responsible for the improvement in the MHAQ score from the data obtained in this study. Almost all patients had mild leukopenia although the incidence of leukopenia higher than Grade 1 increased from 11.8% to 23.5% throughout the study. Moreover, there were no severe adverse effects in 17 patients.

From these results, it was demonstrated that MTX chronotherapy is safe and markedly improves the disease activity and functional capacity of RA patients.

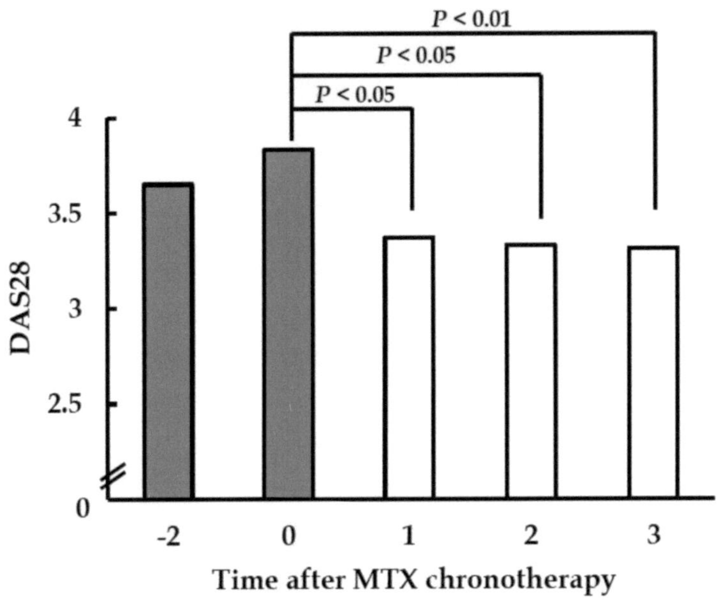


Fig. 13. Efficacy of 3 months MTX treatment in Japanese RA patients (redrawn from the data of To et al., 2011)

## 4. Conclusion

RA is an autoimmune disorder of unknown etiology, and morning stiffness is a well-known characteristic of the condition. Inflammatory responses show circadian rhythms in RA patients, and these rhythms correspond to that of morning stiffness. Moreover, it is considered that cytokine rhythms contribute to the rhythm of inflammatory responses since the circadian rhythms of inflammatory responses and cytokines are similar. The symptoms of RA such as disease activity and the patients' functional capacity, arthritis, pain, etc. were relieved after the administration of anti-antirheumatic drugs such as MTX, steroids, NSAID, etc. at specific times in synchronization with the circadian rhythm of cytokines and the inflammatory response. Choosing an optimal dosing time that is associated with the circadian rhythms of RA symptoms is, therefore, expected to lead to more effective medical therapy for RA (Fig. 14).

Presently, we are performing basic and clinical studies to prove the utility of chronotherapy involving various anti-antirheumatic drugs. From these studies, we hope to be able to propose safe and effective RA therapies. Furthermore, the mechanism regulating the generation of circadian rhythms in RA is being studied. It is expected that new drugs targeting RA will be discovered and that new RA therapies that regulate the abovementioned circadian rhythms will be developed once the mechanism responsible for their generation has been clarified.

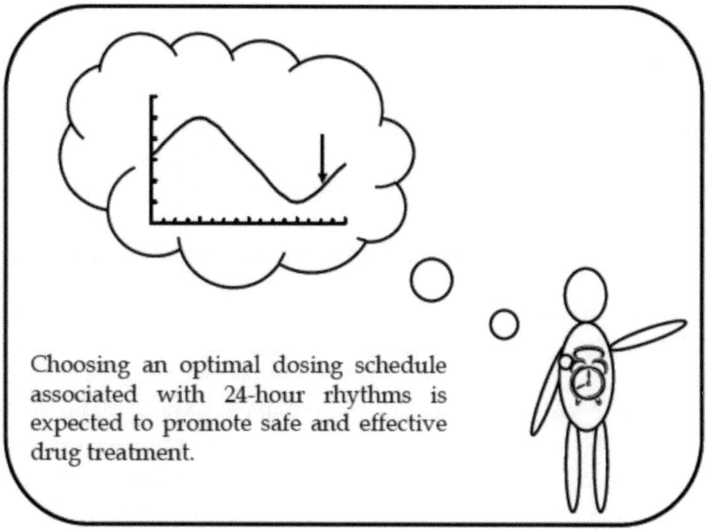


Fig. 14. Concept of chronotherapy

## 5. References


Abe C, Mitsunaga K, Shiokawa Y., Spontaneous polyarthritis in MRL/1 mice. Ryumachi ., 1980; 20: 233- 9.

Alten R, Döring G, Cutolo M, Gromnica-Ihle E, Witte S, Straub R, Buttgereit F., Hypothalamus-pituitary-adrenal axis function in patients with rheumatoid arthritis treated with nighttime-release prednisone. J Rheumatol., 2010; 37: 2025-31.

Argentino C, Toni D, Rasura M, Violi F, Sacchetti ML, Allegretta A, Balsano F, Fieschi C., Circadian variation in the frequency of ischemic stroke. Stroke., 1990; 21: 387-9.

Arnett FC, Edworthy SM, Bloch DA, McShane DJ, Fries JF, Cooper NS., The American Rheumatism Association 1987 revised criteria for the classification of rheumatoid arthritis. Arthritis Rheum., 1988; 31: 315-24.

Arvidson NG, Gudbjörnsson B, Elfman L, Rydén AC, Tötterman TH, Hällgren R., Circadian rhythm of serum interleukin-6 in rheumatoid arthritis. Ann Rheum Dis., 1994; 53: 521-4.

Arvidson NG, Gudbjornsson B, Larsson A, Hallgren R., The timing of glucocorticoid administration in rheumatoid arthritis. Ann. Rheum. Dis., 1997; 56: 27-31.

Balis FM, Jeffries SL, Lange B, Murphy RF, Doherty KM, Arndt CA, Luery N, Poplack DG., Chronopharmacokinetics of oral methotrexate and 6-mercaptopurine: is there diurnal variation in the disposition of antileukemic therapy? Am J Pediatr Hematol Oncol., 1989; 11: 324-6.

Baumann H, Gauldie J., The acute phase response. Immunol Today., 1994; 15: 74- 80.

Becker C, Barbulescu K, Hildner K, Meyer zum Büschenfelde KH, Neurath MF., Activation and methotrexate-mediated suppression of the TNFα promoter in T cells and macrophages. Ann. N. Y. Acad. Sci., 1998; 859: 219-22.

Bellamy N, Sothern RB, Campbell J, Buchanan WW., Circadian rhythm in pain, stiffness, and manual dexterity in rheumatoid arthritis: relation between discomfort and disability. Ann Rheum Dis., 1991; 50: 243-8.

Buchi KN, Moore JG, Hrushesky WJ, Sothern RB, Rubin NH., Circadian rhythm of cellular proliferation in the human rectal mucosa. Gastroenterology., 1991; 101: 410-5.

Buttgereit F, Doering G, Schaeffler A, Witte S, Sierakowski S, Gromnica-Ihle E, Jeka S, Krueger K, Szechinski J, Alten R., Efficacy of modified-release versus standard prednisone to reduce duration of morning stiffness of the joints in rheumatoid arthritis (CAPRA-1): a double-blind, randomised controlled trial. Lancet., 2008; 371: 205-14.

Carpentier N, Bertin P, Marquet P, Sabot C, Bonnet C, Debord J, Lachâtre G, Trèves R., Is there an optimal time to administer methotrexate in the treatment of rheumatoid arthritis? J Rheumatol., 1998; 25: 1270-5.

Choi HK, Hernán MA, Seeger JD, Robins JM, Wolfe F., Methotrexate and mortality in patients with rheumatoid arthritis: a prospective study. Lancet., 2002; 359: 1173-7.

Chu CQ, Field M, Feldmann M, Maini RN., Localization of tumor necrosis factor alpha in synovial tissues and at the cartilage-pannus junction in patients with rheumatoid arthritis. Arthritis Rheum., 1991; 34: 1125-32.

Clarke JM, Hamer J, Shelton JR, Taylor S, Venning GR. The rhythm of the normal human heart. Lancet., 1976; 1: 508-12.

Conti A, Maestroni GJ., Melatonin rhythms in mice: role in autoimmune and lymphoproliferative diseases. Ann N Y Acad Sci., 1998; 840: 395-410.

Crofford LJ, Kalogeras KT, Mastorakos G, Magiakou MA, Wells J, Kanik KS, Gold PW, Chrousos GP, Wilder RL., Circadian relationships between interleukin (IL)-6 and hypothalamic-pituitary-adrenal axis hormones: failure of IL-6 to cause sustained hypercortisolism in patients with early untreated rheumatoid arthritis. J Clin Endocrinol Metab., 1997; 82: 1279-83.

Cutolo M, Seriolo B, Craviotto C, Pizzorni C, Sulli A., Circadian rhythms in RA. Ann Rheum Dis., 2003; 62: 593-6.

D'Alonzo GE, Smolensky MH, Feldman S, Gnosspelius Y, Karlsson K., Bambuterol in the treatment of asthma: A placebo-controlled comparison of once-daily morning vs. evening administration. Chest., 1995; 107: 406-12.

De Silva M, Binder A, Hazleman BL., The timing of prednisolone dosage and its effect on morning stiffness in rheumatoid arthritis. Ann Rheum Dis., 1984; 43: 790-3.

Degaute JP, van de Borne P, Linkowski P, Van Cauter E. Quantitative analysis of the 24-hour blood pressure and heart rate patterns in young men. Hypertension., 1991; 18: 199-210.

Dethlefsen U, Repges R., Ein neues therapieprinzip bei nachtlichem asthma. Med. Klin., 1985; 80: 44–7.

Dolhain RJ, Tak PP, Dijkmans BA, De Kuiper P, Breedveld FC, Miltenburg AM., Methotrexate reduces inflammatory cell numbers, expression of monokines and of adhesion molecules in synovial tissue of patients with rheumatoid arthritis. Br J Rheumatol., 1998; 37: 502-8.

Egstrup K., Attenuation of circadian variation by combined antianginal therapy with suppression of morning and evening increases in transient myocardial ischemia. Am Heart J., 1991; 122: 648-55.

Feldmann M, Brennan FM, Maini RN., Role of cytokines in rheumatoid arthritis. Ann Rev Immunol., 1996; 14: 397- 440.

Fox AW, Davis RL., Migraine chronobiology. Headache., 1998; 38: 436-41.

Fransen J, van Riel PL., The Disease Activity Score and the EULAR response criteria. Clin. Exp. Rheumatol., 2005; 23: S93-S99.

Gabay C, Kushner I., Acute-phase proteins and other systemic responses to inflammation. New Engl J Med., 1999; 340: 448- 54.

Gabriel SE., The epidemiology of rheumatoid arthritis. Rheum Dis Clin North Am., 2001; 27: 269-81.

Gallerani M, Portaluppi F, Grandi E, Manfredini R., Circadian rhythmicity in the occurrence of spontaneous acute dissection and rupture of thoracic aorta. J Thorac Cardiovasc Surg., 1997 ;113: 603-4.

Garcia-Mauriño S, Gonzalez-Haba MG, Calvo JR, Rafii-El-Idrissi M, Sanchez-Margalet V, Goberna R, Guerrero JM., Melatonin enhances IL-2, IL-6, and IFN-gamma production by human circulating CD4+ cells: a possible nuclear receptor-mediated mechanism involving T helper type 1 lymphocytes and monocytes. J Immunol., 1997; 159: 574-81.

Gavrila A, Peng CK, Chan JL, Mietus JE, Goldberger AL, Mantzoros CS., Diurnal and ultradian dynamics of serum adiponectin in healthy men: comparison with leptin, circulating soluble leptin receptor, and cortisol patterns. J Clin Endocrinol Metab., 2003; 88: 2838-43.

Gerards AH, de Lathouder S, de Groot ER, Dijkmans BA, Aarden LA., Inhibition of cytokine production by methotrexate. Studies in healthy volunteers and patients with rheumatoid arthritis., Rheumatology., 2003; 42: 1189-96.

Harris ED Jr., Rheumatoid arthritis. Pathophysiology and implications for therapy. New Engl J Med., 1990; 322: 1277-89.

Hashiramoto A, Yamane T, Tsumiyama K, Yoshida K, Komai K, Yamada H, Yamazaki F, Doi M, Okamura H, Shiozawa S., Mammalian clock gene Cryptochrome regulates arthritis via proinflammatory cytokine TNF-alpha. J Immunol., 2010; 184: 1560-5.

Haus E., Chronobiology in the endocrine system. Adv. Drug Deliv. Rev. 2007; 59: 985-1014.

Holmdahl R, Andersson ME, Goldschmidt TJ, Jansson L, Karlsson M, Malmstrom V. , Collagen induced arthritis as an experimental model for rheumatoid arthritis. Immunogenetics, pathogenesis and autoimmunity. APMIS., 1989; 97:575- 84.

Hermida RC, Ayala DE, Mojón, Fernández JR., Infleunce of circadian time of hypertension treatment on cardiovascular risk: Results of the MAPEC Study. Chronobiol. Int., 2010; 27: 1629-51.

Herold M, Günther R., Circadian rhythm of C-reactive protein in patients with rheumatoid arthritis. Prog Clin Biol Res., 1987: 227B: 271-9.

Iurisci I, Filipski E, Reinhardt J, Bach S, Gianella-Borradori A, Iacobelli S, Meijer L, Lévi F. Improved tumor control through circadian clock induction by Seliciclib, a cyclin-dependent kinase inhibitor. Cancer Res., 2006; 66: 10720- 8.

Jones PJ, Pappu AS, Illingworth DR, Leitch CA., Correspondence between plasma mevalonic acid levels and deuterium uptake in measuring human cholesterol synthesis. Eur J Clin Invest., 1992; 22: 609-13.

Kennaway DJ, Voultsios A., Circadian rhythm of free melatonin in human plasma. J Clin Endocrinol Metab., 1998; 83: 1013-5.

Kobayashi M, To H, Tokue A, Fujimura A, Kobayashi E., Cisplatin-induced vomiting depends on circadian timing. Chronobiol Int., 2001; 18: 851-63.

Koopman MG, Koomen GC, Krediet RT, de Moor EA, Hoek FJ, Arisz L., Circadian rhythm of glomerular filtration rate in normal individuals. Clin Sci., 1989; 77: 105-11.

Koopman WJ, Gay S., The MRL-lpr/lpr mouse. A model for the study of rheumatoid arthritis. Scand J Rheumatol., 1988; 75 (Suppl): 284-9.

Koyanagi S, Suyama H, Kuramoto Y, Matsunaga N, Takane H, Soeda S, Shimeno H, Higuchi S, Ohdo S., Glucocorticoid regulation of 24-hour oscillation in interferon receptor gene expression in mouse liver. Endocrinology., 2006; 147: 5034-40.

Kowanko IC, Knapp MS, Pownall R, Swannell AJ., Domiciliary self-measurement in the rheumatoid arthritis and the demonstration of circadian rhythmicity. Ann Rheum Dis., 1982; 41: 453-5.

Kremer JM, Phelps CT., Long-term prospective study of the use of methotrexate in the treatment of rheumatoid arthritis. Update after a mean of 90 months. Arthritis Rheum., 1992; 35: 138-45.

Lack LC, Gradisar M, Van Someren EJ, Wright HR, Lushington K. The relationship between insomnia and body temperatures. Sleep Med Rev., 2008; 12: 307-17.

Lemmer B, Nold G. Circadian changes in estimated hepatic blood flow in healthy subjects. Br J Clin Pharmacol., 1991; 32: 627-9.

Levi F, Le Louarn C, Reinberg A., Timing optimizes sustained-release indomethacin treatment of osteoarthritis. Clin Pharmacol Ther., 1985; 37: 77-84.

Matsunaga N, Nakamura N, Yoneda N, Qin T, Terazono H, To H, Higuchi S, Ohdo S. Influence of feeding schedule on 24-h rhythm of hepatotoxicity induced by acetaminophen in mice. J. Pharmacol. Exp. Ther., 2004; 311: 594-600.

Marinova-Mutafchieva L, Williams RO, Mason LJ, Mauri C, Feldmann M, Maini RN. , Dynamics of proinflammatory cytokine expression in the joints of mice with collagen-induced arthritis (CIA). Clin Exp Immunol. 1997; 107: 507-12.

McInnes IB, Liew FY., Cytokine networks - towards new therapies for rheumatoid arthritis. Nat Clin Prac Rheumatol., 2005; 1: 31- 9.

Miyatake A, Morimoto Y, Oishi T, Hanasaki N, Sugita Y, Iijima S, Teshima Y, Hishikawa Y, Yamamura Y., Circadian rhythm of serum testosterone and its relation to sleep: comparison with the variation in serum luteinizing hormone, prolactin, and cortisol in normal men. J Clin Endocrinol Metab., 1980; 51: 1365-71.

Miyawaki T, Taga K, Nagaoki T, Seki H, Suzuki Y, Taniguchi N., Circadian changes of T lymphocyte subsets in human peripheral blood. Clin Exp Immunol., 1984; 55: 618-22.

Morrey KM, McLachlan JA, Serkin CD, Bakouche O., Activation of human monocytes by the pineal hormone melatonin. J Immunol., 1994; 153: 2671-80.

Mussener A, Litton MJ, Lindroos E, Klareskog L., Cytokine production in synovial tissue of mice with collagen-induced arthritis (CIA). Clin Exp Immunol., 1997; 107: 485-93.

Neeck G, Federlin K, Graef V, Rusch D, Schmidt KL., Adrenal secretion of cortisol in patients with rheumatoid arthritis. J Rheumatol., 1990; 17: 24-9.

Ohdo S, Inoue K, Yukawa E, Higuchi S, Nakano S, Ogawa N., Chronotoxicity of methotrexate in mice and its relation to circadian rhythm of DNA synthesis and pharmacokinetics. Jpn J Pharmacol., 1997; 75: 283-90.

Perry MG, Kirwan JR, Jessop DS, Hunt LP., Overnight variations in cortisol, interleukin 6, tumour necrosis factor α and other cytokines in people with rheumatoid arthritis. Ann Rheum Dis., 2009; 68: 63-8.

Pincus T, Summey JA, Soraci SA Jr, Wallston KA, Hummon NP., Assessment of patient satisfaction in activities of daily living using a modified Stanford Health Assessment Questionnaire. Arthritis Rheum., 1983; 26: 1346-53.

Pöllmann L, Harris PH., Rhythmic changes in pain sensitivity in teeth. Int J Chronobiol., 1978; 5: 459-64.

Quigg M, Straume M, Menaker M, Bertram EH 3rd., Temporal distribution of partial seizures: comparison of an animal model with human partial epilepsy. Ann Neurol., 1998; 43: 748-55.

Robinson BA, Begg EJ, Colls BM, Jeffery GM, Sharman JR., Circadian pharmacokinetics of methotrexate. Cancer Chemother Pharmacol., 1989; 24: 397-9.

Saito Y, Yoshida S, Nakaya N, Hata Y, Goto Y., Comparison between morning and evening doses of simvastatin in hyperlipidemic subjects. A double-blind comparative study. Arterioscler. Thromb., 1991; 11: 816-26.

Sato TK, Yamada RG, Ukai H, Baggs JE, Miraglia LJ, Kobayashi TJ, Welsh DK, Kay SA, Ueda HR, Hogenesch JB., Feedback repression is required for mammalian circadian clock function. Nat Genet., 2006; 38: 312-9.

Smaaland R, Laerum OD, Lote K, Sletvold O, Sothern RB, Bjerknes R., DNA synthesis in human bone marrow is circadian stage dependent. Blood., 1991; 77: 2603-11.

Smolensky MH, Lemmer B, Reinberg AE., Chronobiology and chronotherapy of allergic disease and bronchial asthma. Adv. Drug Deliv. Rev., 2007; 59: 828-51.

Straub RH, Cutolo M., Circadian rhythms in rheumatoid arthritis: implications for pathophysiology and therapeutic management. Arthritis Rheum., 2007; 56: 399-408.

Sulli A, Maestroni GJ, Villaggio B, Hertens E, Craviotto C, Pizzorni C, Briata M, Seriolo B, Cutolo M., Melatonin serum levels in rheumatoid arthritis. Ann N Y Acad Sci., 2002; 966: 276-83.

Tabuchi M, To H, Sakaguchi H, Goto N, Takeuchi A, Higuchi S, Ohdo S. Therapeutic index by combination of adriamycin and docetaxel depends on dosing time in mice. Cancer Res., 2005; 65: 8448-54.

Tampellini M, Filipski E, Liu XH, Lemaigre G, Li XM, Vrignaud P, François E, Bissery MC, Lévi F. Docetaxel chronopharmacology in mice. Cancer Res., 1998; 58: 3896-904.

To H, Irie S, Tomonari M, WatanabeY, Kitahara T, Sasaki H., Therapeutic index of methotrexate depends on circadian cycling of tumor necrosis factor-α in collagen-induced arthritis rats and mice. J Pharm Pharmacol., 2009; 61: 1333-8.

To H, Yoshimatsu H, Tomonari M, Ida H, Tsurumoto T, Tsuji Y, Sonemoto E, Shimasaki N, Koyanagi S, Sasaki H, Ieiri I, Higuchi S, Kawakami A, Ueki Y, Eguchi K., Methotrexate chronotherapy is effective against rheumatoid arthritis. Chronobiol Int., 2011; 28: 267-74.

Ushijima K, Sakaguchi H, Sato Y, To H, Koyanagi S, Higuchi S, Ohdo S. Chronopharmacological study of antidepressants in forced swimming test of mice. J. Pharmacol. Exp. Ther., 2005; 315: 764-70.

van Gestel AM, Prevoo ML, van 't Hof MA, van Rijswijk MH, van de Putte LB, van Riel PL., Development and validation of the European League Against Rheumatism response criteria for rheumatoid arthritis. Comparison with the preliminary

American College of Rheumatology and the World Health Organization/International League Against Rheumatism Criteria. Arthritis Rheum., 1996; 39: 34-40.

Vermeer SE, Rinkel G JE, Algra A., Circadian fluctuations in onset of subarachnoid hemorrhage. New Data on Aneurysmal and Perimesencephalic Hemorrhage and a Systematic Review. Stroke., 1997; 28: 805-8.

Weinblatt ME, Weissman BN, Holdsworth DE, Fraser PA, Maier AL, Falchuk KR, Coblyn JS., Long-term prospective study of methotrexate in the treatment of rheumatoid arthritis. 84-month update. Arthritis Rheum., 1992; 35: 129-37.

Williams AS, Topley N, Dojcinov S, Richards PJ, Williams BD., Amelioration of rat antigen-induced arthritis by liposomally conjugated methotrexate is accompanied by down-regulation of cytokine mRNA expression. Rheumatology., 2001; 40: 375-83.

Wooley PH, Luthra HS, Krco CJ, Stuart JM, David CS., Type II collagen-induced arthritis in mice. II. Passive transfer and suppression by intravenous injection of anti-type II collagen antibody or free native type II collagen. Arthritis Rheum., 1984; 27: 1010-7.

# 28

# Four Aspects of Autoimmunity and How to Regain Tolerance to Self from an Autoimmune Disease Utilizing the Modified Vaccination Technique

Arpad Z. Barabas[1], Chad D. Cole[2], Arpad D. Barabas[1], Rene Lafreniere[1] and Donald M. Weir[3]

[1]*Department of Surgery, University of Calgary, Calgary, Alberta,*
[2]*Department of Neurosurgery, University of Utah, Salt Lake City, Utah,*
[3]*University of Edinburgh Medical School, Edinburgh,*
[1]*Canada*
[2]*USA*
[3]*Scotland*

## 1. Introduction

The cells of the immune system are exposed to two broad types of antigenic challenges – challenges from the external environment (bacteria, viruses, etc.), and challenges from the internal environment of the host (from both normal and abnormal self). The immune system functions throughout life to preserve the integrity of the organism, allowing its various organs and systems to carry out their intended functions, and maintaining normal health. The cells of the immune system have intimate knowledge of self and non-self. Normal self is allowed to live and function, whereas abnormal self or non-self, e.g. degraded cellular products or abnormal cells, are recognized as non-self and removed by the cells and products of the immune system and processed into reusable small MW peptides (Manson et al., 2005; Quartier et al., 2005; Wermeling et al., 2009). Occasionally, modified self will affect the normally functioning immune system and stimulate a pathogenic immune response causing an autoimmune disease (Barabas et al., 2004c; Heymann et al., 1959). In other instances, because of the minimal antigenicity of cancer specific antigens (ags) on cancer cell surfaces, cancer is not recognized as non-self and is allowed to grow and cause harm (Berinstein, 2007; Engelhard et al., 2002).

The question of how to correct immunological mishaps that not only compromise the normal functioning of an affected organ but can even threaten the life of the host has engaged numerous investigators in the search for curative solutions. So far the options available for treating ailments caused by autoimmune disorders have been mainly limited to drugs (Cattran, 1988; Matsukawa et al., 1992; Penny et al., 1998), which in general have undesirably over-broad effects. Yet there are encouraging signs that targeted, specific cures might be achieved by immunological means (Andreakos et al., 2002; Berinstein, 2007;

Hasegawa et al., 2001; Lollini & Forni, 2002; Yokoyama et al., 1999). Studies have shown that the method of presentation of the ag - whether it be exogenous or endogenous - to the cells of the immune system determines the immune response outcome.

Medical science has learned, over the course of the developmental history of vaccination, how to present antigenic components in an inoculate to stimulate protective immune responses in the vaccinated host against exogenous ags. However, the possibility of using vaccination to achieve protective or curative outcomes in patients with disorders caused by endogenous ags, without causing side effects, has remained elusive (Ben Yehuda et al., 1988; Fox & McCune, 1994; Golbus & McCune, 1994; Hu et al., 2009; Nepom, 2002; Perosa et al., 2005; Thaiss et al., 1989).

Our investigations into the etiology and pathogenesis of an experimental autoimmune kidney disease have resulted in a new immunological approach involving the presentation of native autoimmune disease related ags to evoke a predetermined corrective immune response in the host (Barabas et al., 2004b; Barabas et al., 2006c; Barabas et al., 2006b; Barabas & Lafreniere, 2005). The approach consists of a new vaccination method called modified vaccination technique (MVT) (Barabas et al., 2007b; Barabas et al., 2007a; Barabas et al., 2008a; Barabas et al., 2009a; Barabas et al., 2009b). The MVT involves the injection of a mixture of antibody (ab) inducing components which are predetermined based on the required outcome. So far the MVT has been implemented:

- to prevent an experimental autoimmune kidney disease, and to terminate the already present disease (Barabas et al., 2004b; Barabas et al., 2006c; Barabas et al., 2006b; Barabas & Lafreniere, 2005); and
- to achieve a powerful immune response against an exogenous ag (Barabas et al., 2007d);

Below we give a detailed account of how and why the MVT has the potential of specifically preventing and curing certain chronic disorders such as autoimmune disease and disease caused by chronic infection.

## 2. Vaccination

Vaccination is the most cost-effective way to protect the public against undesirable medical conditions that can result in acute or chronic ailments. Vaccination by active immunization can prevent serious infectious and contagious diseases from occurring; and vaccination by passive immunization can neutralize existing disease causing/contributing agents (Hjelm et al., 2006; Imbach et al., 1981; Leandro & de, I, 2009; Levesque, 2009; Pirofsky & Kinzey, 1992; Segal et al., 1999). However, neither vaccination technique has been successfully implemented to date to achieve preventative or curative immune response outcomes in endogenous ag initiated and maintained disorders. It has been evident for a number of years that a technique other than those applied to diseases caused by exogenous ags is needed. The danger of using components derived from endogenous ags and causing added complications (e.g. autoimmune disease) has presented obstacles in the search for solutions (Finn & Forni, 2002; Peakman & Dayan, 2001). However, a better understanding of naturally occurring immune events, particularly pathogenic and non-pathogenic immune responses against self (Barabas et al., 2008b) - where the terms "pathogenic" and "non-pathogenic" do not equate with the terms "harmful" and "beneficial" - within the concept of autoimmunity promises to provide a framework for creating new possibilities for designing prophylactic and therapeutic vaccines for mishaps caused by or involving endogenous ags.

## 3. Autoimmunity conventional definition

Autoimmunity is conventionally defined in the scientific literature as abnormal immune response against self resulting in autoimmune disease. As such, autoimmunity is viewed as a self-destructive process, involving aberrant immune responses against self by the cells and products of the immune system, along with the wide spectrum of resulting autoimmune diseases which are generally chronic and progressive in nature. An autoimmune process is often irreversible, and currently the only readily available treatment is with drugs. In most cases the prognosis is guarded at best; even with the best medical care the symptoms of autoimmune conditions can generally only be minimized. Autoimmunity can result in morphological changes, including structural alterations in affected organs, that compromise and even destroy the normal functioning of the affected part. For example, in an experimental autoimmune kidney disease called Heymann nephritis (HN), we observe: a collection of symptoms including proteinuria, the presence in the circulation of pathogenic IgG autoantibodies (aabs) directed against the brush border (BB) region of the proximal renal tubules, massive deposition of immune complexes (ICs) in the glomeruli, and overall morphological and functional changes in affected regions of the kidney (Alousi et al., 1969; Andres et al., 1986; Edgington et al., 1967; Farquhar et al., 1995; Heymann et al., 1959; Kerjaschki, 1993; Kerjaschki & Farquhar, 1982; Singh & Kasinath, 1993). As in the case of HN, if the affected part is vitally important to the host and can no longer contribute to health, then premature death due to organ failure can ensue.

It is a common belief that once an autoimmune response is triggered it continues *in perpetuum* (Manz et al., 2002). However, many autoimmune diseases exhibit remission or exacerbation of disease processes, with or without drug treatment. Generally speaking it is not understood why. Autoimmune diseases are treated with immunosuppressive agents (Cattran, 1988; Fox & McCune, 1994; Fox & Ransohoff, 2004; Matsukawa et al., 1992) that have side effects and do not act specifically to terminate disease processes (Perna et al., 2004). In addition, as a result of their non-selective inhibition of the overall function of the immune system, these immunosuppressants expose patients to infection and related complications. The conventional understanding of how immunopathological processes cause autoimmune diseases (Davidson & Diamond, 2001; Feldmann & Steinman, 2005; Hill & Sarvetnick, 2002) does not allow for the possibility of reversing disease processes and re-establishing normalcy (Dorner et al., 2009) by the application of a vaccination technique.

## 4. Autoimmunity within the concept of beneficial and harmful aspects of immune responses against self in the light of new evidence

Autoimmunity properly understood denotes a complex interconnected network of immune responses against self that are not pathological in the first instance, but rather are designed to maintain the structural and functional integrity of the host's internal environment throughout life. The cells and products of the autoimmune system keep the internal environment of the host in a state of homeostasis. As a result of the proper functioning of the autoimmune system, intracytoplasmic components released from damaged cells (by burns, drugs, infectious agents, ischemia, toxic compounds, etc.) and from normal cells at the end of their life span are assisted in their removal by non-pathogenic IgM aabs (Avrameas, 1991; Casali & Notkins, 1989; Chen et al., 1995; Weir et al., 1966; Weir, 1966) and phagocytic cells (Barabas et al., 2004a; Helmy et al., 2006; Mevorach et al., 1998; UytdeHaag et al., 1991; Wermeling et al., 2009). Likewise, abnormal cells and cell lines having non-self antigenic surface markers (e.g. cancer cells) are also recognized and removed (Cheent & Khakoo, 2009; Foss, 2002; Topham & Hewitt, 2009). These are the two beneficial aspects of autoimmunity, by which it endeavours to keep the internal environment, composed as it is of endogenous ags, free of change. It is a major undertaking since several factors, both internal and external, have the potential to create an imbalance and cause harmful pathogenic immune responses against self, especially if the right triggers are present.

A well functioning autoimmune system averts most attempts by internal and external agents to create a harmful autoimmune response resulting in autoimmune disorders such as autoimmune disease and cancer (which themselves may be considered the two negative aspects of autoimmunity). It stands to reason that in order to protect against the kinds of insults that could lead to autoimmune disorders, we should engage in healthful consumption and healthful avoidance, eating healthy diets (consisting of fruits, vegetables, etc.) that contain chemicals or trace elements that boost the immune system or contribute to the prevention of cancer, and minimizing exposure to noxious agents (cigarette smoke, legal and illegal drugs, alcohol, and other toxic or infectious agents) that can chemically alter autoantigens (aags) and initiate autoimmune diseases (Greenwald et al., 2001; Howells et al., 2007; Nair et al., 2007). However it would also be advantageous to know more about the workings of the beneficial aspects of the autoimmune system, how it operates, how it maintains tolerance to self, how it might be influenced by naturally occurring or medically induced events to correct harmful immune responses and restore the organism to a normal state of health.

Observation tells us that the autoimmune system has the inbuilt ability to self-correct - with or without medical intervention - and restore the host to health, provided the correction occurs prior to overwhelming injury to the host's immune system and/or organs, tissues, or cells. We have conducted several recent experiments in this area, and have observed through these experiments that corrective immune responses can in fact be initiated by providing the right "information" to the cells of the autoimmune system. We have shown that with a vaccination technique that induces a predetermined immune response, autoimmune diseases can not only be prevented, but also, when present, terminated (Barabas et al., 2004b; Barabas et al., 2006c; Barabas et al., 2006b).

### 4.1 Beneficial aspects of autoimmunity resulting in tolerance to self

There are two beneficial aspects of autoimmunity, both characterized by maintenance of the integrity of the host's internal environment (homeostasis/healthy state) and involving the clearing and elimination of cellular waste and abnormal cell lines that are not conducive to the morphological and functional unity of the organism. Immunological cell lines are dedicated to surveyance and recognition of self and difference, or self and non-self (Kreuwel & Sherman, 2001; Sakaguchi, 2000). When difference is recognized there is usually enough time for the host to mount an immune response to avoid the establishment of an autoimmune disorder. Such protective immune responses are carried out by the normally functioning autoimmune system and as such the host is not aware of them. On the other hand, if the autoimmune system's natural ability to correct mishaps is compromised by age, dysfunction, suppression, misinformation, etc. then there exists a stronger likelihood of the host not being able to regain tolerance to self, and the host has a greater chance of experiencing ill health in the form of an autoimmune disorder.

### 4.1.1 Removal of cellular waste

Cells damaged by various agents or events (e.g. chemicals, drugs, ischemia, trauma, toxic compounds, UV irradiation, etc.) release their intracytoplasmic components into intra- and extravascular spaces. These cellular wastes are assisted in their removal by specific non-pathogenic IgM aabs (Avrameas, 1991; Weir, 1964; Weir et al., 1966; Weir, 1969; Zwart et al., 2004) and subsequently phagocytosed and broken down into reusable small MW peptides (Ciurana et al., 2004; Manson et al., 2005; Ogden et al., 2005; Quartier et al., 2005). It was shown by Weir and associates that in a physiological sense we are not *per se* tolerant to our own intracytoplasmic components, and specific IgM aabs are present in the circulation throughout life to clear the system of cellular breakdown products (Weir et al., 1966; Weir & Elson, 1969; Weir & Pinckard, 1967). Specific IgM aab production increases following excessive release of aags (secondary ab response) from an organ damaged by toxic agents, pathogenic IgG aabs, or ischemia at the site of rapid tumour growth etc. (Barabas et al., 2003; Pinckard & Weir, 1966; Weir, 1966). Circulating specific IgM aabs also contribute to rapid and efficient removal of cellular wastes to prevent not only their toxic accumulation in the system but also their possible chemical modification, which could trigger a tissue to be targeted and damaged by a pathogenic IgG aab response, an event which has the potential to initiate an autoimmune disease (Weir, 1969; Weir & Elson, 1969). IgM aabs are able to assist in the removal from the intracytoplasmic space not only of normal native aags released into the intra- and extravascular spaces but also of native-like ags (molecular mimicry) and native aags that are chemically or otherwise modified (Barabas et al., 2004b). Specific IgM aabs in the circulation are present with high titres measurable during the chronic phase of an autoimmune disease, as they assist in the removal of both disease causing and maintaining aags (modified aags that stimulate pathogenic IgG aab production) and disease contributing aags (target aags from the targeted organ) (Barabas et al., 2003; Barabas et al., 2004b). These cross-reactive specific IgM aabs are greatly responsible for the maintenance of tolerance to self during life by efficiently clearing the system of native and modified aags. If they can effectively clear the system of both native and modified aags during an autoimmune disease, then remission will occur, as manifested in signs of improvement and diminished symptoms (Barabas et al., 2004b; Barabas et al., 2006c; Barabas et al., 2006b; Barabas & Lafreniere, 2005). If the stimulus agent – that produces the modified self – ceases to be present in the system then spontaneous remission and termination of the autoimmune disease process will follow. However, as long as the modifying agent remains present in the system and is able to alter the chemical nature of self into non-self, the immune responses that cause the disease will continue, and the condition will be exacerbated and will manifest in a chronic progressive disease.

The autoimmune system's specific IgM aab production cell line will lose its ability to carry out its intended beneficial function in such circumstances where the modifying agent is continuously present in the system and maintains a pathogenic immune response. Its work may also be compromised in cases where the immune system is dysfunctional or has low IgM aab production because of old age, ill health, genetic predisposition, malnutrition, immune suppression, ineffective phagocytosis, etc. (Schulze et al., 2008; Wermeling et al., 2009).

### 4.1.2 Removal of abnormal cell lines

Just as intracytoplasmic waste is recognized as unwanted self and assisted in its removal by physiological non-pathogenic IgM aabs, cells with non-self markers, i.e., cancer cells, are also recognized by lymphocytes and their products – NK cells, cytolytic IgG aabs, etc. – and are eliminated from the system (Cheent & Khakoo, 2009; Kim et al., 2007; Topham & Hewitt, 2009). Such naturally occurring autoimmune responses are necessary to maintain the morphological and functional integrity of the host's organs, tissues, cells, etc. Without this beneficial aspect of autoimmunity, normal cells exposed to carcinogens, genetic influences, or even to normal aging could become cancerous, non-functional tissue, infiltrating the body and compromising its health. It is well documented that the incidence of cancer in the young is considerably lower than in the elderly, presumably because in the young a more efficient autoimmune system recognizes and responds to changes more readily, and/or cell cycles are more precisely regulated. (However, the autoimmune system's beneficial function of recognizing and eliminating cancer can be compromised at any age by a hazardous lifestyle [diets known to cause cancer, smoking, drinking, excessive exposure to the sun], genetic predisposition, exposure to certain infectious agents, malnutrition, immune suppression, etc. (Arver et al., 2000; Baniyash, 2006; Beral et al., 1991; Birkeland et al., 1995; Greenwald et al., 2001; Khuder et al., 1998).

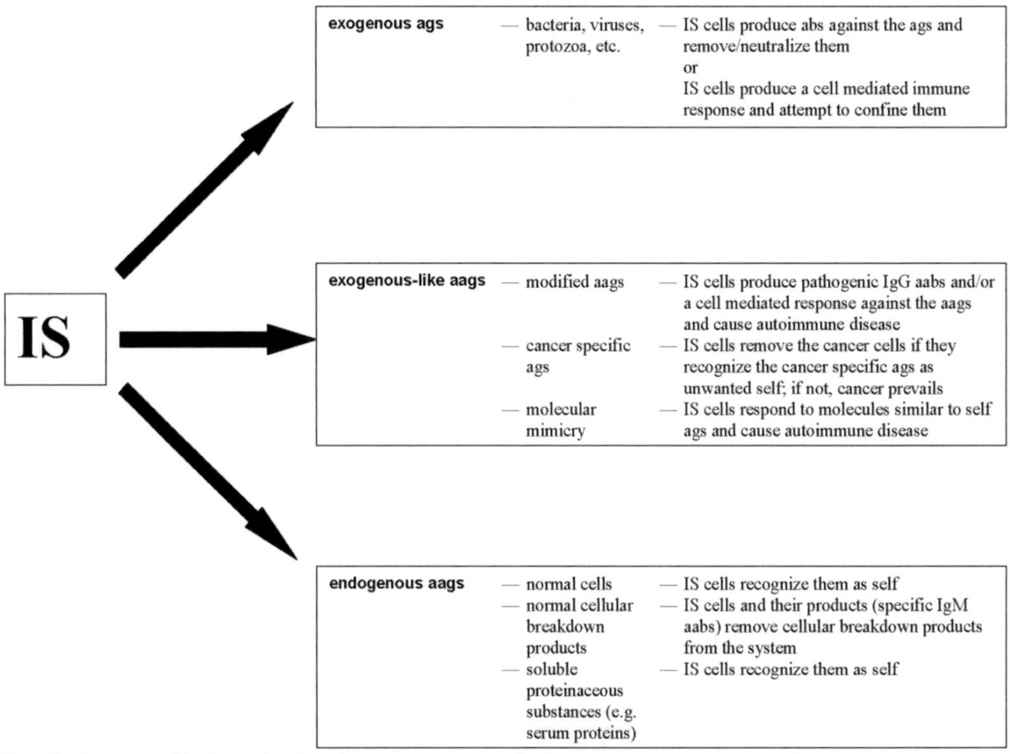


Fig. 1. A normally functioning immune system's immune responses against exogenous ags, exogenous-like and endogenous aags.
The IS is designed to remove exogenous ags, exogenous-like aags, and cellular breakdown products of normal cells from the system to maintain homeostasis and tolerance to self. However, prolonged exposure to exogenous ags can result in chronic infections, exogenous-like aags can induce autoimmune diseases, and deficient processing of cancer specific aags on the surface of cancer cells can permit the growth of cancer.
Abbreviations: aabs, autoantibodies; aags, autoantigens; abs, antibodies; ags, antigens; IgG, immunoglobulin G; IgM, immunoglobulin M; IS, immune system

In order for the autoimmune system to respond for the benefit of the host, the cancer specific ags on cancer cell surfaces must be readily available for immune processing. In this regard, the cancer specific ag must be somehow detached, chemically degraded, and made available separately from normal cell membrane components or other normal self molecules shared with normal cells to stimulate immune cell lines to produce pathogenic lytic IgG aabs (primary ab response) against the cancer cell line bearing that specific ag. If this process occurs and pathogenic lytic IgG aabs are produced, then regardless of where those cancer cells are located in the body they will be lysed and the cellular breakdown products eliminated by non-pathogenic IgM aabs (secondary ab response).

It is noteworthy that in cancer defence one of the most important aspects of autoimmunity is manifested in a pathogenic IgG aab response against a self-like group of cells (Jager et al., 1999; Tureci et al., 2006) (Figure 1).

Pathogenic autoimmune response against altered self (i.e., cancer specific ag on cancer cells) is clearly a highly beneficial aspect of autoimmunity. In such circumstances tolerance to self (to a self-like group of cells) is lost, but the host's internal environment is protected from possible changes that could result in tumour growth. However, pathogenic lytic IgG ab response may fail to occur for the following reasons:

- the cancer specific ag is minimally antigenic (Foss, 2002; Lollini & Forni, 2002) (and a small MW protein), is closely associated with normal cell surface components, and does not detach easily to allow its recognition as non-self for pathogenic immune response inducement; or
- the host's immune system is prevented from functioning against an apparent self ag by inbuilt protective regulatory cells and molecules (Cheent & Khakoo, 2009; Musiani et al., 1997).

### 4.2 Harmful aspects of autoimmunity resulting in autoimmune disorders

There are two harmful aspects of autoimmunity, both of which have the potential to manifest in disease states, one being an adverse immune response against normal self, causing an autoimmune disease; and the other being tolerance of an abnormal cell line, so that cancer growth is permitted. These disease states, or autoimmune disorders, come about when the immune system's surveying ability is mislead into situations of improper response or non-response to changes in self. It is observed in many autoimmune diseases that modified self initiates and/or maintains pathogenic aab responses against a target ag, causing a disease state (Barabas et al., 2004c; Heymann et al., 1959), whereas in cancer, ags identifiable as cancer specific are minimally antigenic and not recognized as unwanted self, and therefore fail to induce an immune response that eliminates the cancer cells (Foss, 2002; Kim et al., 2007).

In many respects the autoimmune system responds correctly during the development and maintenance of autoimmune disorders. In fact, the immune system does what it is instructed to do or not to do by the "information" it receives. In the case of self reaction, for instance, the cells and the products of the cells of the autoimmune system are virtually predestined to react against altered self, in that altered self is non-self and non-self should provoke a pathogenic immune response. Unfortunately, such an immune response against altered self can cause an autoimmune disease, as the developing pathogenic aabs are cross-reactive, i.e., in addition to reacting against the modified self ag that initiates and maintains their production, they also react with normal self, causing harm to the tissue and providing more substrate for the reaction to continue. In the case of cancer, on the other hand, the cells and the products of the autoimmune system do not react with the minimally altered self on cancer cell surfaces and the cancer cells are not be eliminated, therefore allowing the cancer to prevail (Foss, 2002).

### 4.2.1 Initiation and maintenance of an autoimmune disease

The induction and maintenance of autoimmune diseases, as well as the associated immunopathological and functional changes, have been extremely well studied in experimental animals (Andres et al., 1986; Barabas et al., 1969; Barabas & Lannigan, 1969; Grupe & Kaplan, 1969; Heymann et al., 1959; Kerjaschki, 1993; Kerjaschki, 2000b; Kerjaschki & Farquhar, 1982); and by comparative study the etiology and pathogenesis of human autoimmune diseases are equally well understood (Davidson & Diamond, 2001; Kretz-Rommel et al., 1997; Kretz-Rommel & Rubin, 1999; Sinha et al., 1990; Theofilopoulos, 1995; Tung, 1994; Von Herrath & Oldstone, 1995). In most instances for an autoimmune disease to begin, a modified self (Barabas et al., 2004c) or self-like (molecular mimicry) (Ebringer et al., 1997; Ebringer, 2003; Mokhtarian et al., 1999; Orbach & Shoenfeld, 2007) ag has to present itself as a foreign-like, exogenous-like ag to the cells of the immune system. There are numerous agents that are able to modify self ags (toxins, chemicals, infectious agents, drugs, adjuvants, vaccines, smoking, chemical dyes, UV irradiation, etc.) and initiate a pathogenic IgG aab response (Barabas et al., 2004c; Conti et al., 2008; Davidson & Diamond, 2001; Hess, 1999; Heymann et al., 1959; Rao & Richardson, 1999; ten Veen & Feltkamp, 1972) (initially a primary immune response, as the immune system has not previously been exposed to the modified ag). If the modifying agent is continuously present in the system, then the modified self ag will continue to stimulate the appropriate T and B cells to maintain the production of pathogenic IgG aabs by the plasma cells (secondary ab response) (Barabas et al., 2003). The developing pathogenic IgG aabs are cross-reactive (Barabas & Lafreniere, 2005). They react with the modified self ag and the normal target ag in an organ. ICs made up of modified self and anti-modified self IgG aab form as a result. The fate of these ICs is twofold. In part they are neutralized and eliminated. However, insofar as they are not fully or quickly enough removed from the body they operate to maintain the pathogenic IgG aab production.

The pathogenic IgG aabs also react with the target ag not just as it appears in the circulation, but also *in situ* within the organ where it originates; e.g. in HN circulating anti-nephritogenic IgG aabs attack renal tubular BB localized nephritogenic ags and release them into the circulation (Barabas et al., 2003; Barabas et al., 2006c). Released aags will join IC deposits on the epithelial side of the glomerular basement membrane enlarging the deposits and thus causing morphological and functional injury to the kidney (Barabas et al., 2003). Continuously produced pathogenic IgG aabs and aags continually released from the damaged normal renal tubules will continue to enlarge the deposits in the glomeruli together with complement components, causing a chronic progressive autoimmune kidney disease (Barabas et al., 2003). The progression of disease processes or diminution of disease intensity depends mainly on the presence of the modifying agent in the system, because as stated above the immune response outcome depends on the presentation of the ag to the cells of the immune system. The continuous alteration of self by the modifying agent in the system drives the pathogenic autoimmune response to produce high levels of circulating pathogenic IgG aabs. As long as a pathogenic IgG aab is present in the circulation, the disease process will continue. The level of pathogenic IgG aab must be at zero for no autoimmune disease process to be detectable in the host (Barabas et al., 2004b).

In contrast to the common belief, we and a few other scientists believe that the normal target ag on its own will not under normal circumstances initiate a pathogenic IgG aab response (Barabas et al., 2004c; Barabas et al., 2006a; Rich, 1996; Totoritis & Rubin, 1985; Weir & Elson, 1969; Weir & Pinckard, 1967). Administration of native ags during autoimmune disease states, e.g. during slowly progressive Heymann nephritis (SPHN), other experimental situations, do not make the disease process progress more intense (Barabas et al., 2006a; Bielekova et al., 2000; Peakman & Dayan, 2001; Prakken et al., 2004). Rather the opposite, in most instances they reduce the pathogenic immune response (Barabas et al., 2004c; Barabas et al., 2006a). It seems that even during a disease state the native target ag preferentially stimulates IgM aab production. The IgM aabs being cross-reactive, their increased levels remove from the circulation both the disease contributing native target ag and the disease causing modified target ag (Barabas et al., 2007a), contributing to remission.

It is worth noting, in reference to a broader context, that the initiation and intensification of an autoimmune disease are undoubtedly complex, and may involve numerous factors or processes besides those described above, such as:

- genetic predisposition;
- dysfunctional autoimmune system response (e.g. reduced phagocytosis and reduced specific IgM aab production due to age, malnutrition, vitamin deficiency, overwhelming infection, etc.);
- presentation of modified self aags or exogenous self-like ags to dendritic cells prior to antigenic information being processed by T and B cells for plasma cells to produce pathogenic IgG aabs;
- regulatory molecules (cytokines, chemokines, etc.) attempting to accelerate or decelerate autoimmune processes;
- complement systems or components playing dominant roles in aag and aab reactions during an autoimmune disease (in both pathogenic and non-pathogenic immune responses) (Blom, 2010):
  a. assisting in the complement-dependent clearance of modified/unmodified self that causes the autoimmune disease (Gaipl et al., 2001; Taylor et al., 2000; Zwart et al., 2004);
  b. in contributing to the continuously layered aag/aab depositions, e.g. in the glomeruli (Barabas et al., 2003; Barabas et al., 2004b; Barabas et al., 2004c) (pathogenic immune response) causing complement mediated C3, $C_5 9_b$ injury (Barabas et al., 2003; Barabas et al., 2004c) resulting in compromised glomerular filtration;
- overwhelming infection by an infectious agent presenting a whole range of potentially antigenic peptides that may initiate autoimmune disease by molecular mimicry;
- environmental factors;
- potentially self reactive clones of T cells can react with self because of immune regulation failure;
- in a few instances self ags can act to initiate and maintain pathogenic autoimmune responses against self, e.g. when regulatory T cells are out of control.

Notwithstanding the influence of such other factors, the set of processes described above appear to be fundamental to autoimmune disease involving misdirected auto-reaction, and understanding them has assisted in the development of a powerful technique to deal with autoimmune disease, as we will describe further below.

#### 4.2.2 Inability to recognize and remove abnormal cell lines

Throughout life abnormal cell lines (some being cancerous) can emerge. They are most often recognized as non-self and removed by the cells of the autoimmune system. NK cells play a dominant role in this regard (Cheent & Khakoo, 2009; Foss, 2002; Topham & Hewitt, 2009).
Cancer specific non-self antigenic markers on the cell surfaces of emerging cancer cells are sometimes weakly antigenic; for this reason, they do not lend themselves to immune recognition and provoke immune response (Foss, 2002; Kim et al., 2007). In addition, tumour ags associated with cancer cell surfaces are camouflaged or protected on the cell membranes of these self-like cancer cells. The combination of minimal antigenicity and firm integration into and protection by the cell surface membrane means that even after cell death, these cancer specific ags do not detach to form individual small MW antigenic fragments that might be recognized as non-self for immune response processing. Further, if these cells are growing in a well vascularised space and allowed to spread into secondary sites without undermining influences such as ischemia, lack of nutrients, vitamins, or trace minerals, immune attack, etc. then the emerging cancer cells are more readily accepted as self. Several factors, such as old age, compromised immune system function (e.g. from treatment with immunosuppressive agents), overwhelming infections, exposure to harmful substances (smoking, alcohol, chemicals, drugs, etc.), and tumour derived soluble factors, can interfere with the normal functioning of the cells of the immune system in carrying out the surveillance of the somatic cells of our internal environments (Kim et al., 2007).
The lack of adjuvant in a mixture of the disintegrated components of dead cancer cells which include cell membrane associated ags has been shown to prevent pathogenic immune response against cancer specific ags, though it also prevented immune response against normal cell membrane associated ags (Ichim, 2005). And as we have noted elsewhere, normal self ags administered in adjuvants can induce pathogenic autoimmune responses, causing autoimmune disease – especially in the case of experimental autoimmune diseases (Barabas et al., 2004c; Heymann et al., 1959). Therefore, although a pathogenic autoimmune response is required against the cancer specific ag in order to kill (lyse) the cancer cells in the system, the use of an adjuvant to induce such an autoimmune response would likely have a deleterious effect against normal self as well. The question is how to overcome the immune system's inability to respond only against the non-self parts of cancer cells without causing harm to their normal functioning counterparts either in the organ where the primary tumour originated or elsewhere.

## 5. MVT for the prevention and cure of diseases caused by chronic immune disorders

Our MVT, which involves the administration of IC formed with condition-specific components that initiate and maintain a predetermined immune response, has the potential to prevent chronic ailments, and to cure already present diseases (Barabas et al., 2004b; Barabas et al., 2006c; Barabas et al., 2006b; Barabas et al., 2009a). This is the first time that the promise has existed to prevent, treat, and cure endogenous ag induced mishaps in humans specifically and without side effects.
The study of the affects of injection of ag:ab ICs at different ratios is not new, nor is the use of ICs in increasing ab production (Klaus, 1978; Kunkl & Klaus, 1981; Nie et al., 1997; Stoner et al., 1975; Stoner & Terres, 1963; Terres et al., 1972; Terres & Stoner, 1962; Terres & Wolins, 1959; Terres & Wolins, 1961) and even in vaccination (Haddad et al., 1997; Jeurissen et al.,

1998; Whitfill et al., 1995; Xu et al., 2005; Yao et al., 2007). So far most of the pertinent investigations have described the role that ag:ab ICs play in immune response upon injection of such complexes at various ratios, and how enhanced ab production occurs during primary and secondary ab responses (Barabas et al., 2007d; Heyman, 2000; Stoner & Terres, 1963; Xu et al., 2005; Yao et al., 2007).

To date, we are the only group to have described how specifically composed ag:ab complexes can redirect the immune response for the health benefit of the vaccinated host (Barabas et al., 2004b; Barabas et al., 2006c; Barabas et al., 2006b; Barabas et al., 2007c; Barabas et al., 2009a; Barabas & Lafreniere, 2005). The possibility of such an approach has just recently become a reality, following the categorization of autoimmunity into four clearly definable functioning immunological responses (Figure 2) against self (Barabas et al., 2008a;

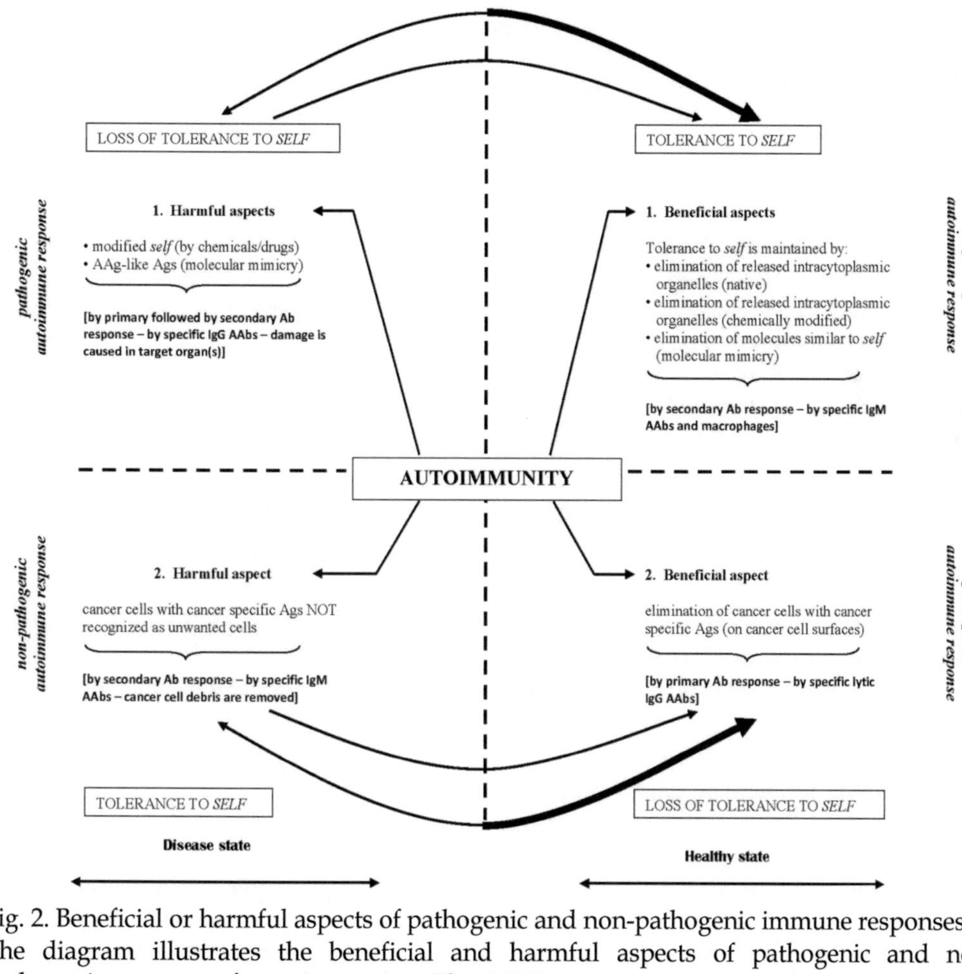


Fig. 2. Beneficial or harmful aspects of pathogenic and non-pathogenic immune responses. The diagram illustrates the beneficial and harmful aspects of pathogenic and non-pathogenic aspects of autoimmunity. The MVT can restore non-pathogenic tolerance, ending an autoimmune disease. [Figure reproduced by permission from BioProcessing Journal, 2007 Winter;6(4):12-18.]

Abbreviations: AAb, autoantibody; AAg, autoantigen; Ab, antibody; Ag, antigen; MVT, modified vaccination technique

Barabas et al., 2009a), and the development of our understanding of autoimmune disease etiology and pathogenesis, in particular the role of non-pathogenic and pathogenic aabs (Figure 1) in both disease development and in its prevention and cure (Barabas et al., 2004b; Barabas et al., 2006c; Barabas et al., 2006b) (e.g. in autoimmune disease).

NOTE:

- The concept of autoimmunity is presently understood as pathogenic immune response against self, causing autoimmune disease.
- Autoimmune anomalies cannot be specifically prevented or treated by any of the presently available vaccination techniques.
- The concept of autoimmunity, according to our definition, encompasses four possible immune responses against self: two beneficial and two harmful ones.
- The harmful aspects of autoimmunity manifest in autoimmune diseases and cancer.

The immune system's natural ability can be utilized to bring about corrective immune responses which can cure/terminate chronic ailments by proper presentation of the target ag. In other words, the ag that causes or contributes to the disease can also terminate it, provided the antigenic information is presented to the cells of the immune system in the proper format.

The vaccination method we have developed - which is essentially the third vaccination rubric to have arisen, coming as it has after the conventional active and passive immunization techniques - promises to be able to deal with chronic ailments that are presently only treatable with drugs. Called MVT, it is so named because every time a vaccine is produced it must be formulated of components that are tailor-made to induce a specific corrective immune response. In order to achieve specificity - and to avoid collateral damage to normal body constituents - the production of absolutely pure and specific target ags and their abs is required. This can be done by present techniques, and soon more sophisticated methodologies will be available.

## 6. Components of the modified vaccine and how it works

### 6.1 Target ag against which the desired ab response is required

- For application in an autoimmune disease: ag prepared *ex vivo* that is identical in molecular composition to, and therefore the specific equivalent of, the host's target ag (native aag) (Kerjaschki, 2000a; Kerjaschki & Farquhar, 1982);
- For application in a chronic infection: ag derived from the causative organism, prepared *ex vivo*.

### 6.2 Ab against the disease causing/contributing target ag

- For application in an autoimmune disease: homologous non-pathogenic IgM ab directed against the target ag(s), prepared *ex vivo* by monoclonal ab technology;
- For application in a chronic infection: homologous pathogenic neutralizing IgG ab against target ags on the surface of infectious agents, prepared *ex vivo*.

The modified vaccine is composed of an IC mixture made up of the target ag and ab against the target ag in slight ag excess. E.g. in an experimental autoimmune kidney disease (Barabas et al., 2003; Barabas et al., 2004b; Barabas et al., 2006c; Barabas et al., 2006b) it was observed that:

- immunization with suitable IC (rat kidney fraction 3 X rat anti-rat kidney fraction 3 IgM ab) at slight ag excess prior and subsequent to disease-inducing inoculation prevented

the occurrence of the autoimmune kidney disease (Barabas et al., 2004b; Barabas et al., 2006b) (prophylactic vaccination);
- immunization post-disease-induction with the same IC, when the autoimmune disease was in its chronic progressive phase, terminated the disease causing immune events (Barabas et al., 2004b; Barabas et al., 2006b) (increased levels of specific IgM aabs removed both the pathogenic immune response inducing modified ag and the disease contributing native aag from the system, thereby terminating pathogenic immune response; therapeutic vaccination);
- corrective immune response induction was immediate (similar to secondary ab response);
- there was no need for adjuvant application as immune response was quick, specific, and powerful;
- the MVT was not a mere supplementary therapeutic option for prevention or treatment of the endogenous ag induced disorder; rather, it was key; by ab information transfer, utilizing the immune system's natural abilities. We achieved production in the vaccinated host of the same ab (i.e., the corrective immune response), with the same specificity against the target ag, as was present in the injected IC; and
- tolerance to self was accomplished specifically and without side effects (utilizing the MVT) by downregulating and terminating pathogenic immune events.

## 7. Conclusion

There are several reasons why up to now chronic disorders have been mainly treated with drugs and not by immune intervention. Perhaps the most important reason was that we were unable to present the offending ag(s) (i.e., the antigenic information) to the cells of the immune system in a suitable form to elicit corrective immune response outcomes. However, we have learned how to prepare and present exogenous ags such as bacterial/viral products to the body in attenuated or inactivated forms - usually in adjuvants - to elicit protective immune responses.

We have developed a new vaccination methodology called MVT that is able to downregulate immunopathological events in an experimental autoimmune kidney disease in animals and is also able to upregulate immune responses against an exogenous ag. This method, which is the third method of vaccination to be developed, has the potential not only to prevent but with equal effectiveness cure certain autoimmune diseases and chronic infections in humans.

Autoimmunity encompasses four possible immunological events against self, two beneficial and two harmful aspects (Figure 2). The two beneficial aspects of autoimmunity function throughout life to preserve the internal integrity of the organism by maintaining tolerance to normal self while preventing corrupted self from taking hold. The maintenance of antigenic homeostasis is the most important function of the autoimmune system.

The autoimmune system achieves its aim on one hand (the first beneficial aspect of autoimmunity) by degrading cellular debris - from cells damaged by various agents (e.g. chemicals, drugs, smoke, toxins, etc.) and from cells which have come to the end of their lifespan - into reusable small MW peptides. The efficient clearance of cellular waste is assisted by non-pathogenic IgM aabs prior to their degradation by phagocytic cells. These specific IgM aabs are the main agents of the maintenance of tolerance to self, and fulfill a continuous physiological role throughout life. In a physiological sense, we are not *per se* tolerant to normal self components within cells.

On the other hand (the second beneficial aspect of autoimmunity) the autoimmune system works to eliminate abnormal cell lines that emerge as a result of external (e.g. drugs, radiation, smoking, etc.) and internal (e.g. genetic) influences. Emerging cancer cells are recognized and eliminated by NK cells. In addition, cancer specific ags can stimulate a pathogenic lytic IgG aab response, particularly when presented to the system with an adjuvant. These aabs may lyse cancer cells in the presence of complement and eliminate them from the system.

The two harmful aspects of autoimmunity, i.e., autoimmune disease and cancer, will manifest only if external (e.g. carcinogens, chemicals, infectious agents, UV irradiation, drugs, smoking) or internal (e.g. genetic) influences cause changes in the structural makeup of cells or cell products containing native ags. Such changes could result in harmful immune events leading to functional disturbance of the affected cells, tissues and organs.

Taking advantage of recent insight into the workings of the immune system, our MVT has proved itself to be effective in preventing the development of an experimental autoimmune kidney disease, and when the disease was in its progressive phase, in terminating it altogether, by halting immunopathological events that were causing the symptomatic, morphological and functional changes.

The immune system has a natural ability to correct immunological mishaps and restore the body to normalcy, provided the right information is presented to it for processing. The MVT is a way of presenting that information, in the form of specific ICs, and triggering or enhancing the body's own ability to counteract autoimmune disease, cancer, and chronic infection. We have observed that by injecting ICs - made up of a given endogenous or exogenous ag and a specific ab against it at slight ag excess - into experimental animals, the recipient's immune system produced the same ab, with the same specificity against the target ag, as was present in the IC (ab information transfer).

We have shown in experimental situations that corrective immune responses can be induced by the application of the MVT. We remain convinced that by the proper application of the MVT in humans, chronic diseases such as cancer, autoimmune disease, and chronic infections will be prevented and cured as well.

## 8. Acknowledgement

We acknowledge the assistance of our research associate, Zoltan B. Kovacs, in computer and laboratory-related work.

## 9. References

Alousi, M.A., Post, R.S. & Heymann, W. (1969). Experimental autoimmune nephrosis in rats. Morphogenesis of the glomerular lesion: immunohistochemical and electron microscopic studies. *Am J Pathol*, 54(1): 47-71.

Andreakos, E., Taylor, P.C. & Feldmann, M. (2002). Monoclonal antibodies in immune and inflammatory diseases. *Curr Opin Biotechnol*, 13(6): 615-20.

Andres, G., Brentjens, J.R., Caldwell, P.R., Camussi, G. & Matsuo, S. (1986). Formation of immune deposits and disease. *Lab Invest*, 55(5): 510-20.

Arver, B., Du, Q., Chen, J., Luo, L. & Lindblom, A. (2000). Hereditary breast cancer: a review. *Semin Cancer Biol*, 10(4): 271-88.

Avrameas, S. (1991). Natural autoantibodies: from 'horror autotoxicus' to 'gnothi seauton'. *Immunol Today*, 12(5): 154-9.

Baniyash, M. (2006). Chronic inflammation, immunosuppression and cancer: new insights and outlook. *Semin Cancer Biol*, 16(1): 80-8.

Barabas, A.Z., Cole, C.D., Barabas, A.D., Bahlis, N.J. & Lafreniere, R. (2008a). New vaccination technology for endogenous antigen-derived ailments. *IDrugs*, 11(2): 111-5.

Barabas, A.Z., Cole, C.D., Barabas, A.D., Bahlis, N.J. & Lafreniere, R. (2007a). A vaccination technique to combat presently untreatable chronic ailments. *BioProcessing Journal*, 6(4): 12-8.

Barabas, A.Z., Cole, C.D., Barabas, A.D., Barabas, A.N. & Lafreniere, R. (2006a). Effect of rat kidney fraction 3 (rKF3) antigen and specific IgM antibody against rKF3 on the progression of slowly progressive Heymann nephritis. *Pathol Int*, 56(9): 516-29.

Barabas, A.Z., Cole, C.D., Barabas, A.D., Barabas, A.N. & Lafreniere, R. (2006b). Reduced incidence of slowly progressive Heymann nephritis in rats immunized with a modified vaccination technique. *Clin Dev Immunol*, 13(1): 17-24.

Barabas, A.Z., Cole, C.D., Barabas, A.D., Cowan, J.M., Yoon, C.S., Waisman, D.M. & Lafreniere, R. (2004a). Presence of immunoglobulin M antibodies around the glomerular capillaries and in the mesangium of normal and passive Heymann nephritis rats. *Int J Exp Pathol*, 85(4): 201-12.

Barabas, A.Z., Cole, C.D., Barabas, A.D., Graeff, R.M., Lafreniere, R. & Weir, D.M. (2009a). Correcting autoimmune anomalies in autoimmune disorders by immunological means, employing the modified vaccination technique. *Autoimmun Rev*, 8(7): 552-7.

Barabas, A.Z., Cole, C.D., Barabas, A.D. & Lafreniere, R. (2003). Production of a new model of slowly progressive Heymann nephritis. *Int J Exp Pathol*, 84(6): 245-58.

Barabas, A.Z., Cole, C.D., Barabas, A.D. & Lafreniere, R. (2004b). Down-regulation of pathogenic autoantibody response in a slowly progressive Heymann nephritis kidney disease model. *Int J Exp Pathol*, 85(6): 321-34.

Barabas, A.Z., Cole, C.D., Barabas, A.D. & Lafreniere, R. (2004c). Production of Heymann nephritis by a chemically modified renal antigen. *Int J Exp Pathol*, 85(5): 277-85.

Barabas, A.Z., Cole, C.D., Barabas, A.D. & Lafreniere, R. (2006c). Downregulation of a pathogenic autoantibody response by IgM autoantibodies directed against the nephritogenic antigen in slowly progressive Heymann nephritis. *Pathol Int*, 56(4): 181-90.

Barabas, A.Z., Cole, C.D., Barabas, A.D. & Lafreniere, R. (2007b). A modified vaccination technique for the prevention and treatment of an experimental autoimmune kidney disease. *Ann N Y Acad Sci*, 1110 619-29.

Barabas, A.Z., Cole, C.D., Barabas, A.D. & Lafreniere, R. (2007c). Preventative and therapeutic vaccination to combat an experimental autoimmune kidney disease. *Biologics: Targets & Therapy*, 1(1): 59-68.

Barabas, A.Z., Cole, C.D., Barabas, A.D. & Lafreniere, R. 2008b. Pathogenic and nonpathogenic autoimmune events – the good and/or the bad?, In: *Autoantibodies research progress*, Dubois, Q., (ed), Nova Science Publishers, Inc., Hauppauge NY, 9-18.

Barabas, A.Z., Cole, C.D., Kovacs, Z.B. & Lafreniere, R. (2007d). Elevated antibody response by antigen presentation in immune complexes. *Med Sci Monit*, 13(5): BR119-BR124.

Barabas, A.Z., Elson, C.J. & Weir, D.M. (1969). The serology of autologous immune complex nephritis in the rat. *Clin Exp Immunol*, 4(3): 345-51.

Barabas, A.Z. & Lafreniere, R. (2005). Antigen-specific down-regulation of immunopathological events in an experimental autoimmune kidney disease. *Autoimmun Rev*, 4(8): 565-70.

Barabas, A.Z. & Lannigan, R. (1969). Auto-immune nephritis in rats. *J Pathol*, 97(3): 537-43.

Barabas, A.Z., Weir, D.M., Cole, C.D., Barabas, A.D., Bahlis, N.J., Graeff, R.M. & Lafreniere, R. (2009b). Preventing and treating chronic disorders using the modified vaccination technique. *Front Biosci*, 14 3892-8.

Ben Yehuda, O., Tomer, Y. & Shoenfeld, Y. (1988). Advances in therapy of autoimmune diseases. *Semin Arthritis Rheum*, 17(3): 206-20.

Beral, V., Jaffe, H. & Weiss, R. (1991). Cancer surveys: cancer, HIV and AIDS. *Eur J Cancer*, 27(8): 1057-8.

Berinstein, N.L. (2007). Enhancing cancer vaccines with immunomodulators. *Vaccine*, 25 Suppl 2 B72-B88.

Bielekova, B., Goodwin, B., Richert, N., Cortese, I., Kondo, T., Afshar, G., Gran, B., Eaton, J., Antel, J., Frank, J.A., McFarland, H.F. & Martin, R. (2000). Encephalitogenic potential of the myelin basic protein peptide (amino acids 83-99) in multiple sclerosis: results of a phase II clinical trial with an altered peptide ligand. *Nat Med*, 6(10): 1167-75.

Birkeland, S.A., Storm, H.H., Lamm, L.U., Barlow, L., Blohme, I., Forsberg, B., Eklund, B., Fjeldborg, O., Friedberg, M., Frodin, L. & . (1995). Cancer risk after renal transplantation in the Nordic countries, 1964-1986. *Int J Cancer*, 60(2): 183-9.

Blom, A.M. 2010. Complement: deficiency diseases, In: *Encyclopedia of life sciences*, John Wiley & Sons, Ltd., Chichester GB, 1-8.

Casali, P. & Notkins, A.L. (1989). CD5+ B lymphocytes, polyreactive antibodies and the human B-cell repertoire. *Immunol Today*, 10(11): 364-8.

Cattran, D.C. (1988). Effect of ciclosporin on active Heymann nephritis. *Nephron*, 48(2): 142-8.

Cheent, K. & Khakoo, S.I. (2009). Natural killer cells: integrating diversity with function. *Immunology*, 126(4): 449-57.

Chen, Z.J., Wheeler, J. & Notkins, A.L. (1995). Antigen-binding B cells and polyreactive antibodies. *Eur J Immunol*, 25(2): 579-86.

Ciurana, C.L., Zwart, B., van Mierlo, G. & Hack, C.E. (2004). Complement activation by necrotic cells in normal plasma environment compares to that by late apoptotic cells and involves predominantly IgM. *Eur J Immunol*, 34(9): 2609-19.

Conti, F., Rezai, S. & Valesini, G. (2008). Vaccination and autoimmune rheumatic diseases. *Autoimmun Rev*, 8(2): 124-8.

Davidson, A. & Diamond, B. (2001). Autoimmune diseases. *N Engl J Med*, 345(5): 340-50.

Dorner, T., Radbruch, A. & Burmester, G.R. (2009). B-cell-directed therapies for autoimmune disease. *Nat Rev Rheumatol*, 5(8): 433-41.

Ebringer, A. 2003. Molecular mimicry as the basis of a new theory of autoimmunity, In: *Frontiers in Autoimmunity: fundamental aspects and clinical perspectives*, Zouali, M., (ed), IOS Press, Amsterdam Netherlands, 79-99.

Ebringer, A., Thorpe, C., Pirt, J., Wilson, C., Cunningham, P. & Ettelaie, C. (1997). Bovine spongiform encephalopathy: is it an autoimmune disease due to bacteria showing molecular mimicry with brain antigens? *Environ Health Perspect*, 105(11): 1172-4.

Edgington, T.S., Glassock, R.J. & Dixon, F.J. (1967). Autologous immune-complex pathogenesis of experimental allergic glomerulonephritis. *Science*, 155(768): 1432-4.

Engelhard, V.H., Bullock, T.N., Colella, T.A., Sheasley, S.L. & Mullins, D.W. (2002). Antigens derived from melanocyte differentiation proteins: self-tolerance, autoimmunity, and use for cancer immunotherapy. *Immunol Rev*, 188 136-46.

Farquhar, M.G., Saito, A., Kerjaschki, D. & Orlando, R.A. (1995). The Heymann nephritis antigenic complex: megalin (gp330) and RAP. *J Am Soc Nephrol*, 6(1): 35-47.

Feldmann, M. & Steinman, L. (2005). Design of effective immunotherapy for human autoimmunity. *Nature*, 435(7042): 612-9.

Finn, O.J. & Forni, G. (2002). Prophylactic cancer vaccines. *Curr Opin Immunol*, 14(2): 172-7.

Foss, F.M. (2002). Immunologic mechanisms of antitumor activity. *Semin Oncol*, 29(3 Suppl 7): 5-11.

Fox, D.A. & McCune, W.J. (1994). Immunosuppressive drug therapy of systemic lupus erythematosus. *Rheum Dis Clin North Am*, 20(1): 265-99.

Fox, R.J. & Ransohoff, R.M. (2004). New directions in MS therapeutics: vehicles of hope. *Trends Immunol*, 25(12): 632-6.

Gaipl, U.S., Kuenkele, S., Voll, R.E., Beyer, T.D., Kolowos, W., Heyder, P., Kalden, J.R. & Herrmann, M. (2001). Complement binding is an early feature of necrotic and a rather late event during apoptotic cell death. *Cell Death Differ*, 8(4): 327-34.

Golbus, J. & McCune, W.J. (1994). Lupus nephritis. Classification, prognosis, immunopathogenesis, and treatment. *Rheum Dis Clin North Am*, 20(1): 213-42.

Greenwald, P., Clifford, C.K. & Milner, J.A. (2001). Diet and cancer prevention. *Eur J Cancer*, 37(8): 948-65.

Grupe, W.E. & Kaplan, M.H. (1969). Demonstration of an antibody to proximal tubular antigen in the pathogenesis of experimental autoimmune nephrosis in rats. *J Lab Clin Med*, 74(3): 400-9.

Haddad, E.E., Whitfill, C.E., Avakian, A.P., Ricks, C.A., Andrews, P.D., Thoma, J.A. & Wakenell, P.S. (1997). Efficacy of a novel infectious bursal disease virus immune complex vaccine in broiler chickens. *Avian Dis*, 41(4): 882-9.

Hasegawa, Y., Kaneoka, H., Tanaka, T., Ogahara, S., Matsumae, T., Noda, R., Yoshitake, K., Murata, T. & Naito, S. (2001). Suppression of experimental membranous glomerulonephritis in rats by an anti-MHC class II antibody. *Nephron*, 88(3): 233-40.

Helmy, K.Y., Katschke, K.J., Jr., Gorgani, N.N., Kljavin, N.M., Elliott, J.M., Diehl, L., Scales, S.J., Ghilardi, N. & van Lookeren, C.M. (2006). CRIg: a macrophage complement receptor required for phagocytosis of circulating pathogens. *Cell*, 124(5): 915-27.

Hess, E.V. (1999). Are there environmental forms of systemic autoimmune diseases? *Environ Health Perspect*, 107 Suppl 5 709-11.

Heyman, B. (2000). Regulation of antibody responses via antibodies, complement, and Fc receptors. *Annu Rev Immunol*, 18 709-37.

Heymann, W., Hackel, D.B., Harwood, S., Wilson, S.G. & Hunter, J.L.P. (1959). Production of the nephritic syndrome in rat by Freund's adjuvant and rat kidney suspension. *Proc Soc Exp Biol Med*, 100 660-4.

Hill, N. & Sarvetnick, N. (2002). Cytokines: promoters and dampeners of autoimmunity. *Curr Opin Immunol*, 14(6): 791-7.

Hjelm, F., Carlsson, F., Getahun, A. & Heyman, B. (2006). Antibody-mediated regulation of the immune response. *Scand J Immunol*, 64(3): 177-84.

Howells, L.M., Moiseeva, E.P., Neal, C.P., Foreman, B.E., Andreadi, C.K., Sun, Y.Y., Hudson, E.A. & Manson, M.M. (2007). Predicting the physiological relevance of in vitro cancer preventive activities of phytochemicals. *Acta Pharmacol Sin*, 28(9): 1274-304.

Hu, C., Wong, F.S. & Wen, L. (2009). Translational Mini-Review Series on B Cell-Directed Therapies: B cell-directed therapy for autoimmune diseases. *Clin Exp Immunol*, 157(2): 181-90.

Ichim, C.V. (2005). Revisiting immunosurveillance and immunostimulation: Implications for cancer immunotherapy. *J Transl Med*, 3(1): 8.

Imbach, P., Barandun, S., d'Apuzzo, V., Baumgartner, C., Hirt, A., Morell, A., Rossi, E., Schoni, M., Vest, M. & Wagner, H.P. (1981). High-dose intravenous gammaglobulin for idiopathic thrombocytopenic purpura in childhood. *Lancet*, 1(8232): 1228-31.

Jager, E., Stockert, E., Zidianakis, Z., Chen, Y.T., Karbach, J., Jager, D., Arand, M., Ritter, G., Old, L.J. & Knuth, A. (1999). Humoral immune responses of cancer patients against "Cancer-Testis" antigen NY-ESO-1: correlation with clinical events. *Int J Cancer*, 84(5): 506-10.

Jeurissen, S.H., Janse, E.M., Lehrbach, P.R., Haddad, E.E., Avakian, A. & Whitfill, C.E. (1998). The working mechanism of an immune complex vaccine that protects chickens against infectious bursal disease. *Immunology*, 95(3): 494-500.

Kerjaschki, D. (1993). Molecular development of immune deposits and proteinuria in Heymann nephritis. *Clin Investig*, 71(10): 817-21.

Kerjaschki, D. (2000a). Megalin/GP330 and pathogenetic concepts of membranous glomerulopathy (MGN). *Kidney Blood Press Res*, 23(3-5): 163-6.

Kerjaschki, D. (2000b). Pathogenetic concepts of membranous glomerulopathy (MGN). *J Nephrol 2000*, 13(Suppl 3): S96-100.

Kerjaschki, D. & Farquhar, M.G. (1982). The pathogenic antigen of Heymann nephritis is a membrane glycoprotein of the renal proximal tubule brush border. *Proc Natl Acad Sci U S A*, 79(18): 5557-81.

Khuder, S.A., Dayal, H.H., Mutgi, A.B., Willey, J.C. & Dayal, G. (1998). Effect of cigarette smoking on major histological types of lung cancer in men. *Lung Cancer*, 22(1): 15-21.

Kim, R., Emi, M. & Tanabe, K. (2007). Cancer immunoediting from immune surveillance to immune escape. *Immunology*, 121(1): 1-14.

Klaus, G.G. (1978). The generation of memory cells. II. Generation of B memory cells with preformed antigen-antibody complexes. *Immunology*, 34(4): 643-52.

Kretz-Rommel, A., Duncan, S.R. & Rubin, R.L. (1997). Autoimmunity caused by disruption of central T cell tolerance. A murine model of drug-induced lupus. *J Clin Invest*, 99(8): 1888-96.

Kretz-Rommel, A. & Rubin, R.L. (1999). Persistence of autoreactive T cell drive is required to elicit anti-chromatin antibodies in a murine model of drug-induced lupus. *J Immunol*, 162(2): 813-20.

Kreuwel, H.T. & Sherman, L.A. (2001). The T-cell repertoire available for recognition of self-antigens. *Curr Opin Immunol*, 13(6): 639-43.

Kunkl, A. & Klaus, G.G. (1981). The generation of memory cells. IV. Immunization with antigen-antibody complexes accelerates the development of B-memory cells, the formation of germinal centres and the maturation of antibody affinity in the secondary response. *Immunology*, 43(2): 371-8.

Leandro, M.J. & de, I.T., I (2009). Translational Mini-Review Series on B Cell-Directed Therapies: The pathogenic role of B cells in autoantibody-associated autoimmune diseases--lessons from B cell-depletion therapy. *Clin Exp Immunol*, 157(2): 191-7.

Levesque, M.C. (2009). Translational Mini-Review Series on B Cell-Directed Therapies: Recent advances in B cell-directed biological therapies for autoimmune disorders. *Clin Exp Immunol*, 157(2): 198-208.

Lollini, P.L. & Forni, G. (2002). Antitumor vaccines: is it possible to prevent a tumor? *Cancer Immunol Immunother*, 51(8): 409-16.

Manson, J.J., Mauri, C. & Ehrenstein, M.R. (2005). Natural serum IgM maintains immunological homeostasis and prevents autoimmunity. *Springer Semin Immunopathol*, 26(4): 425-32.

Manz, R.A., Arce, S., Cassese, G., Hauser, A.E., Hiepe, F. & Radbruch, A. (2002). Humoral immunity and long-lived plasma cells. *Curr Opin Immunol*, 14(4): 517-21.

Matsukawa, W., Hara, S., Yoshida, F., Suzuki, N., Fukatsu, A., Yuzawa, Y., Sakamoto, N. & Matsuo, S. (1992). Effects of a new immunosuppressive agent, FK506, in rats with active Heymann nephritis. *J Lab Clin Med*, 119(2): 116-23.

Mevorach, D., Mascarenhas, J.O., Gershov, D. & Elkon, K.B. (1998). Complement-dependent clearance of apoptotic cells by human macrophages. *J Exp Med*, 188(12): 2313-20.

Mokhtarian, F., Zhang, Z., Shi, Y., Gonzales, E. & Sobel, R.A. (1999). Molecular mimicry between a viral peptide and a myelin oligodendrocyte glycoprotein peptide induces autoimmune demyelinating disease in mice. *J Neuroimmunol*, 95(1-2): 43-54.

Musiani, P., Modesti, A., Giovarelli, M., Cavallo, F., Colombo, M.P., Lollini, P.L. & Forni, G. (1997). Cytokines, tumour-cell death and immunogenicity: a question of choice. *Immunol Today*, 18(1): 32-6.

Nair, S., Li, W. & Kong, A.N. (2007). Natural dietary anti-cancer chemopreventive compounds: redox-mediated differential signaling mechanisms in cytoprotection of normal cells versus cytotoxicity in tumor cells. *Acta Pharmacol Sin*, 28(4): 459-72.

Nepom, G.T. (2002). Therapy of autoimmune diseases: clinical trials and new biologics. *Curr Opin Immunol*, 14(6): 812-5.

Nie, X., Basu, S. & Cerny, J. (1997). Immunization with immune complex alters the repertoire of antigen-reactive B cells in the germinal centers. *Eur J Immunol*, 27(12): 3517-25.

Ogden, C.A., Kowalewski, R., Peng, Y., Montenegro, V. & Elkon, K.B. (2005). IGM is required for efficient complement mediated phagocytosis of apoptotic cells in vivo. *Autoimmunity*, 38(4): 259-64.

Orbach, H. & Shoenfeld, Y. (2007). Vaccination infection and autoimmunity: myth and reality VIAMR 2005-10-26-28, Beau-Rivage Palace Hotel, Lausanne, Switzerland. *Autoimmun Rev*, 6(5): 261-6.

Peakman, M. & Dayan, C.M. (2001). Antigen-specific immunotherapy for autoimmune disease: fighting fire with fire? *Immunology*, 104(4): 361-6.

Penny, M.J., Boyd, R.A. & Hall, B.M. (1998). Permanent CD8(+) T cell depletion prevents proteinuria in active Heymann nephritis. *J Exp Med*, 188(10): 1775-84.

Perna, A., Schieppati, A., Zamora, J., Giuliano, G.A., Braun, N. & Remuzzi, G. (2004). Immunosuppressive treatment for idiopathic membranous nephropathy: a systematic review. *Am J Kidney Dis*, 44(3): 385-401.

Perosa, F., Favoino, E., Caragnano, M.A., Prete, M. & Dammacco, F. (2005). CD20: a target antigen for immunotherapy of autoimmune diseases. *Autoimmun Rev*, 4(8): 526-31.

Pinckard, R.N. & Weir, D.M. (1966). Antibodies against the mitochondrial fraction of liver after toxic liver damage in rats. *Clin Exp Immunol*, 1(1): 33-43.

Pirofsky, B. & Kinzey, D.M. (1992). Intravenous immune globulins. A review of their uses in selected immunodeficiency and autoimmune diseases. *Drugs*, 43(1): 6-14.

Prakken, B.J., Samodal, R., Le, T.D., Giannoni, F., Yung, G.P., Scavulli, J., Amox, D., Roord, S., de, K., I, Bonnin, D., Lanza, P., Berry, C., Massa, M., Billetta, R. & Albani, S. (2004). Epitope-specific immunotherapy induces immune deviation of proinflammatory T cells in rheumatoid arthritis. *Proc Natl Acad Sci U S A*, 101(12): 4228-33.

Quartier, P., Potter, P.K., Ehrenstein, M.R., Walport, M.J. & Botto, M. (2005). Predominant role of IgM-dependent activation of the classical pathway in the clearance of dying cells by murine bone marrow-derived macrophages in vitro. *Eur J Immunol*, 35(1): 252-60.

Rao, T. & Richardson, B. (1999). Environmentally induced autoimmune diseases: potential mechanisms. *Environ Health Perspect*, 107 Suppl 5 737-42.

Rich, M.W. (1996). Drug-induced lupus. The list of culprits grows. *Postgrad Med*, 100(3): 299-8.

Sakaguchi, S. (2000). Regulatory T cells: key controllers of immunologic self-tolerance. *Cell*, 101(5): 455-8.

Schulze, C., Munoz, L.E., Franz, S., Sarter, K., Chaurio, R.A., Gaipl, U.S. & Herrmann, M. (2008). Clearance deficiency--a potential link between infections and autoimmunity. *Autoimmun Rev*, 8(1): 5-8.

Segal, D.M., Weiner, G.J. & Weiner, L.M. (1999). Bispecific antibodies in cancer therapy. *Curr Opin Immunol*, 11(5): 558-62.

Singh, A.K. & Kasinath, B.S. (1993). Metabolic fate of monovalent and multivalent antibodies of Heymann nephritis following formation of surface immune complexes on glomerular epithelial cells. *Clin Exp Immunol*, 94(3): 403-11.

Sinha, A.A., Lopez, M.T. & McDevitt, H.O. (1990). Autoimmune diseases: the failure of self tolerance. *Science*, 248(4961): 1380-8.

Stoner, R.D. & Terres, G. (1963). Enhanced antitoxin responses in irradiated mice elicited by complexes of tetanus toxoid and specific antibody. *J Immunol*, 91 761-70.

Stoner, R.D., Terres, G. & Hess, M.W. (1975). Early and enhanced antioxin responses elicited with complexes of tetanus toxoid and specific mouse and human antibodies. *J Infect Dis*, 131(3): 230-8.

Taylor, P.R., Carugati, A., Fadok, V.A., Cook, H.T., Andrews, M., Carroll, M.C., Savill, J.S., Henson, P.M., Botto, M. & Walport, M.J. (2000). A hierarchical role for classical pathway complement proteins in the clearance of apoptotic cells in vivo. *J Exp Med*, 192(3): 359-66.

ten Veen, J.H. & Feltkamp, T.E. (1972). Studies on drug induced lupus erythematosus in mice. I. Drug induced antinuclear antibodies (ANA). *Clin Exp Immunol*, 11(2): 265-76.

Terres, G., Morrison, S.L., Habicht, G.S. & Stoner, R.D. (1972). Appearance of an early "primed state" in mice following the concomitant injections of antigen and specific antiserum. *J Immunol*, 108(6): 1473-81.

Terres, G. & Stoner, R.D. (1962). Specificity of enhanced immunological sensitization of mice following injections of antigens and specific antisera. *Proc Soc Exp Biol Med*, 109 88-91.

Terres, G. & Wolins, W. (1959). Enhanced sensitization in mice by simultaneous injection of antigen and specific rabbit antiserum. *Proc Soc Exp Biol Med*, 102 632-5.

Terres, G. & Wolins, W. (1961). Enhanced immunological sensitization of mice by the simultaneous injection of antigen and specific antiserum. I. Effect of varying the amount of antigen used relative to the antiserum. *J Immunol*, 86 361-8.

Thaiss, F., Schoeppe, W., Willaredt-Stoll, J.G., Batsford, S. & Mihatsch, M.J. (1989). Cyclosporin A prevents proteinuria in an active model of membranous nephropathy in rats. *Lab Invest*, 61(6): 661-9.

Theofilopoulos, A.N. (1995). The basis of autoimmunity: Part I. Mechanisms of aberrant self-recognition. *Immunol Today*, 16(2): 90-8.

Topham, N.J. & Hewitt, E.W. (2009). Natural killer cell cytotoxicity: how do they pull the trigger? *Immunology*, 128(1): 7-15.

Totoritis, M.C. & Rubin, R.L. (1985). Drug-induced lupus. Genetic, clinical, and laboratory features. *Postgrad Med*, 78(3): 149-61.

Tung, K.S. (1994). Mechanism of self-tolerance and events leading to autoimmune disease and autoantibody response. *Clin Immunol Immunopathol*, 73(3): 275-82.

Tureci, O., Mack, U., Luxemburger, U., Heinen, H., Krummenauer, F., Sester, M., Sester, U., Sybrecht, G.W. & Sahin, U. (2006). Humoral immune responses of lung cancer patients against tumor antigen NY-ESO-1. *Cancer Lett*, 236(1): 64-71.

UytdeHaag, F., van der, H.R. & Osterhaus, A. (1991). Maintenance of immunological memory: a role for CD5+ B cells? *Immunol Today*, 12(12): 439-42.

Von Herrath, M.G. & Oldstone, M.B. (1995). Role of viruses in the loss of tolerance to self-antigens and in autoimmune diseases. *Trends Microbiol*, 3(11): 424-30.

Weir, D.M. (1964). Immunological reaction after tissue injury. *Lancet*, 1 749-50.

Weir, D.M. (1966). The immune response after tissue injury. *Pathol Eur*, 1(1): 108-18.

Weir, D.M. (1969). Altered antigens and autoimmunity. *Vox Sang*, 16(4): 304-13.

Weir, D.M. & Elson, C.J. (1969). Antitissue antibodies and immunological tolerance to self. *Arthritis Rheum*, 12(3): 254-60.

Weir, D.M. & Pinckard, R.N. (1967). Failure to induce tolerance to rat tissue antigens. *Immunology*, 13(4): 373-80.

Weir, D.M., Pinckard, R.N., Elson, C.J. & Suckling, D.E. (1966). Naturally occurring anti-tissue antibodies in rat sera. *Clin Exp Immunol*, 1(4): 433-42.

Wermeling, F., Karlsson, M.C. & McGaha, T.L. (2009). An anatomical view on macrophages in tolerance. *Autoimmun Rev*, 9(1): 49-52.

Whitfill, C.E., Haddad, E.E., Ricks, C.A., Skeeles, J.K., Newberry, L.A., Beasley, J.N., Andrews, P.D., Thoma, J.A. & Wakenell, P.S. (1995). Determination of optimum formulation of a novel infectious bursal disease virus (IBDV) vaccine constructed by mixing bursal disease antibody with IBDV. *Avian Dis*, 39(4): 687-99.

Xu, D.Z., Huang, K.L., Zhao, K., Xu, L.F., Shi, N., Yuan, Z.H. & Wen, Y.M. (2005). Vaccination with recombinant HBsAg-HBIG complex in healthy adults. *Vaccine*, 23(20): 2658-64.

Yao, X., Zheng, B., Zhou, J., Xu, D.Z., Zhao, K., Sun, S.H., Yuan, Z.H. & Wen, Y.M. (2007). Therapeutic effect of hepatitis B surface antigen-antibody complex is associated with cytolytic and non-cytolytic immune responses in hepatitis B patients. *Vaccine*, 25(10): 1771-9.

Yokoyama, H., Goshima, S., Wada, T., Takaeda, M., Furuichi, K., Kobayashi, K. & Kida, H. (1999). The short- and long-term outcomes of membranous nephropathy treated with intravenous immune globulin therapy. Kanazawa Study Group for Renal Diseases and Hypertension. *Nephrol Dial Transplant*, 14(10): 2379-86.

Zwart, B., Ciurana, C., Rensink, I., Manoe, R., Hack, C.E. & Aarden, L.A. (2004). Complement activation by apoptotic cells occurs predominantly via IgM and is limited to late apoptotic (secondary necrotic) cells. *Autoimmunity*, 37(2): 95-102.

# 29

# Parasitic Helminths as Potential Therapeutic Agents Against Autoimmune Disorders

Yoshio Osada
*University of Occupational and Environmental Health, Japan*
*Japan*

## 1. Introduction

In developed countries, the prevalence of both allergic disease (asthma) and autoimmune disorders such as Crohn's disease (CD), multiple sclerosis (MS), and type 1 diabetes (T1D) is increasing. This trend seems to be inversely correlated to prominent decreases in infectious diseases such as measles, tuberculosis, and hepatitis A (Bach, 2002). Based on such epidemiological observations, the "hygiene hypothesis", that exposure to infectious agents; i.e. bacteria, viruses, and parasites, especially in childhood, lowers the risk of later onset of immunological disorders, has attracted much attention. According to the hypothesis, a reduced exposure to infectious agents due to improved hygienic conditions in developed countries, urbanized areas, and/or a westernized lifestyle is responsible for the higher incidence of autoimmunity and allergies in modern society. A number of epidemiological and experimental studies have demonstrated the plausibility of this hypothesis. However, there is also considerable evidence that does not support or contradicts the hypothesis. In this chapter, conflicting reports are introduced and discussed.

Most studies trying to elucidate the mechanisms involved have been conducted using rodent models. In various models of autoimmune or allergic diseases, effects of bacterial, viral or parasitic infections were tested. Consequently, in many cases, preventive or ameliorating effects of infectious agents have been confirmed. In the main part of this chapter, the influence of parasitic helminths on autoimmune disorders will be introduced.

Although the mechanisms underlying the amelioration and/or prevention of immunological disorders by infectious agents have been studied extensively, they are not yet fully understood. As both Th1-polarizing (bacteria and viruses) and Th2-polarizing (parasitic helminths) infectious agents have anti-autoimmune/anti-allergic activities (Zaccone & Cooke, 2011), the "Th1/Th2 paradigm" is not enough to explain the mechanisms involved. Additionally, some autoimmune diseases have been shown to be dependent on a pathogenic T helper subset (Th17), and not on the Th1 subset. The suppressive mechanisms of infectious agents have been attributed to various regulatory/suppressive cell populations, such as Treg cells, Breg cells, NKT cells and alternatively activated macrophages (AA MΦs). In addition, the involvement of suppressive cytokines (e.g. IL-4, IL-10 or TGF-β) has been studied and demonstrated. Focusing on helminth infections, the possible involvement of regulatory cells and cytokines is discussed.

Some autoimmune diseases are being treated successfully with recently developed biological products (mainly humanized monoclonal antibodies against pro-inflammatory cytokines). These products have outstanding therapeutic effects on autoimmune diseases (Nixon et al., 2007; Jones & Ding, 2010) compared to traditional immunomodulatory agents such as disease modifying anti-rheumatic drugs (DMARDs). However, they can cause severe adverse effects such as opportunistic infections. Helminths or their excretory/secretary products might solve the problems of monoclonal antibody therapy (Puneet et al, 2011). Therefore, at the end of this chapter, clinical trials of viable parasitic helminths for the treatment of immunological disorders are briefly introduced.

## 2. Evidence of the hygiene hypothesis

As described in Introduction, the prevalence of asthma, T1D, MS, and inflammatory bowel diseases (IBD) has been increasing in developed countries in an inverse relation to the declining prevalence of infectious diseases (Bach, 2002). In addition to the chronological trend, the geographical distribution of some autoimmune diseases seems to support the hygiene hypothesis. MS and T1D have a similar geographical distribution pattern known as a "North-south gradient", with a high prevalence in northern European (Scandinavian) countries (= relatively hygienic) and low prevalence in southern European countries (= relatively non-hygienic) (Bach, 2002; Shapira et al., 2010a). This pattern could be explained by the hygiene hypothesis, but also attributable to differences in genetic background. For example, the single nucleotide polymorphism (SNP) PTPN22 is associated with high risk of T1D and distributed more in the northern regions than southern regions of Europe (Shapira et al., 2010a). Another factor that might explain the "North-south gradient" of MS and T1D is the amount of sun exposure. Vitamin D, production of which is dependent on exposure to UV, has been reported to have immunomodulatory effects, and insufficient production of vitamin D might be responsible for the higher incidence of autoimmune disorders in northern European countries (Shoenfeld et al., 2009; Ponsonby et al., 2002).

There is epidemiological evidence of the importance of non-hygienic conditions in the prevention of autoimmune or atopic disorders. For instance, a significant difference in allergen-specific IgE level was reported between people of neighboring regions sharing the same ethnic background; Finland (relatively hygienic) and Russian Karelia (relatively non-hygienic) (Seiskari et al., 2007). Enteroviral infections were found to protect the children in Karelia from atopy. Moreover, there are reports that offspring of immigrants from developing countries acquire a higher incidence of autoimmune diseases, such as T1D and MS, than the population of their parents' motherland countries (Bach, 2002; Bodansky, 1992). These findings clearly indicate the importance of environmental factors (including hygienic standards) rather than genetic background in the pathogenesis of autoimmune disorders.

The "sibling effect", that children with more siblings have a lower risk of developing atopic disorders (Strachan, 1989), is the basic finding that the hygiene hypothesis comes from. The sibling effect on atopic disorders has been demonstrated in cohort studies (Benn et al., 2004; Matheson et al., 2009; Cullinan et al., 2003). A similar effect was reported in case of T1D (Cardwell et al., 2008a) and IBD (Koloski et al., 2008). From the viewpoint of the hygiene hypothesis, the decrease of the disease risk can be explained by the increased exposure to pathogens from elder siblings. Regarding atopic disorders, a meta-analysis of atopic dermatitis (AD) has shown inverse relationships with exposure to endotoxins, early day care, and contact with animals (Flohr et al., 2005). The risk of the early onset of allergic rhinitis (AR) was inversely correlated with viral infections during childhood, in addition to cumulative exposure to siblings before the age of 2 years (Matheson et al., 2009). Not only overt infections but also non-invasive exposure to pathogen-derived products, such as endotoxins (Gereda et al., 2000), are considered responsible for prevention of atopy (von Mutius, 2007). In the case of autoimmune diseases, the risk of T1D is reduced in children living with siblings, sharing a bedroom and of households that often move (Cardwell et al., 2008b). A population-based study in Canada demonstrated correlations between IBD and high socioeconomic status and low rates of enteric infections (Green et al., 2006). The report also revealed a positive correlation between IBD and MS.

## 3. Evidence that does not match the hygiene hypothesis

In great contrast to T1D and MS, rheumatoid arthritis (RA) has been declining in prevalence in recent decades (Gabriel &Michaud, 2009). Moreover, its geographical distribution is very different from that of T1D or MS. That is, RA is generally evenly distributed in the world and does not have a "North-south gradient". (Shapira et al., 2010b). The geographical distribution of systemic sclerosis (SSc) seems to be contrast to those of T1D and MS. Within Europe, SSc is less frequent in the north than south (Shapira et al., 2010b). In the case of ankylosing spondylitis (AS), a genetic factor (HLA-B27) rather than environmental factors seems to explain the prevalence of the disease (Shapira et al., 2010b). Therefore, the geographical distribution and/or chronological transition of some autoimmune diseases cannot be explained by the hygiene hypothesis.

For atopic disorders, the sibling effect itself has been confirmed (Benn et al, 2004; Matheson et al., 2009; Cullinan et al., 2003). However, some authors suggest that infections in early life do not explain the observed sibling effect (Benn et al., 2004; Cullinan et al., 2003). In a report on the preventive effects of endotoxins against AD (Flohr et al., 2005), apparent infections in early life were shown to increase the risk of AD. In a meta-analysis of relationships between exposure to furry pets and asthma and allergic rhinitis, there were different effects in different species of animals. That is, exposure to dogs increases the risk but exposure to cats decreases it (Takkouche et al., 2008). Moreover, in a meta-analysis of interrelationships between vaccinations with bacterial products (BCG and pertussis vaccine) and the incidence of asthma, no statistical association was found (Balicer et al., 2007). For T1D, there was no association between routinely recorded infections in early life and subsequent risk of the disease (Cardwell et al., 2008a). In addition, T1D had inverse relationships with asthma (Cardwell et al., 2003). These finding do not match the hypothesis that infections and exposure to pathogens protect against both atopy and autoimmunity. A systematic review of mycobacterial infections and atopy (Obihara et al., 2007) found that the negative correlations between them were mainly based on cross-sectional studies. The authors, therefore, claimed that population-based prospective studies would be needed.

Regarding etiology of MS, two hypotheses have been proposed (Milo & Kahana, 2010). The "prevalence hypothesis" postulates that MS is caused by a pathogen common in high-incidence areas. In contrast, according to the more accepted "poliomyelitis-hygiene hypothesis", certain infections in early childhood protect against MS whereas infections with the same infectious agents later in life (e.g. adolescence) cause the disease, as in the cases of poliomyelitis. This concept is different from that of the "original" hygiene hypothesis, in that people living in hygienic conditions (= non-infected people) are protected from the disease. Epstein-Barr virus (EBV) is one of the infectious agents suspected to be causative of MS. Individuals infected with EBV in early childhood have a lower risk of MS than those infected in adolescence and as a consequence, suffer from infectious mononucleosis (IM). Additionally, non-infected people are known to have the lowest risk of MS (Ascheiro & Munger, 2010), suggesting the plausibility of the poliomyelitis-hygiene hypothesis. In addition to the causal relationship betwen EBV and MS, a number of infectious agents (HCV, rotavirus, Coxsackie virus, HHV-6, *Helicobacter pylori, Trypanosoma cruzi* etc.) were reported to have an association with autoimmunity (Kivity et al., 2009; Getts & Miller 2010).

Collectively, numerous reports seem to contradict the hygiene hypothesis. In the 99th Dahlem Conference on Infection, Dr. Matricardi tried to reconcile the conflicting evidence (Matricardi, 2010). For instance, infections with orofecal pathogens like hepatitis A virus (HAV) were shown to be inversely correlated with atopy whereas infections of airborne viruses (measles virus, mumps virus, rubella virus etc.) were not (Matricardi et al., 1997; Matricardi et al., 2000). He proposes gastrointestinal infections that stimulate immunological changes in gut-associated lymphoid tissue (GALT) to be important for protective effects against atopic diseases (Matricardi, 2010, Matricardi et al., 2000). Likewise, to explain why some microorganisms protect against immunological disorders and others do not, a refined version of the hygiene hypothesis, the "old friends hypothesis" has been proposed (Rook, 2009). According to this hypothesis, immunological disorders develop if "old friends" (=microorganisms present in humans for a long time on the evolutionary time scale) are expelled from the body. Parasitic helminths and saprophytic bacteria are representative "old friends". To avoid having to fight the host's immune systems long term, they become relatively harmless and continuously activate regulatory dendritic cells (DCs) and regulatory T cells (Treg) at background levels. Consequently, the presence of "old friends" renders hosts resistant to immune dysregulation. This hypothesis seems very attractive, especially to explain immunoregulatory mechanisms by parasitic helminths.

## 4. Influence of helminth infections on human autoimmune disorders

There have been a few papers on the interrelationships between helminth infections and autoimmune diseases in humans. Correale and colleagues have reported the influence of helminth infections on MS. In a prospective, double-cohort study, they found that MS patients infected with helminths (*Hymenolepis nana, Trichuris trichiura, Ascaris lumbricoides, Strongyloides stercolaris* or *Enterobius vermicularis*) showed fewer exacerbations, reduced disability scores, and lower MRI activity compared with uninfected MS patients (Correale & Farez, 2007). Furthermore, the infected MS patients showed an increase in myelin basic protein (MBP)-specific IL-10 and TGF-$\beta$ - producing cells and a decrease in IL-12 and IFN-$\gamma$ - producing cells. B cells from helminth-infected MS patients tend to produce high levels of IL-10, brain-derived neurotropic factor (BDNF), and nerve growth factor (NGF) (Correale et al., 2008). More importantly, some MS patients who received anti-parasite treatment, due to an exacerbation of helminth-derived symptoms, showed an increase in MS activity (Correale & Farez, 2011). The authors also showed that both B cells and DCs from intestinal helminth-infected MS patients had increased expression of TLR2 and some of immunological changes observed in helminth Ag-exposed cells were TLR2-dependent (Correale & Farez, 2009). Collectively, these results suggest that parasitic helminths have anti-MS activity in humans. Fleming & Cook (2006) summarized the relationship between prevalence of *T. trichiura* and MS at the country / regional level. According to the data, MS is prevalent only in *T. trichiura*-free countries. Regarding other autoimmune diseases, in a case-control study in Okinawa (Japan), *S. stercolaris* was less frequent in the autoimmune liver disease group than control group, suggesting that the parasite might protect against autoimmune liver diseases (Aoyama et al., 2007). Most recently, Mutapi et al. (2011) reported epidemiological study in Zimbabwe on the interrelationships between *Schistosoma haematobium* infection and auto-reactive antibody levels. They found an inverse relationship between infection intensity and anti-nuclear antibody (ANA) levels in schistosome- endemic areas. According to the study, anti-helminthic treatment significantly increased ANA levels.

## 5. Influence of helminth infections on human atopic disorders

Compared to studies on human helminth infections and autoimmunity, reports on the interrelationships between helminth infections and atopic disorders are much more common. However, as there is considerable variation in results among the reports, systematic reviews and meta-analyses are important. According to reviews of cross-sectional studies on the relationships between current parasitic infections and athma and atopy (Leonardi-Bee et al., 2006; Flohr et al., 2009; Feary et al., 2011), both intestinal helminths (Hookworms, *Ascaris, Trichuris, Strongyloides, Enterobius*) and schistosomes significantly lowered reactivity in the skin prick test. In contrast, only hookworm infections lowered the risk of asthma significantly; odds ratio (OR) = 0.50 (Leonardi-Bee et al., 2006). It is worth noting that *Ascaris* infections heightened the risk of asthma (OR = 1.34). Other geohelminths had no significant effects on the risk of asthma.
The evidence obtained in cross-sectional studies is indirect. Direct evidence of ameliorating effects of helminths can be obtained by intervention studies. According to the review literature above (Flohr et al., 2009), in some intervention studies, allergic skin sensitization increased after de-worming treatment. This finding was reproducibly observed in independent studies in Venezuela (Lynch et al., 1993), Gabon (van den Biggelaar et al., 2004) and Vietnam (Flohr et al., 2010). However, in a study in Ecuador (Cooper et al., 2006), there was no increase in the prevalence of atopy or clinical allergies after de-worming treatment. Furthermore, in the study in Vietnam (Flohr et al., 2010), the clinical symptoms of allergy did not worsen in the treated group despite the increased sensitization. Remarkably, a study in Venezuela (Lynch et al., 1997) showed a clinical *improvement* in asthma after regular anti-helminthic treatment. Taken together with cross-sectional studies of allergies in helminth-infected individuals, the overall results could be summarized as follows: 1) In general, parasitic helminths suppress skin sensitization. 2) However, parasitic helminths do not always suppress clinical allergies and can sometimes worsen allergic symptoms. Regarding the timing of helminth infections, a study in Brazil is especially noteworthy (Rodrigues et al., 2008). In the study, heavy infections with *T. trichiura* in early childhood were shown to reduce reactivity to allergens in later childhood. Even if the child was not infected at the time of the skin test, this protective effect was observed. Cooper et al. (2009) summarized studies on helminth infections and clinical allergies in a review, in which he stated that different helminths have different effects on allergies depending on the timing of exposure. According to the review, *Trichuris* and hookworms are protective, whereas *Ascaris* and *Toxocara* may be risk factors in certain situations. Further studies, especially de-worming intervention studies or therapeutic clinical trials using helminths, may be necessary to establish a general view of the anti-allergic effects of helminths.

## 6. T cell subsets and autoimmunity

Until several years ago, major autoimmune diseases such as MS, T1D, RA and CD and animal models thereof had been classified as Th1-dependent diseases. Recently, however, the finding of a critical role for IL-23 in the pathogenesis of some experimental forms of autoimmune diseases (Cua et al., 2003; Murphy et al., 2003) and subsequent discovery of a pathogenic T cell subset producing IL-17 (Th17) (Langrish et al., 2005; Park et al., 2005) has led us to revisit the "Th1/Th2 paradigm". The simplified "Th1/Th2 paradigm" still explains many immunological phenomena, but there is accumulating evidence of the importance of Th17 in the pathogenesis of autoimmunity. By using IL-17-deficient mice, essential roles of IL-17 in the pathogenesis of autoimmune disease have been demonstrated directly (Nakae et al., 2003a, 2003b; Komiyama et al., 2003). Development of the Th17 lineage is antagonized by both Th1-related cytokines (IL-12 and IFN-γ) and a Th2 cytokine (IL-4) (Park et al., 2005; Nakae et al., 2007). Conversely, IL-23 and IL-17 negatively regulate Th1 differentiation (Nakae et al., 2007). Therefore, the balance of these Th subsets is much more complex than previously believed. Complicating the situation further is the recent finding that Th17 is not a stable subset and can be changed to the Th1 phenotype; i.e. plasticity of Th17 (Kurschus et al., 2010; Dong, 2011). The fate of Th17 cells depends on their surrounding environment (Dong, 2011; Lee et al., 2009) and Th17's pathogenic nature depends on the conversion to Th1 cells, in the case of experimental T1D (Martin-Orozco et al., 2009; Bending et al., 2009). The relative importance of each Th subset to the pathogenesis may differ with the disease model, however in most cases, the pathogenicity of Th1 and Th17 is still under debate. There is a report that a transcription factor, T-bet, is essential for the encephalitogenicity of T cells rather than cytokine production (Yang et al., 2009). In contrast, T-bet seems to be a negative regulator in experimental autoimmune myocariditis (Rangachari et al., 2006). Given the unstable nature of the Th17 subset and disease heterogeneity of individual patients, antagonism of both the Th1 and Th17 subsets would be a better choice for the successful suppression of autoimmune diseases. From this viewpoint, parasitic helminths may have ideal immunomodulatory activities for treatment of autoimmunity.

## 7. Effect of helminths on experimental autoimmunity

### 7.1 Experimental autoimmune encephalomyelitis (EAE)

EAE in rodents has been widely used as an animal model of MS. In EAE, both Th1 and Th17 have been reported to be encephalitogenic and their relative importance depends on the mouse strain and MOG epitope used for immunization (El-behi et al., 2010). In addition, Th1 and Th17 have different encephalitogenic roles as demonstrated by pathological observations; e.g., distinct cellular infiltrates (macrophage predominant or neutrophil predominant) and distinct sites of inflammation (mainly in the spinal cord or mainly in the brain) (El-behi et al., 2010; Domingues et al., 2010). These observations reinforce the necessity for an antagonistic effect against both Th1 and Th17 for ideal immunomodulatory medicines.

Studies of therapeutic effects of helminths on EAE are summarized in Table 1. Anti-encephalitogenic effects have been observed in all three groups of parasitic helminths; i.e. nematodes (*Heligmosomoides polygyrus* (Wilson et al., 2010), *Trichinella spiralis* (Gruden-Movsesijan et al., 2008), *Trichinella pseudospiralis* (Wu et al., 2010) ), trematodes (*Schistosoma japonicum* (Zheng et al., 2008), *Schistosoma mansoni* (Sewell et al., 2003; La Flamme et al., 2003), *Fasciola hepatica* (Walsh et al., 2009)) and cestodes (*Taenia crassiceps*) (Reyes et al., 2011). Among them, there are some distinct results in the effects of schistosomes. According to Sewell et al. (2003), the intra-peritoneal injection of schistosome eggs protected mice from EAE, whereas La Flamme et al. (2003), reported that a similar injection did not have protective effect. In general, a down-regulation of both Th17 and Th1 cytokine expression has been demonstrated (Walsh et al., 2009; Wu et al., 2010; Reyes et al., 2011) except in papers published before the emergence of the Th17 concept (Sewell et al., 2003; La Flamme et al., 2003). Regarding cellular involvement in the suppression, B cells highly expressing CD23 were shown to be responsible for EAE suppression (Wilson et al., 2010) in adoptive transfer experiments. In that study, B cells from IL-10-deficient mice as well as from wild-type mice conferred protection against EAE. The involvement of AAMΦ is also plausible, because AAMΦ markers are increased in the brain in *T. crassiceps*-infected EAE mice (Reyes et al., 2011). In addition, abrogation of schistosome-induced anti- encephalitogenic effects in STAT6-deficient mice (Sewell et al., 2003) might support the importance of AAM Φ.

| Helminth | Treatment | Proposed mechanism | Refs |
|---|---|---|---|
| *Heligmosomoides polygyrus* | Adoptive transfer of infected mouse cells | B cells, Independent of IL-10 | Wilson et al., 2010 |
| *Trichinella spiralis* | Infection | | Gruden-Movsesijan et al., 2008 |
| *Trichinella pseudospiralis* | Infection | IL-17↓, IL-6↓, IL-1β↓, IFN-γ↓, TNF-α↓ | Wu et al., 2010 |
| *Schistosoma japonicum* | Egg Ag i.p. | IFN-γ↓, IL-4↑ | Zheng et al., 2008 |
| *Schistosoma mansoni* | Egg i.p. | IFN-γ↓, IL-4↑, TGF-β↑, IL-10↑, Dependent on STAT6 | Sewell et al., 2003 |
| | Infection | IL-12/23 p40↓, IFN-γ↓, TNF-α↓, IL-4↑ | La Flamme et al., 2003 |
| *Fasciola hepatica* | Infection | IFN-γ↓, IL-17↓, Dependent on TGF-β, Independent of IL-10 | Walsh et al., 2009 |
| *Taenia crassiceps* | Infection | IL-17↓, TNF-α↓, IL-4↑, IL-10↑ AAMΦ markers↑ | Reyes et al., 2011 |

↓ : down-regulation, ↑ : up-regulation

Table 1. Suppressive effect of parasitic helminths on EAE.

### 7.2 Experimental T1D

Non-obese diabetic (NOD) mice have been used widely as an animal model of T1D. Spontaneous destruction of pancreatic β-cells and subsequent hyperglycemia are observed in NOD mice. The pathogenesis of T1D in this mouse has been studied extensively, however, there is still considerable controversy over the relative contribution of Th1 (or IFN-γ) and Th17 (or IL-17). Anti-IFN-γ treatment rendered NOD mice resistant to cyclophosphamide (CY)-accelerated diabetes (Debray-Sachs et al., 1991). In contrast, in IFN-γ deficient NOD mice, neither insulitis nor diabetes was prevented although the onset was delayed (Hultgren et al., 1996; Gysemans et al., 2008). These findings suggest that IFN-γ is involved in, but not essential to, the pathogenesis. IFN-γ is not itself detrimental to β-cells, but induces apoptosis when acting with IL-1β or TNF-α (Gysemans et al., 2008). Regarding this pro-apoptotic effect, dual roles of IFN-γ in NOD mice have been indicated; i.e. IFN-γ induces β-cell destruction via STAT-1 but protects β-cells via IRF-1 (Gysemans et al., 2008). On the other hand, pathological roles of IL-17 have been also suggested in mice (Miljkovic et al., 2005: Emamaullee et al., 2009) and humans (Honkanen et al., 2010). Anti-IL-17 antibody prevented diabetes in NOD mice when administered around the time of onset (Emamaullee et al., 2009). At present, it is reasonable to conclude that both Th1 and Th17 play some role in diabetogenesis in NOD mice.

Along with NOD mice, inducible T1D models have been used for diabetes research. One of them is streptozotocin (STZ)-induced diabetes. STZ is a glucosamine- nitrosourea compound specifically toxic to pancreatic islet β-cells (Yamamoto et al., 1981). Multiple low-dose administrations of STZ cause immune mechanism-mediated β-cell destruction and diabetes in mice (Kantwerk-Funke et al., 1991). In this T1D model, pathogenic roles of both IL-12/IFN-γ axis (Herold et al., 1996; Müller et al., 2002; Gysemans et al., 2005; Cetkovic-Cvrlje & Uckun, 2005) and IL-23/IL-17 axis (Miljkovic et al., 2005, Mensah-Brown et al., 2006) have been suggested, as in NOD mice.

| T1D model | Helminth | Treatment | Proposed mechanism | Refs |
|---|---|---|---|---|
| Spontaneous T1D in NOD mice | *Litomosoides sigmodontis* | Infection, Worm Ag | IL-4↑, IL-5↑, Treg | Hübner et al., 2009 |
| | *Heligmosomoides polygyrus* | Infection | Independent of IL-10 and Treg | Liu et al., 2009 |
| | *Trichinella spiralis* | Infection | IL-4↑, IL-10↑ | Saunders et al., 2007 |
| | *Schistosoma mansoni* | Infection / Egg i.p. | Anti-insulin IgG↓ | Cooke et al., 1999 |
| | | Eggs, Egg Ag, Worm Ag i.p. | NKT cells↑ | Zaccone et al., 2003 |
| | | Egg Ag i.p. | Treg | Zaccone et al., 2009 |
| Streptozotocin-induced diabetes in mice (Multiple low dose model) | *Schistosoma mansoni* | Infection | | EL-Wakil et al., 2002 |
| | *Taenia crassiceps* | Infection | AAMΦ | Espinoza-Jiménez et al., 2010 |

↓ : down-regulation, ↑ : up-regulation

Table 2. Suppressive effects of parasitic helminths on experimental T1D.

Studies of the therapeutic effects of helminths on experimental T1D models are summarized in Table 2. As in the case of EAE, all three groups of helminths (nematodes, trematodes and cestodes) have preventive effects against experimental T1D models. As Treg cells play an important regulatory role against diabetogenesis (Brode et al., 2006; Ott et al., 2005), some authors suggest that they are also responsible for the anti-diabetogenic effects of helminths (Hübner et al., 2009; Zaccone et al., 2009). However, other reports do not support the importance of Treg cells (Liu et al., 2009; Espinoza-Jiménez et al., 2010). This inconsistency probably suggests the presence of distinct suppressive mechanisms in each parasite species. In our recent study, intestinal helminth infection protected mice from diabetes induced by multiple low-doses of STZ in a STAT6-independent manner (unpublished observation). This finding suggests that immune polarization from Th1 to Th2 induced by helminths cannot explain the anti-diabetogenic effect. Further studies using gene-targeted mice are needed to elucidate the anti-diabetogenic mechanisms of helminths.

### 7.3 Experimental autoimmune arthritis

There are various models of autoimmune arthritis in rodents. Collagen-induced arthritis (CIA) is one of the most widely used classical models of RA (Stuart et al., 1982). In this model, anti-collagen antibodies are responsible for the destruction of cartilage (Terato et al., 1992). Regarding cytokines, TNF-α, IL-1β and IL-6 are crucial to the inflammatory bone destruction in autoimmune arthritis (Ferraccioli et al., 2010; Möller & Villiger, 2006). However, the most important factor in the bone destruction is receptor activator of NFκB ligand (RANKL). This cytokine is induced to express on osteoblasts and synovial fibroblasts by IL-17 and acts on osteoclast precursors to stimulate their differentiation into multinucleated osteoclasts (Okamoto & Takayanagi, 2010). An essential role for IL-17 in the pathogenesis of CIA has been demonstrated directly by using IL-17-deficient mice (Nakae et al., 2003a). IL-17 is an essential pathological factor also in other models of arthritis; e.g. IL-1 receptor antagonist-deficient mice (Nakae et al., 2003b), Ag-induced arthritis (AIA) (Irmler et al., 2007) and glucose 6-phosphate isomerase (GPI)- induced arthritis (Iwanami et al., 2008). Thus, these models could be considered Th17-dependent. In contrast, IFN-γ is now considered an ameliorating factor in CIA (Kelchtermans et al., 2009; Chu et al., 2007) and in AIA (Irmler et al., 2007). However, in proteoglycan-induced arthritis, IFN-γ (not IL-17) is responsible for the pathogenesis (Doodes et al., 2008). Taken together, models of autoimmune arthritis are mainly dependent on Th17 but exceptions do exist. In human RA, the pathological importance of TNF-α, IL-1 β, IL-6 and IL-17 has been demonstrated directly by the striking efficacy of biological drugs targeting those cytokines (Nixon et al., 2007; Jones & Ding, 2010; Genovese et al., 2010). In addition, an anti-RANKL monoclonal antibody has been approved for osteoporosis and is now under clinical development for RA (Pageau, 2009).

As described in section 3, the global distribution and trends of RA do not match the hygiene hypothesis (Gabriel & Michaud, 2009; Shapira et al., 2010b). In addition, to our knowledge, there is no report of anti-RA effects of parasitic helminths in humans. Nonetheless, several investigators (including us) have found anti-arthritic effects of helminths or helminth-derived products in rodents. Those studies are summarized in Table 3. We ourselves have reported suppressive effects of a blood fluke, *S. mansoni,* on mouse CIA (Osada et al., 2009). In that study, the *S. mansoni* infection reduced the severity of CIA as evaluated using scores of arthritis and numbers of arthritic paws. Histopathological observation revealed the prevention of bone destruction in the infected mice. According to an analysis of splenic cytokine production pattern, production of IL-17A, TNF-α and IFN-γ were down-regulated and that of IL-4 and IL-10 was up-regulated. The real-time PCR analysis of inflamed paws showed the striking augmentation of the gene expression of bone-absorptive pro-inflammatory mediators (IL-1β, IL-6 and RANKL) observed in non-infected arthritic mice to be abrogated in infected mice. *S. mansoni* is a gonochoristic worm and forms a pair in the portal vein. Egg deposition in the infected host organs is the major stimulus of Th2-polarization (Grzych et al., 1991) and other immunomodulatory events such as Treg induction (Taylor et al., 2006). In our experiments, the severity of CIA correlated inversely with the numbers of worm pairs, theoretically proportional to the number of eggs produced (Osada et al., 2009). In addition, in a time-course experiment, the splenic cytokine modulation (including down-modulation of IL-17 and TNF-α) was observed from 6 to 8 week post-infection, which corresponds to the beginning of egg deposition (unpublished observation). However, repeated intra-peritoneal injections of soluble egg antigen (SEA) did not protect mice from CIA and viable eggs lost their ability to suppress IL-17 production by freeze-thawing and subsequent crushing treatment (Osada et al., 2010). Therefore, a viable infection, which supplies viable eggs continuously, may be essential for the schistosome-induced anti-arthritic effects. By plotting the relationship between infection intensity and severity levels, we have found that a single pair of worms was enough to abrogate the augmentation of pro-inflammatory mediators and approximately 4 pairs were enough to suppress the onset of arthritis (Osada et al., 2009).

| Arthritis model | Helminth | Treatment | Proposed mechanism | Refs |
|---|---|---|---|---|
| Collagen-induced arthritis (CIA) in mice | *Ascaris suum* | Worm Ag i.p. | | Rocha et al., 2008 |
| | *Acanthocheilonema viteae* | ES-62 i.p. | IFN-γ↓, TNF-α↓, IL-6↓, Anti-collagen IgG↓ | McInnes et al., 2003 |
| | *Schistosoma mansoni* | Infection | IL-17↓, TNF-α↓, IL-6↓, RANKL ↓, Anti-collagen IgG↓ | Osada et al., 2009 |
| | *Schistosoma japonicum* | Infection | IL-4↑, Anti-collagen IgG↓ | He et al., 2010 |
| Zymosan-induced arthritis (ZYA) in mice/rats | *Ascaris suum* | Worm Ag i.p./p.o. | NO↓, IL-1β↓ | Rocha et al., 2008 |
| Adjuvant-induced arthritis (AIA) in rats | *Schistosoma japonicum* | rSj16 i.p. | TNF-α↓, IL-1β↓,NO↓, IL-10↑ | Sun et al., 2010 |
| Spontaneous arthritis in MRL/lpr mice | *Nippostrongylus brasiliensis* | Infection | | Salinas-Carmona et al., 2009 |
| | *Heligmosomoides polygyrus* | Infection | | |
| FCA-induced monoarthritis in rats | *Hymenolepis diminuta* | Infection | IL-10 from CD4+ cells | Shi et al., 2011 |

↓ : down-regulation, ↑ : up-regulation

Table 3. Suppressive effects of parasitic helminths on experimental arthritis.

In addition to the down-regulation of pro-inflammatory cytokines, pathogenic anti-collagen IgG levels were lowered in the infected mice. Since our publication, other investigators also have demonstrated therapeutic effects of schistosomes on arthritis models. He et al. (2010) showed that *S.japonicum* suppressed CIA. However, infection at 2 weeks before CIA induction resulted in an exacerbation of the disease, whereas infection at 7 weeks before induction prevented the disease. This is in contrast to our study in which infection at 2 weeks before induction reduced the severity of CIA. The reason of this discrepancy is not clear, but as speculated by He et al., the difference in parasite species (*S.mansoni* and *S.japonicum*) might have affected the outcome. Sun et al. (2010) demonstrated that a recombinant protein of *S. japonicum* (rSj16) ameliorated adjuvant-induced arthritis in rats. The authors observed a suppression of IL-12 production and augmentation of IL-10 production in rSj16-treated bone marrow-derived dendritic cells (BMDCs). A filarial nematode-derived phosphorylcholine- containing glycoprotein, ES-62, was proven to suppress ongoing CIA (McInnes et al., 2003). In vitro, ES-62 suppressed LPS-induced production of TNF-α and IL-6 from RA synovial cells. Moreover, ES-62 also inhibited TNF-α production in human T cells and macrophages. Regarding the involvement of regulatory cytokines and cells, Shi et al. (2011) reported that IL-10 from CD4+ cells of infected mice was important for anti-arthritic effects of the rat tapeworm *Hymenolepis diminuta*. They also found that the absence of IL-4Rα chain signaling in mice cancelled the anti-arthritic effects of the worm. These findings seem to suggest the importance of Th2-polarization by the parasite, however, we recently found that the Th2-polarizing intestinal parasite *H. polygyrus* did not protect mice from CIA but rather, exacerbated the disease (unpublished observation). The anti-arthritic mechanisms of helminths seem complicated, probably because of the heterogeneity of both experimental models and parasites.

### 7.4 Experimental colitis as a model of IBD

Human IBD includes heterogeneous inflammatory diseases of the intestines. For instance, in terms of T cell subset, CD had been considered a "Th1 disease", but at present, the importance of the Th17 subset in the pathogenesis of CD is emphasized (Sarra et al., 2010).

Increases in both IL-17 and IL-12 mRNA in CD and UC patients has been reported (Nielsen et al., 2003). The most striking evidence of the involvement of IL-23/Th17 axis is the finding of Th17-related genes (including IL-23R gene) as susceptibility genes for CD (Brand, 2009). In contrast, Th2-related cytokines are dominant in UC (Sarra et al., 2010). Likewise, models of colitis are also composed of diseases with a distinct pathogenesis (Strober et al., 2002). Experimental colitis induced by the intra-rectal injection of hapten, such as TNBS or DNBS, resembles human CD and its development seems independent of IFN-γR (Camoglio et al., 2000) and dependent on IL-17R signaling (Zhang et al., 2006). Colitis can be also induced by causing dysfunction in epithelial cell barrier. Supply of drinking water containing dextran sulfate sodium (DSS) induces this type of colitis. In this model, T and B cells are dispensable (Dieleman et al., 1994) and macrophages seem to play both a pathological role (Bauer et al., 2010) and a regulatory role (Qualls et al., 2006; Smith et al., 2007). Considering predominant expression of Th2-related cytokines in the chronic phase, DSS-induced colitis resembles UC (Alex et al., 2009). Interestingly, neutralization of IL-17 aggravates the model (Ogawa et al., 2004), suggesting that IL-17 plays a protective role against DSS-induced colitis. By contrast, another study demonstrated that the colitis was alleviated in IL-17A deficient mice (Ito et al., 2008). The reason for this discrepancy is not clear, but might be due to different mouse strains used in their experiments as indicated by Ito et al.

Using these models of colitis, a number of studies on helminth effects have been conducted (Table 4). Generally, helminths seem to ameliorate TNBS/DNBS- induced colitis. It is worth noting that even worms that usually cause intestinal pathology by laying a large number of eggs in the mesenteric vein (i.e. *Schistosoma* spp.) have anti-colitic effects (Moreels et al., 2004; Ruyssers et al., 2009; Elliott et al., 2003; Mo et al., 2007; Zhao et al., 2009; Bodammer et al., 2011; Smith et al., 2007). A down-regulation of Th1/Th17-related cytokines and up-regulation of anti-inflammatory cytokines are observed in most studies. However, only a few papers have provided direct evidence of the involvement of certain cells or cytokines. For instance, anti-colitic effects of *S.mansoni* (Elliott et al., 2003) and *H.diminuta* (Hunter et al., 2005) were demonstrated to be STAT6-dependent. The latter authors also a showed the anti-colitic effect of the worms to be dependent on IL-10 and the presence of macrophages (Hunter et al., 2010). In contrast to the regularly observed helminths' ameliorating effects on Th1/Th17 dominant (TNBS/DNBS- induced) models, macrophage-mediated or Th2-dominant (DSS-induced or oxazolone- induced) colitis was not alleviated or rather worsened by some helminth infections (Table 4). This exacerbation seems due to the robust Th2-polarization by the helminths; e.g. *H. diminuta* infection worsened oxazolone-induced colitis via IL-5 induction and consequently caused eosinophila (Wang et al., 2010), demonstrated by a loss of exacerbation in eotaxin-deficient mice or anti-IL-5 antibody-treated mice. The finding that anti-colitic effects of schistosome male worms were lost in DSS-induced colitis when mice were infected with worms of mixed sex (Smith et al., 2007) may support the speculation, because the Th2-polarizing ability of schsitosome eggs (produced in mixed sex infection) is more potent than that of adult worms (Grzych et al., 1991). Weinstock's group has been studying anti-colitic mechanisms of the intestinal helminth *H.polygyrus* by using colitis in IL-10-deficient or TGF-βRII dominant negative (DN) mice (Elliott et al., 2004, 2008; Ince et al., 2009). According to the studies, the helminth's anti-colitic effect depends not on IL-10 but on TGF-β signaling. This finding does not mean that host-derived TGF-β is necessary, because it has been recently shown that *H. polygyrus*-derived "TGF-β-like molecules" mobilize host TGF-β signaling and induce subsequent Treg cell development (McSorley et al., 2010; Grainger et al., 2010).

| Colitis model | Helminth | Treatment | Effect | Proposed mechanism | Refs |
|---|---|---|---|---|---|
| TNBS/DNBS-induced colitis | *Ancylostoma caninum* | Worm Ag i.p. | A | | Ruyssers et al., 2009 |
| | *Heligmosomoides polygyrus* | Infection | A | Mast cell-mediated, Neural control of secretory function | Sutton et al., 2008 |
| | *Trichinella spiralis* | Worm Ag i.r. | A | IL-1β↓, iNOS↓, IL-13↑, TGF-β↑ | Motomura et al., 2009 |
| | *Schistosoma mansoni* | Infection | A | IL-2↑, IL-4↑ | Moreels et al., 2004 |
| | | Egg i.p. | A | IFN-γ↓, IL-4↑, STAT6 dependent | Elliott et al., 2003 |
| | | Worm Ag i.p. | A | IFN-γ↓, IL-17↓, TGF-β↑, IL-10↑ | Ruyssers et al., 2009 |
| | *Schistosoma japonicum* | Egg i.p. | A | IFN-γ↓, IL-4↑, IL-10↑, Treg↑ | Mo et al., 2007 |
| | | Egg i.p. | A | IFN-γ↓, IL-10↑, TLR4↓ | Zhao et al., 2009 |
| | *Hymenolepis diminuta* | Infection | A | TNF-α↓, IL-10↑, IL-4↑, AAMΦ-dependent, IL-10/STAT6 dependent | Hunter et al., 2005; Hunter et al., 2010; Johnston et al., 2010 |
| DSS-induced colitis | *Ancylostoma ceylanicum* | Worm Ag / ES Ag i.p. | A | IFN-γ↓, IL-17↓, TNF-α↓ | Cançado et al., 2011 |
| | *Acanthocheilonema viteae* | Cystatin i.p. | A | IL-10 producing MΦ | Schnoeller et al., 2008 |
| | *Toxascaris leonina* | Galectin homologue i.p. | A | TGF-β↑, IL-10↑ | Kim et al., 2010 |
| | *Schistosoma mansoni* | Infection (male only) | A | MΦ dependent, Treg/IL-10/IL-4/IL-13/TGF-β independent | Smith et al., 2007 |
| | | Infection (mixed) | N | | |
| | | Egg Ag i.p. | N | | |
| | | Infection (mixed) | A | TNF-α↓ | Bodammer et al., 2011 |
| | | Egg Ag i.p. | N | | |
| | *Hymenolepis diminuta* | Infection | E | | Reardon et al., 2001 |
| Oxazolone colitis | *Hymenolepis diminuta* | Infection | E | IL-5↑, Eosinophils↑ | Wang et al., 2010 |
| Piroxicam-induced colitis in IL-10 deficient mice | *Heligmosomoides polygylus* | Infection | A | IL-17↓, IL-10 independent | Elliott et al., 2004; Elliott et al., 2008 |
| Colitis in TGF-βRII DN mice | *Heligmosomoides polygylus* | Infection | N | TGF-β signal dependent | Ince et al., 2009 |
| Rag/IL-10-/- Tcell transfer | *Heligmosomoides polygylus* | Infection | A | Modulation of DC function | Hang et al., 2010 |

↓ : down-regulation, ↑ : up-regulation     A: Amelioration, E: Exacerbation, N: No effect

Table 4. Effects of parasitic helminths on experimental colitis.

## 8. Clinical trials of parasitic helminths against immunological disorders

The administration of non-pathogenic or hypo-virulent parasitic worms could be considered for the treatment of immunological disorders. Several clinical trials using parasitic worms have been and are currently being conducted. Significant therapeutic effects have been confirmed in some of these studies. Weinstock's group conducted trials with *Trichuris suis* (porcine whipworm) ova (TSO) against CD (Summers et al., 2005a) and UC (Summers et al., 2005b), and demonstrated significant efficacy. TSO is also being tested for MS and promising results have been obtained in a phase I trial (Fleming et al., 2011). Regarding allergic disorders, Bager et al. (2010) found no therapeutic effect of TSO on allergic rhinitis. However, Summers et al. (2010) critically commented on the report that it was premature to conclude that TSO is ineffective on allergic rhinitis because the TSO treatment was too late and not sufficient. *Necator americanus* (Hookworm) is also under clinical trials for asthma (Feary et al., 2010) and CD (Croese et al., 2006). The advantage of this worm is its long life in the host (at least 6 years) and no need for repeated inoculation (Elliott and Weinstock, 2009). The parasite was well-tolerated without severe adverse effects on asthmatic patients, but a safe dosage of the parasites (10 infective larvae) did not show significant therapeutic efficacy (Feary et al., 2010).

## 9. Concluding remarks

There are two ways of developing parasite-based biomedicines for clinical use. One approach is the direct applications of non-pathogenic/hypo-virulent viable helminths to patients, as introduced in section 8. In addition to TSO and hookworms, other hypo-virulent helminths could be considered for human application. However, before clinical trials, sufficient accumulation of epidemiological and experimental evidence of their therapeutic efficacy is required. Hypo-virulent intestinal nematodes (e.g. *Trichostrongylus* spp.), intestinal trematodes (e.g. *Metagonimus* sp.) and intestinal tapeworms (e.g. *Hymenolepis diminuta*) may become candidates for such studies in the future. It is also essential that the parasites can be maintained in domestic or experimental animals. This is because parasites that infect only humans cannot be maintained and expanded efficiently for clinical use. Another way of developing parasite-based biomedicines comes from the identification of effector molecules of parasites. Considerable numbers of immunomodulatory molecules have been identified from helminths (Harnett W & Harnett MM, 2010). The majority have shown therapeutic effects on experimental autoimmunity or allergy. Some investigators reported that viable parasites were superior to administration of the antigens of parasites (Hunter et al., 2010; Bodammer et al., 2011; Osada et al., 2010) in therapeutic efficacy. In addition, there is still considerable controversy over the roles of regulatory cells (e.g. Treg, Breg or AAMΦ) and regulatory cytokines (e.g. IL-4, IL-10, TGF-$\beta$) in helminth-induced immunomodulation. Therefore, further investigation is needed to elucidate the immunomodulatory mechanisms of viable parasite infections, and new findings obtained there should help to establish an optimal screening system for anti-autoimmune/anti-allergic substances from parasitic helminths.

## 10. Acknowledgements

Our studies introduced in this chapter were supported by Grants-in-aid for Scientific Research from the Japan Society for the Promotion of Science (nos. 20590435, 22590386) and Health and Labour Sciences Research Grants from the Ministry of Health, Labor and Welfare of Japan (H22-Kokui-Shitei-004). I am grateful to Prof. Tamotsu Kanazawa and other laboratory members for their valuable scientific advice. I also acknowledge the technical assistance of Ms. Yukari Horie and the clerical assistance of Ms. Tomoko Fujitomi.

## 11. References

Alex, P., Zachos, N.C., Nguyen, T., Gonzales, L., Chen, T.E., Conklin, L.S., Centola, M. & Li, X. (2009). Distinct cytokine patterns identified from multiplex profiles of murine DSS and TNBS-induced colitis. *Inflamm Bowel Dis.* 15 (3):341-352.

Aoyama, H., Hirata, T., Sakugawa, H., Watanabe, T., Miyagi, S., Maeshiro, T., Chinen, T., Kawane, M., Zaha, O., Nakayoshi, T., Kinjo, F. & Fujita, J. (2007). An inverse relationship between autoimmune liver diseases and *Strongyloides stercoralis* infection. *Am J Trop Med Hyg.* 76 (5):972-976.

Ascherio, A. & Munger, K. L. (2010). 99th Dahlem conference on infection, inflammation and chronic inflammatory disorders: Epstein-Barr virus and multiple sclerosis: epidemiological evidence. *Clin Exp Immunol.* 160 (1):120-124.

Bach, J.F. (2002). The effect of infections on susceptibility to autoimmune and allergic diseases. *N Engl J Med.* 347(12):911-920.

Bager, P., Arnved, J., Rønborg, S., Wohlfahrt, J., Poulsen, L.K., Westergaard, T., Petersen, H. W., Kristensen, B., Thamsborg, S., Roepstorff, A., Kapel, C. & Melbye, M. (2010) *Trichuris suis* ova therapy for allergic rhinitis: a randomized, double-blind, placebo-controlled clinical trial. *J Allergy Clin Immunol.* 125 (1):123-130.e1-3.

Balicer, R. D., Grotto, I., Mimouni, M. & Mimouni, D. (2007). Is childhood vaccination associated with asthma? A meta-analysis of observational studies. *Pediatrics.* 120 (5):e1269-1277.

Bauer, C., Duewell, P., Mayer, C., Lehr, H. A., Fitzgerald, K. A., Dauer, M., Tschopp, J., Endres, S., Latz, E. & Schnurr, M. (2010). Colitis induced in mice with dextran sulfate sodium (DSS) is mediated by the NLRP3 inflammasome. *Gut.* 59 (9):1192-1199.

Bending, D., De La Peña, H., Veldhoen, M., Phillips, J. M., Uyttenhove, C., Stockinger, B. & Cooke, A. (2009). Highly purified Th17 cells from BDC2.5NOD mice convert into Th1-like cells in NOD/SCID recipient mice. *Clin Invest.* 119 (3):565-572.

Benn, C. S., Melbye, M., Wohlfahrt, J., Björkstén, B. & Aaby, P. (2004). Cohort study of sibling effect, infectious diseases, and risk of atopic dermatitis during first 18 months of life. *BMJ.* 328 (7450):1223.

Bodammer, P., Waitz, G., Loebermann, M., Holtfreter, M. C., Maletzki, C., Krueger, M. R., Nizze, H., Emmrich, J. & Reisinger, E. C. (2011). *Schistosoma mansoni* infection but not egg antigen promotes recovery from colitis in outbred NMRI mice. *Dig Dis Sci.* 56 (1):70-78.

Bodansky, H. J., Staines, A., Stephenson, C., Haigh, D. & Cartwright, R. (1992). Evidence for an environmental effect in the aetiology of insulin dependent diabetes in a transmigratory population. *BMJ.* 304 (6833):1020-1022.

Brand, S. (2009). Crohn's disease: Th1, Th17 or both? The change of a paradigm: new immunological and genetic insights implicate Th17 cells in the pathogenesis of Crohn's disease. *Gut.* 58 (8):1152-1167.

Brode, S., Raine, T., Zaccone, P. & Cooke, A. (2006). Cyclophosphamide-induced type-1 diabetes in the NOD mouse is associated with a reduction of CD4+CD25+Foxp3+ regulatory T cells. *J Immunol.* 177 (10):6603-6612.

Camoglio, L., te Velde, A. A., de Boer, A., ten Kate, F. J., Kopf, M. & van Deventer, S.J. (2000). Hapten-induced colitis associated with maintained Th1 and inflammatory responses in IFN-gamma receptor-deficient mice. *Eur J Immunol.* 30 (5):1486-1495.

Cançado, G. G., Fiuza, J. A., de Paiva, N. C., Lemos, L. D., Ricci, N. D., Gazzinelli-Guimarães, P. H., Martins, V. G., Bartholomeu, D. C., Negrão-Corrêa, D. A., Carneiro, C. M. & Fujiwara, R. T. (2011). Hookworm products ameliorate dextran sodium sulfate-induced colitis in BALB/c mice. *Inflamm Bowel Dis.* 2011 Feb 2. doi: 10.1002/ibd.21629. [Epub ahead of print]

Cardwell, C. R., Carson, D. J. & Patterson, C. C. (2008a). No association between routinely recorded infections in early life and subsequent risk of childhood-onset Type 1 diabetes: a matched case-control study using the UK General Practice Research Database. *Diabet Med.* 25 (3):261-267.

Cardwell, C. R., Carson, D. J., Yarnell, J., Shields, M. D. & Patterson, C. C. (2008b). Atopy, home environment and the risk of childhood-onset type 1 diabetes: a population-based case-control study. *Pediatr Diabetes.* 9 (3 Pt 1):191-196.

Cardwell, C. R., Shields, M. D., Carson, D. J. & Patterson, C. C. (2003). A meta-analysis of the association between childhood type 1 diabetes and atopic disease. *Diabetes Care*. 26 (9):2568-2574.

Cetkovic-Cvrlje, M. & Uckun, F. M. (2005). Effect of targeted disruption of signal transducer and activator of transcription (Stat)4 and Stat6 genes on the autoimmune diabetes development induced by multiple low doses of streptozotocin. *Clin Immunol.* 114 (3):299-306.

Chu, C. Q., Swart, D., Alcorn, D., Tocker, J. & Elkon, K. B. (2007). Interferon-gamma regulates susceptibility to collagen-induced arthritis through suppression of interleukin-17. *Arthritis Rheum.* 56 (4):1145-1151.

Cooke, A., Tonks, P., Jones, F. M., O'Shea, H., Hutchings, P., Fulford, A. J. & Dunne, D. W. (1999). Infection with *Schistosoma mansoni* prevents insulin dependent diabetes mellitus in non-obese diabetic mice. *Parasite Immunol.* 21 (4):169-176.

Cooper, P. J., Chico, M. E., Vaca, M. G., Moncayo, A. L., Bland, J. M., Mafla, E., Sanchez, F., Rodrigues, L. C., Strachan, D. P. & Griffin, G. E. (2006). Effect of albendazole treatments on the prevalence of atopy in children living in communities endemic for geohelminth parasites: a cluster-randomised trial. *Lancet.* 367 (9522):1598-1603.

Cooper, P. J. (2009). Interactions between helminth parasites and allergy. *Curr Opin Allergy Clin Immunol.* 9 (1):29-37.

Correale, J. & Farez, M. (2007). Association between parasite infection and immune responses in multiple sclerosis. *Ann Neurol.* 61 (2):97-108.

Correale, J. & Farez, M. (2009). Helminth antigens modulate immune responses in cells from multiple sclerosis patients through TLR2-dependent mechanisms. *J Immunol.* 183 (9):5999-6012.

Correale, J. & Farez, M. F. (2011). The impact of parasite infections on the course of multiple sclerosis. *J Neuroimmunol.* 233 (1-2):6-11.

Correale, J., Farez, M. & Razzitte, G. (2008). Helminth infections associated with multiple sclerosis induce regulatory B cells. *Ann Neurol.* 64 (2):187-199.

Croese, J., O'neil, J., Masson, J., Cooke, S., Melrose, W., Pritchard, D. & Speare, R. (2006). A proof of concept study establishing *Necator americanus* in Crohn's patients and reservoir donors. *Gut.* 55 (1):136-137.

Cua, D. J., Sherlock, J., Chen, Y., Murphy, C. A., Joyce, B., Seymour, B., Lucian, L., To, W., Kwan, S., Churakova, T., Zurawski, S., Wiekowski, M., Lira, S. A., Gorman, D., Kastelein, R. A. & Sedgwick, J. D. (2003). Interleukin-23 rather than interleukin-12 is the critical cytokine for autoimmune inflammation of the brain. *Nature.* 421 (6924):744-748.

Cullinan, P., Harris, J. M., Newman Taylor, A. J., Jones, M., Taylor, P., Dave, J. R., Mills, P., Moffat, S. A., White, C. W., Figg, J. K., Moon, A. M. & Barnes, M. C. (2003). Can early infection explain the sibling effect in adult atopy? *Eur Respir J.* 22 (6):956-961.

Debray-Sachs, M., Carnaud, C., Boitard, C., Cohen, H., Gresser, I., Bedossa, P. & Bach, J. F. (1991). Prevention of diabetes in NOD mice treated with antibody to murine IFN gamma. *J Autoimmun.* 4 (2):237-248.

Dieleman, L. A., Ridwan, B. U., Tennyson, G. S., Beagley, K. W., Bucy, R. P. & Elson, C. O. (1994). Dextran sulfate sodium-induced colitis occurs in severe combined immunodeficient mice. *Gastroenterology.* 107 (6):1643-1652.

Domingues, H. S., Mues, M., Lassmann, H., Wekerle, H. & Krishnamoorthy, G. (2010). Functional and pathogenic differences of Th1 and Th17 cells in experimental autoimmune encephalomyelitis. *PLoS One*. 5 (11):e15531.

Dong, C. (2011). Genetic controls of Th17 cell differentiation and plasticity. *Exp Mol Med*. 43 (1):1-6.

Doodes, P. D., Cao, Y., Hamel, K. M., Wang, Y., Farkas, B., Iwakura, Y. & Finnegan, A. (2008). Development of proteoglycan-induced arthritis is independent of IL-17. *J Immunol*. 181 (1):329-37.

El-behi, M., Rostami, A. & Ciric, B. (2010). Current views on the roles of Th1 and Th17 cells in experimental autoimmune encephalomyelitis. *J Neuroimmune Pharmacol*. 5 (2):189-197.

El-Wakil, H. S., Aboushousha, T. S., El Haddad, O., Gamil, N. B., Mansour, T. & El-Said, H. (2002). Effect of *Schistosoma mansoni* egg deposition on multiple low doses streptozotocin induced insulin dependent diabetes. *J Egypt Soc Parasitol*. 32 (3):987-1002.

Elliott, D. E., Li, J., Blum, A., Metwali, A., Qadir, K., Urban, J. F. Jr & Weinstock, J. V. (2003). Exposure to schistosome eggs protects mice from TNBS-induced colitis. *Am J Physiol Gastrointest Liver Physiol*. 284 (3):G385-91.

Elliott, D. E., Metwali, A., Leung, J., Setiawan, T., Blum, A. M., Ince, M. N., Bazzone, L. E., Stadecker, M. J., Urban, J. F. Jr & Weinstock, J. V. (2008). Colonization with *Heligmosomoides polygyrus* suppresses mucosal IL-17 production. *J Immunol*. 181 (4):2414-2419.

Elliott, D. E., Setiawan, T., Metwali, A., Blum, A., Urban, J. F. Jr & Weinstock, J. V. (2004). *Heligmosomoides polygyrus* inhibits established colitis in IL-10-deficient mice. *Eur J Immunol*. 34 (10):2690-2698.

Elliott, D. E. & Weinstock, J. V. (2009). Helminthic therapy: using worms to treat immune-mediated disease. *Adv Exp Med Biol*. 666:157-166.

Emamaullee, J. A., Davis, J., Merani, S., Toso, C., Elliott, J. F., Thiesen, A. & Shapiro, A. M. (2009). Inhibition of Th17 cells regulates autoimmune diabetes in NOD mice. *Diabetes*. 58 (6):1302-11.

Espinoza-Jiménez, A., Rivera-Montoya, I., Cárdenas-Arreola, R., Morán, L. & Terrazas, L. I. (2010). *Taenia crassiceps* infection attenuates multiple low-dose streptozotocin-induced diabetes. *J Biomed Biotechnol*. 2010:850541.

Feary, J., Britton, J. & Leonardi-Bee, J. (2011) Atopy and current intestinal parasite infection: a systematic review and meta-analysis. *Allergy*. 66: 569-578.

Feary, J. R., Venn, A. J., Mortimer, K., Brown, A. P., Hooi, D., Falcone, F. H., Pritchard, D. I. & Britton, J. R. (2010). Experimental hookworm infection: a randomized placebo-controlled trial in asthma. *Clin Exp Allergy*. 40 (2):299-306.

Ferraccioli, G., Bracci-Laudiero, L., Alivernini, S., Gremese, E., Tolusso, B. & De Benedetti, F. (2010). Interleukin-1β and interleukin-6 in arthritis animal models: roles in the early phase of transition from acute to chronic inflammation and relevance for human rheumatoid arthritis. *Mol Med*. 16 (11-12):552-557.

Fleming, J. O. & Cook, T. D. (2006). Multiple sclerosis and the hygiene hypothesis. *Neurology*. 67 (11):2085-6.

Fleming, J., Isaak, A., Lee, J., Luzzio, C., Carrithers, M., Cook, T., Field, A., Boland, J. & Fabry, Z. (2011). Probiotic helminth administration in relapsing-remitting multiple sclerosis: a phase 1 study. *Mult Scler*. 2011 Mar 3. [Epub ahead of print]

Flohr, C., Pascoe, D. & Williams, H. C. (2005). Atopic dermatitis and the 'hygiene hypothesis': too clean to be true? *Br J Dermatol.* 152 (2):202-216.

Flohr, C., Quinnell, R. J. & Britton, J. (2009). Do helminth parasites protect against atopy and allergic disease? *Clin Exp Allergy.* 39 (1):20-32.

Flohr, C., Tuyen, L. N., Quinnell, R. J., Lewis, S., Minh, T. T., Campbell, J., Simmons, C., Telford, G., Brown, A., Hien, T. T., Farrar, J., Williams, H., Pritchard, D. I. & Britton, J. (2010). Reduced helminth burden increases allergen skin sensitization but not clinical allergy: a randomized, double-blind, placebo-controlled trial in Vietnam. *Clin Exp Allergy.* 40 (1):131-142.

Gabriel, S. E. & Michaud, K. (2009). Epidemiological studies in incidence, prevalence, mortality, and comorbidity of the rheumatic diseases. *Arthritis Res Ther.* 11 (3):229.

Genovese, M. C., Van den Bosch, F., Roberson, S. A., Bojin, S., Biagini, I. M., Ryan, P. & Sloan-Lancaster, J. (2010). LY2439821, a humanized anti-interleukin-17 monoclonal antibody, in the treatment of patients with rheumatoid arthritis: A phase I randomized, double-blind, placebo-controlled, proof-of-concept study. *Arthritis Rheum.* 62 (4):929-939.

Gereda, J. E., Leung, D. Y., Thatayatikom, A., Streib, J. E., Price, M. R., Klinnert, M. D. & Liu, A. H. (2000). Relation between house-dust endotoxin exposure, type 1 T-cell development, and allergen sensitisation in infants at high risk of asthma. *Lancet.* 355 (9216):1680-1683.

Getts, M. T. & Miller, S. D. (2010). 99th Dahlem conference on infection, inflammation and chronic inflammatory disorders: triggering of autoimmune diseases by infections. *Clin Exp Immunol.* 160 (1):15-21.

Grainger, J. R., Smith, K. A., Hewitson, J. P., McSorley, H. J., Harcus, Y., Filbey, K. J., Finney, C. A., Greenwood, E. J., Knox, D. P., Wilson, M. S., Belkaid, Y., Rudensky, A. Y. & Maizels, R. M. (2010). Helminth secretions induce de novo T cell Foxp3 expression and regulatory function through the TGF-β pathway. *J Exp Med.* 207 (11):2331-2341.

Green, C., Elliott, L., Beaudoin, C. & Bernstein, C. N. (2006). A population-based ecologic study of inflammatory bowel disease: searching for etiologic clues. *Am J Epidemiol.* 164 (7):615-623

Gruden-Movsesijan, A., Ilic, N., Mostarica-Stojkovic, M., Stosic-Grujicic, S., Milic, M. & Sofronic-Milosavljevic, Lj. (2008). *Trichinella spiralis*: modulation of experimental autoimmune encephalomyelitis in DA rats. *Exp Parasitol.* 118 (4):641-647.

Grzych, J. M., Pearce, E., Cheever, A., Caulada, Z. A., Caspar, P., Heiny, S., Lewis, F. & Sher. A. (1991) Egg deposition is the major stimulus for the production of Th2 cytokines in murine schistosomiasis mansoni. *J Immunol.* 146 (4):1322-1327.

Gysemans, C., Callewaert, H., Overbergh, L. & Mathieu, C. (2008). Cytokine signalling in the beta-cell: a dual role for IFNgamma. *Biochem Soc Trans.* 36 (Pt 3):328-333.

Gysemans, C. A., Ladrière, L., Callewaert, H., Rasschaert, J., Flamez, D., Levy, D. E., Matthys, P., Eizirik, D. L. & Mathieu, C. (2005). Disruption of the gamma-interferon signaling pathway at the level of signal transducer and activator of transcription-1 prevents immune destruction of beta-cells. *Diabetes.* 54 (8):2396-2403.

Hang, L., Setiawan, T., Blum, A. M., Urban, J., Stoyanoff, K., Arihiro, S., Reinecker, H. C. & Weinstock, J. V. (2010). *Heligmosomoides polygyrus* infection can inhibit colitis through direct interaction with innate immunity. *J Immunol.* 185 (6):3184-3189.

Harnett, W. & Harnett, M. M. (2010). Helminth-derived immunomodulators: can understanding the worm produce the pill? *Nat Rev Immunol.* 10 (4):278-284.

He, Y., Li, J., Zhuang, W., Yin, L., Chen, C., Li, J., Chi, F., Bai, Y. & Chen, X. P. (2010). The inhibitory effect against collagen-induced arthritis by *Schistosoma japonicum* infection is infection stage-dependent. *BMC Immunol.* 11:28.

Herold, K. C., Vezys, V., Sun, Q., Viktora, D., Seung, E., Reiner, S. & Brown, D. R. (1996). Regulation of cytokine production during development of autoimmune diabetes induced with multiple low doses of streptozotocin. *J Immunol.* 156 (9):3521-3527.

Honkanen, J., Nieminen, J. K., Gao, R., Luopajarvi, K., Salo, H. M., Ilonen, J., Knip, M., Otonkoski, T. & Vaarala, O. (2010). IL-17 immunity in human type 1 diabetes. *J Immunol.* 185 (3):1959-1967.

Hübner, M. P., Stocker, J. T. & Mitre, E. (2009). Inhibition of type 1 diabetes in filaria-infected non-obese diabetic mice is associated with a T helper type 2 shift and induction of FoxP3+ regulatory T cells. *Immunology.* 127 (4):512-522.

Hultgren, B., Huang, X., Dybdal, N. & Stewart, T. A. (1996). Genetic absence of gamma-interferon delays but does not prevent diabetes in NOD mice. *Diabetes.* 45 (6):812-817.

Hunter, M. M, Wang, A., Hirota, C. L. & McKay, D. M. (2005). Neutralizing anti-IL-10 antibody blocks the protective effect of tapeworm infection in a murine model of chemically induced colitis. *J Immunol.* 174 (11):7368-7375.

Hunter, M. M., Wang, A., Parhar, K. S., Johnston, M. J., Van Rooijen, N., Beck, P. L. & McKay, D. M. (2010). In vitro-derived alternatively activated macrophages reduce colonic inflammation in mice. *Gastroenterology.* 138 (4):1395-1405.

Ince, M. N., Elliott, D. E., Setiawan, T., Metwali, A., Blum, A., Chen, H. L., Urban, J. F., Flavell, R. A. & Weinstock, J. V. (2009). Role of T cell TGF-beta signaling in intestinal cytokine responses and helminthic immune modulation. *Eur J Immunol.* 39 (7):1870-1878.

Irmler, I. M., Gajda, M. & Bräuer, R. (2007). Exacerbation of antigen-induced arthritis in IFN-gamma-deficient mice as a result of unrestricted IL-17 response. *J Immunol.* 179 (9):6228-6236.

Ito, R., Kita, M., Shin-Ya, M., Kishida, T., Urano, A., Takada, R., Sakagami, J., Imanishi, J., Iwakura, Y., Okanoue, T., Yoshikawa, T., Kataoka, K. & Mazda, O. (2008). Involvement of IL-17A in the pathogenesis of DSS-induced colitis in mice. *Biochem Biophys Res Commun.* 377 (1):12-16.

Iwanami, K., Matsumoto, I., Tanaka-Watanabe, Y., Inoue, A., Mihara, M., Ohsugi, Y., Mamura, M., Goto, D., Ito, S., Tsutsumi, A., Kishimoto, T. & Sumida, T. (2008). Crucial role of the interleukin-6/interleukin-17 cytokine axis in the induction of arthritis by glucose-6-phosphate isomerase. *Arthritis Rheum.* 58 (3):754-763.

Johnston, M. J., Wang, A., Catarino, M. E., Ball, L., Phan, V. C., MacDonald, J. A. & McKay, D. M. (2010). Extracts of the rat tapeworm, *Hymenolepis diminuta*, suppress macrophage activation in vitro and alleviate chemically induced colitis in mice. *Infect Immun.* 78 (3):1364-1375.

Jones, G & Ding, C. (2010). Tocilizumab: a review of its safety and efficacy in rheumatoid arthritis. *Clin Med Insights Arthritis Musculoskelet Disord.* 3:81-9.

Kantwerk-Funke, G., Burkart, V. & Kolb, H. (1991). Low dose streptozotocin causes stimulation of the immune system and of anti-islet cytotoxicity in mice. *Clin Exp Immunol.* 86 (2):266-270.

Kelchtermans, H., Schurgers, E., Geboes, L., Mitera, T., Van Damme, J., Van Snick, J., Uyttenhove, C. & Matthys, P. (2009). Effector mechanisms of interleukin-17 in collagen-induced arthritis in the absence of interferon-gamma and counteraction by interferon-gamma. *Arthritis Res Ther.* 11 (4):R122.

Kim, J. Y., Cho, M. K., Choi, S. H., Lee, K. H., Ahn, S. C., Kim, D. H. & Yu, H. S. (2010). Inhibition of dextran sulfate sodium (DSS)-induced intestinal inflammation via enhanced IL-10 and TGF-beta production by galectin-9 homologues isolated from intestinal parasites. *Mol Biochem Parasitol.* 174 (1):53-61.

Kivity, S., Agmon-Levin, N., Blank, M. & Shoenfeld, Y. (2009). Infections and autoimmunity--friends or foes? *Trends Immunol.* 30 (8):409-414.

Koloski, N. A., Bret, L. & Radford-Smith, G. (2008). Hygiene hypothesis in inflammatory bowel disease: a critical review of the literature. *World J Gastroenterol.* 14 (2):165-173.

Komiyama, Y., Nakae, S., Matsuki, T., Nambu, A., Ishigame, H., Kakuta, S., Sudo, K. & Iwakura, Y. (2006). IL-17 plays an important role in the development of experimental autoimmune encephalomyelitis. *J Immunol.* 177 (1):566-573.

Kurschus, F. C., Croxford, A. L., Heinen, A. P., Wörtge, S., Ielo, D. & Waisman, A.Genetic proof for the transient nature of the Th17 phenotype. *Eur J Immunol.* 40 (12):3336-3346.

La Flamme, A. C., Ruddenklau, K. & Bäckström, B. T. (2003). Schistosomiasis decreases central nervous system inflammation and alters the progression of experimental autoimmune encephalomyelitis. *Infect Immun.* 71 (9):4996-5004.

Langrish, C. L., Chen, Y., Blumenschein, W. M., Mattson, J., Basham, B., Sedgwick, J. D., McClanahan, T., Kastelein, R. A. & Cua, D. J. (2005). IL-23 drives a pathogenic T cell population that induces autoimmune inflammation. *J Exp Med.* 201 (2):233-240.

Lee, Y. K., Turner, H., Maynard, C. L., Oliver, J. R., Chen, D., Elson, C. O. & Weaver, C. T. (2009). Late developmental plasticity in the T helper 17 lineage. Immunity. 30 (1):92-107.

Leonardi-Bee, J., Pritchard, D. & Britton, J. (2006). Asthma and current intestinal parasite infection: systematic review and meta-analysis. *Am J Respir Crit Care Med.* 174 (5):514-523.

Liu, Q., Sundar, K., Mishra, P. K., Mousavi, G., Liu, Z., Gaydo, A., Alem, F., Lagunoff, D., Bleich, D. & Gause, W. C. (2009). Helminth infection can reduce insulitis and type 1 diabetes through CD25- and IL-10-independent mechanisms. *Infect Immun.* 77 (12):5347-5358.

Lynch, N. R., Hagel, I., Perez, M., Di Prisco, M. C., Lopez, R. & Alvarez, N. (1993). Effect of anthelmintic treatment on the allergic reactivity of children in a tropical slum. *J Allergy Clin Immunol.* 92 (3):404-411.

Lynch, N. R., Palenque, M., Hagel, I. & DiPrisco, M. C. (1997). Clinical improvement of asthma after anthelminthic treatment in a tropical situation. *Am J Respir Crit Care Med.* 156 (1):50-54.

Martin-Orozco, N., Chung, Y., Chang, S. H., Wang, Y. H. & Dong, C. (2009). Th17 cells promote pancreatic inflammation but only induce diabetes efficiently in lymphopenic hosts after conversion into Th1 cells. *Eur J Immunol.* 39 (1):216-224.

Matheson, M. C., Walters, E. H., Simpson, J. A., Wharton, C. L., Ponsonby, A. L., Johns, D. P., Jenkins, M. A., Giles, G. G., Hopper, J. L., Abramson, M. J. & Dharmage, S. C. (2009). Relevance of the hygiene hypothesis to early vs. late onset allergic rhinitis. *Clin Exp Allergy.* 39 (3):370-8.

Matricardi, P. M. (2010). 99th Dahlem conference on infection, inflammation and chronic inflammatory disorders: controversial aspects of the 'hygiene hypothesis'. *Clin Exp Immunol.* 160 (1):98-105.

Matricardi, P. M., Rosmini, F., Ferrigno, L., Nisini, R., Rapicetta, M., Chionne, P., Stroffolini, T., Pasquini, P. & D'Amelio, R. (1997). Cross sectional retrospective study of prevalence of atopy among Italian military students with antibodies against hepatitis A virus. *BMJ.* 314 (7086):999-1003.

Matricardi, P. M., Rosmini, F., Riondino, S., Fortini, M., Ferrigno, L., Rapicetta, M. & Bonini, S. (2000). Exposure to foodborne and orofecal microbes versus airborne viruses in relation to atopy and allergic asthma: epidemiological study. *BMJ.* 320 (7232):412-417.

McInnes, I. B., Leung, B. P., Harnett, M., Gracie, J. A., Liew, F. Y. & Harnett, W. (2003). A novel therapeutic approach targeting articular inflammation using the filarial nematode-derived phosphorylcholine-containing glycoprotein ES-62. *J Immunol.* 171 (4):2127-33.

McSorley, H. J., Grainger, J. R., Harcus, Y., Murray, J., Nisbet, A. J., Knox, D. P. & Maizels, R. M. (2010). daf-7-related TGF-beta homologues from Trichostrongyloid nematodes show contrasting life-cycle expression patterns. *Parasitology.* 137 (1):159-171.

Mensah-Brown, E. P., Shahin, A., Al-Shamisi, M., Wei, X. & Lukic, M. L. (2006). IL-23 leads to diabetes induction after subdiabetogenic treatment with multiple low doses of streptozotocin. *Eur J Immunol.* 36 (1):216-223.

Miljkovic, D., Cvetkovic, I., Momcilovic, M., Maksimovic-Ivanic, D., Stosic-Grujicic, S. & Trajkovic, V. (2005). Interleukin-17 stimulates inducible nitric oxide synthase-dependent toxicity in mouse beta cells. *Cell Mol Life Sci.* 62 (22):2658-2668.

Milo, R. & Kahana, E. (2010). Multiple sclerosis: geoepidemiology, genetics and the environment. *Autoimmun Rev.* 9 (5):A387-394.

Mo, H. M., Liu, W. Q., Lei, J.H., Cheng, Y. L., Wang, C. Z. & Li, Y. L. (2007). *Schistosoma japonicum* eggs modulate the activity of CD4+ CD25+ Tregs and prevent development of colitis in mice. *Exp Parasitol.* 116 (4):385-389.

Möller, B.& Villiger, P. M. (2006). Inhibition of IL-1, IL-6, and TNF-alpha in immune-mediated inflammatory diseases. *Springer Semin Immunopathol.* 27 (4):391-408.

Moreels, T. G., Nieuwendijk, R. J., De Man, J. G., De Winter, B. Y., Herman, A. G., Van Marck, E. A.& Pelckmans, P. A. (2004). Concurrent infection with *Schistosoma mansoni* attenuates inflammation induced changes in colonic morphology, cytokine levels, and smooth muscle contractility of trinitrobenzene sulphonic acid induced colitis in rats. *Gut.* 53 (1):99-107.

Motomura, Y., Wang, H., Deng, Y., El-Sharkawy, R. T., Verdu, E. F. & Khan, W. I. (2009). Helminth antigen-based strategy to ameliorate inflammation in an experimental model of colitis. *Clin Exp Immunol.* 155 (1):88-95.

Müller, A., Schott-Ohly, P., Dohle, C. & Gleichmann, H. (2002). Differential regulation of Th1-type and Th2-type cytokine profiles in pancreatic islets of C57BL/6 and BALB/c mice by multiple low doses of streptozotocin. *Immunobiology.* 205 (1):35-50.

Murphy, C. A., Langrish, C. L., Chen, Y., Blumenschein, W., McClanahan, T., Kastelein, R. A., Sedgwick, J. D. & Cua, D. J. (2003). Divergent pro- and antiinflammatory roles for IL-23 and IL-12 in joint autoimmune inflammation. *J Exp Med.* 198 (12):1951-1957.

Mutapi, F., Imai, N., Nausch, N., Bourke, C. D., Rujeni, N., Mitchell, K. M., Midzi, N., Woolhouse, M. E., Maizels, R. M. & Mduluza, T. (2011). Schistosome infection intensity is inversely related to auto-reactive antibody levels. *PLoS One.* 6 (5):e19149.

Nakae, S., Iwakura, Y., Suto, H. & Galli, S. J. (2007). Phenotypic differences between Th1 and Th17 cells and negative regulation of Th1 cell differentiation by IL-17. *J Leukoc Biol.* 81 (5):1258-1268.

Nakae, S., Nambu, A., Sudo, K. & Iwakura, Y. (2003a). Suppression of immune induction of collagen-induced arthritis in IL-17-deficient mice. *J Immunol.* 171 (11):6173-6177.

Nakae, S., Saijo, S., Horai, R., Sudo, K., Mori, S. & Iwakura, Y. (2003b). IL-17 production from activated T cells is required for the spontaneous development of destructive arthritis in mice deficient in IL-1 receptor antagonist. *Proc Natl Acad Sci U S A.* 100 (10):5986-5990.

Nielsen, O. H., Kirman, I., Rüdiger, N., Hendel, J. & Vainer, B. (2003). Upregulation of interleukin-12 and -17 in active inflammatory bowel disease. *Scand J Gastroenterol.* 38 (2):180-185.

Nixon, R., Bansback, N. & Brennan, A. (2007). The efficacy of inhibiting tumour necrosis factor alpha and interleukin 1 in patients with rheumatoid arthritis: a meta-analysis and adjusted indirect comparisons. *Rheumatology (Oxford).* 46 (7):1140-1147.

Obihara, C. C., Bollen, C. W., Beyers, N. & Kimpen, J. L. (2007). Mycobacterial infection and atopy in childhood: a systematic review. *Pediatr Allergy Immunol.* 18 (7):551-9.

Ogawa, A., Andoh, A., Araki, Y., Bamba, T. & Fujiyama. Y. (2004). Neutralization of interleukin-17 aggravates dextran sulfate sodium-induced colitis in mice. *Clin Immunol.* 110 (1):55-62.

Okamoto, K. & Takayanagi, H. (2011). Osteoclasts in arthritis and Th17 cell development. *Int Immunopharmacol.* 11 (5):543-548.

Osada, Y., Shimizu, S., Kumagai, T., Yamada, S. & Kanazawa, T. (2009). *Schistosoma mansoni* infection reduces severity of collagen-induced arthritis via down-regulation of pro-inflammatory mediators. *Int J Parasitol.* 39 (4):457-464.

Osada, Y., Shimizu, S., Kumagai, T., Yamada, S. & Kanazawa, T. (2010). *Schistosoma mansoni* has anti-arthritic effects accompanied with IL-17's down-modulation dependent on viable eggs. *Proceedings of XIIth International Congress of Parasitology.* Medimond srl, Melbourne, pp.113-116.

Ott, P. A., Anderson, M. R., Tary-Lehmann, M. & Lehmann, P. V. (2005). CD4+CD25+ regulatory T cells control the progression from periinsulitis to destructive insulitis in murine autoimmune diabetes. *Cell Immunol.* 235 (1):1-11.

Pageau, S. C. (2009). Denosumab. *MAbs.* 1 (3):210-215.

Park, H., Li, Z., Yang, X. O., Chang, S. H., Nurieva, R., Wang, Y. H., Wang, Y., Hood, L., Zhu, Z., Tian, Q. & Dong, C. (2005). A distinct lineage of CD4 T cells regulates tissue inflammation by producing interleukin 17. *Nat Immunol.* 6 (11):1133-1141.

Ponsonby, A. L., McMichael, A. & van der Mei, I. (2002). Ultraviolet radiation and autoimmune disease: insights from epidemiological research. *Toxicology.* 181-182:71-78.

Puneet, P., McGrath, M. A., Tay, H. K., Al-Riyami, L., Rzepecka, J., Moochhala, S. M., Pervaiz, S., Harnett, M. M., Harnett, W. & Melendez, A. J. (2011). The helminth product ES-62 protects against septic shock via Toll-like receptor 4-dependent autophagosomal degradation of the adaptor MyD88. *Nat Immunol.* 12(4):344-351.

Qualls, J. E., Kaplan, A. M., van Rooijen, N. & Cohen, D. A. (2006). Suppression of experimental colitis by intestinal mononuclear phagocytes. *J Leukoc Biol.* 80 (4):802-815.

Rangachari, M., Mauermann, N., Marty, R.R., Dirnhofer, S., Kurrer, M. O., Komnenovic, V., Penninger, J. M. & Eriksson, U. (2006). T-bet negatively regulates autoimmune myocarditis by suppressing local production of interleukin 17. *J Exp Med.* 203 (8):2009-2019.

Reardon, C., Sanchez, A., Hogaboam, C. M. & McKay, D. M. (2001). Tapeworm infection reduces epithelial ion transport abnormalities in murine dextran sulfate sodium-induced colitis. *Infect Immun.* 69 (7):4417-4423.

Reyes, J. L., Espinoza-Jiménez, A. F., González, M. I., Verdin, L. & Terrazas, L. I. (2011). *Taenia crassiceps* infection abrogates experimental autoimmune encephalomyelitis. *Cell Immunol.* 267 (2):77-87.

Rocha, F. A., Leite, A. K., Pompeu, M. M., Cunha, T. M., Verri, W. A. Jr, Soares, F. M., Castro, R. R. & Cunha, F. Q. (2008). Protective effect of an extract from *Ascaris suum* in experimental arthritis models. Infect Immun. 76 (6):2736-2745.

Rodrigues, L. C., Newcombe, P. J., Cunha, S. S., Alcantara-Neves, N. M., Genser, B., Cruz, A. A., Simoes, S. M., Fiaccone, R., Amorim, L., Cooper, P. J. & Barreto, M. L.: Social Change, Asthma and Allergy in Latin America.(2008). Early infection with *Trichuris trichiura* and allergen skin test reactivity in later childhood. *Clin Exp Allergy.* 38 (11):1769-1777.

Rook, G. A. (2009). Review series on helminths, immune modulation and the hygiene hypothesis: the broader implications of the hygiene hypothesis. *Immunology.* 126 (1):3-11.

Ruyssers, N. E., De Winter, B. Y., De Man, J. G., Loukas, A., Pearson, M. S., Weinstock, J. V., Van den Bossche, R. M., Martinet, W., Pelckmans, P. A. & Moreels, T. G. (2009). Therapeutic potential of helminth soluble proteins in TNBS-induced colitis in mice. *Inflamm Bowel Dis.* 15 (4):491-500.

Salinas-Carmona, M. C., de la Cruz-Galicia, G., Pérez-Rivera, I., Solís-Soto, J. M., Segoviano-Ramirez, J. C., Vázquez, A. V. & Garza, M. A. (2009). Spontaneous arthritis in MRL/lpr mice is aggravated by *Staphylococcus aureus* and ameliorated by *Nippostrongylus brasiliensis* infections. *Autoimmunity.* 42 (1):25-32.

Sarra, M., Pallone, F., Macdonald, T. T. & Monteleone, G. (2010). IL-23/IL-17 axis in IBD. *Inflamm Bowel Dis.* 16 (10):1808-1813.

Saunders, K. A., Raine, T., Cooke, A. & Lawrence, C. E. (2007). Inhibition of autoimmune type 1 diabetes by gastrointestinal helminth infection. *Infect Immun.* 75 (1):397-407.

Schnoeller, C., Rausch, S., Pillai, S., Avagyan, A., Wittig, B. M., Loddenkemper, C., Hamann, A., Hamelmann, E., Lucius, R. & Hartmann, S. (2008). A helminth immunomodulator reduces allergic and inflammatory responses by induction of IL-10-producing macrophages. *J Immunol.* 180 (6):4265-4272.

Seiskari, T., Kondrashova, A., Viskari, H., Kaila, M., Haapala, A. M., Aittoniemi, J., Virta, M., Hurme, M., Uibo, R., Knip, M. & Hyöty, H.; EPIVIR study group. (2007). Allergic sensitization and microbial load--a comparison between Finland and Russian Karelia. *Clin Exp Immunol.* 148 (1):47-52.

Sewell, D., Qing, Z., Reinke, E., Elliot, D., Weinstock, J., Sandor, M. & Fabry, Z. (2003). Immunomodulation of experimental autoimmune encephalomyelitis by helminth ova immunization. *Int Immunol.* 15 (1):59-69.

Shapira, Y., Agmon-Levin, N. & Shoenfeld, Y. (2010a). Defining and analyzing geoepidemiology and human autoimmunity. *J Autoimmun.* 34 (3):J168-177.

Shapira, Y., Agmon-Levin, N. & Shoenfeld, Y. (2010b). Geoepidemiology of autoimmune rheumatic diseases. *Nat Rev Rheumatol.* 6 (8):468-76.

Shi, M., Wang, A., Prescott, D., Waterhouse, C. C., Zhang, S., McDougall, J. J., Sharkey, K. A. & McKay, D. M. (2011). Infection with an intestinal helminth parasite reduces Freund's complete adjuvant-induced monoarthritis in mice. *Arthritis Rheum.* 63 (2):434-444.

Shoenfeld, N., Amital, H. & Shoenfeld, Y. (2009). The effect of melanism and vitamin D synthesis on the incidence of autoimmune disease. *Nat Clin Pract Rheumatol.* 5 (2):99-105.

Smith, P., Mangan, N. E., Walsh, C. M., Fallon, R. E., McKenzie, A. N., van Rooijen, N. & Fallon, P. G. (2007). Infection with a helminth parasite prevents experimental colitis via a macrophage-mediated mechanism. *J Immunol.* 178 (7):4557-4566.

Strachan, D. P. (1989). Hay fever, hygiene, and household size. *BMJ.* 299 (6710):1259-1260.

Strober, W., Fuss, I. J. & Blumberg, R. S. (2002). The immunology of mucosal models of inflammation. *Annu Rev Immunol.* 20: 495-549.

Stuart, J. M., Townes, A. S. & Kang, A. H. (1982). Nature and specificity of the immune response to collagen in type II collagen-induced arthritis in mice. *J Clin Invest.* 69 (3):673-683.

Summers, R. W., Elliott, D. E., Urban, J. F. Jr, Thompson, R. & Weinstock, J. V. (2005a). *Trichuris suis* therapy in Crohn's disease. *Gut.* 54 (1):87-90.

Summers, R. W., Elliott, D. E., Urban, J. F. Jr, Thompson, R. & Weinstock, J. V. (2005b). *Trichuris suis* therapy for active ulcerative colitis: a randomized controlled trial. *Gastroenterology.* 128 (4):825-832.

Summers, R. W., Elliott, D. E. & Weinstock, J. V. (2010). *Trichuris suis* might be effective in treating allergic rhinitis. *J Allergy Clin Immunol.* 125 (3):766-767.

Sun, X., Liu, Y. H., Lv, Z. Y., Yang, L. L., Hu, S. M., Zheng, H. Q., Hu, W., Cao, J. P., Fung, M. Q. & Wu, Z. D. (2010). rSj16, a recombinant protein of *Schistosoma japonicum*-derived molecule, reduces severity of the complete Freund's adjuvant-induced adjuvant arthritis in rats' model. *Parasite Immunol.* 32 (11-12):739-748.

Sutton, T. L., Zhao, A., Madden, K. B., Elfrey, J. E., Tuft, B. A., Sullivan, C. A., Urban, J. F. Jr & Shea-Donohue, T. (2008). Anti-Inflammatory mechanisms of enteric *Heligmosomoides polygyrus* infection against trinitrobenzene sulfonic acid-induced colitis in a murine model. *Infect Immun.* 76 (10):4772-4782.

Takkouche, B., González-Barcala, F. J., Etminan, M. & Fitzgerald, M.(2008). Exposure to furry pets and the risk of asthma and allergic rhinitis: a meta-analysis. *Allergy.* 63 (7):857-864.

Taylor, J. J., Mohrs, M. & Pearce, E. J. (2006). Regulatory T cell responses develop in parallel to Th responses and control the magnitude and phenotype of the Th effector population. *J Immunol.* 176 (10):5839-5847.

Terato, K., Hasty, K. A., Reife, R. A., Cremer, M. A., Kang, A. H. & Stuart, J. M.(1992). Induction of arthritis with monoclonal antibodies to collagen. *J Immunol.* 148 (7):2103-2108.

van den Biggelaar, A. H., Rodrigues, L. C., van Ree, R., van der Zee, J. S., Hoeksma-Kruize, Y. C., Souverijn, J. H., Missinou, M. A., Borrmann, S., Kremsner, P. G. &

Yazdanbakhsh, M. (2004). Long-term treatment of intestinal helminths increases mite skin-test reactivity in Gabonese schoolchildren. *J Infect Dis.* 189 (5):892-900.

von Mutius, E. (2007). Allergies, infections and the hygiene hypothesis--the epidemiological evidence. *Immunobiology.* 212 (6):433-439.

Walsh, K. P., Brady, M. T., Finlay, C. M., Boon, L. & Mills, K. H. (2009). Infection with a helminth parasite attenuates autoimmunity through TGF-beta-mediated suppression of Th17 and Th1 responses. *J Immunol.* 183 (3):1577-1586.

Wang, A., Fernando, M., Leung, G., Phan, V., Smyth, D. & McKay, D. M. (2010). Exacerbation of oxazolone colitis by infection with the helminth *Hymenolepis diminuta*: involvement of IL-5 and eosinophils. *Am J Pathol.* 177 (6):2850-2859.

Wilson, M. S., Taylor, M. D., O'Gorman, M. T., Balic, A., Barr, T. A., Filbey, K., Anderton, S. M. & Maizels, R. M. (2010). Helminth-induced CD19+CD23hi B cells modulate experimental allergic and autoimmune inflammation. *Eur J Immunol.* 40 (6):1682-1696.

Wu, Z., Nagano, I., Asano, K. & Takahashi, Y. (2010). Infection of non-encapsulated species of *Trichinella* ameliorates experimental autoimmune encephalomyelitis involving suppression of Th17 and Th1 response. *Parasitol Res.* 107 (5):1173-1188.

Yamamoto, H., Uchigata, Y. & Okamoto, H. (1981). Streptozotocin and alloxan induce DNA strand breaks and poly (ADP-ribose) synthetase in pancreatic islets. *Nature.* 294 (5838):284-286.

Yang, Y., Weiner, J., Liu, Y., Smith, A. J., Huss, D. J., Winger, R., Peng, H., Cravens, P. D., Racke, M. K. & Lovett-Racke, A. E. (2009). T-bet is essential for encephalitogenicity of both Th1 and Th17 cells. *J Exp Med.* 206 (7):1549-1564.

Zaccone, P., Burton, O., Miller, N., Jones, F. M., Dunne, D. W. & Cooke, A. (2009). *Schistosoma mansoni* egg antigens induce Treg that participate in diabetes prevention in NOD mice. *Eur J Immunol.* 39 (4):1098-1107.

Zaccone, P. & Cooke, A. (2011). Infectious triggers protect from autoimmunity. *Semin Immunol.* 23:122-129.

Zaccone, P., Fehérvári, Z., Jones, F. M., Sidobre, S., Kronenberg, M., Dunne, D. W. & Cooke, A. (2003). *Schistosoma mansoni* antigens modulate the activity of the innate immune response and prevent onset of type 1 diabetes. *Eur J Immunol.* 33 (5):1439-1449.

Zhang, Z., Zheng, M., Bindas, J., Schwarzenberger, P. & Kolls, J. K. (2006). Critical role of IL-17 receptor signaling in acute TNBS-induced colitis. *Inflamm Bowel Dis.* 12 (5):382-388.

Zhao, Y., Zhang, S., Jiang, L., Jiang, J. & Liu, H. (2009). Preventive effects of *Schistosoma japonicum* ova on trinitrobenzenesulfonic acid-induced colitis and bacterial translocation in mice. *J Gastroenterol Hepatol.* 24 (11):1775-1780.

Zheng, X., Hu, X., Zhou, G., Lu, Z., Qiu, W., Bao, J. & Dai, Y. (2008). Soluble egg antigen from *Schistosoma japonicum* modulates the progression of chronic progressive experimental autoimmune encephalomyelitis via Th2-shift response. *J Neuroimmunol.* 194 (1-2):107-114.